Concepts in DRUG METABOLISM

DRUGS AND THE PHARMACEUTICAL SCIENCES

A Series of Textbooks and Monographs

Edited by

James Swarbrick
School of Pharmacy
University of Southern California
Los Angeles, California

Volume 1. PHARMACOKINETICS, *Milo Gibaldi and Donald Perrier*

Volume 2. GOOD MANUFACTURING PRACTICES FOR PHARMACEUTICALS: A PLAN FOR TOTAL QUALITY CONTROL, *Sidney H. Willig, Murray M. Tuckerman, and William S. Hitchings IV*

Volume 3. MICROENCAPSULATION, *edited by J. R. Nixon*

Volume 4. DRUG METABOLISM: CHEMICAL AND BIOCHEMICAL ASPECTS, *Bernard Testa and Peter Jenner*

Volume 5. NEW DRUGS: DISCOVERY AND DEVELOPMENT, *edited by Alan A. Rubin*

Volume 6. SUSTAINED AND CONTROLLED RELEASE DRUG DELIVERY SYSTEMS, *edited by Joseph R. Robinson*

Volume 7. MODERN PHARMACEUTICS, *edited by Gilbert S. Banker and Christopher T. Rhodes*

Volume 8. PRESCRIPTION DRUGS IN SHORT SUPPLY: CASE HISTORIES, *Michael A. Schwartz*

Volume 9. ACTIVATED CHARCOAL: ANTIDOTAL AND OTHER MEDICAL USES, *David O. Cooney*

Volume 10. CONCEPTS IN DRUG METABOLISM (in two parts), *edited by Peter Jenner and Bernard Testa*

Other Volumes in Preparation

Concepts in DRUG METABOLISM

(IN TWO PARTS)

Part B

EDITED BY

PETER JENNER

University Department of Neurology
Institute of Psychiatry and
King's College Hospital Medical School
London, England

BERNARD TESTA

Department of Medicinal Chemistry
School of Pharmacy
University of Lausanne
Lausanne, Switzerland

MARCEL DEKKER, INC. New York and Basel

Library of Congress Cataloging in Publication Data (Revised)

Main entry under title:

Concepts in drug metabolism.

(Drugs and the pharmaceutical sciences ; v. 10) Part B
Includes bibliographical references and indexes.
1. Drug metabolism. I. Jenner, Peter, [date]
II. Testa, Bernard. III. Series. [DNLM: 1. Drugs--
Metabolism. W1 DR893B v. 10 pt. A etc.]
RM301.55.C66 615'.7 80-12792
ISBN 0-8247-6906-6 (pt. A) AACR2
ISBN 0-8247-1323-0 (pt. B)

MARCEL DEKKER, INC.
270 Madison Avenue, New York, New York 10016

Current printing (last digit):
10 9 8 7 6 5 4 3 2 1

PRINTED IN THE UNITED STATES OF AMERICA

PREFACE

The Development of Concepts in Drug Metabolism

At least a century ago it was recognized that ingested drugs or other foreign compounds are excreted either unchanged or chemically modified.* At that time, however, the chemical alteration of drugs by living tissues was regarded mainly as a curiosity of little importance in terms of mainstream scientific advances, which saw the establishment of the fundamentals of modern chemistry, biochemistry, and pharmacology. Although preoccupation with the early development of these three disciplines caused a neglect of research into drug metabolism per se, ironically the same disciplines were later to provide the basis of its methodology and the foundation of its principles. Despite the neglect just mentioned, a considerable body of information was generated during the later part of the nineteenth century and the beginning of the twentieth century, leading to the initial concept of drugs undergoing a number of distinct chemical changes within the intact organism. Truly, many major pathways of drug metabolism that are readily accepted today were first reported during this era.

What then formed the major advances that have caused the study of drug metabolism to evolve from its embryonic existence and to distinguish itself from its parent sciences of chemistry, biochemistry, pharmacology, and toxicology?

First, there was a realization that the processes of drug metabolism might be of importance in determining the pharmacological activity, clinical efficacy, and toxicological profile of drug molecules. The increased effort put into the subsequent investigation of drug metabolism processes led to the emergence of specialists in this area of research. The significance of this human factor cannot be overestimated, since it is the ultimate limiting factor in the development of any science, as it is in fact in human progress generally.

This realization would have had a comparatively limited impact were it not for the concurrent improvement that occurred in analytical technology.

---

*A. Conti and M. H. Bickel, Drug Metab. Rev. 6:1 (1977).

Thus, advances in the selectivity, sensitivity, and accuracy of the analytical tools, as well as the development of methods specifically designed for drug metabolism studies, have played a major role in formulating the science of drug metabolism as we understand it.

It was during the 1940s that the work of pioneers such as the late R. T. Williams and B. B. Brodie, whose ideas were far ahead of their time, led to the opening of the road to modern progress.* Indeed, it was during this period that the concepts of drug metabolism were extended to establish principles such as Phase I and Phase II metabolism, which remain viable today.

Following this lead a rapid maturation of drug metabolism research occurred in the 1950s, and development has continued exponentially until the present day. In fact, the last two decades have seen the field of drug metabolism gain a reputable status and establish itself as a new science. The importance of drug metabolism and disposition on biological activity has become universally recognized. As a result of stringent legal requirements governing the use of novel drug molecules in humans, many countries have made metabolism studies compulsory. This in turn has done much to increase the amount of energy (both human and financial) applied to the adolescent science.

The increased necessity for such drug metabolism studies has led to a rapid growth in the relevant literature. Indeed, the current flood of data threatens to overwhelm researchers. They must feel the need to walk uphill in search of original approaches and generalizing concepts.† This situation presents difficulties and, in our opinion, must only be transitional if drug metabolism is to mature into a full science. The need for unifying concepts exists and is perceived by many, if not yet clearly. For example, a number of reviews and monographs have appeared in recent years that have attempted to bring some semblance of order to drug metabolism or its subfields by classifying and organizing the mass of available data.

We feel the time is now ripe for the members of the drug metabolism community to once again focus on the concepts which govern their science. A <u>concept</u>, the dictionary informs us, is "the idea of the attributes common to a class of things." With this as a goal we have invited a number of our colleagues to undertake an uphill contemplation of an area of drug metabolism research and to present the reader with a wide-ranging and conceptual approach to major topics in drug metabolism and allied fields. This has led to some overlap between contributions—which we have encouraged, since the relationships and interdependence between topics thus become more evident and the confrontation of viewpoints is often provocative and refreshing.

---

*L. Young, in <u>Drug Metabolism: From Microbe to Man</u> (D. V. Parke and R. L. Smith, eds.), Taylor & Francis, London, 1977, pp. 1-11.

†B. Testa, Drug Metab. Rev. <u>5</u>(2):i (1976).

Due to the very requirements of the conceptual approach, the various chapters in the present work reflect the personalities and views of their authors more than do ordinary reviews. The reader will find some chapters to be quite philosophical in their approach, whereas others make use of a large body of factual examples to illustrate the underlying concepts. In either case, however, we hope to show how vital is the generation of concepts and generalizing theories if the study of drug metabolism is to become a mature science—a science in which results can be predicted and not guessed, and which can in turn fertilize other sciences through its own discoveries.

Peter Jenner
Bernard Testa

CONTRIBUTORS

JOHANNES BIRCHER, M.D. Professor of Pharmacology and Medicine, Department of Clinical Pharmacology, University of Berne, Berne, Switzerland.

FREDERICK J. DI CARLO, Ph.D. Consultant, Health Review Division, U.S. Environmental Protection Agency, Washington, D.C.

SHARAT D. GANGOLLI, Ph.D., F.R.S.C., M.R.C.P. Assistant Director, The British Industrial Biological Research Association, Carshalton, Surrey, England

HELMUT A. GREIM, M.D. Professor of Pharmacology and Toxicology, Department of Toxicology, Munich Society for Radiation and Environment Research, Neuherberg, Federal Republic of Germany

PETER JENNER, Ph.D., M.P.S. Senior Lecturer in Biochemistry, University Department of Neurology, Institute of Psychiatry and King's College Hospital Medical School, London, England

W. ROBERT JONDORF, Ph.D. Department of Pharmacology, University of Berne, Berne, Switzerland

ARMANDA JORI, Ph.D. Special Projects Unit, "Mario Negri" Institute for Pharmacological Research, Milan, Italy

BRIAN G. LAKE, Ph.D. Biochemistry Section, The British Industrial Biological Research Association, Carshalton, Surrey, England

GILBERT J. MANNERING, Ph.D. Professor of Pharmacology, Department of Pharmacology, University of Minnesota School of Medicine, Minneapolis, Minnesota

DENNIS V. PARKE, Ph.D., DSc., FRCS, CChem, FIBiol., FRCPath
Head of Department, Biochemistry Department, University of Surrey, Guildford, Surrey, England

RUDOLF PREISIG, M.D. Professor of Pharmacology and Medicine, Department of Clinical Pharmacology, University of Berne, Berne, Switzerland

BERNARD TESTA, Ph.D. Professor and Chairman of Medicinal Chemistry, Department of Medicinal Chemistry, School of Pharmacy, University of Lausanne, Lausanne, Switzerland

CONTENTS

CONTENTS OF PART A

Chapter 1

THE ENDOPLASMIC RETICULUM: ITS ROLE IN PHYSIOLOGICAL FUNCTIONS AND PATHOLOGICAL SITUATIONS

Dennis V. Parke

Biochemistry Department
University of Surrey
Guildford, Surrey, England

The endoplasmic reticulum of the eukaryotic cell fulfills a number of vital roles in the regulation of carbohydrate and lipid metabolism, in the biosynthesis of many essential biochemical entities such as cholesterol and steroids, and in the metabolism of xenobiotics. Its most important function, however, is probably the synthesis of glycoproteins which subsequently are incorporated into the cytocavitary network of the cell or are secreted for extracellular and intercellular functions. The glycoproteins and steroid hormones appear to constitute a fundamental integrated system for the regulation of cellular division, growth, and function, and intercellular communication in the multicellular organism.

A major component of the endoplasmic reticulum is the enzyme cytochrome P-450, a monooxygenase concerned with the insertion of oxygen into specific molecular sites required for the biosynthesis and catabolism of cholesterol and steroid hormones, and for the detoxication of environmental chemicals and molecular oxygen. In natural environments this enzyme system can usually deal effectively with nutrient xenobiotic chemicals, and if overwhelmed is augmented by regulatory mechanisms which bring about enzyme induction. Exposure of the organism to environmental chemicals which are metabolized with difficulty, or which are metabolized into reactive intermediates, such as halogenated or polycyclic chemicals, can result in the formation of complexes with cytochrome P-450 and damage to the endoplasmic reticulum. This in turn may lead to loss of enzymic activity of cytochrome P-450, the appearance of cytochrome P-448, autoxidation, lipid peroxidation, autophagocytosis, destruction of cytochrome P-450, and cellular necrosis.

These processes of autoxidation and autophagocytosis, which occur spontaneously at a slow rate in the normal healthy cell, also become augmented with age, possibly due to changes in the nature of the phospholipid coupling of the monooxygenases. As might be expected, damage of this vital system for intra- and intercellular regulation may result in intra- and intercellular disorganization, with consequent disfunction of the organism. Evidence is now accumulating to indicate that these changes in the endoplasmic reticulum and monooxygenase activity, whether the result of age or environmental chemicals, may result in cellular pathology associated with carcinogenesis, cardiovascular disease, and arthritis.

I. INTRODUCTION

The endoplasmic reticulum of mammalian cells is primarily associated with the function of drug metabolism by the pharmacologist and with protein synthesis by the biochemist. In recent years, the concept of microsomal drug metabolism has been extended from the earlier ideas of detoxication to embrace the antithesis of this, namely, the metabolic activation of chemicals, and particularly those chemicals which are mutagens and carcinogens. The microsomal monooxygenases which catalyze the oxygenation of these drugs and environmental chemicals are also concerned with the oxygenation of many endogenous substrates including the metabolism of fatty acids, cholesterol, and steroid hormones. Whereas much attention has been given to the effects of the microsomal enzymes on exogenous chemicals, less has been accorded to the effects of these chemicals and their metabolites on the endoplasmic reticulum. Carcinogens and other toxic chemicals are known to cause the shedding of ribosomes from the rough endoplasmic reticulum (degranulation) which may have serious consequences for the synthesis of glycoproteins, and consequently may affect the synthesis of intracellular membranes, lysosomal enzymes, mucins, and immunoglobulins, with changes in the nature of the cell glycocalyx, the rate of DNA synthesis, and mitosis. Damage, by chemicals, of the endoplasmic reticulum is known to be associated with various pathological changes in the cells including lipid peroxidation, and is possibly fundamental to malignant transformation and carcinogenesis. Accumulation of lipophilic chemicals, and certain lipids, within the lipid milieu of the endoplasmic reticulum may also result in changes of the normal pattern of oxygenation, modulating the metabolism of exogenous and endogenous substrates with consequent aberrations in lipid and cholesterol homeostasis, which may be associated with cardiovascular disease and premature aging.

II. NORMAL PHYSIOLOGICAL FUNCTION

The endoplasmic reticulum is an intracellular membrane, richly endowed with numerous enzymes, which carries out a large number of essential cellular functions and plays an important role in the biosynthesis, modification, and transport of various classes of proteins and lipids. Certain regions of the endoplasmic reticulum bear ribosomes bound to the cytoplasmic surface (rough endoplasmic reticulum, RER) and these are concerned in the synthesis of proteins secreted from the cell and of proteins destined for incorporation into the endoplasmic reticulum and other subcellular membranes. Other regions are devoid of ribosomes (smooth endoplasmic reticulum, SER) and although not capable of synthesizing proteins are, like the RER, involved in numerous aspects of lipid metabolism and monooxygenations of steroids and environmental chemicals (xenobiotics) (see Table 1). The endoplasmic reticulum is readily ruptured into vesicular fragments (rough

TABLE 1
Comparison of Rough and Smooth Endoplasmic Reticulum

Rough ER	Smooth ER
Ribosomes are bound.	No ribosomes present.
Synthesis of proteins for secretion of intracellular membranes occurs.	No protein synthesis, but contains newly synthesized secretory proteins.
Sugar dolichol phosphates formed, but no significant glycosyltransferase activity present.	Glycosyltransferase activity present, synthesis of glycoproteins begins.
Monooxygenase system elaborated.	Monooxygenase system has higher activity.

and smooth microsomes) which may be separated from other cellular organelles, and from each other, for the detailed study of the enzymic and other components.

A. Protein Synthesis

The most widely studied endoplasmic reticulum is that of rat liver, and this rough endoplasmic reticulum, like that of other organs and tissues, is primarily concerned with the synthesis of secretory proteins, which are normally discharged into the lumen of the endoplasmic reticulum and thence to the exterior of the cell. Serum albumin, a major protein synthesized in the hepatocyte, first appears in the rough then the smooth endoplasmic reticulum, and finally the Golgi apparatus, to be secreted from the cell without passing into the cytosol. Nevertheless, this classical model of protein secretion has been criticized and it has been shown that proteins and glycoproteins may pass through the membranes into the cytosol, especially for the elaboration of new membranes of the endoplasmic reticulum [1]. The secretion of proteins from the pancreas probably does involve transfer into the cytoplasm, where modification and mixing of the proteins may occur before their secretion from the cell. With the questionable exception of serum albumin, most secreted proteins are glycoproteins in which carbohydrate moieties are covalently bound to the polypeptide in the smooth ER and Golgi complex before leaving the cell [2]. However, although it may not be strictly obligatory for ribosomes to be bound to the ER for the synthesis of secretory proteins, this undoubtedly increases the efficiency of such synthesis and, since the glycosyltransferases appear to be confined to the ER and Golgi complex, it would seem a prerequisite for the synthesis of glycoproteins to be initiated by polypeptide synthesis on the rough ER. Apart from secretory proteins, other types of protein may be synthesized on the rough ER, although the intracellular proteins are believed to be synthesized preferentially on the free polyribosomes [2]. From morphological and cell fractionation studies the concept has arisen that the ratio of free to bound microsomes decreases as the cell differentiates, thus reflecting the greater need for the synthesis of intracellular proteins in rapidly growing embryonic cells compared to the corresponding mature differentiated cells engaged in their normal physiological role of protein secretion [2]. The protein complement of free and bound ribosomal subunits of rat liver are identical, suggesting that there is no structural difference between free and bound ribosomes and that the two populations are interchangeable [3]. Selective labeling studies with ^{14}C-fluoro-orotic acid has shown that labeled m-RNA, although found, as expected, in the free polyribosomes, is not particularly associated with the bound ribosomes but instead is found on the membranes of the rough ER which is consistent with the suggestion of membrane-mediated transport of m-RNA to the cytoplasm [4].

Using techniques specifically designed to exclude contamination by nuclear and mitochondrial material, Bond and collaborators [5] have demonstrated the existence of microsomal DNA. The role of this unique form of DNA is not known but it is tempting to speculate that it may have a role in regulation of the synthesis of glycoproteins. Rabin and his co-workers [6] have suggested that certain steroids are implicated in the binding of ribosomes to the endoplasmic reticulum and, although this concept has not gained wide acceptance, the control of tissue proliferation and differentiation, mediated by regulation of the binding of ribosomes to the ER by steroid hormones, is an attractive hypothesis which accords with many physiological and biochemical observations. Corticosterone was found to promote RER formation in liver and to increase the ability of smooth microsomes to bind polyribosomes; estradiol, but not testosterone, produces the same effect with male SER and polyribosomes, whereas the converse effect is found for the SER and ribosomes from female rat liver [7]. Further studies by these workers showed that aflatoxin and a number of chemically unrelated carcinogens were able to cause shedding of the polyribosomes from the endoplasmic reticulum membrane (degranulation) [8,9], and on the basis of these observations it has been suggested that a primary lesion in carcinogenesis may be the degranulation of the endoplasmic reticulum.

Glycoproteins function either as secreted proteins or as components of the plasma membrane, other intracellular membranes, and lysosomal enzymes. These proteins play an essential and fundamental role in the structure and functions of the cell, being integral components of the endoplasmic reticulum, with all that implies in intermediary metabolism; they are also components of the plasma membrane and as such appear to determine cell-cell recognition, the immune character of the cell, and the rate of mitosis; and also comprise the lysosomal enzymes which probably determine the rate of turnover of all cellular components. As secretory materials, glycoproteins comprise some plasma proteins, the immunoglobulins, hormones such as thyroglobulin, and the various mucins, which recently have been shown to provide so many essential services to the mammalian organism (see Table 2) (cf. Ref. 10). The synthesis of glycoproteins is complex and occurs sequentially at different locations (RER, SER, Golgi) during a transport process. The regulation of these syntheses is largely unknown but sugar transfer may be regulated by the specificity of individual polyprenyl phosphates and by the specificity of the individual glycosyltransferases. There are two major types of amino acid-sugar linkage involved, namely, asparagine-N-acetylglucosamine and serine(threonine)-N-acetylgalactosamine; other linkages include hydroxylysine-galactose and serine-xylose [11].

B. Enzyme Components of the Endoplasmic Reticulum

The endoplasmic reticulum, both SER and RER, contain the monooxygenase system which, following detergent solubilization and partial purification, has

TABLE 2
The Nature of Some Glycoproteins

Tissue	Product	Role	Linkage
All cells	Plasma membrane components	Cell-cell interactions	?
All cells	Lysosomal enzymes	Turnover of cellular components	?
Mucous gland	Mucins	Protection, lubrication, transport	Ser(Thr)-GalNAc
Cartilage cells	Collagen		HydroxyLys-Gal
Lymphocytes and plasma cells	IgA, IgG, IgM	Immune surveillance	Asn-GlcNAc
Liver	Plasma glycoproteins	Transport etc.	Asn-GlcNAc
Thyroid	Thyroglobulin	Hormone	Asn-GlcNAc

been shown by reconstitution studies to require cytochrome P-450 (a hemoprotein), NADPH-cytochrome P-450 reductase (a FAD- and FMN-containing flavoprotein) [12,13], and phosphatidylcholine. This lipid component, which is essential for monooxygenase activity, is obviously not an electron carrier but in reconstituted systems is essential for electron transport from NADPH to cytochrome P-450 [14]. Dilauroyl phosphatidylcholine was found to be the most active lipid in this respect, comparable to the natural membrane lipid. For some monooxygenations certain nonionic detergents, such as Triton X-100, were found to have 70-80% of the activity of natural lipid in reconstituted microsomal enzyme systems. This suggests that the role of the lipid is a physical one and that phosphatidylcholine and certain other lipids and detergents form micelles of appropriate dimension to allow the coupling of the cytochrome with its reductase [14]. In support of this concept Stier [15] has reported studies which suggest that the phospholipid in the immediate vicinity of cytochrome P-450 is more highly organized than the bulk membrane phospholipids, and encloses the cytochrome and its reductase in a lipid halo which may regulate the monooxygenase activity.

The normal physiological role(s) of cytochrome P-450 and the monooxygenase system is probably still unknown. Undoubtedly, the protection of the organism against the progressive accumulation of lipophilic xenobiotics or anutrients (detoxication) is a major function essential to the biological economics, and probably to the survival, of the organism. The synthesis and catabolism of cholesterol and the steroid hormones is another area of essential physiological function, but even these two important roles together do not seem to suffice for the observed complexity of the structure of this system. Cytochrome P-450 is an unusual hemoprotein found in animals, plants, and microorganisms. In Pseudomonas it is a soluble enzyme; in yeasts [16] it is membrane-bound, as it is also in the animal kingdom where it occurs as a major constituent of certain tissues, like liver, in which it comprises 20% of the microsomal protein and some 2% of the total hepatic protein. It may act as a monooxygenase, a dioxygenase, or peroxidase and has, like iron-sulfur proteins, a very low redox potential which would have enabled it to function in the earliest evolutionary times when the Earth's atmosphere was largely free from molecular oxygen. Its earliest, and consequently most fundamental, function could therefore have been the protection of the primitive living organism from the toxic effects of oxygen [17]. The consequent occasional production of peroxides and superoxide anion would have been taken care of subsequently by the emergence of the enzymes catalase and superoxide dismutase. When the protective value in detoxicating oxygen was superseded by the development of aerobic organisms and respiratory cytochromes, the hydroxylase function of cytochrome P-450 was probably retained because of its value in numerous biosyntheses and in the degradation of complex molecules [17]. The recent observation that cytochrome P-450 is possibly the site of binding of the ribosomes to the endoplasmic reticulum [18] suggests that this enzyme system might also be involved in the synthesis of glycoproteins, such as in post-translational hydroxylation of certain amino acids, although there is no firm evidence for this.

The microsomal cytochrome b_5 system, which catalyzes fatty acid desaturation, has also been solubilized and purified, and for effective reconstitution requires NADH, NADH-cytochrome b_5 reductase, cytochrome b_5, the desaturase enzyme, stearyl CoA, molecular oxygen, and the presence of phospholipid [14].

Glucose 6-phosphatase is a complex, multifunctional enzyme of the endoplasmic reticulum of liver and kidney which not only hydrolyzes glucose 6-phosphate but can also synthesize this compound from glucose and inorganic pyrophosphate or from high-energy phosphates. This enzyme occupies a unique and strategic position in carbohydrate metabolism in that it catalyzes the terminal reactions of gluconeogenesis and glycogenolysis and thus is important in maintaining blood glucose homeostasis. Glucose 6-phosphatase is inhibited by phospholipases, and partially purified preparations of the enzyme protein(s) require phosphatidylcholine containing one unsaturated fatty acid for effective restoration of enzymic activity.

In contrast to glucose 6-phosphatase, and also to the cytochrome b_5 fatty acid desaturase and the cytochrome P-450 oxygenase, the microsomal enzyme uridine diphosphate (UDP) glucuronyltransferase is normally constrained by the membrane phospholipids and is enhanced by detergents and phospholipases which perturb membrane structure. Such contrast may be important in regulating the activity, and possibly also the substrate specificity, of UDP-glucuronyltransferase.

Apart from the phospholipids which regulate the enzymic activity in the endoplasmic reticulum, two other classes of lipids, namely, derivatives of dolichol and retinol phosphates, are involved as lipid carriers of monosaccharides to the microsomal glycosyltransferases for the addition of the carbohydrate moieties to the nascent polypeptide in the synthesis of glycoproteins [14].

C. Lipid Metabolism

1. Fatty Acids

The endoplasmic reticulum plays a major role in the metabolism of lipids, with a diversity of enzyme functions [19], and contains the enzyme acyl CoA-synthetase which is responsible for removing lipids from these membranes and for initiation of the synthesis and transformation of fatty acids by activation of exogenous and endogenous acids to acyl-CoA derivatives. The oxidation of fatty acids occurs primarily in the mitochondria, and the de novo synthesis of saturated fatty acids occurs in the cytosol, but it is the endoplasmic reticulum which is concerned with the desaturation of fatty acids and with the conversion of unsaturated acyl CoA derivatives to higher homologs with increased chain length and an increased number of double bonds. Moreover, microsomal cytochrome P-450 can also effect ω- and certain other hydroxylations of fatty acids. The Δ^9-desaturation of fatty acids, e.g., stearic acid ⟶ stearyl CoA ⟶ oleyl CoA, which can occur in both animal and plant microsomes, requires NADH or NADPH, a flavoprotein reductase, cytochrome b_5, and the terminal oxidase (desaturase) which is a nonheme iron protein [19,20].

Polyunsaturated fatty acids are essential components of phospholipids and cholesteryl esters and play important roles in intracellular membranes, in the transport of plasma lipoproteins, and as precursors of prostaglandins. The biosynthesis of these polyunsaturated acids is different in plants and animals and in the latter occurs by the insertion of a new double bond between the preexisting double bond and the carboxyl group. Four families of polyunsaturated fatty acids are synthesized in the endoplasmic reticulum of animal cells, namely, palmitoleic, oleic, linoleic, and linolenic; the first two may be formed by microsomal desaturase from palmitic and stearic acids, but the latter two are essential fatty acids obtained from plants. The Δ^6, Δ^5, and Δ^4-desaturases are microsomal enzymes, very similar to the Δ^9-desaturase in that they involve the cytochrome b_5 system and form double bonds between the 6,7-; 5,6-; and 4,5-carbon atoms. The Δ^6-desaturase is the first enzyme in the sequence of microsomal reactions which synthesizes polyunsaturated acids and is usually followed by chain elongation to 20-carbon acids and then further desaturation by Δ^5-desaturase, further extension to 22-carbon acids, and desaturation by Δ^4-desaturase [19]. The fatty acid elongation process may occur in the mitochondria or the microsomes; the mitochondrial reaction requires condensation with acetyl CoA and reversal of β-oxidation, while the microsomal reaction requires condensation with malonyl CoA (see Fig. 1).

Fatty acids may also undergo hydroxylation at the ω, ω-1 and α positions catalyzed by the microsomal cytochrome P-450 monooxygenase system. ω-Hydroxylation of the hydrocarbon chain of fatty acids is followed by oxidation to a dicarboxylic acid which involves soluble enzymes of the cytosol and NAD. ω-Hydroxylation of fatty acids is important in the production of succinyl-CoA from fatty acids and in the regulation of carbohydrate metabolism. In starving or diabetic rats, significant ω-oxidation and subsequent β-oxidation of fatty acids occurs, and the dicarboxylic acids are more readily converted into blood glucose than are monocarboxylic acids [21]. α-Hydroxylation by cytochrome P-450 yields 2-hydroxyacids which are important in the biosynthesis of cerebrosides, e.g., 2-hydroxylignoceric acid. These fatty acid oxygenations occur in microsomes of liver and kidney cortex, and the kidney cytochrome P-450k system has a preference for the hydroxylation of fatty acids, such as lauric acid, to the hydroxylation of drugs and xenobiotics [22].

Microsomal enzymes are also involved in the biosynthesis of phosphatidic acid, the phosphatidyl-cholines, -serines, -ethanolamines, and -inositols, the sphingolipids, and other lipid molecules [19].

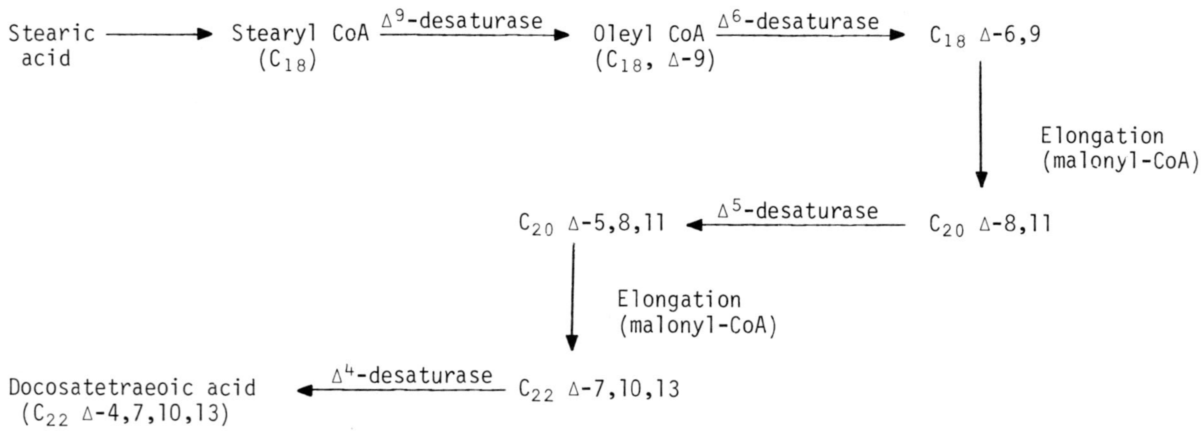

FIGURE 1 Microsomal biosynthesis of polyunsaturated fatty acids. Similar pathways occur for the other families of polyunsaturated acids, namely, palmitic, linoleic, and linolenic.

2. Prostaglandins

The enzyme system which converts the polyunsaturated fatty acids to prostaglandins, namely, prostaglandin synthetase, is a microsomal enzyme which has been shown to occur in a wide variety of tissues including liver, kidney, intestines, prostate, uterus, and the eye. The biosynthesis requires monooxygenation and dioxygenation via a transient peroxide species and a five-membered cyclic endoperoxide and, since both prostaglandins ($F_{1\alpha}$, E_1, and E_2) and their fatty acid precursors have high affinities for cytochrome P-450 of the adrenal microsomes, it has been suggested that cytochrome P-450 may play a role in both the synthesis and metabolism of these compounds [23]. It has also been shown that prostaglandins PGA_1 and PGE_2 are hydroxylated by kidney cortex microsomal monooxygenase [24]. Furthermore, inhibition and spectral studies of blood platelet microsomal cytochrome P-450 and arachidonate suggest that the microsomal monooxygenases may play a role in the complex enzyme system which converts arachidonate to cyclic endoperoxides, thromboxane A_2, and platelet-aggregating factors [25].

3. Cholesterol

The contribution of microsomal enzymes, particularly those of the liver, to the biosynthesis of cholesterol is substantial and includes the conversion of β-hydroxymethylglutaryl-CoA into mevalonate, the conversion of farnesyl pyrophosphate into presqualene pyrophosphate and its reduction to squalene, the monooxygenation of squalene to form squalene 2,3-epoxide, and the cyclization of this into lanosterol. The alternative pathways of conversion of lanosterol into cholesterol also involve the participation of microsomal enzymes.

The principal fate of cholesterol is its conversion into bile acids; hydroxyl groups may be introduced into the 6α, 6β, 7α, 12α, 16α, 23, 24, 25, and 26 positions all of which, with the exception of C-24 and C-26 hydroxylations which are mitochondrial processes, are catalyzed by microsomal monooxygenases requiring NADPH and molecular oxygen (see Fig. 2) [19]. Cytochrome P-450, cytochrome P-450 reductase, and phosphatidylcholine are required in many of these hydroxylations and free cholesterol, but not its esters, is first hydroxylated to 7α-hydroxycholesterol, which is the rate-limiting step in the biosynthesis of the bile acids. Cholesterol 7α-hydroxylase, although cytochrome P-450-dependent, is a unique monooxygenase which is distinctly different from that which catalyzes drug oxygenations [26]. The 26-hydroxylase has also been shown to be a cytochrome P-450-dependent enzyme, but this monooxygenase is located in the mitochondria of the liver [27]. The activity of 7α-hydroxylase is regulated by the concentrations of bile and cholesterol in the liver; the enzyme is inhibited by the catatoxic steroid, PCN, by high bile acid concentrations and consequently by a high degree of enterohepatic recirculation of these acids, but

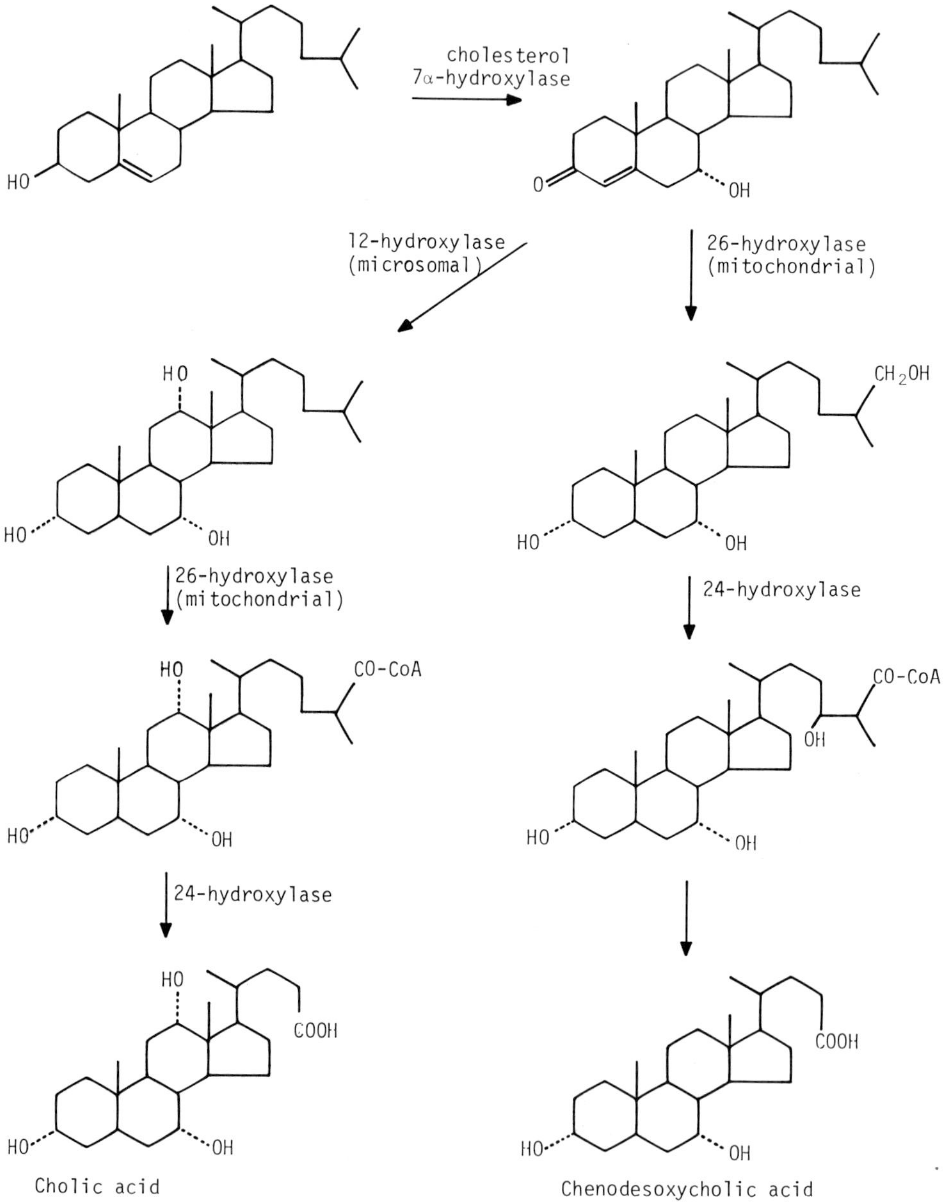

FIGURE 2 Hydroxylations involved in biosynthesis of bile acids.

is induced by administration of D-thyroxine and cholesterol and by the retention of the bile acids in the intestine by the administration of cholestryramine [26,28]. Unlike the hepatic microsomal monooxygenase(s) concerned with drug metabolism, cholesterol 7α-hydroxylase activity in rat liver also shows a marked circadian rhythm which parallels the plasma corticosterone concentration, and administration of natural or synthetic glucocorticoids similarly increases the enzymic activity [29].

4. Steroid Hormones

The biosynthesis of steroid hormones occurs in the ovary, testis, adrenal, and placenta, and proceeds from cholesterol via progesterone to androgens and thence to estrogens. The conversion of cholesterol by hydroxylations and side chain cleavage to pregnenolone occurs in the adrenal, testis, corpus luteum, and placenta but the enzymes are mitochondrial. The further metabolism of pregnenolone to progesterone is catalyzed by Δ5-3β-hydroxysteroid dehydrogenase which occurs in the microsomes of the adrenals, testis, and corpus luteum.

In the conversion of progesterone to androgens the first hydroxylation is effected by a 17α-hydroxylase which is a cytochrome P-450 enzyme found in the microsomal fraction of testis [30], and the subsequent metabolism of 17α-hydroxyprogesterone to androstene-3,17-dione and the reduction of this to testosterone are also catalyzed by microsomal enzymes of testis. The conversion of androgens into estrogens occurs readily in the placenta and involves elimination of the C-19 methyl group and aromatization of ring A. This complex reaction involves three hydroxylation reactions, two at C-19 and a third at C-1; all three hydroxylations require $NADPH_2$ and O_2 and appear to be mediated by microsomal cytochrome P-450 and its reductase [31,32]. Androstene-3,17-dione and testosterone are converted into estrone and estradiol, respectively. This placental microsomal cytochrome P-450 hydroxylase is anomalous in that although it is highly active as an aromatase in the conversion of androgens into estrogens, it exhibits but little drug-metabolizing activity.

In the biosynthesis of the corticosteroids by the adrenal cortex, progesterone is converted by the 21- and 11β-hydroxylases into corticosterone, or by the 17α-, 21-, and 11β-hydroxylases into cortisol. Corticosterone is further hydroxylated at C-18 to 18-hydroxycorticosterone and aldosterone. The 17α-, 21-, and 11β-hydroxylations involve cytochrome P-450 and a flavoprotein of both the microsomal and mitochondrial fractions, and may involve the formation of hydroperoxide intermediates and the formation of superoxide anion radicals from adrenodoxin and adrenodoxin reductase. In recent studies two distinctive cytochrome P-450 proteins have been isolated from bovine adrenal cortex mitochondria and purified to homogeneity [33]. The first of these, P-450_{sec}, catalyzes the formation of pregnenolone from cholesterol and the second, P-$450_{11\beta}$, hydroxylates deoxycorticosterone at the 11β and 18 positions, in addition to hydroxylating 4-androstene-3,17-dione and several other steroids.

Not only are the microsomal enzymes involved in the biogenesis of the steroid hormones, but they also play an important role in their metabolic deactivation. For example, testosterone is metabolized into the polar, saturated 2β-, 6β-, 7α-, and 16α-hydroxy-5α-dihydrotestosterone by rat liver microsomal preparations [34] (see Fig. 3).

5. Vitamin D

The activation of vitamin D_3 to 25-hydroxycholecalciferol by hepatic microsomal hydroxylation, then further hydroxylation to 1,25- or 24,25-dihydroxycholecalciferol in kidney mitochondria, yields the active hormone(s) concerned in calcium and phosphate metabolism. The 25-hydroxylation of cholecalciferol in the liver is catalyzed by a microsomal monooxygenase [35]. The biosynthesis of 1,25-dihydroxycholecalciferol in kidney is catalyzed by a multienzyme system in which cytochrome P-450 serves as the terminal oxidase for an iron-sulfur-protein reductase requiring NADPH and O_2 [36]. The demonstration that long-term administration of phenobarbital or diphenylhydantoin to rats decreases the activity of calciferol 25-hydroxylase suggests that if cytochrome P-450 is involved in the hydroxylation of vitamin D, it is probably an atypical form of this enzyme which is inhibited, rather than induced, by these drugs [37].

D. Heterogeneous Nature of Cytochrome P-450

The great multiplicity of substrates which undergo hydroxylations involving this enzyme has raised innumerable doubts concerning its homogeneity. How else could one single substrate, such as testosterone, undergo several hydroxylations at different C-atoms which change their relative magnitudes following pretreatment of the animal with different inducing agents? Three different concepts of enzymology may account for this phenomenon, namely:

i. Heterogeneity of the apoenzyme, by which there exists a multiplicity of enzyme proteins, all with overlapping substrate selectivities, but each with a preference for a particular class of substrate
ii. Structural changes of the cytochrome, brought about by the substrate and by pretreatment, which may produce allosteric or conformational changes in the apoenzyme, or in its relationship to the heme, which results in changes in the selectivity and/or availability of the enzyme site(s)
iii. Changes in the mode of hydroxylation and mechanism of oxygen transfer, due to changes in the structure or conformation of the cytochrome itself, or in its relationships with cytochrome P-450 reductase or other components of the endoplasmic reticulum, which would modulate the hydroxylation process between the various alternative available mechanisms, including epoxidation, dioxygenation,

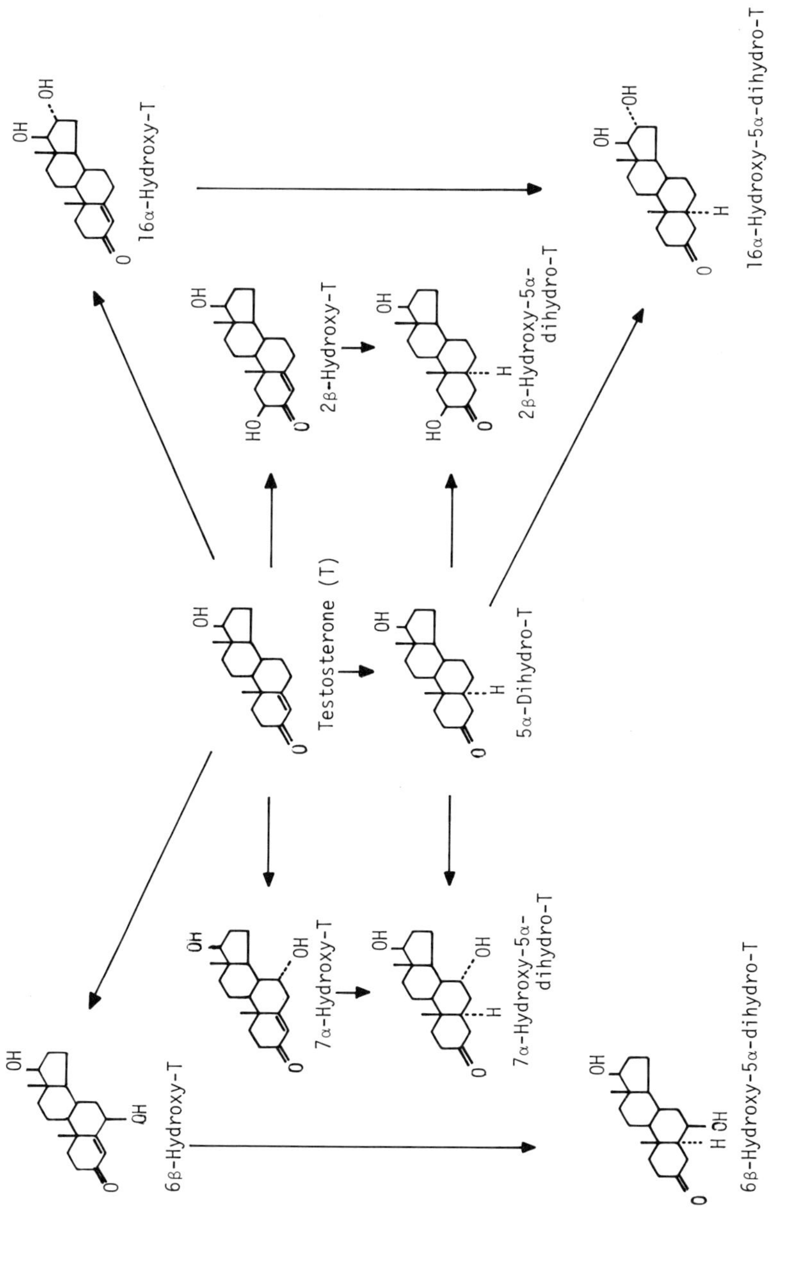

FIGURE 3 Hydroxylation products of testosterone.

hydroperoxidation, direct insertion of singlet oxygen, superoxide anion mediation, etc. [38].

The fact that the microsomal monooxygenase system is a multicomponent, membrane-bound enzyme makes possible all of these alternative postulates, and the combination of these phenomena could result in an almost infinite variety of hydroxylations, applicable to a great diversity of substrates yet each with a high degree of substrate and product selectivity. The existence of multiple forms of the terminal oxidase cytochrome P-450 was predicted by Conney [39] and has been recently established on the basis of spectrophotometric, electrophoretic, immunological, and structural evidence obtained with detergent-solubilized preparations of the hemoprotein. These multiple forms have differing substrate selectivities, with varying degrees of overlap, and although genetically determined, appear to be individually substrate-inducible. Induction of rat liver microsomal hemoprotein with phenobarbital and 3-methylcholanthrene gives two spectrally different enzymes, namely, cytochrome P-450 and cytochrome P-448, respectively [40], but more recent studies with the mouse have shown that, based on density subfractionation and different spectral behavior, a total of seven cytochromes are necessary to explain the response to the two types of inducing agent [41]. Using immunochemical methods, Thomas and colleagues [42,43] have presented evidence of the existence of six different cytochrome P-450s in the endoplasmic reticulum of rat liver. However, spectral differences could be due to differences in associated ligands, enzyme conformation, or membrane structure, as well as to structural differences in the apoenzyme, and immunological differences could be due merely to the presence of different sugar moieties in the cytochrome P-450 glycoprotein.

Using gel electrophoresis methods, Bell and Hodgson [44] have demonstrated the existence of four cytochrome P-450 proteins in mouse liver microsomal preparations; one increases following 3-methylcholanthrene administration, two increase with phenobarbital, and the fourth decreases following treatment with either of these inducing agents. However, SDS polyacrylamide gel electrophoresis will not separate component polypeptides of similar molecular weight, so that a greater number of different cytochromes than four is possible. Anion-exchange chromatography of detergent-solubilized cytochrome P-450 from livers of untreated rats also yielded four fractions with 70-80% recovery and no significant denaturation to cytochrome P-420 [45]. Each of the four fractions was further resolved by electrofocusing in polyacrylamide into numerous protein bands, more than eight of which contained heme. These results indicate potential extensive heterogeneity, but the authors [45] rightly advise cautious interpretation in view of the possible effects of the detergents used.

As a contribution to the clarification and rationalization of this rather confused state of knowledge, a number of cytochrome P-450s have been purified to apparent homogeneity [46]. One fraction from the liver microsomes of methylcholanthrene-treated rats and two fractions from phenobarbital-treated rats have been purified to homogeneity as judged by the following criteria: polyacrylamide gel electrophoresis in six systems, immunological activity, NH_2-terminal analysis, specific activity, and the kinetics of 7-ethoxycoumarin deethylase with reconstituted enzyme systems. A third fraction from phenobarbital-treated rats was heterogeneous only in one of the gel electrophoresis systems and from this and the other criteria was judged to be a mixture of two proteins. The three homogeneous cytochrome P-450s are distinguished by different electrophoretic mobilities, amino acid compositions, NH_2- and -COOH terminal amino acid sequences, and immunological characteristics. Yet, although Ouchterlony double diffusion analysis in the presence of two antibodies shows that the three purified cytochrome P-450s are distinct from each other, there are indications that the three proteins are immunochemically related [46]. Further evidence of the distinctiveness of these three homogeneous cytochrome P-450s has been obtained by their enzymic hydrolysis with α-chymotrypsin, papain, or with a protease from Staph. aureus, followed by peptide mapping in acrylamide gel [47]. The results confirm that these three cytochrome P-450s are different proteins whose differences in electrophoretic mobilities, immunological properties, and substrate selectivities are not due to minor variations of basic polypeptide structure. Thus from these rigorous biochemical studies there is indication of the existence of at least three and possibly five distinctive cytochrome P-450s in the endoplasmic reticulum of rat liver.

Similar heterogeneity has been observed in the NADPH-cytochrome P-450 reductase, although the flavoproteins isolated from different tissues, and even from different species, exhibit much similarity in their peptide maps [47], suggesting a closer relationship than exists for the cytochrome P-450s.

Evidence also exists for the existence of two different substrate-selective liver microsomal enzyme systems for UDP-glucuronyltransferase, one of which is stimulated by phenobarbital and the other by 3-methylcholanthrene [48]. However, without isolation and purification of these enzymes to homogeneity, it is not possible to decide whether the two different enzyme systems are due to distinct enzyme proteins or result from a single enzyme protein subject to differential regulation.

Changes in the nature of the enzyme activity of cytochrome P-450 not resulting from enzyme induction and de novo synthesis of new hemoproteins have been seen in the shift from 4-hydroxylation of biphenyl (cytochrome P-450) to 2-hydroxylation (cytochrome P-448) following the in vitro treatment of rat liver microsomes with corticosteroids or carcinogens [49-52]. This phenomenon of "activation" has been observed by other workers and possibly results from a conformational change of the enzyme. A similar phenomenon has been observed following the administration of certain chlorophenols when the flavoprotein reductase appears to take over the function of monooxygenase and switches the C-hydroxylation of N,N-dimethylaniline to predominantly N-oxidation [53]. Similarly, repeated administration of 2-acetamidofluorene results in a 12-fold increase in the N-hydroxylation of this substrate in rat liver, but with no increase in the synthesis of microsomal protein [54]. Stier [15] has suggested that changes in the lipid milieu of the endoplasmic reticulum could lead to decoupling of the cytochrome P-450 from its flavoprotein reductase resulting in changes in the mode of hydroxylation with the cytochrome functioning as a dioxygenase and the flavoprotein as a monooxygenase. Varying degrees of change to the lipid envelope could result in a continuous modulation of the different types of oxygenase activity which, from examination of the products of the reaction, could give the erroneous impression of a multiplicity of enzymes. Since this modulation could, to some extent, be induced by the lipophilic substrates themselves, this might result in a substrate-induced specificity of the enzymic reaction and of the product(s).

As liver microsomes may produce superoxide anion radicals and hydrogen peroxide from both the cytochrome and the flavoprotein moieties [55], structural changes in the cytochrome itself, and/or modulation of the lipid milieu, might result in an infinite variation of the operative mode of hydroxylation, which could add to the possible variety of hydroxylation products. These dynamic concepts of heterogeneity of the monooxygenases, which arise from the intrinsic dynamic heterogeneity of the biological membrane, have the virtue of almost infinite versatility which is difficult to envisage solely from the chemical concepts of multiple enzyme proteins.

III. PHYSIOLOGICAL CHANGES

A. Regulation of Protein Synthesis by Steroid Hormones

The binding of the ribosomes to the endoplasmic reticulum requires corticosteroid and/or appropriate sex hormones. Male rat liver smooth microsomes associate with ribosomes to form rough microsomes only under the influence of corticosterone or estradiol and female rat liver smooth microsomes require corticosterone or androgenic hormones for combination with ribosomes [56]. These steroid hormones also exert a protective effect against the degranulation of RER by the carcinogen aflatoxin. The regulation of the pattern of protein synthesis, that is, the ratio of secretory proteins (glycoproteins) synthesized on the RER to intracellular proteins synthesized by free polyribosomes, thus appears to be under the control of steroid hormones. There is evidence that this also pertains to tissues other than the liver, for cortisol and other glucocorticoids inhibit the biosynthesis of glycosaminoglycans by human fibroblasts [57], the synthesis of rat gastric mucus [58], and the formation of collagen, together with the activities of the prolyl and lysyl hydroxylases, of rat dermis [59]. Presumably, glucocorticoid hormone inhibition of glycoprotein synthesis in the lymphocyte and plasma cell could result in a diminution of immunoglobulin formation and thus account for the immunosuppressive action of corticosteroid hormones.

Similarly, it could explain the regulation of cellular proliferation and tissue growth by the corticosteroid and sex hormones.

B. Regulation of Monooxygenase Activity

The coupling of cytochrome P-450 with its flavoprotein reductase by the membrane phospholipid may be affected by drugs and environmental chemicals in two ways [15]. They could bring about phase separation and decoupling of the monooxygenase components by binding to cytochrome P-450, or by interactions with the bulk of membrane lipids, thus resulting in changes in the nature of the oxygenase activity from hydroxylation (coupled cytochrome P-450 and flavoprotein reductase) to hydroxylation (decoupled flavoprotein) and peroxidation (decoupled cytochrome P-450).

C. Induction and Inhibition of the Microsomal Monooxygenases

Repeated dosing with certain drugs or environmental chemicals leads to enhanced activity of the microsomal monooxygenases as a result of increased synthesis of these enzymes. It is believed that high substrate concentration is responsible for enzyme induction; for if a drug is slowly metabolized, or is present at high concentration, the enzyme active site will be occupied by substrate for long periods of time, and may lead to competitive inhibition of the enzyme, which in turn leads to genomal derepression, accelerated synthesis of the enzyme protein, and enhanced enzymic activity. Hence, substrates which are only slowly metabolized (phenobarbital) or metabolized with difficulty (DDT, polychlorobiphenyls) are generally found to be inducing agents of the monooxygenases in the endoplasmic reticulum.

Inhibition of the drug-metabolizing enzymes may result from the competitive inhibition of high concentrations of substrate, which is followed by enzyme induction, or may be noncompetitive inhibition in which the inhibitor is firmly bound to the enzyme, as for example the inhibition by methylenedioxyaryl compounds [60] and thiono sulfur-containing compounds [61].

The various microsomal enzyme activities may be induced to different extents by different enzyme-inducing agents, but three major classes of inducers of the drug-metabolizing enzyme have been recognized:

i. Drugs—which lead to an increase of cytochrome P-450 and of the coupled reductase(s)
ii. Carcinogenic polycyclic hydrocarbons—which result in an increase of cytochrome P-448 but not to any significant increase of reductase(s).

iii. Catatoxic steroids—which give no increase of cytochrome(s) but lead to a substantial increase in NADPH-cytochrome c reductase

1. Differences Between Drugs and Carcinogens as Enzyme Inducers

The carcinogenic polycyclic aromatic hydrocarbons, such as benzo[a]-pyrene and 3-methylcholanthrene, are rather slow inducers of the microsomal enzymes compared with drugs like phenobarbital. The carcinogens result in the appearance of cytochrome P-448 instead of cytochrome P-450, with no increase in the reductase; the increase in de novo protein synthesis is relatively slow and with methylcholanthrene does not reach a maximum for several days, whereas with phenobarbital the maximum increase in enzyme synthesis occurs within 2 or 3 days.

In contrast to drugs, the carcinogenic polycyclic hydrocarbons lead to no significant hepatic hypertrophy, no marked inhibition of microsomal ribonuclease, and to little or no increase in microsomal phospholipid, all suggesting lesser increases in de novo synthesis. In addition there are substantial differences between drug and carcinogen inducers in the changed preference for substrate, and of the products of oxygenation, which has been associated with the preferential synthesis of different cytochrome P-450s. Whereas phenobarbital increases the binding of both type I and type II substrates, carcinogens increase primarily the binding of type II substrates; for example, the hydroxylation of hexobarbital and phenobarbital are increased by drugs but show no marked increase following treatment with carcinogen inducers. An even more fundamental difference is seen with the metabolism of biphenyl, for whereas drugs enhance the 4-hydroxylation of biphenyl, the 2-hydroxylation is increased only by carcinogens. This distinct difference between these two types of enzyme-inducing agent has been suggested as the basis of a short-term test for chemical carcinogenicity [51].

Many persistent environmental chemicals, especially when halogenated are highly potent inducers of the microsomal monooxygenases (e.g., tetrachlorodibenzodioxins, polyhalogenated biphenyls). The polychlorinated biphenyl isomers have been shown to fall into the category of "drug" or "carcinogen" inducers according to the positions of the halogen substituents [62]. Biphenyls chlorinated symmetrically in both the meta and para positions (3,4,3',4'-tetra and 3,4,5,3',4',5'-hexa-chlorophenyls), like carcinogens, increase cytochrome P-448 and are the most toxic. In contrast, biphenyl isomers chlorinated in both para and ortho positions (2,4,2',4'-tetra- and 2,4,5,2',4',5'-, 2,3,4,2',3',4'-, and 2,4,6,2',4',6'-hexa-chlorobiphenyls) act like drugs and increase cytochrome P-450. Other chlorinated biphenyls have little or no enzyme-inducing activity.

Many naturally occurring substances are both inhibitors and inducers of the microsomal drug-metabolizing enzymes, and none of these has been studied more than alcohol. There are many claims that ethanol induces the drug-metabolizing enzymes of the liver and specifically increases one particular form of cytochrome P-450 [63,64]. However, this is a matter of considerable controversy and many laboratories, including our own [65], have been unable to demonstrate enzyme induction except after very high dosage (>12 g/kg body wt per day) [66].

2. Effects of Enzyme Induction and Inhibition on Toxicity

Induction of the microsomal monooxygenases decreases the toxic actions of those chemicals which are toxic per se and are detoxicated by metabolism. For example, pretreatment with various drugs increases the 2-hydroxylation and conjugation of strychnine and thus decreases its toxicity [67]. Similarly, the catatoxic steroid inducing agent pregnenolone-16α-carbonitrile (PCN) decreases the acute hepatotoxicity of dimethylnitrosamine. When toxic chemicals are activated instead of being detoxicated by metabolism, enzyme induction leads to increased toxicity. For example, pretreatment with phenobarbital markedly increases the hepatotoxicity of carbon tetrachloride and the centrilobular hepatic necrosis produced by bromobenzene. In contrast, pretreatment with 3-methylcholanthrene does not markedly accelerate the metabolism of bromobenzene but shifts the pattern of metabolism away from the more toxic pathways, increasing the amounts of bromophenyldihydrodiol and 2-bromophenol formed but decreasing the amount of 4-bromophenol and bromophenylmercapturic acid [68]. Similarly, in contrast to pretreatment with phenobarbital, treatment of rats with methylcholanthrene decreases the hepatotoxicity of carbon tetrachloride [69,70], and this has been attributed to the absence of any increase in the flavoprotein reductase and the replacement of cytochrome P-450 by cytochrome P-448. The activation of CCl_4 to the toxic CCl_3 free radical probably requires reductive dechlorination by cytochrome P-450, but the consequent lipid peroxidation appears to result from a leakage of electrons from the flavoprotein reductase.

Microsomal enzyme induction may also affect testosterone biosynthesis, and, contrary to the effect on the liver cytochrome, pretreatment of rats with 3-methylcholanthrene leads to a <u>decrease</u> of global cytochrome P-450s in the testis (50%), decreased progesterone 17α-hydroxylase activity (40%), decreased testosterone biosynthesis (40%), and decreased weight of the seminal vesicles [71]. In contrast, pretreatment with phenobarbital had no effect on testicular cytochrome P-450 or any other of these parameters affecting male fertility.

Many studies have been made of the effects of microsomal enzyme inhibitors on the activation of carcinogens, obviously with a view to decreasing their potential carcinogenicity. 7,8-Benzoflavone, an inhibitor of aryl hydrocarbon hydroxylase, inhibits the hydroxylation of benzo[a]pyrene in rat liver and decreases the extent of covalent binding of the activated metabolites to DNA [72]. Retinol and various vitamin A derivatives and the antioxidant butylated hydroxytoluene (BHT) also inhibit epoxidation of benzo[a]pyrene and other carcinogenic hydrocarbons, and result in decreased binding of the carcinogen active metabolites to DNA [73]. Inhibition may also increase the activity of certain carcinogens; for example, piperonyl butoxide administered to hamsters inhibits the 7-hydroxylation of 2-acetamidofluorene (detoxication) by 61% but simultaneously stimulates the N-hydroxylation (activation) 10-fold leading to a marked increase in the binding of this carcinogenic amide to RNA and DNA [74]. Inhibition of metabolic pathways, other than hydroxylation, may also result in changes in the activity of carcinogens. Pretreatment of rats with para-hydroxyacetanilide leads to no significant change in microsomal aryl hydroxylase but increases the glucuronyltransferase activity threefold, resulting in a marked decrease in tumor induction by 2-acetamidofluorene or its N-hydroxy metabolite [75].

3. Enzyme Induction in Extrahepatic Tissues

Enzyme induction and inhibition are not confined to the microsomal enzymes of the liver but have also been shown to occur in the lungs, the gastrointestinal tract, and several other tissues, and may lead to increased or decreased toxicity as with the liver enzymes.

One unusual aspect of extrahepatic enzyme induction concerns the induction of the monooxygenases of the mammalian placenta. For although the placenta contains only a very small amount of cytochrome P-450, it exhibits high monooxygenase activity, especially that concerning the synthesis of estrogens by the aromatization of androgens. Attempts to induce this cytochrome P-450 system by the administration of various drugs have been largely unsuccessful, but benzopyrene hydroxylase, 3-methyl-4-monomethylaminoazobenzene-N-demethylase, phenacetin deethylase, and the metabolism of cholesterol to pregnenolone are markedly affected by administration of carcinogenic polycyclic hydrocarbons to the mother, or as the result of the mother smoking cigarettes. Benzopyrene hydroxylation in placental tissue is increased, and cholesterol metabolism decreased, as the number of cigarettes smoked per day increases [76]. What effect this has on the unborn infant is a matter for conjecture, but it is well known that low weight for date babies are associated with heavy cigarette smoking. As smoking decreases the metabolism of cholesterol to pregnenolone, it is possible that this would also decrease the placental synthesis of progestational steroids and estrogens, hormones which are essential for the maintenance of the pregnancy.

4. Long-term Drug Therapy and Folate Deficiency

One of the adverse effects of enzyme induction, which is observed in long-term drug therapy, is the depletion of folate. In pregnant rats maintained on a limited folate diet, the long-term administration of phenobarbital plus phenytoin results in offspring with low birth weights and marked deformities of the bones and soft tissues, whereas rats maintained on a folate-supplemented diet and also given phenobarbital and phenytoin long-term, delivered perfectly normal progeny [77].

The prolonged administration of enzyme-inducing drugs, such as the anticonvulsants phenobarbital, phenytoin, primidone, and pheneturide, may also result in vitamin D deficiency and osteomalacia. This has been attributed to an enhancement of the microsomal deactivation of 1,25-dihydroxycholecalciferol, since inducers such as phenobarbital may accelerate the hepatic 25-hydroxylation of cholecalciferol (vitamin D_3) and do not alter the rate of the subsequent conversion to 1,25-dihydroxycholecalciferol, the biologically active coenzyme [78].

D. Changes in Phospholipids

Phospholipids are intrinsic components of the endoplasmic reticulum and phosphatidylcholine has been demonstrated as an essential component of the hepatic microsomal monooxygenase system [79]. In reconstitution of the solubilized liver microsomal monooxygenases, phosphatidylcholine is essential to the hydroxylation activity of purified cytochrome P-450 plus NADPH-cytochrome P-450 reductase. Moreover, treatment of microsomal preparations with phospholipase results in a significant decrease of the N-demethylation of benzphetamine or aminopyrine, although aniline hydroxylation is unaffected [80], and peroxidative destruction of the unsaturated fatty acids of the phospholipids of the endoplasmic reticulum also causes a marked decrease in oxidative demethylation [81]. Pretreatment with phenobarbital increased the contents of phosphatidylcholine and phosphatidylethanolamine of rat liver endoplasmic reticulum, and also increased the linoleic acid of phosphatidylcholine in a manner which paralleled the increases in cytochrome P-450, NADPH-cytochrome P-450 reductase, and aminopyrine N-demethylase and biphenyl hydroxylase activities [82]. These authors therefore consider that a distinct species of phosphatidylcholine, or phosphatidylethanolamine, containing linoleic acid in the β position is essential for hepatic microsomal oxidative demethylation.

The ratio of phosphatidylcholine to phosphatidylethanolamine ($\sim$2.5) would appear to be of importance in the normal functioning of the endoplasmic reticulum, and is disturbed by deficiencies in choline, vitamin B_{12}, or methyl group donors. The stepwise methylation of phosphatidylethanolamine to phosphatidylcholine is catalyzed by an enzyme(s) of the endoplasmic reticulum, and is regulated by the existing ratio of these two phospholipids [83]. Phosphatidylcholine may also be synthesized by the direct incorporation of choline, via CDP-choline. The female rat, like choline-deficient animals, preferentially synthesizes phosphatidylcholine via the indirect, methylation pathway, and if given dietary supplements of choline shows a marked increase in hepatic smooth endoplasmic reticulum and the associated microsomal monooxygenase activities [83a]. The male rat shows no similar changes when given choline, so that the well-known sex difference of microsomal oxidase activities in the rat may be due, at least in part, to the deficiency of phosphatidylcholine in the female, and to the greater dependence of this sex on the methylation pathway for lecithin synthesis. Administration of choline increased the metabolic activation and acute hepatotoxicity of dimethylnitrosamine in female rats [84], and dietary depletion of choline to male rats changed the organ susceptibility of the direct-acting carcinogen azaserine, increasing its hepatocarcinogenic effect with simultaneous decrease in its pancreatic carcinogenicity [85].

The total phospholipid content of mouse hepatic microsomal fraction declines with age. The choline-containing phospholipids (phosphatidylcholine, lysophosphatidylcholine, and sphingomyelin) are maximal at 100-300 days of age after which they decline to 50% or less of these levels at 600 days of age. The noncholine phospholipids (phosphatidylethanolamine, phosphatidylserine, and phosphatidic acid) increase, to partially compensate for the loss of the choline phospholipids. Since phosphatidylethanolamine is an antagonist for phosphatidylcholine, an essential component for hydroxylation by the reconstituted microsomal system [79], these age-related changes might be expected to result in marked changes in the rates and patterns of microsomal hydroxylation in older animals.

IV. PATHOLOGICAL CHANGES

A. Ligand-complex Formation, Inhibition of Cytochrome P-450, and Cytotoxicity

In recent years a new facet of microsomal oxidation has been revealed, in which an intermediate of the enzymic reaction, or the reaction product, remains tightly bound to the enzyme system, usually in the form of a ligand complex with cytochrome P-450. The results of this binding of reaction products may include inhibition of microsomal monooxygenase activity [86], lipid peroxidation, loss of cytochrome P-450 activity with increase in cytochrome P-448-type hydroxylations [87], and denaturation and degradation of cytochrome P-450 [88]. For example, the weak hepatocarcinogen safrole when repeatedly administered to rats leads to induction of the hepatic microsomal monooxygenases and increased total cytochrome P-450s, but results in a decrease of the activities of these enzymes, except biphenyl 2-hydroxylase (P-448), because of the ligand binding of an oxidative product of safrole to cytochrome P-450 forming a carbene complex [89] (see Fig. 4). There is further evidence that long-term administration of this chemical to rats results in a continued increase in synthesis of the microsomal monooxygenase but, paradoxically, with the loss of normal cytochrome P-450 activity, and an accompanying degranulation of the endoplasmic reticulum and increase in cytochrome P-448 enzymic activity [90].

Similar ligand complexes are formed by other methylenedioxyaryl compounds (e.g., piperonyl butoxide), amphetamines, and other lipophilic

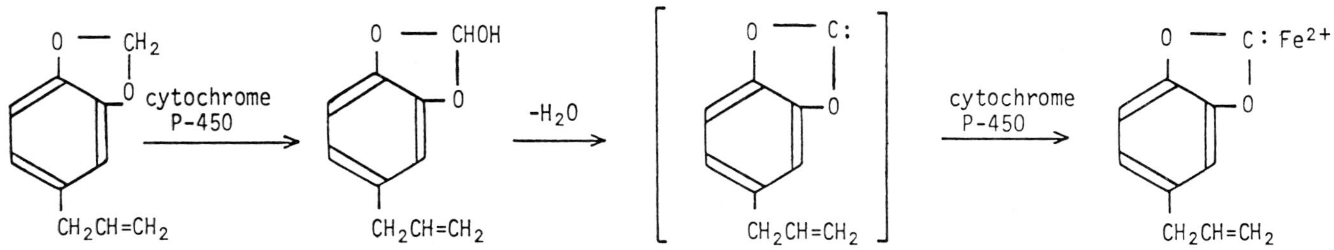

Safrole

Safrole carbene

Safrole carbene complex with cytochrome P-450

FIGURE 4 Ligand complex formation of safrole with cytochrome P-450.

amines [91], hydroxylamines [92], carbanions, carbenes, organic thiols and sulfides, phosphines, etc. Moreover, it is not only the cytochrome P-450 of the liver which is affected, for cytochrome P-450 of the lung, intestines, and probably other extrahepatic tissues have also been shown to form ligand complexes with these substrates [93]. The formation of ligand complexes is higher with the species of cytochrome P-450 resulting from induction with phenobarbital, but is almost abolished following enzyme induction with 3-methylcholanthrene, which yields predominantly cytochrome P-448 [94]. Of the mammalian species examined, ligand complex formation is highest in the mouse [91], as might have been predicted, since microsomal oxidation is a prerequisite of ligand complex formation and the rates of monooxygenation are highest in the smallest animals [87].

Many halogenated compounds such as carbon tetrachloride, chloroform, halothane, Freons [95,96], and polychlorobiphenyls [97] are known to result in ligand complex formation with cytochrome P-450. It has been shown by various workers that these halogenated compounds are dehalogenated by cytochrome P-450, operating in the anaerobic mode, giving rise to highly reactive, dehalogenated radicals which bind to cytochrome P-450 to form a carbene ligand complex (see Fig. 5). The mechanism by which carbon tetrachloride, and other haloalkanes, undergo covalent binding to lipid and protein, and initiate lipid peroxidation and hepatic necrosis, is still not agreed. Slater and Sawyer [98] have suggested that CCl_4 is converted to $\dot{C}Cl_3$ by the microsomal flavoprotein reductase, whereas other investigators have proposed that the site of activation of the CCl_4 is cytochrome P-450/cytochrome P-450 reductase. More recent studies [99] have shown that cytochrome P-450 is the site of bioactivation of CCl_4 and other halomethanes, and that whereas the activation of CCl_4 proceeds by cytochrome P-450-dependent reductive pathways, the activation of $CHCl_3$ proceeds by cytochrome P-450–dependent oxidative pathways. However, the work of Suarez and coworkers [70] and Masuda and Murano [100] has revealed that the microsomal flavoprotein NADPH-cytochrome P-450 reductase is also involved in the lipid peroxidation/cytotoxic effects of CCl_4. This is possibly because the ligand complexing and inhibition of the terminal cytochrome P-450 leads to decoupling of the cytochrome from the flavoprotein [15] when the flavoprotein then functions as a nonspecific oxygenase leading to lipid peroxidation [86]. This phenomenon has been observed with pentachlorophenol and other halogenated phenols and pesticides, which have been shown to interfere with the functional coupling of cytochrome P-450 to the flavoprotein reductase, switching the C-hydroxylation by cytochrome P-450 of secondary and tertiary amines to their N-oxidation by the flavoprotein [53].

Numerous thiocarbonyl compounds (carbon disulfide, [101]; disulfiram, [102]) and thiophosphonyl compounds (parathion) are converted into their oxygen analogs by the microsomal monooxygenases. As a consequence of this process the sulfur atom is transferred onto the apocytochrome P-450,

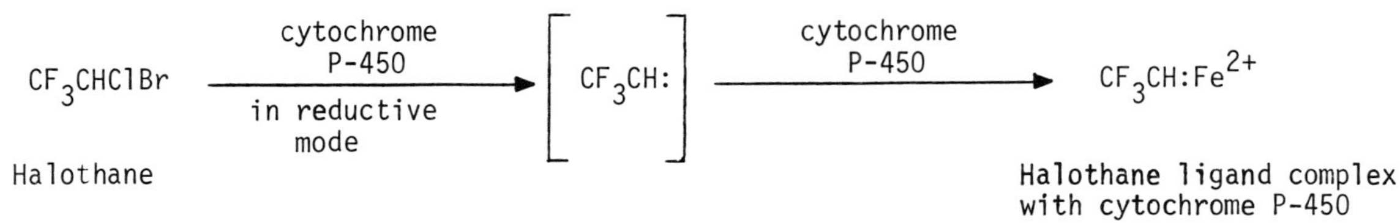

FIGURE 5 Ligand complex formation of halothane with cytochrome P-450.

resulting in inhibition of hydroxylase activity, lipid peroxidation, and destruction of the cytochrome P-450. Recent studies have shown that carbon disulfide is progressively oxidized to carbon dioxide with transfer of S to cytochrome P-450 [103] which becomes denatured to cytochrome P-420, leads to lipid peroxidation and to the ultimate destruction of cytochrome P-450 and cytochrome P-448 [88]. It is suggested that the sulfur atom may become covalently bound to the thiol of the fifth ligand of cytochrome P-450, forming a disulfide bond and leading to destabilization of the cytochrome [88] (see Fig. 6).

Microsomal preparations undergoing NADPH-dependent lipid peroxidation exhibit a loss of heme from cytochrome P-450, production of green pigment (porphyrins) as degradation products of heme, and formation of small amounts of CO. Similar phenomena are seen in the heme degradation resulting from the administration of 2-allyl-2-isopropylacetamide. In contrast to its natural degradation by the liver heme oxygenase system, the CO produced in the lipid peroxidative destruction of cytochrome P-450 is not derived from peroxidative cleavage of one of its methene bridges and may arise from the lipid itself [104]. Similarly, a number of acetylenic-substituted steroids (e.g., norethindrone) and other acetylenic compounds (e.g., dipropargylacetamide) also results in a decrease in liver microsomal cytochrome P-450, abnormal heme degradation, and formation of the characteristic green pigments by a process involving the oxidation of the acetylenic group [105].

When microsomal preparations incubated with ascorbate or NADPH undergo lipid peroxidation, the polyunsaturated fatty acids of the membrane phospholipids are degraded, leading to the formation of malondialdehyde, the destruction of membrane architecture, and the breakdown of membrane-bound enzymes including cytochrome P-450.

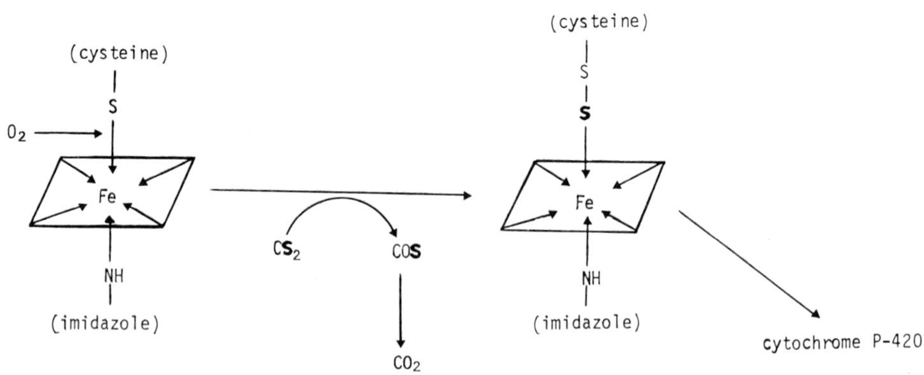

FIGURE 6 Proposed mechanism for desulfuration of carbon disulfide and simultaneous degradation of cytochrome P-450.

B. Lipid Peroxidation

Lipid peroxidation is the degradative oxidation of polyunsaturated fatty acids of intracellular lipids, often chemically induced, which leads to the formation of free radical intermediates and autocatalysis of the process. It leads to the destruction of membrane architecture, the degradation of membrane-bound enzymes, and eventually to cell death, and has been associated with aging, atherosclerosis, liver toxicity, and lung tissue injury. The etiology and mechanisms of action of lipid peroxidation have recently been reviewed by Plaa and Witschi [106]. Since the lipid peroxides undergo degradation to malondialdehyde, the extent of lipid peroxidation is frequently determined in biological material by the measurement of a colored complex with thiobarbituric acid, but this and other methods, such as the detection of conjugated dienes by UV spectrometry, have been criticized for lack of sensitivity, which is probably responsible for the paucity of firm knowledge concerning this phenomenon.

Rat liver microsomal preparations, as well as whole homogenates and subcellular fractions of many other tissues, when incubated in the presence of NADPH and ADP, or ascorbate, result in lipid peroxidation, which can be inhibited by antioxidants. Cytochrome P-450 does not seem to be involved in this process as it is not inhibited by carbon monoxide, and may even be increased, but nonheme iron in the form of a complex Fe^{2+} with phosphate appears to be essential. The unsaturated fatty acids of the endoplasmic reticulum and other membranes form the substrate for peroxidation which subsequently leads to the degradation of cytochrome P-450 and to loss of monooxygenase activity. Antioxidants such as butylated hydroxytoluene, chelating agents (EDTA), and free-radical trapping agents, inhibit microsomal lipid peroxidation. Simultaneously, these compounds inhibit the loss of microsomal unsaturated lipids and of cytochrome P-450, as well as the formation of malondialdehyde. The drug tinoridine, a potent lipid-antioxidant and an antiinflammatory drug, effectively inhibits peroxidation with an activity about 50 times greater than α-tocopherol [107]. Superoxide dismutase also inhibits microsomal lipid peroxidation in vitro which suggests that superoxide anion may be involved in this reaction. This peroxidative impairment of the integrity of the endoplasmic reticulum is normally minimized by the presence of antioxidants, such as α-tocopherol (Vitamin E) and selenium, although a low rate of lipid peroxidation may be responsible for the natural turnover of the endoplasmic reticulum and its component enzymes. In selenium deficiency, impaired activity of glutathione peroxidase may occur which will enhance lipid peroxidation. Selenium deficiency also leads to defective incorporation of heme into hemoproteins such as cytochrome P-450 and tryptophan pyrrolase, with a consequent increase in size of the pool of "free heme" and in the activity of microsomal heme oxygenase [108]. Singlet oxygen ($^1O_2$) is also generated as a transient by-product of the peroxidative decomposition of microsomal lipid [109].

The microsomal flavoprotein NADPH-cytochrome c reductase (NADPH-cytochrome P-450 reductase) has a critical role in lipid peroxidation, and antibodies to this enzyme completely inhibit the NADPH-dependent reaction. Another microsomal flavoprotein, cytochrome b_5 reductase, may also initiate liver microsomal lipid peroxidation.

Whereas microsomal lipid peroxidation may lead to a marked loss of cytochrome P-450 [110] and drug-metabolizing enzyme activity such as ethylmorphine demethylase, many substrates of these enzymes, such as aminopyrine and codeine, will inhibit NADPH-mediated peroxidation. The nonlinearity of enzyme kinetics in the rat liver microsomal oxidative metabolism of drugs in vitro has been attributed, at least in part, to lipid peroxidation and the consequent degradation of cytochrome P-450 [111]. However, the in vitro lipid peroxidation of liver microsomes varies widely with animal species, being highest in rat > guinea pig > mouse > rabbit. The degradation of microsomal lipids, cytochrome P-450, and of the microsomal membrane itself, would be expected to lead to an accelerated de novo synthesis of the membrane and its components, and is probably the natural mechanism for the biological turnover of the endoplasmic reticulum. This would explain the observation by Paine [38] that singlet oxygen is responsible for microsomal enzyme induction and proliferation of the endoplasmic reticulum.

Singlet oxygen may also be responsible for the toxic action of the herbicide paraquat upon the lung, since paraquat poisoning results in peroxidation of the lipids of lung tissue, and both poisoning and lipid peroxidation can be partially inhibited by treatment with superoxide dismutase [112]. Lipid peroxidation in lung tissue might similarly occur with drugs and other chemicals ingested orally, but which reach the lungs via the bloodstream.

Lipid peroxidation is one of the principal causes of the hepatotoxicity resulting from carbon tetrachloride ingestion. CCl_4 toxicity has been attributed to homolytic dehalogenation to yield a CCl_3 free radical, with subsequent lipid peroxidation, covalent binding to microsomal protein, and loss of cytochrome P-450 and microsomal enzyme activities. Both cytochrome P-450 and NADPH-cytochrome c reductase seem to be involved and it has been suggested that the dehalogenation is initiated by cytochrome P-450 with the CCl_3 radical binding to cytochrome P-450 and/or damaging the phospholipid milieu of the endoplasmic reticulum, with consequent lipid peroxidation mediated by the NADPH-cytochrome c reductase [86]. Antioxidants such as α-tocopherol, and selenium because of its enhancement of glutathione peroxidase, as well as free radical scavengers, act protectively against CCl_4-induced lipid peroxidation. Chloroform, halothane, and Freon 11 also produce hepatotoxicity to varying degrees and all undergo covalent binding to microsomal protein, though to a much lesser extent than CCl_4, which may account for the apparent absence of lipid peroxidation with these halogenohydrocarbons. It has been proposed that reductive dehalogenation of these compounds occurs with covalent binding to microsomal cytochrome P-450 to form ligand complexes. The consequent loss of monooxygenase activity could lead to decoupling of the cytochrome from its flavoprotein reductase (NADPH-cytochrome c reductase) which would then result in an electron leak from the flavoprotein culminating in lipid peroxidation [86].

Lipid peroxidation has also been proposed as an important factor in the alcohol-induced fatty degeneration of the liver, and rats treated with alcohol at high dosage show increased lipid peroxidation in the liver, possibly by destruction of endogenous antioxidants, with damage to both mitochondrial and microsomal membranes. Deficiency in dietary choline, which has also been associated with accumulation of lipid in the liver, may also enhance lipid peroxidation because of decreased availability of phosphatidylcholine with consequent easier decoupling of the cytochrome and flavoprotein reductase. Hence, under appropriate conditions, microsomal membranes in particular, but also mitochondrial and lysosomal membranes, may show loss of functional integrity with simultaneous manifestation of lipid peroxidation. When peroxidation proceeds at a high rate, as in CCl_4 poisoning, this leads to the death of the cell and to necrosis. At slower rates, the loss of integrity of the endoplasmic reticulum and the shedding of the bound ribosomes, with consequent alterations in glycoprotein synthesis, may result in changes in the structures/function of plasma, mitochondrial, lysosomal, and microsomal membranes, as well as to more chronic changes associated with malignancy, to degenerative diseases such as rheumatoid arthritis, and to aging.

C. Adjuvant Arthritis

The development of adjuvant arthritis lesions in the rat has been shown to be accompanied by a loss of hepatic cytochrome P-450 and drug-metabolizing enzyme activity (see Table 3) [114,115]. The loss of cytochrome P-450 activity precedes the development of the arthritic lesion [113] and different types of adjuvant may have varying effects on the drug-metabolizing enzyme activities [116]. The adjuvant treatment has no inhibitory effect on cytochrome P-450-specific enzyme activities and does not inhibit the synthesis of microsomal heme, nor is microsomal cytochrome b_5 decreased. However, a high total tryptophan oxygenase activity in the arthritic animals is suggestive of a diminution in the heme pool [113]. The most probable explanation of this phenomenon appears to be an increased degradation of cytochrome P-450, and although this is comparable to the degradation produced by allylisopropylacetamide, it is a much slower process. This has been confirmed by the recent studies of Mathur and coworkers [117] who have shown that the cytochrome P-450 is degraded to cytochrome P-420 which is present in increased amounts. This phenomenon is not confined to hepatic cytochrome P-450 and Carlson and Ciaccio [118] have shown that a similar loss of P-450 occurs in the lung of rats with adjuvant-induced arthritis.

TABLE 3
Changes Observed in Hepatic Cytochrome P-450 and Related Parameters in Adjuvant Arthritic Rats[a]

	Control	Arthritic
Cytochrome P-450 (nmol/mg protein)	0.41 ± 0.04	0.15 ± 0.06
Aminopyrine N-demethylase (μmol HCHO hr^{-1} per g liver)	9.8 ± 0.6	2.0 ± 0.7
Microsomal heme synthesis (incorporation of ^{14}C-glycine, dpm/mg protein)	24 ± 2.5	20 ± 5.3
5-Aminolevulinate synthetase (μmol hr^{-1} per g liver)	9.2	7.6
Tryptophan oxygenase[b] (nmol hr^{-1} per g liver)		
haloenzyme	6.1 ± 1.2	3.1 ± 0.4
total enzyme (+ heme)	18 ± 3	32 ± 7
Serum α_2-globulin[c] (% total serum proteins)	12 ± 1	19 ± 1

[a]Data are for rats 18 days after treatment with adjuvant.
[b]14 days after treatment with adjuvant.
[c]Mycoplasma-induced arthritis.
Source: From Ref. 113.

Rats with mycoplasma-induced arthritis also exhibit a similar loss of hepatic microsomal drug-metabolizing enzyme activity as compared to the adjuvant-treated rats and, as with human arthritis cases, show a marked increase (60-80%) in the serum α_2-globulin (see Table 3). This has led to the suggestion that a defect in cytochrome P-450 may occur in human rheumatoid patients [113] and would account for the changes seen in the composition of the serum proteins. The molecular mechanism(s) involved in this phenomenon are largely unknown, but the activation of macrophages, which results from the immunological response to adjuvant treatment, leads to increased production of hydrogen peroxide and superoxide with subsequent damage of microsomal membrane phospholipids, cytochrome P-450, and other components of the monooxygenase system [119]. The degradation of cytochrome P-450 would be expected to result in changes in the synthesis of glycoproteins and other secretory proteins and this is reflected in the changes observed in the serum proteins. This loss of cytochrome P-450 may also be expected to result in changes to the lysosomal membranes and lysosomal enzymes, which are synthesized on the endoplasmic reticulum, and these have both been implicated in the production of the arthritic lesions.

Treatment of adjuvant-arthritic rats with fenclorac, a new nonsteroidal antiinflammatory drug, reduced the polyarthritic syndrome but did not restore the hepatic concentration of cytochrome P-450 to normal [119].

D. Atherosclerosis

Atherosclerosis, which vies with cancer for premier place in the fatal diseases of modern society, has been variously attributed to the excessive consumption of animal fats or refined carbohydrates, to a dietary lack of fiber or antioxidants like ascorbic acid, and to the lack of exercise, to excessive smoking, or to environmental stress.

It has been suggested that human atherosclerotic plaques are monoclonal in origin and that a necessary requirement for the genesis of atherosclerosis is the focal proliferation of smooth muscle cells in the intima of the aorta [120]. This would imply that one or more of the smooth muscle cells of the aorta undergoes some kind of cellular transformation which results in the subsequent atherosclerotic lesions. Bond and coworkers [121] have suggested that environmental mutagens in the circulating blood could become activated by enzymes in the wall of the aorta and consequently initiate local somatic cell mutations and subsequent atherosclerotic lesions. This mechanism alone is unlikely to account for the complete clinical syndrome of atherosclerosis, which is obviously multifactorial with its involvement of genetic, dietary, and environmental factors, but might be an initiating event which is exacerbated by these other factors into the typical clinical condition.

The walls of the aortas of humans, monkeys, and rabbits have been shown to possess a microsomal monooxygenase system [122], and the treatment of chickens with the environmental promutagens, benzo[a]-pyrene and 7,12-dimethylbenz[a]anthracene, led to increases in the number and rate of development of aortic plaques with no concomitant increase in blood cholesterol concentration [123]. The monooxygenase present in the aorta wall of rabbits has been more fully characterized. It hydroxylates benzo[a]pyrene, is induced by polycyclic carcinogenic aromatic hydrocarbons and by polychlorinated biphenyls and, rather surprisingly, is markedly activated in vitro by the addition of heme [121].

Another facet of this problem may be seen from a consideration of the role of lipid metabolism. Cardiovascular disease is associated with raised concentrations of plasma cholesterol [124] and with a lowering of the cholesterol-transporting high-density lipoproteins [125,126]. The metabolism of cholesterol is known to be dependent upon a number of microsomal hydroxylations, including the very important cholesterol 7α-hydroxylation,

TABLE 4
Possible Role of Endoplasmic Reticulum in Etiology of Cardiovascular Disease

Biochemical pathology	Reference
1. Unsaturated fatty acids reduce the risk of cardiovascular disease; the hepatic endoplasmic reticulum contains a fatty acid desaturase system.	127
2. Cholesterol-regulating enzyme, cholesterol 7α-hydroxylase, is a monooxygenase, involving cytochrome P-450.	26
3. Ascorbic acid deficiency predisposes to hypercholesteremia and cardiovascular disease, and to decreased liver monooxygenase activity.	128 129 130
4. Vitamin D_2, associated with vascular calcification and experimental atherosclerosis, has a high affinity for cytochrome P-450 and decreases cholesterol 7α-hydroxylase.	90
5. Aorta wall contains monooxygenases which activate promutagens, to cause primary lesion.	122
6. Blood platelets contain monooxygenases involved in synthesis of thromboxanes; thromboxanes and prostaglandins are involved in blood clotting and vasodilation.	25
7. High concentrations of carbon monoxide inhibit cytochrome P-450 and are associated with increased incidence of atherosclerosis.	131

the first step in the catabolic conversion of cholesterol into the bile acids. Impaired 7α-hydroxylation of cholesterol, as might occur through excessive enterohepatic recirculation of bile acids, because of a lack of dietary fiber to retain the bile acids and facilitate their fecal excretion, could lead to a progressive accumulation of cholesterol in liver and other tissues. A number of other aspects of the role of lipids in the etiology of cardiovascular disease appear to involve the endoplasmic reticulum and especially the function of cytochrome P-450 (see Table 4).

In the early stages of experimental lipid induction of atherosclerosis in rabbits the synthesis of prostacyclin (PGI_2) by heart, aorta, and mesenteric arteries was strongly suppressed, whereas the generation of thromboxane A_2 by blood platelets was later enhanced. It is suggested that the generation of lipid peroxides by the atherogenic diet damages the endothelial PGI_2 synthetase, which thus contributes to the pathogenesis of the lesion [132] (see Fig. 7).

The lipids also play an important role in regulating the enzymic function of the endoplasmic reticulum, and an excessive concentration of triglycerides, cholesterol, or lipophilic chemicals would be expected to disturb the normal fluidity of the membrane, decoupling the monooxygenase system with an increase in nonspecific hydxylation and peroxidation by the flavoprotein reductase. This in turn might lead to the pathological hydroxylation of tissue components, as has been seen in diabetic nephropathy and old age where there is an increased hydroxylation of protein with an associated increase in glycoprotein content and thickening of the glomerula basement membrane [133]. The endoplasmic reticulum would therefore appear to be fundamentally involved in the etiology of cardiovascular disease, and this multifactorial syndrome would appear to be primarily a series of lesions arising from unregulated biological oxygenation.

E. Carcinogenesis

Most adult mammalian cancer arises in epithelial tissues, namely, the skin, the gastrointestinal, respiratory, and genitourinary tracts, the breasts, and the liver. These epithelial tissues are characterized by their synthesis of extracellular proteins and their cells contain a well-developed endoplasmic reticulum where this protein synthesis occurs. This endoplasmic reticulum is also concerned with the detoxication and activation of chemical carcinogens.

It has recently been suggested that the substrate selectivity and product regio- and stereoselectivity of the various forms of cytochrome P-450 may determine the balance between detoxication and activation pathways, and thus decide the susceptibility of individual species and strains of animals, and different tissues, to the toxic and carcinogenic effects of chemicals [134]. Other microsomal enzymes, concerned primarily with detoxication, but in specific cases also with activation, are epoxide hydrase, glucuronyltransferase, and the glutathione transferases which further metabolize the oxygenated metabolites, converting arene oxides into dihydrodiols and mercapturic acids, and conjugating the diols, phenols, etc. to form the corresponding glucuronides.

It has generally been presumed that the lipophilic procarcinogens (e.g., benzo[a]pyrene) enter the cell, migrate to the endoplasmic reticulum where they undergo oxygenation (detoxication/activation), and the proximate carcinogens migrate to the nucleus where they become covalently bound to the DNA of the chromatin and to nuclear RNA and regulatory proteins. However, both the endoplasmic reticulum and the nuclear membrane have similar monooxygenase activities and both are important in the activation of carcinogens [135]. Nevertheless, there are differences, and whereas the

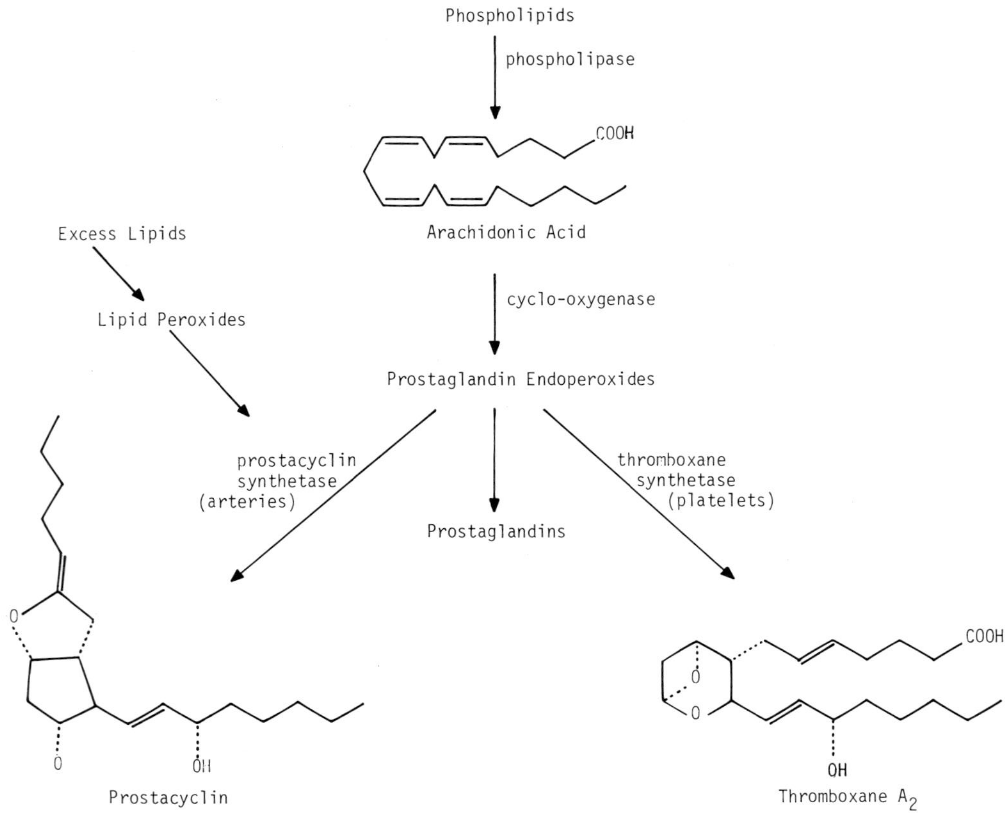

FIGURE 7 Effects of lipid peroxidation of prostacyclin and thromboxane synthesis in experimental atherosclerosis. (From Ref. 132.)

rate of activation of benzo[a]pyrene by the enzymes of the nuclear envelope is much lower than that of the endoplasmic reticulum, it is greatly induced by pretreatment with 3-methylcholanthrene, but not by phenobarbital [136]. The relative proportions of the various forms of cytochrome P-450 in the nuclear envelope therefore differ from those in the endoplasmic reticulum.

The carcinogenic polycyclic hydrocarbons, such as benzo[a]pyrene and benzo[a]anthracene, are characterized by the presence of the phenanthrene nucleus within the chemical structure, and Jerina [137,138] has proposed that activation of polycyclic hydrocarbons to the proximate or ultimate carcinogens necessitates "bay region" epoxidation of this phenanthrene nucleus. Other workers [139-141] have found that a diol-epoxide is the active carcinogen, with the initial polycyclic hydrocarbon 7,8-epoxide being converted into the corresponding dihydrodiol by epoxide hydrase, then further oxygenated to yield the 7,8-diol-9,10-epoxide (see Fig. 8). These diol epoxides do not appear to be suitable substrates for epoxide hydrase, and form stabilized internal ion-pair compounds which react as carbonium ions with DNA, even in the presence of glutathione and proteins, so that no threshold concentration of the diol epoxide need exist for DNA arylation and consequent damage of DNA and carcinogenesis [142]. A more detailed study of the interaction of the various metabolic products of the microsomal oxidation of benzo[a]pyrene has shown that this polycyclic hydrocarbon may be metabolized to four different types of reactive intermediates capable of binding to DNA, namely, (1) primary arene oxides, (2) diol epoxides, (3) oxygenated phenols, and (4) oxygenated quinones [143]. Microsomal oxygenation is also known to be involved in the activation of other carcinogens, including aromatic amines such as 2-naphthylamine [144], amides such as 2-acetamidofluorene [145], and nitrosamines such as dimethylnitrosamine [146].

The metabolic activation of carcinogens has an interesting model system in the microsomal oxygenation of the substrate biphenyl, which yields two major products, namely, 2-hydroxy- and 4-hydroxy-biphenyl. It is of mechanistic interest that although both the 2- and 4-hydroxylations of biphenyl are catalyzed by cytochrome P-448, cytochrome P-450 is able to catalyze only the 4-hydroxylation [147,148]. This specificity of cytochrome P-448 for the 2-hydroxylation, and the known induction of cytochrome P-448 by carcinogens, have suggested a correlation between the effect of carcinogens on the endoplasmic reticulum and an increase in the enzymic 2-hydroxylation of biphenyl [52,149]. Furthermore, the irreversible displacement of ribosomes from the endoplasmic reticulum (degranulation) by carcinogens [8,150], has suggested that a further relationship may exist between the degranulation of the endoplasmic reticulum and the expression of the enzyme biphenyl 2-hydroxylase [151]. The biphenyl structure contains the spatial arrangement of the phenanthrene nucleus, and the 2-hydroxylation, but not 4-hydroxylation, may be considered as "bay region" oxygenation.

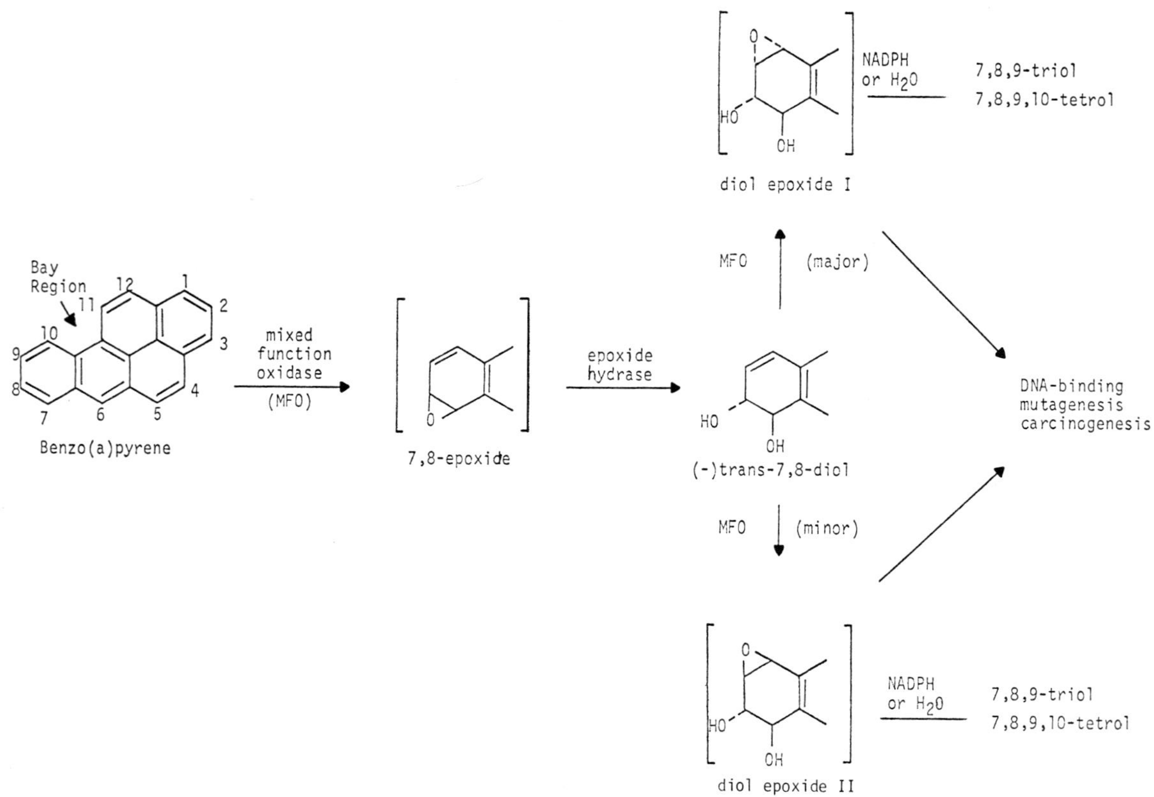

FIGURE 8 Activation of benzo[a]pyrene by epoxidation.

The interaction of activated carcinogens, namely, the electrophilic or carbonium ion ultimate carcinogens, with DNA to form alkylated or arylated derivatives, seems to be fundamental to mutagenesis and to the initiation of chemical carcinogenesis [152]. However, not all mutagens are carcinogenic and it would appear that some biological damage additional to DNA alkylation is requisite for the expression of carcinogenesis. The essential requirements are for an increased rate of DNA synthesis, increased mitosis, and decreased immune surveillance, to ensure the replication of the damaged DNA and the establishment of a clone of malignantly transformed cells before DNA repair can be effected [152].

Carcinogenesis is a complex process but in the most simple concept comprises two major phases, namely, initiation—a genetic mechanism which involves the alkylation of DNA; and promotion—probably epigenetic which concerns the development of the genetic damage into a viable clone of malignantly transformed cells. The mechanisms of these two processes are probably quite different and although the processes of initiation and DNA alkylation are reasonably well understood, the processes of promotion are still vaguely envisaged, and may include the actions of hormones, enzyme-inducing agents, and phorbol esters. The various known properties of these different agents are shown in Table 5.

Although the role of promoting agents and their mechanisms of action have been neglected, these may be just as important, or even more important, than the initiating agents [151-153,154] since they may stimulate the replication of dormant initiated cells which in the absence of promotion would not have undergone proliferation to form a viable malignancy. Stimulation of mitosis, e.g., by partial hepatectomy [155], and stimulation of

TABLE 5
Biological Properties of Initiating and Promoting Agents of Malignancy

Initiating agents	Promoting agents
1. Electrophiles or carbonium ions, or capable of forming these	1. Diverse chemical structures including hormones, phorbol esters, enzyme inducers
2. Genotoxic, alkylate DNA, RNA, protein - mutagenic	2. Epigenetic, nonalkylating, nonmutagenic
3. Single exposure often sufficient; threshold questioned	3. Prolonged exposure required; threshold probable
4. Reversible only by DNA repair	4. Probably readily reversible
5. Required before promoting agent	5. Required after initiating agent

Source: After Ref. 153.

protein synthesis by the administration of enzyme-inducing agents such as phenobarbital [156,157] may greatly potentiate the malignant effects of threshold doses of carcinogens such as diethylnitrosamines, and Pitot and his colleagues have used this system to provide enzymic evidence to distinguish two distinct stages in the genesis of liver cancer in rats [158]. Several other workers similarly have concluded that mutagenesis is responsible for the initiation of carcinogenesis while an epigenetic mechanism is responsible for its promotion [152,159].

One of the consistently observable ultrastructural changes produced by carcinogens is an apparent detachment of ribosomes from the endoplasmic reticulum (degranulation) [160] which generally requires microsomal metabolic activation of the carcinogen [8] and is associated with the phenomenon of autophagocytosis [161] and lipoperoxidation [162]. This effect of carcinogens on degranulation of the endoplasmic reticulum has recently been disputed [162] but this may be because only a specific subpopulation of ribosomes, comprising about 20% of the total, are removed by carcinogen treatment [163].

A number of chemicals which have been identified as weak carcinogens or cocarcinogens, such as chloroform, safrole, tetrachlorodibenzo-para-dioxin (TCDD), and polychlorobiphenyls (PCBs), are now known to undergo metabolism to form highly reactive intermediates such as radicals or carbenes and, consequent upon this, to form ligand complexes with cytochrome P-450. This results in loss of typical cytochrome P-450 oxygenase activity with the appearance of cytochrome P-448 and cytochrome P-448 oxygenase activity (aryl hydrocarbon hydroxylation). The prolonged administration of safrole to rats has been shown to lead to these changes in cytochrome P-450 of the liver, and this is accompanied by degranulation of the endoplasmic reticulum, and neoplastic liver nodule formation [90]. In the consideration of a number of inducing agents of the liver microsomal enzymes and carcinogens, these authors conclude that chemicals which enhance cytochrome P-450 activity do not generally show carcinogenic activity, whereas those chemicals which inhibit or damage cytochrome P-450, with enhancement of cytochrome P-448 activity, result in cytotoxic processes which may lead to neoplasia and carcinogenesis. More recently, nitrosamines have been shown to bind to cytochrome P-450 [164] and, whereas noncarcinogenic nitrosamines lead to induction of cytochrome P-450 activity, the carcinogenic nitrosamines result in inhibition of this cytochrome [165]. It would thus appear that the irreversible binding of reactive metabolites to cytochrome P-450 may result in degranulation of the endoplasmic reticulum, and a marked change in microsomal monooxygenase activity, possibly with accompanying lipid peroxidation and damage to the microsomal and other cellular membranes which may potentiate or even initiate carcinogenesis.

It is now well recognized that one of the most essential biological functions of the endoplasmic reticulum is the synthesis of glycoproteins.

Indeed, the initiation of glycoprotein synthesis appears to be exclusive to membrane-bound ribosomes [166], and the glycosyltransferases are found only in the membranes of the endoplasmic reticulum, Golgi complex, and plasma membrane [11]. Glycoproteins play a vital role in the overall function and economy of the cell, and in the regulation of the whole eukaryotic organism [167]. They are secreted into the plasma membrane glycocalyx, they regulate cell division, and those glycoproteins which are secreted from the cell, such as the immunoglobulins, play a major role in immune surveillance. The nature of the carbohydrate moieties of these glycoproteins appears to be the critical feature determining the rate of mitosis, the immune characteristics of the cell, and the immune surveillance within the living organism. However, the mechanism by which the various glycosyltransferases within the endoplasmic reticulum are regulated is as yet unknown [11].

The binding of the ribosomes to the endoplasmic reticulum, which is necessary for the formation of the glycoprotein polypeptide backbone, appears to directly involve cytochrome P-450. An increase in cytochrome P-450 produced by phenobarbital or 3-methylcholanthrene leads to enhancement of polysome binding, whereas loss of cytochrome P-450 by administration of cobalt salts diminishes binding. Purified cytochrome P-450 and P-448 also bind polysomes, so that it is likely that it is the destruction of this cytochrome, or the loss of the activity of this enzyme, which leads to degranulation [18].

The degranulation of the endoplasmic reticulum which accompanies carcinogenesis [150] must of consequence be accompanied by interference with glycoprotein synthesis [152]. Indeed, in malignantly transformed cells, one of the earliest and most significant changes observed is the loss of a high-molecular-weight glycoprotein (fibronectin) from the cell surface [168,169] and changes occur in the nature of the terminal sugar moieties of the glycoproteins of the glycocalyx [167,170]. When a cell becomes malignant, marked changes are found in the carbohydrate components of all cellular membranes and many glycoproteins contain altered oligosaccharide chains [167]. Since these carbohydrate moieties of the glycoproteins are regulators of intercellular reactions governing the social harmony of the different tissues and organs of the multicellular organism, the extensive changes in the carbohydrate moieties of glycoproteins (and glycolipids) which affect every biological membrane of the organism may thus account for the pleiotypic nature of the malignant cell, and for its unregulated and antisocial behavior [167]. Elevated levels of certain glycosyltransferases have been observed in the plasma of cancer patients, raised levels of serum sialyltransferase have been seen in breast cancer patients [171], and high levels of fucosyltransferase with correspondingly low levels of sialyltransferase and galactosyltransferase were demonstrated in various human metastasizing tumors [172,173]. The rate of glycoprotein synthesis has been shown to be significantly decreased in human colonic cancer [174], and significant reductions in glycoprotein carbohydrate content, and reductions in several glycosyltransferase activities and in two hexosamididases, were observed in dimethylhydrazine-induced rat colonic tumors [175]. Similarly, we have shown a marked inhibition of glycosyltransferase in the synthesis of gastric mucus in patients with gastric carcinoma [58].

An increased concentration of serum sialic acid has been associated with malignant melanoma [176], changes in the normal variants of sialic acid have been demonstrated in malignant human bowel mucosa [177], and increased microsomal sialyltransferase activity has been observed in human kidney cells infected with oncogenic adenovirus [178]. Terminal sialic acid plays a major role in determining the survival of serum glycoproteins [179], as sialic acid on glycoproteins prevents their uptake and degradation by the liver and phagocytic cells and decreases their immunogenicity [167]. The serum glycoproteins of cancer patients are glycosylated in a different manner from those of healthy subjects [180] and hence have increased stability and decreased immunogenicity [179,181]. Similarly, the lysosomal enzyme β-glucuronidase isolated from malignant tissue has been shown to be immunologically different from the normal enzyme due to a marked increase in sialic acid content, and may be related to the increased activity of β-glucuronidase associated with malignant invasion [182].

It would therefore appear that both the quantitative and qualitative aspects of glycoprotein synthesis are profoundly affected by malignant transformation, and that the changes occurring in the glycoprotein of the cell surface are associated with many of the characteristics of the malignant cell, namely, loss of adhesiveness, accelerated cell division, and altered antigenicity [168]. Furthermore, degranulation of the endoplasmic reticulum might lead to an increased synthesis of intracellular proteins by the cytoplasmic ribosomes which, as in the neonate or in regenerating tissues [183], leads to accelerated cellular and tissue growth which parallels the decreased synthesis of extracellular glycoproteins. Hence, degranulation would result in a switchover of the economy of the cell from a predominance of synthesis of glycoproteins for export (glycocalyx, immunoglobulins, mucus) to the fetal/neonatal state of predominantly intracellular protein synthesis, with accelerated cell growth and mitosis.

As fetal and neonatal tissues have a characteristic high ratio of free to bound ribosomes and a high rate of cellular growth and division, it is interesting to note that the human trophoblast shows other features commonly associated with neoplasia, including cell proliferation and invasion. Furthermore, the appearance of many fetal proteins in the blood plasma is frequently characteristic of malignancy. From a study of the surface glycosylation of the trophoblast and fetal cells it has been suggested that two species of glycoprotein may be involved in atypical cellular behavior. The first of these, associated with cellular growth and invasion, contains sialic acid and other sugars, but not fucose. The second, characteristic of neoplastic cells, contains both sialic acid and fucose, as well as other sugars [184].

The determination of fucosyltransferase activity has been shown to be valuable in the diagnosis of malignancy, and in assessment of the success of surgical treatment, chemotherapy, and irradiation [185]. Indeed, surgical removal of colon carcinomas has been shown to decrease the rate of incorporation of $[^{14}C]$fucose into its endogenous acceptor in human serum, and a similar correlation has been seen between fucosyltransferase activity and the therapeutic response of patients with breast cancer. These changes in the nature of glycoproteins and alterations in the activities of the glycosyltransferases, probably consequent to damage of the endoplasmic reticulum and cytochrome P-450, including degranulation, are obviously fundamental to the pathobiology of carcinogenesis.

F. Adverse Effects on Reproduction

The effects of environmental chemicals on the endoplasmic reticulum of the gonads are potentially much greater than for other tissues, since the gonads have a number of different roles in the biology of the mammalian organism and may affect both the exposed individual and its progeny. These are the organs which produce the sex hormones, the androgens, estrogens, and progestogens. These hormones, produced by the stroma, are responsible not only for sexual maturation and the physiological regulation of reproduction, but also play a significant role in the regulation of many fundamental metabolic processes. For example, in the liver of rat, the attachment of ribosomes to the endoplasmic reticulum, the microsomal monooxygenase activities, and lipid metabolism all exhibit sex differences. In addition to these functions, the gonads also contain the germ cells, which hold and propagate the genetic information requisite for the continued survival of the species. Environmental chemicals reaching the gonads may therefore affect the synthesis of the sex hormones, resulting in changes in basal metabolism, sexual development, or reproductive function, or could lead to damage of the germinal epithelia and genetic mutations which might result in gonadal tumors, impaired fertility, and somatic and genetic mutations of the progeny.

Carcinogenic polycyclic hydrocarbons have been shown to result in premature sterility, development of ovarian tumors [186], and altered sperm morphology [187]. However, there are considerable species differences in both the testicular and ovarian microsomal oxidases which metabolically detoxicate and activate environmental chemicals, and consequently there are also differences in the germ cell toxicity of these chemicals, such as the differences seen in the oocyte toxicity of 3-methylcholanthrene in mice and rats [188]. Chemicals such as the pesticides DDT and dieldrin have been reported to cause decreased reproductive activity in male dogs, and impotence in farm workers, which has been attributed to induction of the hepatic microsomal hydroxylases which deactivate testosterone [189]. More recently it has been shown that treatment of rats

TABLE 6
Effect of Chronic Treatment of Rats with Phenobarbital or 3-Methylcholanthrene on Cytochrome P-450 and Testosterone Synthesis

	Hepatic cytochrome P-450 (nmol/mg protein)	Testicular cytochrome P-450 (nmol/mg protein)	Testicular testosterone synthesis (nmol/mg protein per 30 min)
Control (saline)	0.94	0.065	0.30
Phenobarbital	1.79	0.068	0.31
3-Methylcholanthrene	1.41	0.036	0.14

Source: From Ref. 71.

with 3-methylcholanthrene results in severe weight loss of the seminal vesicles due to impaired testicular testosterone formation [71]; however, treatment with phenobarbital had no similar effect. It is also significant that whereas both phenobarbital and 3-methylcholanthrene increase the cytochrome P-450 content of the rat liver, the cytochrome P-450 content of the testes was unaffected by phenobarbital treatment and even decreased by 3-methylcholanthrene (see Table 6).

The administration of carcinogens to pregnant animals may result in the development of fetal tumors, as with the triazenes [190] or to subsequent development of malignancies or gonadal abnormalities, as with the clear-cell adenocarcinoma and testicular impairment observed with diethylstilbestrol [191,192]. Additionally, the administration of toxic chemicals to pregnant animals may lead to fetal death, impaired development, or to teratogenic effects, as first seen with thalidomide [191,192]. More recently, the anticonvulsant drug phenytoin has been associated with harelip and cleft palate in children born to mothers taking the drug long-term, and has been shown to increase the frequency of fetal resorptions and incidence of cleft lip/palate in fetuses of mice dosed with the drug. This embryopathic effect has been ascribed to the metabolism of phenytoin to an arene oxide which covalently binds to target tissue macromolecules to exert a teratogenic effect [193], but other workers have shown that the effect is associated with maternal folate deficiency due to the prolonged enzyme-inductive effects of the drug, and that the same phenomenon is observed with a variety of enzyme-inducing drugs when administered long-term [194].

REFERENCES

1. A. Elhammer, H. Svensson, F. Autuori and G. Dallner, J. Cell. Biol. 67:715 (1975).
2. P. R. McIntosh and K. O'Toole, Biochim. Biophys. Acta 457:171 (1976).
3. J. A. Lewis and D. D. Sabatini, Biochim. Biophys. Acta 478:331 (1977).
4. S. N. Alam and T. K. Shires, Biochem. Biophys. Res. Commun. 74: 1441 (1977).
5. H. E. Bond, J. A. Cooper II, D. P. Courington, and J. S. Wood, Science 165:705 (1969).
6. D. J. Williams, D. Gurari, and B. R. Rabin, FEBS Lett. 2:133 (1968).
7. G. H. Sunshine, D. J. Williams, and B. R. Rabin, Nature, New Biol. 230:133 (1971).
8. D. J. Williams and B. R. Rabin, Nature 232:102 (1971).
9. I. F. H. Purchase and P. A. Le Fevre, Chem. Ind. 415 (1975).
10. M. Elstein and D. V. Parke (Eds.), Mucus in Health and Disease. Plenum, New York, 1977.

11. H. Schachter, Biochem. Soc. Symp. 40:57 (1974).
12. J. L. Vermilion and M. J. Coon, J. Biol. Chem. 253:8812 (1978).
13. T. Iyanagi, F. K. Anan, Y. Imai, and H. S. Mason, Biochemistry 17: 2224 (1978).
14. J. W. DePierre and G. Dallner, Biochim. Biophys. Acta 415:411 (1975).
15. A. Stier, Biochem. Pharmacol. 25:109 (1976).
16. W.-H. Schunck, P. Riege, and R. Kuhl, Pharmazie 33:412 (1978).
17. R. H. Wickramasinghe and C. A. Villee, Nature 256:509 (1975).
18. M. Takagi, J. Biochem. 82:1077 (1977).
19. R. R. Brenner, Drug Metab. Rev. 6:155 (1977).
20. J. B. Schenkman, I. Jansson, and K. M. Robie-Suh, Life Sci. 19:611 (1976).
21. F. Wada and M. Usami, Biochim. Biophys. Acta 487:261 (1977).
22. A. Ellin, S. Orrenius, A. Pilotti, and C.-G. Swahn, Arch. Biochem. Biophys. 158:597 (1973).
23. L. Tan, H. M. Wang, and J. G. Lehoux, Prostaglandins 4:9 (1973).
24. J. Navarro, D. E. Piccolo, and D. Kupfer, Arch. Biochem. Biophys. 191:125 (1978).
25. D. L. Cinti and M. B. Feinstein, Biochem. Biophys. Res. Commun. 73:171 (1976).
26. W. S. Mellon, D. T. Witiak, and D. R. Feller, Biochem. Pharmacol. 27:1055 (1978).
27. K. Okuda, H.-H. Ruf, V. Ullrich, Hoppe-Seyler's Z. Physiol. Chem. 358:689 (1977).
28. J. I. Mason and G. S. Boyd, Steroids 31:849 (1978).
29. J. E. Gielen, J. V. Cantfort, and P. Kremers, Arch. Toxicol. 36: 255 (1976).
30. G. Betz, P. Tsai, and R. Weakley, Steroids 25:791 (1975).
31. E. A. Thompson, Jr. and P. K. Siiteri, J. Steroid Biochem. 7:635 (1976).
32. P. K. Zachariah, Q. P. Lee, K. G. Symms, and M. R. Juchau, Biochem. Pharmacol. 25:793 (1976).
33. K. Suhara, T. Gomi, H. Sato, E. Itagaki, S. Takemori, and M. Katagiri, Arch. Biochem. Biophys. 190:290 (1978).
34. J.-A. Gustafsson, B. P. Lisboa, and J. Sjövall, Eur. J. Biochem. 5: 437 (1968).
35. T. C. Madhok, H. K. Schnoes, and H. F. DeLuca, Biochem. J. 175: 479 (1978).
36. J. G. Ghazarian, P.-Y. Hsu, and B. L. Peterson, Arch. Biochem. Biophys. 184:596 (1977).
37. S. Sulimovici and M. S. Roginsky, Life Sci. 21:1317 (1978).
38. A. J. Paine, Biochem. Pharmacol. 27:1805 (1978).
39. A. H. Conney, Pharmacol. Rev. 19:317 (1967).

40. A. P. Alvares, G. Schilling, W. Levin, and R. Kuntzman, J. Pharmacol. Exp. Ther. 163:417 (1968).
41. R. B. Mailman, W. Edmundson, K. Muse, and E. Hodgson, Gen. Pharmacol. 8:281 (1977).
42. P. E. Thomas, A. Y. H. Lu, D. Ryan, S. B. West, J. Kawalek, and W. Levin, Molec. Pharmacol. 12:746 (1976).
43. P. E. Thomas, A. Y. H. Lu, D. Ryan, S. B. West, J. Kawalek, and W. Levin, J. Biol. Chem. 251:1385 (1976).
44. D. Y. Bell and E. Hodgson, Gen. Pharmacol. 8:121 (1977).
45. M. Warner, M. V. La Marca, and A. H. Neims, Drug Metab. Disp. 6:353 (1978).
46. F. P. Guengerich, J. Biol. Chem. 253:7931 (1978).
47. F. P. Guengerich, Biochem. Biophys. Res. Commun. 82:820 (1978).
48. G. J. Wishart, Biochem. J. 174:671 (1978).
49. J. M. Tredger, J. Chakraborty, and D. V. Parke, Biochem. Soc. Trans. 1:998 (1973).
50. J. M. Tredger, J. Chakraborty, and D. V. Parke, Biochem. Soc. Trans. 1:1000 (1973).
51. F. McPherson, J. W. Bridges, and D. V. Parke, Nature 252:488 (1974).
52. F. J. McPherson, J. W. Bridges, and D. V. Parke, Biochem. Pharmacol. 25:1345 (1976).
53. E. Arrhenius, L. Renberg, L. Johansson, and M-A. Zetterqvist, Chem.-Biol. Interact. 18:35 (1977).
54. D. Malejka-Giganti, R. C. McIver, A. L. Glasebrook, and H. R. Gutmann, Biochem. Pharmacol. 27:61 (1978).
55. G. M. Bartoli, T. Galeotti, G. Palombini, G. Parisi, and A. Azzi, Arch. Biochem. Biophys. 184:276 (1977).
56. D. W. James, B. R. Rabin, and D. J. Williams, Nature 224:371 (1969).
57. H. Saarni, Biochem. Pharmacol. 27:1029 (1978).
58. D. V. Parke and A. M. Symons, in Mucus in Health and Disease (M. Elstein and D. V. Parke, Eds.). Plenum, New York, 1977, p. 423.
59. R. A. Newman and K. R. Cutroneo, Mol. Pharmacol. 14:185 (1978).
60. K. Fujii, H. Jaffe, Y. Bishop, E. Arnold, D. Mackintosh, and S. S. Epstein, Toxicol. Appl. Pharmacol. 16:482 (1970).
61. A. L. Hunter and R. A. Neal, Biochem. Pharmacol. 24:2199 (1975).
62. J. A. Goldstein, P. Hickmann, H. Bergman, J. D. McKinney, and M. P. Walker, Chem-Biol. Interact. 17:69 (1977).
63. J. M. Khanna, H. Kalant, Y. Yee, S. Chung, and A. J. Siemens, Biochem. Pharmacol. 25:329 (1976).
64. H. Kalant, J. M. Khanna, G. Y. Lin, and S. Chung, Biochem. Pharmacol., 25:337 (1976).

65. C. Ioannides, B. G. Lake, and D. V. Parke, Xenobiotica 5:665 (1975).
66. D. V. Parke, in Enzyme Induction (D. V. Parke, Ed.). Plenum, New York, 1975, p. 207.
67. R. Kato, Arzneim.-Forsch. 11:797 (1961).
68. N. G. Zampaglione, D. J. Jollow, J. R. Mitchell, B. Stripp, M. Hamrick, and J. R. Gillette, J. Pharmacol. Exp. Ther. 187:218 (1973).
69. K. A. Suarez, G. P. Carlson, G. C. Fuller, and N. Fausto, Toxicol. Appl. Pharmacol. 23:171 (1972).
70. K. A. Suarez, G. P. Carlson, and G. C. Fuller, Toxicol. Appl. Pharmacol. 34:314 (1975).
71. B. Stripp, R. H. Menard, and J. R. Gillette, Life Sci. 14:2121 (1974).
72. J. K. Selkirk, R. G. Croy, P. P. Roller, and H. V. Gelboin, Cancer Res. 34:3473 (1974).
73. D. L. Hill and T.-W. Shih, Cancer Res. 34:564 (1974).
74. M. A. Friedman and S. Woods, Res. Comm. Chem. Path. Pharmacol. 17:623 (1977).
75. L. C. Mohan, P. H. Grantham, E. K. Weisburger, J. H. Weisburger, and J. Idoine, J. Nat. Cancer Inst. 56:763 (1976).
76. M. R. Juchau, P. K. Zachariah, J. Colson, K. G. Symmy, J. Krasner, and S. J. Yaffe, Drug Metab. Disp. 2:79 (1974).
77. D. Labadarios, Studies on the effects of drugs on nutritional status. Ph.D. Thesis, University of Surrey, 1975.
78. R. Burt, J. W. Freston, and K. G. Tolman, J. Clin. Pharmacol. 16:393 (1976).
79. H. W. Strobel, A. Y. H. Lu, J. Hedema, and M. J. Coon, J. Biol. Chem. 245:4851 (1970).
80. T. E. Eling and R. P. DiAugustine, Biochem. J. 123:539 (1971).
81. E. D. Wills, Biochem. J. 123:983 (1971).
82. S. C. Davison and E. D. Wills, Biochem. J. 140:461 (1974).
83. B. Åkesson, FEBS Lett. 92:173 (1978).
83a. P. Pani, M. Porcu, A. Columbano, S. Dessi, G. M. Ledda, and G. Diaz, Exp. Mol. Pathol. 28:154 (1978).
84. P. Pani, A. Columbano, S. Dessi, M. Porcu, G. M. Ledda, and G. Diaz, Toxicol. Appl. Pharmacol. 42:613 (1977).
85. H. Shinozuka, S. C. Katyal, and B. Lombardi, Int. J. Cancer 22:36 (1978).
86. D. V. Parke, in Drug Toxicity (J. W. Gorrod, Ed.). Taylor & Francis, London, 1979, p. 133.
87. D. V. Parke, in The Principles and Methods in Modern Toxicology (C. L. Galli, S. D. Murphy, and R. Paoletti, Eds.). Elsevier/North Holland, Amsterdam, 1980, p. 102.
88. M. Obrebska, P. Kentish, and D. V. Parke, Biochem. J. 188:107 (1980).
89. V. Ullrich, in Microsomes and Drug Oxidations (V. Ullrich, I. Roots, A. Hildebrandt, R. W. Estabrook, and A. H. Conney, Eds.). Pergamon, Oxford, 1977, p. 192.

90. D. V. Parke and T. J. B. Gray, in Primary Liver Tumours (H. Remmer, H. M. Bolt, P. Bannasch, and H. Popper, Eds.). MTP Press, Lancaster, 1978, p. 335.
91. M. Franklin, Pharmacol. Ther., Ser. A 2:227 (1977).
92. D. Mansuy, E. Rouer, C. Bacot, P. Gans, J. C. Chottard, and J. P. Leroux, Biochem. Pharmacol. 27:1229 (1978).
93. M. K. Buening and M. R. Franklin, Drug Metab. Disp. 4:556 (1976).
94. P. Hlavica and G. Aichinger, Biochem. Biophys. Acta 544:185 (1978).
95. H. Uehleke and S. Poplawski-Tabarelli, Arch. Toxicol. 37:289 (1977).
96. C. R. Wolf, L. J. King, and D. V. Parke, Chem.-Biol. Interact. 21:277 (1978).
97. T. Shimada and R. Sato, Biochem. Pharmacol. 27:585 (1978).
98. T. F. Slater and B. C. Sawyer, Biochem. J. 123:815 (1971).
99. I. G. Sipes, G. Krishna, and J. R. Gillette, Life Sci. 20:1541 (1977).
100. Y. Masuda and T. Murano, Biochem. Pharmacol. 27:1985 (1978).
101. F. DeMatteis, Mol. Pharmacol. 10:849 (1974).
102. K. J. Freundt, Int. J. Clin. Pharmacol. 16:323 (1978).
103. R. R. Dalvi and R. A. Neal, Biochem. Pharmacol. 27:1608 (1978).
104. F. De Matteis, A. H. Gibbs, and A. Unseld, Biochem. J. 168:417 (1977).
105. I. N. H. White, Biochem. J. 174:853 (1978).
106. G. L. Plaa and H. Witschi, An. Rev. Pharmacol. Toxicol. 16:125 (1976).
107. O. Shimada and H. Yasuda, Biochim. Biophys. Acta 489:163 (1977).
108. M. A. Correia and R. F. Burk, J. Biol. Chem. 253:6203 (1978).
109. C. Auclair and M.-C. Lecomte, Biochem. Biophys. Res. Commun. 85:946 (1978).
110. F. P. Guengerich, Biochemistry 17:3633 (1978).
111. M. Jacobson, W. Levin, A. Y. H. Lu, A. H. Conney, and R. Kuntzman, Drug Metab. Disp. 1:766 (1973).
112. A. P. Autor, Life Sci. 14:1309 (1974).
113. M. A. Cawthorne, E. D. Palmer, and J. Green, Biochem. Pharmacol. 25:2683 (1976).
114. D. M. Morton and D. M. Chatfield, Biochem. Pharmacol. 19:473 (1970).
115. M. W. Whitehouse and F. J. Beck, Drug Metab. Disp. 1:251 (1973).
116. F. J. Beck and M. W. Whitehouse, Biochem. Pharmacol. 22:2453 (1973).
117. P. P. Mathur, G. S. Carr, and R. D. Smyth, Biochem. Pharmacol. 27:1279 (1978).
118. R. P. Carlson and E. I. Ciaccio, Biochem. Pharmacol. 24:1893 (1975).
119. P. P. Mathur, R. D. Smyth, C. M. Witmer, and G. S. Carr, Biochem. Pharmacol. 27:1771 (1978).

120. E. P. Benditt and J. M. Benditt, Proc. Nat. Acad. Sci. U.S. 70: 1753 (1973).
121. J. A. Bond, C. J. Omiecinski, and M. R. Juchau, Biochem. Pharmacol. 28:305 (1979).
122. M. R. Juchau, J. A. Bond, and E. P. Benditt, Proc. Nat. Acad. Sci. U.S. 73:3723 (1976).
123. R. E. Albert, M. Vanderlaan, F. S. Burns, and M. Nishizumi, Cancer Res. 37:2232 (1977).
124. A. M. Gotto, D. Yeshurun, and M. E. De Bakey, J. Chron. Dis. 29: 677 (1976).
125. G. J. Miller and N. E. Miller, Lancet 1:16 (1975).
126. T. Gordon, W. P. Castelli, M. C. Hjortland, W. B. Kannel, and T. R. Dawber, Amer. J. Med. 62:707 (1977).
127. P. Hill and E. L. Wynder, J. Amer. Diet. Ass. 68:25 (1976).
128. E. Ginter and L. Mikus, Experientia 33:716 (1977).
129. S. D. Turley, C. E. West, and B. J. Horton, Atherosclerosis 24:1 (1976).
130. V. G. Zannoni, Acta Vitaminol. Enzymol. 31:17 (1977).
131. P. Astrup, K. Kjeldsen, and J. Wanstrup, Ann. N.Y. Acad. Sci. 174:294 (1970).
132. R. J. Gryglewski, A. Dembinska-Kièć, A. Zmuda, and T. Gryglewska, Atherosclerosis 31:385 (1978).
133. A. De Bats, Immunology and biochemistry of normal and diabetic renal basement membrane. Ph.D. Thesis, University of Surrey, 1974.
134. J. Deutsch, J. C. Leutz, S. K. Yang, H. V. Gelboin, Y. L. Chiang, K. P. Vatsis, and M. J. Coon, Proc. Nat. Acad. Sci. U.S. 75:3123 (1978).
135. J. M. Pezzuto, M. A. Lea, and C. S. Yang, Cancer Res. 37:3427 (1977).
136. W. E. Fahl, C. R. Jefcoate, and C. B. Kasper, J. Biol. Chem. 253:3106 (1978).
137. D. M. Jerina and J. W. Daly, in Drug Metabolism: From Microbe to Man (D. V. Parke and R. L. Smith, Eds.). Taylor & Francis, London, 1977, p. 13.
138. D. M. Jerina and R. E. Lehr, in Microsomes and Drug Oxidations (V. Ullrich, I. Roots, A. Hildebrandt, R. W. Estabrook, and A. H. Conney, Eds.). Pergamon, Oxford, 1977, p. 709.
139. P. Sims, P. L. Grover, A. J. Swaisland, K. Pal, and A. Hewer, Nature 252:326 (1974).
140. A. J. Swaisland, A. Hewer, K. Pal, G. R. Keysell, J. Booth, P. L. Grover, and P. Sims, FEBS Lett. 47:34 (1974).
141. W. Levin, A. W. Wood, R. L. Chang, H. Yagi, H. D. Mah, D. M. Jerina, and A. H. Conney, Cancer Res. 38:1831 (1978).

142. P. B. Hulbert, Nature 256:146 (1975).
143. O. Pelkonen, A. R. Boobis, H. Yagi, D. M. Jerina, and D. W. Nebert, Mol. Pharmacol. 14:306 (1978).
144. J. L. Radomski and E. Brill, Science 167:992 (1970).
145. J. H. Weisburger, R. S. Yamamoto, G. M. Williams, P. H. Grantham, T. Matsushima, and E. K. Weisburger, Cancer Res. 32:491 (1972).
146. P. N. Magee and M. J. Barnes, Advan. Cancer Res. 10:163 (1967).
147. M. D. Burke and J. W. Bridges, Xenobiotica 5:357 (1975).
148. S. A. Atlas and D. W. Nebert, Arch. Biochem. Biophys. 175:495 (1976).
149. P. J. Creaven and D. V. Parke, Biochem. Pharmacol. 15:7 (1966).
150. J. Delauney and G. Schapira, Biomedicine 20:327 (1974).
151. D. V. Parke, in Microsomes and Drug Oxidations (V. Ullrich, I. Roots, A. Hildebrandt, R. W. Estabrook, and A. H. Conney, Eds.). Pergamon, Oxford, 1977, p. 721.
152. D. V. Parke, in Principles of Surgical Oncology (R. W. Raven, Ed.). Plenum, London, 1977, p. 113.
153. I. B. Weinstein, Bull. N.Y. Acad. Med. 54:366 (1978).
154. Is cancer irreversible? (editorial), Brit. Med. J. 2:585 (1978).
155. E. Cayama, H. Tsuda, D. S. R. Sarma, and E. Farber, Nature, 275:60 (1978).
156. C. Peraino, R. J. M. Fry, E. Staffeldt, and W. E. Kisieleski, Cancer Res. 33:2701 (1973).
157. C. Peraino, R. J. M. Fry, and E. Staffeldt, Cancer Res. 37:3623 (1977).
158. H. C. Pitot, L. Barsness, T. Goldsworthy, and T. Kitagawa, Nature 271:456 (1978).
159. E. H. Y. Chu, J. E. Trosko, and C.-C. Chang, J. Toxicol. Environ. Health 2:1317 (1978).
160. D. Svoboda and J. Higginson, Cancer Res. 28:1703 (1968).
161. G. Rez, A. Kiss, M. J. Bucsek, and J. Kovacs, Chem.-Biol. Interact. 13:77 (1976).
162. T. K. Shires, Lab. Invest. 38:693 (1978).
163. D. N. Palmer, B. R. Rabin, and D. J. Williams, Biochem. J. 176:9 (1978).
164. K. E. Appel, H. H. Ruf, B. Mahr, M. Schwarz, R. Rickart, and W. Kunz, Chem.-Biol. Interact. 28:17 (1979).
165. W. P. Norred, K. Nishie, and A. C. Keyl, Biochem. Pharmacol. 24:1313 (1975).
166. T. Hallinan, C. N. Murty, and J. H. Grant, Life Sci. 7:225 (1968).
167. L. Warren, C. A. Buck, and G. P. Tuszynski, Biochim. Biophys. Acta 516:97 (1978).

168. L. Warren, J. P. Fuhrer, G. P. Tuszynski, and C. A. Buck, Biochem. Soc. Symp. 40:147 (1974).
169. A. Vaheri and D. F. Mosher, Biochim. Biophys. Acta 516:1 (1978).
170. W. P. Van Beek, L. A. Smets, and P. Emmelot, Cancer Res. 33:2913 (1973).
171. C. Ip and T. Dao, Cancer Res. 38:723 (1978).
172. S. K. Chatterjee and U. Kim, J. Nat. Cancer Inst. 61:151 (1978).
173. D. Kessel, E. Sykes, and M. Henderson, J. Nat. Cancer Inst. 59:29 (1977).
174. T. O'Gorman and J. T. La Mont, Cancer Res. 38:2784 (1978).
175. H. J. Freeman, Y. Kim, and Y. S. Kim, Cancer Res. 38:3385 (1978).
176. H. K. B. Silver, D. M. Rangel, and D. L. Morton, Cancer 41:1497 (1978).
177. C. M. Rogers, K. B. Cooke, and M. I. Filipe, Gut 19:587 (1978).
178. Y. Aoi and M. Yokota, Tohoku J. Exp. Med. 125:177 (1978).
179. G. Ashwell and A. Morell, Biochem. Soc. Symp. 40:117 (1974).
180. I. Rostenberg, J. Guizar-Vasquez, P. Suarez, R. Rico, L. Nungaray, and C. Dominguez, J. Nat. Cancer Inst. 60:83 (1978).
181. G. L. Fisher and M. Shifrine, Oncology 35:22 (1978).
182. R. Harris, D. C. Williams, and D. V. Parke, unpublished data, 1979.
183. Y. Okamoto, E. Ito, and N. Akamatsu, Biochim. Biophys. Acta 542:21 (1978).
184. A. Whyte and Y. W. Loke, J. Exp. Med. 148:1087 (1978).
185. C. H. Bauer, W. G. Reutter, K. P. Erhart, E. Köttgen, and W. Gerok, Science 201:1232 (1978).
186. T. Krarup, Acta Pathol. Microbiol. Scand. 70:241 (1967).
187. A. J. Wyrobek and W. R. Bruce, Proc. Nat. Acad. Sci. U.S. 72:4425 (1975).
188. D. R. Mattison and S. S. Thorgeirsson, Cancer Res. 38:1368 (1978).
189. A. H. Conney, R. M. Welch, R. Kuntzman, and J. J. Burns, Clin. Pharmacol. Ther. 8:2 (1967).
190. H. Druckrey, Xenobiotica 3:271 (1973).
191. D. V. Parke, in Biochemistry of Women: Clinical Concepts (A. S. Curry and J. V. Hewitt, Eds.). CRC Press, Cleveland, 1974, p. 111.
192. D. V. Parke, in Modern Trends in Toxicology, Vol. 2 (E. Boyland and R. Goulding, Eds.). Butterworths, London, 1974, p. 116.
193. F. Martz, C. Failinger, and D. A. Blake, J. Pharmacol. Exp. Ther. 203:231 (1977).
194. D. Labadarios, J. W. T. Dickerson, D. V. Parke, E. G. Lucas, and G. H. Obuwa, Brit. J. Clin. Pharmacol. 5:167 (1978).

Chapter 2

HEPATIC CYTOCHROME P-450-LINKED DRUG-METABOLIZING SYSTEMS

Gilbert J. Mannering

Department of Pharmacology
University of Minnesota School of Medicine
Minneapolis, Minnesota

The present chapter examines and discusses hepatic monooxygenase systems by following two approaches, namely, analytical and synthetic.

In the first approach, the monooxygenase components are considered in turn, with the greatest attention being given to the terminal oxidase, cytochrome P-450. Of special interest is the multiplicity of cytochrome P-450s. The many criteria by which this multiplicity is experimentally revealed are presented at length, allowing attention to be focused to the multivalent nature and manifold functional aspects of cytochrome P-450s. The electron transport chains of the monooxygenase systems are also duly considered.

In the second, synthetic approach, the interplay of the individual components is pictured by following the temporal sequence of events building up the functional cycle of monooxygenases. The binding of the substrate to cytochrome P-450, the binding of oxygen, the reductive steps, the activation of oxygen, and the product formation are all revealing of the intricacies of this capital enzyme system.

The analytical and synthetic approaches are thus complementary in clarifying our rapidly advancing understanding of monooxygenases. Indeed, it is in a synthetic view that the diversity and complexity of the individual components can be put into perspective and acquire their real significance.

I. INTRODUCTION

The early biochemical, spectrophotometric, and electron spin resonance (ESR) studies which led to the discovery of hepatic cytochrome P-450-linked drug-metabolizing systems were published by investigators who at the time had little reason to suspect that they had been performing experiments of mutual interest. In 1949, James Miller, who had been studying the biotransformation of carcinogens for more than a decade at the McArdle Laboratories, University of Wisconsin, and Gerald Mueller observed that an NADPH-linked reductive cleavage of 4-dimethylaminoazobenzene to N,N-dimethyl-para-phenylenediamine and aniline was catalyzed by a microsomal fraction of liver homogenate [1]. Four years later they reported the oxidative N-demethylation of the same aminoazo dye by hepatic microsomes [2]. Molecular oxygen and NADPH were required for the reaction and NADH was needed for optimal activity. It is now known that cytochrome P-450 is involved in both reactions.

At about the same time that Mueller and Miller were experimenting with aminoazo dyes, Bernard B. Brodie and his associates at the Laboratory of Chemical Pharmacology, National Institutes of Health, were studying the biotransformation of drugs by hepatic microsomes. They showed that microsomal enzymes catalyze the side chain oxidation of barbiturates, the N-dealkylation of amines, the deamination of alkylamines, the cleavage of alkyl and aryl ethers, and aromatic hydroxylation [3]. The microsomal system was shown to consist of an NADPH-dependent flavoprotein reductase and an unidentified terminal oxidase, which is now recognized as cytochrome P-450. The reductase had been described previously by Horecker in 1950 [4], but at that time its location in microsomes was not recognized. Strittmatter and Velick [5], Phillips and Langdon [6], and Williams and Kamin [7] documented its microsomal origin and purified the enzyme. During this very active period in Brodie's laboratory, many factors which affect the activity of the system were studied, including the effects of inducing agents, age, sex, hormonal status, and species differences.

The requirement of these oxidative microsomal systems for both molecular oxygen and a reducing agent (NADPH) was enigmatical until Mason [8] and Hayaishi [9] and their associates showed in independent studies published in 1955 that certain oxidases transfer one atom of molecular oxygen to the substrate to form hydroxylated products while the other oxygen atom undergoes two-equivalent reduction to water. These enzymes were designated "mixed-function oxidases" by Mason [10] and "monooxygenases" by Hayaishi [11]. From studies that used $^{18}O_2$ they formulated the overall reaction:

$$XH + NADPH + H^+ + O_2 \longrightarrow XOH + NADP^+ + H_2O \qquad (1)$$

The following events, which led to the identification of cytochrome P-450 as a component of the microsomal drug-metabolizing system, illustrate how a flux of investigators through a distinguished laboratory can give continuity to a scientific endeavor. In 1955, G. R. Williams of the Johnson Foundation for Medical Physics, University of Pennsylvania, observed a difference spectrum with a maximum absorbance at 450 nm when carbon monoxide was added to hepatic microsomes from the rat. He was working in the laboratory of Britton Chance, who had developed a double-beam recording spectrophotometer capable of recording difference spectra of highly turbid samples. This unpublished observation (cited in Ref. 12) led to more detailed studies by M. Klingenberg [12], a visitor to this laboratory from Germany. The binding of carbon monoxide suggested the presence of a heavy metal ion in the chromophore of the pigment, but its spectrum did not resemble that of a cytochrome or of other known metalloproteins. The investigation of this "microsomal carbon monoxide-binding pigment" was resumed by Garfinkel [13] after Klingenberg left the Johnson Foundation. Attempts to solubilize the pigment in pig liver microsomes with sodium cholate or pancreatin resulted in the disappearance of the absorbance peak at 450 nm. Studies of the nature of the pigment were begun by R. Sato in 1960 at the Institute of Protein Research, Osaka University. Sato was once associated with the Johnson Foundation and had visited Chance's laboratory while Klingenberg was there. In 1962 Omura and Sato [14] presented conclusive evidence that the pigment with the unusual absorption spectrum was indeed a cytochrome. Their observation of characteristic α- and β-bands, as well as intense bands in the Soret region of the ethyl isocyanide difference spectrum of reduced microsomes, revealed the hemoprotein nature of the pigment. They named it cytochrome P-450. They also observed that detergent solubilized the pigment and converted it to a CO-combining derivative with a maximum absorption at 420 nm [15].

The reduced-minus-oxidized spectrum of this derivative was typical of a b-type cytochrome.

While these studies of Omura and Sato were in progress, Mason and his associates [16] at the University of Oregon examined the ESR spectrum of hepatic microsomes from the rabbit and observed a new, characteristic absorption in the g = 2 region with a signal at $g_m = 2.25$ as its most prominent feature. They concluded that the substance responsible for these signals was probably a low-spin ferric hemoprotein, which they designated "microsomal Fe_x." The ESR signal was diminished by NADH or NADPH under anaerobic conditions and carbon monoxide enhanced this decrease. The calculated amount of microsomal Fe_x was about equal to the difference between the total protohemin and the cytochrome b_5 protohemin contents of the microsomes. Their suggestion that microsomal Fe_x and cytochrome P-450 are the same enzyme was established later by Yamano and associates [17,18].

Cytochrome P-450 was first observed in hepatic microsomes, but its function was revealed from studies of adrenocortical microsomes (see Ref. 19 for review). At the Harrison Department of Surgical Research, University of Pennsylvania, David Cooper, a surgeon, and Otto Rosenthal, a biochemist, had become interested in the hydroxylation of steroids by adrenocortical microsomes. They observed that CO inhibited the C-21 hydroxylation of 17-hydroxyprogesterone [19]. Ryan and Engle [20] had made the same observation earlier and had also shown that the inhibition was reversed by light. Otto Warburg's discovery in 1926 [21] of the light-reversible CO inhibition of the respiration of yeast led him to recognize the hematin nature of the "respiratory" enzyme; since then, light-reversible inhibition of enzymatic reactions has been one criterion for implicating iron-porphyrin-containing enzymes in reactions involving molecular oxygen. When Cooper bubbled carbon monoxide through a detergent-solubilized preparation of adrenocortical microsomes that had been reduced with dithionite, he observed an absorption maximum at 450 nm. Klingenberg was on the University of Pennsylvania campus at the time. When he saw Cooper's spectrum he agreed that the pigment in the adrenal microsomes was the same pigment he had observed in liver microsomes in 1957 [19]. Cooper and Rosenthal took their problem to Ronald Estabrook's laboratory at the Johnson Foundation, which at that time probably housed the only spectrophotometer that could be used to study turbid solutions. Thus, after six years, the investigation that had begun with Williams' discovery, had returned to the Johnson Foundation. Estabrook, Cooper, and Rosenthal [22] used Warburg's photochemical action spectrum technique [23] to demonstrate the function of cytochrome P-450. They showed that the ratio of CO to O_2 had the same effect on the rate of hydroxylated product formed from 17-hydroxyprogesterone as it had on the formation of the absorbance of the CO-binding pigment at 450 nm. A curve showing the effectiveness of different wavelengths of light in reversing the inhibition of hydroxylation by CO simulated the spectrum of cytochrome P-450 between 400 nm and 500 nm; the maximum effect was seen at 450 nm. The photochemical action spectrum method was used later by Cooper and associates [24,25] to demonstrate the role of cytochrome P-450 in the oxidation of acetanilide, benzo[a]pyrene, codeine, and 4-methylaminoantipyrine by hepatic microsomes.

The coexistence of the cytochrome P-450 and cytochrome b_5 electron-transfer systems in the endoplasmic reticulum of the liver suggested to Hildebrandt and Estabrook [26] that the systems might interact during the oxidation of drug substrates in much the same way cytochrome electron-transfer systems are known to interact in mitochondria. They concluded from studies of the steady-state reduction of cytochrome b_5 and the stoichiometry of NADH and NADPH utilization during the oxidation of ethylmorphine by hepatic microsomes that the first of the two electrons required for monooxygenation must be derived from NADPH, but that the second electron may originate from either NADH or NADPH. Immunochemical studies of Sasame [27] and Mannering [28] and their associates supported the concept of the transfer of the second electron from NADH via cytochrome b_5. Figure 1 shows how cytochromes P-450 and b_5 are believed by many investigators to contribute electrons to NADPH-dependent monooxygenase reactions.

Hepatic cytochrome P-450 was originally thought to be a single molecular entity with an extraordinarily broad substrate selectivity. However, indirect evidence soon began to accumulate that hepatic microsomes contain more than one species of cytochrome P-450. Rates of oxidation of a variety of substrates did not always parallel one another when animals were treated with different inducing agents, and relative rates of oxidation of selected substrates by microsomes from different animal species differed widely. While this suggested the existence of multiple species of cytochrome P-450, it could be argued that the composition of the membrane might differ among animal species or might be altered by inducing agents and that these differences could account for the observed differences in substrate selectivity. The first material basis for the existence of more than one species of hepatic cytochrome P-450 was provided in 1966 by Sladek and Mannering [29], who observed that the administration of 3-methylcholanthrene (3MC) to rats caused a change in the ethyl isocyanide difference spectrum of dithionite-reduced microsomes. This and other evidence led them to conclude that 3MC and certain other polycyclic hydrocarbons caused the induction of a new hemoprotein, which they designated "cytochrome P_1-450" (see Ref. 30 for review). The reduced-CO difference spectrum of cytochrome P_1-450 was observed to have a maximum absorbance at 448 nm rather than at 450 nm [31] and before long the terms "P_1-450" and "P-448" were used interchangeably. Acceptance of cytochrome P_1-450 as a specific molecular entity was not immediate. Some investigators [32,33] argued that observed changes in the ethyl isocyanide and CO spectra were due to the binding of 3MC or its metabolites to cytochrome P-450. Others [34] argued that the inducing agent could change the hydrophobic environment surrounding the

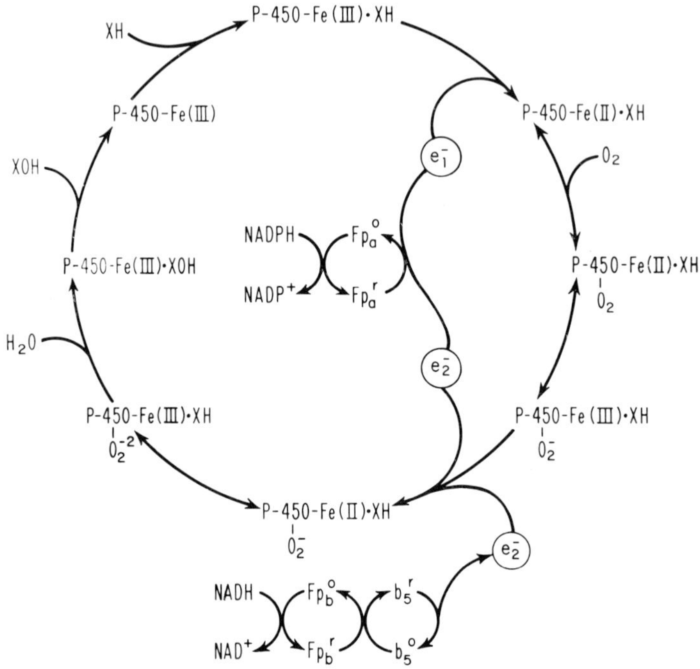

FIGURE 1 Cytochrome P-450- and cytochrome b_5-linked hepatic monooxygenase system. P-450(III) = ferricytochrome P-450; P-450(II) = ferrocytochrome P-450; P-450-Fe(III) with O_2^- = oxyanionferricytochrome P-450; b_5 = cytochrome b_5; Fp_a = NADPH-cytochrome P-450 reductase; Fp_b = NADH-cytochrome b_5 reductase; XH = substrate. (From Ref. 230. Reproduced with kind permission of Pharmacological Therapeutics, Series A.)

cytochrome P-450 in the membrane and thereby alter both its spectral characteristics and its substrate selectivity. Conclusive evidence that cytochrome P_1-450 is indeed a specific P-450 was provided when it was solubilized, partially purified, and shown to possess physical and catalytic properties that distinguish it from the cytochrome P-450 found in microsomes from untreated or phenobarbital (PB)-treated animals [35-38].

Early attempts to solubilize cytochrome P-450 in its native form by conventional procedures failed because the hemoprotein was converted rapidly to its inactive form (P-420). This problem was largely solved when Ichikawa and Yamano [39] discovered the stabilizing effect of glycerol on cytochrome P-450. Miyaki et al. [40] were the first to partially purify a cytochrome that retained the optical and magnetic properties of the membrane bound hemoprotein. They referred to their preparation as "submicrosomal particles." In 1973, Comai and Gaylor [41] provided the first direct evidence for the multiplicity of cytochrome P-450 when they separated solubilized microsomes into three fractions with different affinities for cyanide. Since then, column chromatography, gel electrophoresis, and immunological procedures have been used to isolate and identify multiple forms of cytochrome P-450 in microsomes from several species of laboratory animals [42-55]. In 1974, Imai and Sato [56] and van der Hoeven et al. [57] reported the purification of PB-induced rabbit cytochrome P-450 to electrophoretic homogeneity.

Lu and Coon [58] were the first to reconstitute solubilized components of hepatic microsomes into an active monooxygenase system. Their system consisted of the combination of a cytochrome P-450 fraction, an NADPH-cytochrome c reductase fraction, and microsomal lipid which catalyzed the (ω-1)-hydroxylation of laurate. A great variety of monooxygenase systems has been reconstituted in the decade that has followed their publication (see Refs. 59 and 60 for reviews).

Cytochrome P-450 hemoproteins were originally presumed to be located only in the liver and adrenals, where they are found in the highest concentrations, but they are now known to be widely distributed in nature. In mammals, they have been found in microsomes of the kidney [61], intestinal mucosa [62], lung [22], skin [63], testis [64], placenta [65], and brain [66]. The location of cytochrome P-450 is not limited to microsomes; it is found in the mitochondria of the adrenal cortex [67], testis [68], corpus luteum [69], kidney [70,71], and liver [72,73]. The nuclear envelope of the liver has also been reported to contain the cytochrome [74]. It has been observed in the livers of fish, amphibia, reptiles, and birds [75,76], and plays an important role in the metabolism of pesticides in insects [77-79]. It has been found in a variety of higher plants [80-85] as well as in yeasts, molds, and bacteria [86-95].

Not only are cytochrome P-450 systems widely distributed, but they participate in a remarkable variety of cellular functions. In microsomes of yeast [96] and mammalian liver [97], these systems are involved in the synthesis of ergosterol and cholesterol, respectively. They also catalyze several steps of the conversion of cholesterol to bile acids by hepatic microsomes [98] and mitochondria [72,73]. Adrenocortical mitochondrial cytochrome P-450 is involved in the cleavage of cholesterol to pregnenolone [99], the step common to almost all of the metabolic pathways leading to the synthesis of steroid hormones in various endocrine glands. Placental cytochrome P-450 catalyzes the conversion of androstenedione to estrone [100, 101]. Cytochrome P-450-linked monooxygenase systems in hepatic microsomes and kidney mitochondria convert cholecalciferol (Vitamin D_3) to its physiologically active form [70,71,102]. This involves 25-hydroxylation in the liver followed by 1-hydroxylation in the kidney. Hydroxylation reactions are very prevalent in higher plants and some of these reactions have been shown to involve cytochrome P-450. Wheat germ microsomal cytochrome P-450 catalyzes the hydroxylation of kaurene to kaurenol, an intermediate in the biosynthesis of gibberellin [80]. 4-Hydroxycinnamic acid, a precursor of lignins, tannins, and flavonoids, is produced in microsomes of sorghum seedlings from cinnamic acid by a cytochrome P-450-linked system [81]. In C. roseus seedlings, cytochrome P-450 is involved in indole alkaloid synthesis through mediation of the hydroxylation of geraniol and nerol [84]. Ergot alkaloid biosynthesis by a fungus has also been reported to depend on cytochrome P-450 [89]. The first evidence for the presence of cytochrome P-450 in a bacterium was presented in 1967 by Appleby [87], who showed that the nitrogen fixing bacteroid, Rhizobium japonicum, contained a soluble carbon monoxide-binding pigment with the optical properties of cytochrome P-450. Bacterial cytochrome P-450s that are induced by unusual carbon sources have received the most study. High concentrations of cytochrome P-450 appear in P. putida [88] and in C. tropicalis [90] when camphor or n-octane, respectively, is provided as the sole source of carbon in the medium. The first steps in the oxidative degradations of camphor and n-octane are mediated by the substrate-induced cytochrome P-450 systems. B. megaterium contains a cytochrome P-450 which catalyzes the 15β-hydroxylation of 3-oxo-Δ^4-steroids [95]. This microbial cytochrome P-450 exists without having to be induced by unusual carbon sources.

The story of cytochrome P-450-linked monooxygenase systems began just over 20 years ago with the observation that hepatic microsomes are involved in the oxidative biotransformation of a variety of carcinogens and drugs. Since then, interest in this remarkable enzyme system has been appropriately tuned to society's increasing concern over the hazardous effects of synthetic chemicals on man and his environment. An enzyme system that will detoxify and occasionally activate drugs, pesticides, food additives, and industrial wastes has made "strange bedfellows" of biologists from a variety of fields—pharmacologists, oncologists, toxicologists, environmentalists, and more recently, theoretical biochemists and biophysicists who have begun to recognize that an enzyme system that can both transfer electrons and catalyze the oxidation of a multitude of substrates must possess some very unusual chemical and physical properties. The membrane chemist has begun to accommodate the system to his models. Indeed, cytochrome P-450-linked monooxygenase systems may very well be the most studied enzyme systems of our time.

The cytochrome P-450 "field" has so many components that a decision had to be made as to what was to be included in this chapter. The decision was made easier by the inclusion in this and the preceding volume of several chapters dealing with subjects related to cytochrome P-450. This chapter is concerned primarily with the individual components of the mammalian cytochrome P-450-linked drug-metabolizing systems of hepatic microsomes and their interaction. The reader is forewarned that the author's views and speculations may not always coincide with those of others who labor in this rapidly expanding and sometimes controversial field.

II. COMPONENTS OF THE SYSTEMS

Two cytochrome P-450-linked monooxygenase systems exist in hepatic microsomes. The system consisting of an NADPH reductase and any of several species of cytochrome P-450 is involved predominantly in drug metabolism. The reductase is called NADPH-cytochrome P-450 reductase when it transfers electrons to cytochrome P-450, the natural electron acceptor, and NADPH-cytochrome c reductase when cytochrome c is used experimentally as an electron acceptor. A large number of drugs and other xenobiotics, and a much smaller number of endogenous substances, are substrates for the system. The microsomal membrane may be considered a facilitative component because it implements interaction of the components of the system. The second system consists of NADH-cytochrome b_5 reductase (NADH-ferricyanide reductase), cytochrome b_5, and cytochrome P-450. Although this system is capable of carrying out the monooxygenation of xenobiotics without the participation of the first system, its most important role in drug metabolism is probably that of synergizing the NADPH-linked system (Sec. III.F). Section II of this chapter deals with the components of these systems, Sec. III with their interaction.

A. Cytochrome P-450

1. Multiplicity

This section presents examples from the many studies which have revealed the multiplicity of cytochrome P-450 systems; they may represent heterogeneity of molecular species, or heterogeneity of physical forms of a given species, or they may conceivably reflect heterogeneity due to diverse locations of the hemoprotein in the membrane.

a. Multiplicity revealed by species-, sex-, and age-related differences in drug metabolism: The earliest suggestion that hepatic monooxygenase reactions might be catalyzed by more than one enzyme system came from the observation that the specific activities of the biotransformations of two or more drugs by hepatic microsomes from different sources were not always proportional. These disproportions reflected differences in the age, sex, and species of laboratory animals. This chapter will not review the vast number of studies that have been published on the subject, but will use the metabolism of ethylmorphine to illustrate how studies of species-, sex-, and age-related differences in drug metabolism have been used to reveal the multiple nature of hepatic monooxygenase systems.

Ethylmorphine is both N-demethylated and O-deethylated by hepatic microsomes. The two reactions appear to be catalyzed by different monooxygenase systems. In Table 1 it is seen that the ratios of the rates of O- to N-dealkylation by hepatic microsomes from the rat, mouse, rabbit, and

TABLE 1
O- and N-Dealkylation of Ethylmorphine by Hepatic Microsomes from the Rat, Mouse, Rabbit, and Guinea Pig

Species	Sex	Cytochrome P-450 (nmol/mg protein)	(A) O-deethylation (nmol CH_3CHO/min)		(B) N-demethylation (nmol HCHO/min)		A/B
			Per mg protein	Per nmol cytochrome P-450	Per mg protein	Per nmol cytochrome P-450	
Mature rat	M	0.81	1.72	2.12	7.12	8.79	0.24
(56 days old)	F	0.52	1.25	2.40	1.28	2.47	0.98
Immature rat	M	0.56	1.87	3.33	3.15	5.63	0.59
(21 days old)	F	0.51	1.67	3.27	3.23	6.33	0.52
Mature mouse	M	1.24	2.37	1.91	8.23	6.64	0.29
	F	1.44	3.05	2.12	9.40	6.53	0.32
Mature rabbit	M	0.96	0.68	0.71	2.00	2.08	0.34
	F	0.96	0.88	0.92	2.15	2.24	0.41
Mature guinea	M	1.26	2.90	2.30	3.52	2.79	0.82
pig	F	1.14	3.13	2.75	3.18	2.79	0.98

Sources: Data from Refs. 103 and 104.

guinea pig vary greatly. Moreover, the proportion of O- to N-dealkylation is much larger in the adult female than in the adult male rat. The low ratio of the rates of O- to N-dealkylation seen with male microsomes relative to that observed with female microsomes is due mainly to the greater N-demethylating capacity of male microsomes. A sex-related difference in the N-demethylation of ethylmorphine, which is not observed in sexually immature rats, develops as the animals reach sexual maturity; the rate of N-demethylation increased from 3.15 to 7.12 nmol of HCHO formed/min per mg of protein between the ages of 21 and 56 days while that of female rats decreased from 3.23 to 1.28 nmol of HCHO formed/min per mg of protein. The widening of the difference in rates of N-demethylation between the sexes as they grew older was due more to a change in the quality of cytochrome P-450, as evaluated by the apparent specific activity (nmol product formed per nmol P-450), than to a change in its quantity. Sex-related differences in O- and N-demethylation were not seen in the mouse, rabbit, or guinea pig.

Temporal aspects of the sex difference in drug metabolism were shown by el Masry and colleagues [105] to be similar for the N-demethylation of ethylmorphine, codeine, N-methylaniline, and 3-methyl-4-methylaminoazobenzene (3MMAB) in rats between the ages of 21 and 56 days; i.e., rates of N-demethylation by microsomal preparations were about the same at 21 days in both sexes, but thereafter, rates increased in males and decreased in females. Apparent specific activities of cytochrome P-450 with respect to the N-demethylation of the four substrates increased with age in males, but not in females. Rates of aniline para-hydroxylation declined in both sexes from the 21st to the 56th day. The apparent K_m for the N-demethylation of ethylmorphine decreased in males between the ages of 21 and 56 days, but remained unchanged in females.

b. Multiplicity revealed by inducers and inhibitors of drug metabolism: Richardson and Cunningham [106] observed in 1951 that the incidence and severity of primary liver cell carcinoma caused by 3-methyl-4-dimethylaminoazobenzene was greatly reduced by the coadministration of 3MC, a carcinogen used to produce experimental skin tumors. The explanation for this serendipitous finding was soon forthcoming from the laboratory of James and Elizabeth Miller, who with Allen Conney, a graduate student, showed that 3MC and several other polycyclic aromatic hydrocarbons induced the activities of the hepatic microsomal enzymes that N-demethylate and reduce aminoazo dyes to less carcinogenic products [107]. Both the reduction and the N-demethylation of aminoazo dyes are now known to be catalyzed by cytochrome P-450-linked systems. Two years later Remmer [108] showed that a large part of the tolerance that animals develop to barbiturates can be explained by the ability of these drugs to induce their own metabolism. As more and more drugs and other xenobiotics were tested for their inductive ability it soon became apparent that inducing agents could be divided into two groups: those compounds like PB, which induce the metabolism of a great number of drugs, and those like 3MC, which induce the metabolism of a much smaller number of substrates (see Refs. 109-111 for reviews). This was interpreted to mean that the liver contained at least two monooxygenase systems.

About the same time that inducing agents were being discovered, a versatile in vivo and in vitro inhibitor of drug metabolism known as SKF-525A (2-diethylaminoethyl 2,2-diphenylvalerate) began to attract attention. While SKF-525A was shown to inhibit the metabolism of a great many drugs, that of some drugs was not (see Refs. 110, 112, 113 for reviews). Moreover, the metabolism of a given drug might be inhibited by SKF-525A in one species of animal, but not in another. Pretreatment of animals with certain inducing agents sometimes altered the inhibitory effect of SKF-525A markedly. This last observation led to the discovery of cytochrome P_1-450 [29]. At a concentration of 0.04 mM, SKF-525A inhibited the N-demethylation of ethylmorphine regardless of the source of microsomes, whether from untreated, PB-treated, or 3MC-treated rats, and the degrees of inhibition were similar [114]. However, this same concentration of SKF-525A inhibited the N-demethylation of 3MMAB by control and PB microsomes, but not by 3MC microsomes. Because SKF-525A was thought to produce its inhibitory effect, at least in part, by acting as an alternative substrate [115], these results implied that 3MC administration had caused the appearance of an N-demethylating system that did not exist in microsomes from untreated or PB-treated rats. Subsequent studies using a variety of methodological approaches showed that 3MC and some other polycyclic aromatic hydrocarbons induce a molecular species of cytochrome P-450 (cytochrome P_1-450) with distinctive biochemical and spectral properties (see Ref. 30 for review).

Many substrates yield more than one product, and PB and 3MC often induce different patterns of product formation. Ullrich and Kremers [116] generalize that PB induces hydroxylation of aliphatic substrates whereas polycyclic aromatic hydrocarbons induce hydroxylation of aromatic substrates. Accordingly, hydroxylation of cyclohexane and n-hexane is induced by PB, but not by benzo[a]pyrene (BP) [117,118], and the hydroxylation of 7-ethoxycoumarin, 7-ethoxyresorufin, and acetanilide are greatly induced by BP, but poorly induced by PB [116,118,119]. Steric hindrance plays a more important role in determining the pattern of product formation when PB microsomes are used than when 3MC microsomes are employed [116]. When alkanes are substrates for PB microsomes, the (ω-1)-position is preferentially hydroxylated [117,120]. Steric hindrance restricts the hydroxylation of the (ω-2)- and (ω-3)-positions. Much less stereoselectivity is exhibited with regard to (ω-1)-, (ω-2)-, or (ω-3)-hydroxylation when BP microsomes are used [117]. BP microsomes hydroxylate the ortho and para positions of biphenyl almost equally, but because the ortho position is sterically hindered, PB microsomes hydroxylate biphenyl almost exclusively in the para position [121]. 7-Ethoxycoumarin is preferentially O-dealkylated by PB microsomes and hydroxylated on the ring by 3MC microsomes; steric inhibition at the ring prevents hydroxylation of the ring by PB microsomes [116]. Fischbach and Lenk [122] observed that different patterns of ω-(ω-1)-, (ω-2)-, and (ω-3)-hydroxylation of several compounds were induced by PB and 3MC in several mammalian species.

Selander and colleagues [123] studied the metabolism of chlorobenzene to ortho-, meta-, and para-chlorophenols by perfused rat livers and by cell-free hepatic preparations at progressive stages of resolution of the monooxygenase systems (postmitochondrial supernatant fraction, microsomes, and reconstituted cytochrome P-450 systems). They found a greater loss of formation of meta-chlorophenol than either the ortho- or the para-metabolite with increasing resolution of the monooxygenase system. Administration of PB caused moderate increases in all three metabolites, but 3MC produced a selective increase in ortho-chlorophenol. SKF-525A and 7,8-benzoflavone inhibited the formation of ortho- and para-chlorophenol to a greater extent than that of the meta isomer. NADH greatly potentiated NADPH-dependent formation of para-chlorophenol, potentiated the formation of meta-chlorophenol moderately, and had very little effect on the formation of ortho-chlorophenol. They concluded that chlorophenol formation is catalyzed by three different monooxygenase systems, two of which form arene oxide intermediates and one of which catalyzes the direct formation of a phenol.

Burke and Bridges [124] studied differences in the ratios of the formation of 2- and 4-hydroxybiphenyl from biphenyl by control, PB, and 3MC microsomes from the hamster. PB induced formation of 4-hydroxybiphenyl preferentially, whereas 3MC induced both the formation and the further metabolism of 2- and 4-hydroxybiphenyl. They concluded that at least two enzyme systems were needed to account for their data.

Ullrich and associates [125] have used the inhibition of the O-dealkylation of 7-ethoxycoumarin by metyrapone and 7,8-benzoflavone to demonstrate the difference in the induction of monooxygenase systems by PB and 3MC. Metyrapone is a potent inhibitor of O-dealkylation in PB microsomes, but has no effect on this reaction when BP microsomes are used. Conversely, the reaction is inhibited by 7,8-benzoflavone in BP microsomes, but not in PB microsomes.

The inhibitory effect of metyrapone on the O-dealkylation of 7-ethoxycoumarin is sex-dependent in the rat; metyrapone inhibits O-dealkylation by male, but not by female microsomes. However, it is an effective inhibitor in both male and female PB microsomes. Cytochrome P_1-450 is induced by 3MC in certain strains of mice ("responsive mice"), but not in other strains ("nonresponsive mice"). The comparison of monooxygenase activities of microsomes from responsive and nonresponsive mice is a convenient way of determining which systems involve cytochrome P_1-450. Nebert and associates [126-131] have used these mice to extend our understanding of the role of cytochrome P_1-450 in the modification of the toxicity and carcinogenicity of foreign compounds. They have identified 20 genetically controlled cytochrome P_1-450-linked monooxygenase activities in mice [126,131,132].

Responsive and nonresponsive mice have also been used to show the selectivity of inhibitors of cytochrome P_1-450 systems. A variety of compounds were tested as inhibitors of BP hydroxylation by microsomes from untreated nonresponsive mice and 3MC-treated nonresponsive and responsive mice [126,133]. A group of compounds that included phenylimidazoles, metyrapone, and p,p'-DDT was 5 to 100 times more effective in blocking BP hydroxylase activity in microsomes from untreated and 3MC-treated nonresponsive mice than in microsomes from 3MC-treated responsive mice. Conversely, another group of compounds, which included α- and β-naptho-flavone and lindane, was 5 to 100 times more effective as an inhibitor of BP-hydroxylation when the microsomes were derived from 3MC-treated responsive mice than when they came from either of the other two groups of mice.

Powis and associates [134] have recently published studies of differences in the inductive effects of PB, 3MC, pregnenolone 16α-carbonitrile (PCN), and the mixture of polychlorinated biphenyls, Arochlor 1254, on the metabolism of ethylmorphine, aminopyrine, benzphetamine, caffeine, and BP which reveal qualitative differences in hepatic cytochrome P-450s.

c. Multiplicity revealed by kinetic studies: Alternative-substrate kinetic studies can be used to determine whether one enzyme or more than one enzyme react with two substrates [135]. Using ethylmorphine and 3MMAB as alternative substrates, Sladek and Mannering [29,114,136] showed that the microsomal system responsible for the N-demethylation of 3MMAB in rats treated with 3MC is not the same as that found in untreated or PB-treated rats. Their studies also suggested that a single enzyme was predominantly responsible for the N-demethylations of both ethylmorphine and 3MMAB when microsomes from untreated or PB-treated rats were used, but that when 3MC microsomes were used, at least two N-demethylating systems were involved, one of which reacted poorly with ethylmorphine. Other alternative-substrate studies [137] suggested that different enzyme systems in microsomes from untreated male rats are involved in the N-demethylation of ethylmorphine and morphine. Ethylmorphine and morphine are so similar structurally that it might seem unlikely that different systems could be involved in their N-demethylation. However, morphine is an ampholyte and ethylmorphine is not, and this might account for selective binding of the two drugs to different cytochrome P-450 hemoproteins. Unlike ethylmorphine, morphine does not elicit a type I binding spectrum when added to control microsomes [138]. When PB microsomes rather than control microsomes were used, alternative-substrate kinetics then indicated that ethylmorphine and morphine were N-demethylated by the same system [137], which again suggests that PB induces a cytochrome P-450 that does not predominate in control microsomes. The following observation that there is not an increase in ethylmorphine type I binding concomitant with the increased concentration of cytochrome P-450 in PB microsomes [139] supports the view that the induction of P-450 by PB is selective. The observation that PB induces the N-demethylation of ethylmorphine [140], but not that of morphine [138,141], is compatible with the involvement of different cytochrome P-450s in the N-demethylation of morphine and ethylmorphine, but not with the view that PB induces a cytochrome P-450 that catalyzes the N-demethylation of both morphine and ethylmorphine.

Differences in the apparent K_m may also reflect multiplicity of monooxygenase systems. For example, a K_m of 0.1 mM for 3MMAB N-demethylation was observed with control microsomes, but with 3MC microsomes the K_m was 0.03 mM [142]. A similar decrease in the K_m for BP hydroxylation was observed after the administration of aromatic polycyclic hydrocarbons [143-145]. A sex- and age-related difference in the K_m for N-demethylation of ethylmorphine has also been observed. With microsomes from sexually immature rats of both sexes and sexually mature female rats, the K_m is about half that observed with microsomes from sexually mature male rats [105,146]. No sex difference in the K_m for ethylmorphine N-demethylation was seen with microsomes from the guinea pig, rabbit, or monkey. However, in the rat and in the mouse, the K_m was significantly lower in male than in female microsomes [147]. It is of interest that castration or the administration of sex hormones eliminated the sex differences in the V_{max} for ethylmorphine N-demethylation, but not in the K_m [145]. The K_m for hexobarbital oxidation is also markedly lower in the mature male than in the mature female rat [148].

Nonlinear kinetic data for the microsomal biotransformation of several substrates, including aminopyrine [149], aniline [150], and aldrin [151] suggest the presence of more than one monooxygenase system, although nonlinearity can be explained in other ways.

d. Multiplicity revealed by stereoselectivity of reactions: Although hepatic monooxygenase systems show great versatility in their substrate selectivity, they are frequently stereoselective (see Refs. 152-154 for reviews). Trager and associates [154-158] have used warfarin to show that this stereoselectivity is due in part to the multiplicity of cytochrome P-450. Aromatic hydroxylation of warfarin occurs at the 6, 7, 8, and 4' positions and aliphatic hydroxylation occurs at the benzylic position. With control microsomes from the rat, hydroxylations at the 7, 8, and benzylic positions are stereoselective for the (R)-enantiomer to the extent of 80, 70, and 80%, respectively, whereas little or no stereoselectivity for hydroxylation is seen at the 6 position. On the other hand, hydroxylation at the 4' position is stereoselective for the (S)-enantiomer. The different stereoselectivities for hydroxylation at the 6 and 7 positions indicate that they cannot arise from a common intermediate such as the 6,7-arene oxide and therefore hydroxylations are presumed to be catalyzed by different enzyme systems. Stereoselectivities were altered by the administration of PB or 3MC. The following stereoselectivities for respective 6-, 7-, 8-, 4'-, and benzylic hydroxylations were observed: PB microsomes—52(R), 72(R), 70(R), 56(S), and 70(S); 3MC microsomes—62(R), 70(R), 90(R), 63(S), and no preference [157].

These data were interpreted to mean that the composition of the cytochrome P-450 population had been altered by the inducing agents. Pohl and colleagues [157] postulated from the stereochemical preferences for warfarin hydroxylation displayed by control, PB, and 3MC microsomes that four cytochrome P-450-linked monooxygenase systems (A-D) are contained in control microsomes: A is inducible by PB or 3MC and is stereoselective and regioselective for 7- and benzylic hydroxylation of (R)-warfarin and 4'-hydroxylation of (S)-warfarin; B is inducible only by PB and is regioselective for 6-, 8-, and some 4'-hydroxylation; C, which is present in control microsomes in very low concentration, is inducible by PB only and is regioselective for 7- and benzylic hydroxylation and more stereoselective for (S)-warfarin than A; D, which is also present in control microsomes in limited concentration, is inducible only by 3MC and is stereoselective and regioselective for 6- and 8-hydroxylation of (R)-warfarin.

e. Multiplicity revealed by the ethyl isocyanide-binding spectrum: The ethyl isocyanide difference spectrum of reduced microsomes was the first observation to reveal the hemoprotein nature of cytochrome P-450 [14]. A difference spectrum characteristic of hemoproteins was obtained with a maximum absorption at 430 nm, but in addition, an anomalous peak was observed at 455 nm. As the pH increased, the height of the 455-nm peak increased with an equivalent decrease in the 430-nm peak. Both forms have the same affinity for ethyl isocyanide and both are affected competitively by CO to the same extent at all pH values. Thus, the ethyl isocyanide-cytochrome P-450 complex exists in two pH-dependent, interconvertible forms. Methyl, tert-butyl, and phenyl isocyanide also produce a spectrum with peaks at 455 and 430 nm [159]. The 455-nm peak increases with increasing carbon number of the isocyanides, and the 430-nm maximum decreases accordingly. 3MC microsomes show a much higher ratio of the 455-nm/430-nm peak than PB microsomes or control microsomes. The magnitudes of the two peaks were equal at pH 6.9 with 3MC microsomes, but with PB microsomes or control microsomes at pH 7.5. These observations led to the conclusion that polycyclic aromatic hydrocarbons induce the synthesis of a distinct molecular species of cytochrome P-450 [29]. Purified cytochrome P-450 preparations from 3MC microsomes also show a higher ratio of 455 nm/430 nm than preparations from PB microsomes [45,160].

A sex-related change in the ethyl isocyanide difference spectrum coincides with the increase in the cytochrome P-450 content of microsomes that occurs in male rats as they mature [105]. As male rats aged from 21 to 56 days, the height of the 430-nm peak increased with the increase in cytochrome P-450, but there was little change in the height of the 455-nm peak. Thus, the 455 nm/430 nm ratio with male microsomes was 1.25 at 21 days and 0.70 at 56 days. With female microsomes, little temporal change was seen in the height of either peak, and the ratio remained at about 0.85 throughout the experimental period. With microsomes from female rats, the pH at which the heights of the two peaks were equal remained at about 7.5

throughout the experimental period, but with microsomes from male rats, it increased from pH 7.6 at 21 days to pH 8.1 at 56 days.

f. Multiplicity revealed by the half-lives of cytochrome P-450 heme: The radioactivity of microsomal cytochrome P-450 heme, labelled in vivo with ^{3}H-δ-aminolevulinic acid, was shown by Levin and Kuntzman [161-163] and by Meyer and Marver [164] to decline biphasically. The half-life of the heme of the fast-phase component of the decline was 7-8 hr, that of the slow-phase component 46-48 hr. The administration of 3MC did not change the half-life of either heme component, but it decreased the ratio of the amount of the fast-phase component to the amount of the slow-phase component from 3.8:1 to 1:1. Three possibilities were offered to explain the two half-lives of cytochrome P-450 heme: (1) two species of P-450 may be synthesized independently; (2) a single P-450 may be broken down or converted to a second P-450; (3) a single P-450 may exist in two physical forms, in which case 3MC changes the less stable form to the more stable form; this change could involve a change in the submicrosomal localization of the cytochrome P-450 or a change in its lipid attachment. At the time these studies were published, a number of investigators had expressed the opinion that cytochrome P_1-450 was simply a high-spin form of a single P-450. Accordingly, Levin and Kuntzman suggested that the slow- and fast-phase components might represent the high- and low-spin forms of cytochrome P-450 [161,162]. As will be discussed later, (Sec. II.A.2.e), the various molecular species of cytochrome P-450, including P_1-450, exist in equilibrated high- and low-spin states.

In contrast to 3MC, PB and chlordane did not alter the ratio of the fast-phase heme to the slow-phase heme, but increased the half-life of the fast-phase component to 12 hr [162]. This suggested the possibility that PB and chlordane had induced the synthesis of a new fast-phase cytochrome P-450 or that these agents had stabilized the hemoprotein. The ratio of the fast-phase component to the slow-phase component ranged between 3.4:1 and 4.4:1 in immature and adult female rats and in the immature rat, but in the adult male the ratio was 1.9:1 [163]. These sex- and age-related differences in the half-lives of cytochrome P-450 heme correlate with the sex- and age-dependent difference in drug metabolism discussed in an earlier section (Sec. III.A.1.a).

Two half-lives of cytochrome P-450 heme suggests enzymatic multiplicity, but does not exclude the possibility that the fast and slow phases may be due to heterogeneity of the membrane rather than to heterogeneity of cytochrome P-450. In the preceding studies it was the half-life of the heme moiety rather than the protein moiety of the cytochrome that was determined. Apocytochrome P-450 is believed by some investigators to be in equilibrium with the heme of an unassigned heme pool [165-169] and it cannot be assumed that both moieties have the same half-life. 3MC, PB, or chlordane could change the amounts or proportions of the two phases by changing the proportions of existing species of cytochrome P-450 or their membrane environment, by inducing the synthesis of new species of cytochrome P-450, or by combinations of these mechanisms.

g. Multiplicity revealed by destruction of cytochrome P-450 by lipid hydroperoxides, mercurials, phospholipase C, and detergents: Cytochrome P-450 is destroyed or denatured when microsomes are exposed to lipid hydroperoxides, mercurials, lipases, or detergents. However, about half of the cytochrome P-450 in microsomes is resistant to these agents. This suggests the existence of multiple species or multiple locations of the cytochrome in the membrane.

Levin and associates [170] showed that NADPH-linked lipid peroxidation in microsomes caused cytochrome P-450 to disappear. After 15 min of incubation, only about 37% of the cytochrome P-450 remained in microsomes, but essentially no further loss of the hemoprotein occurred during the next 45 min of incubation. The time course of lipid peroxidation, as determined by the rate of malondialdehyde formation, approximated that of cytochrome P-450 destruction. Lipid peroxidation probably causes the destruction of cytochrome P-450 by two mechanisms acting in concert. Unsaturated fatty acids of membrane phospholipids are the substrates for lipid peroxidation. The membrane immediately surrounding the cytochrome P-450 loses its integrity as its phospholipids are consumed by lipid peroxidation, thus "exposing" and thereby rendering cytochrome P-450 more vulnerable to destruction by the lipid hydroperoxides produced by the reaction. If this is the case, the resistance of some of the cytochrome P-450 to destruction could be due either to properties that make it less susceptible to destruction by lipid hydroperoxides, or it could be due to the absence or unavailability of unsaturated fatty acids in the phospholipids that comprise its immediate environment. The latter possibility is suggested by the simultaneous declines of lipid peroxidation and cytochrome P-450 destruction. The loss of cytochrome P-450 from PB or 3MC microsomes was similar to that from control microsomes, but occurred more slowly. This might suggest that the species of cytochrome P-450 induced by PB or 3MC may react more slowly with lipid hydroperoxides or that the phospholipids with which they are associated are less vulnerable to lipid peroxidation. A third possibility to be considered is that some molecules of cytochrome P-450 are not associated with the NADPH-cytochrome P-450 reductase that catalyzes both lipid peroxidation and the reduction of the oxidase [171], and are therefore not associated with phospholipids that can undergo peroxidation. This possibility seems unlikely in view of our studies [172,173] with linoleic acid hydroperoxide (LAHP).

LAHP, added to control microsomes in increasing concentrations in the absence of NADPH, destroyed cytochrome P-450 biphasically [172,173]. About 50% was destroyed at concentrations of LAHP of 50 μM or less, but only about half of the remainder was lost at concentrations as high as 150 μM (Fig. 2). Cytochrome b_5 and NADPH- and NADH-cytochrome c reductases were not affected by the high concentrations of LAHP. Almost all of

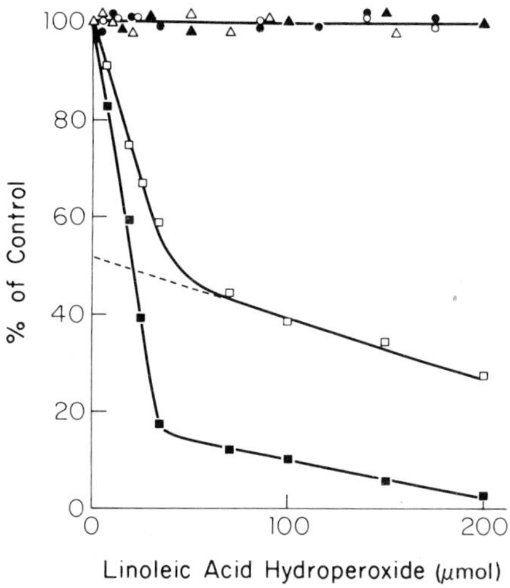

FIGURE 2 Effect of linoleic acid hydroperoxide on microsomal monooxygenase systems. ▲—▲ NADPH oxidation; △—△ cytochrome b_5; ●—● NADH-cytochrome b_5 reductase; ○—○ NADPH-cytochrome c reductase; □—□ cytochrome P-450; ■—■ ethylmorphine N-demethylase. Respective 100% values (nmol or nmol/min per mg of protein): 7.5; 0.37; 1536; 244; 0.56; 4.0. (From Ref. 172. Reproduced by kind permission of Pergamon Press.)

the monooxygenase activity (ethylmorphine N-demethylase, aniline hydroxylase) was associated with the labile cytochrome P-450. Very similar results were obtained with PB microsomes, but the loss of cytochrome P-450 from 3MC microsomes was not biphasic and more of the stable form remained at the high concentrations of LAPH. Of considerable interest was the observation that NADPH-oxidase activity was not affected by LAHP, even at the higher concentrations. It was concluded from these studies that the labile cytochrome P-450 functions in the oxidation of exogenous substrates, that the stable cytochrome P-450 functions in the oxidation of endogenous substrates, and that the two functions are essentially independent of each other.

Indirect evidence [174] suggests that LAHP produces its effect on cytochrome P-450 by stimulating nonenzymatic lipid peroxidation as described by O'Brien and Rahimtula [175].

The studies of Nastainzcyk and associates [176] on the interaction of lipophilic sulfides (thioethers) may provide an explanation as to why LAHP destroys some, but not all of the cytochrome P-450. Spectral and ESR studies showed that certain thioethers interact preferentially with the fifth ligand (mercaptide), whereas others react with the substrate binding site located in a hydrophobic region near the sixth ligand. Only about 50% of the cytochrome P-450 of PB microsomes elicit ligand binding with thioethers. The propensity of thioethers to bind as a substrate was greater in 3MC microsomes than in PB microsomes, probably because of the greater hydrophobicity of the substrate binding site of the cytochrome P-450 of 3MC microsomes. It would be of interest to determine if the stability of microsomal cytochrome P-450 to LAHP relates to thioether ligand formation.

A large number of unrelated compounds convert cytochrome P-450 to cytochrome P-420, an inactive form of the hemoprotein (see Refs. 177 and 178 for reviews). Franklin [179] showed that 50- to 75-nM concentrations of mersalyl (sodium o-[(3-hydroxymercuri-2-mercuri-2-methoxypropyl)carbamoyl]phenoxyacetate), para-chloromercuriphenysulfonic acid, para-chloromercuribenzoate, and $HgCl_2$ convert about 50% of microsomal cytochrome P-450 to cytochrome P-420, but that very little further conversion occurs at higher concentrations of these sulfhydryl reagents. The percentage of mercurial-resistant cytochrome P-450 in microsomes was increased by prior treatment of the animals with PB and decreased by 3MC treatment; it was also greater in rats than in rabbits [180]. Franklin concluded that differences in the susceptibility of cytochrome P-450 to degradation by mercurials probably reflect microsomal enzyme multiplicity.

De Pierre and Ernster [181] showed that when rat hepatic microsomes were incubated with phospholipase C, about 40% of the cytochrome P-450 were converted to cytochrome P-420 during the first 3 min, but that about 80% of the remaining cytochrome P-450 were intact after 30 min of incubation. Bovine serum albumin, which binds fatty acids, stabilized cytochrome P-450 without interfering with phospholipase C activity. This led them to conclude that the diglycerides produced by phospholipase C are acted upon by microsomal diglyceride lipase to yield fatty acids which in turn denature cytochrome P-450. They postulated that the phospholipase C-induced losses of type I binding and monooxygenase activity observed by Chaplin and Mannering [182] are also due to fatty acids produced in situ. The time courses of phospholipid hydrolysis and losses of cytochrome P-450, type I binding, and monooxygenase activity are roughly similar, which suggests that phospholipase C-stable and -unstable cytochrome P-450s are located differently in the membrane, or that they represent different molecular species.

Takeshige and coworkers [183] showed that the addition of Triton X-100 (1%) to hepatic microsomes at 4°C caused an almost instantaneous loss of about 50% of the cytochrome P-450, while the remainder was stable for at least 48 hr. Increasing the concentration of the detergent to 5% did not increase the loss of cytochrome P-450. Similar results were obtained with PB microsomes, 3MC microsomes, and microsomes from untreated rats. Resistance to conversion of cytochrome P-450 to cytochrome P-420 by detergents may relate to the spin state of the hemoprotein. Yamano and Ichikawa [177] showed that the high-spin form of the cytochrome P-450 in rabbit 3MC microsomes is much more susceptible to denaturation by sodium cholate than the low-spin hemoprotein in the same microsomes. The loss of cytochrome P-450 with increasing concentrations of cholate was biphasic; 50% was converted to cytochrome P-420 by a concentration of sodium cholate of less than 5% (w/v), but half of the remainder was still intact at a 20% concentration of the detergent. Reduced cytochrome P-450, which is entirely in the high-spin state, is generally much more unstable than the oxidized hemoprotein. In view of these studies with cholate, it was speculated that the high-spin nature of reduced cytochrome P-450 contributes to its instability [177].

h. Multiplicity revealed by the administration of allylisopropylacetamide and fluroxene: Allylisopropylacetamide (AIA) destroys the heme of hepatic cytochrome P-450, but not that of cytochrome b_5 or other hepatic hemoproteins (see Ref. 184 for review). The destruction is caused by a metabolite of AIA formed at the catalytic site of the enzyme [184]. Predictably, the species of cytochrome P-450 most readily destroyed by AIA would be those most capable of catalyzing the formation of the active metabolite. Bradshaw and associates [185] showed that only 17% of the hepatic cytochrome P-450 of 3MC-treated rats was destroyed by administered AIA, but that 45 and 70%, respectively, were lost in untreated and PB-treated animals. Ethylmorphine, para-nitroanisole, and ethoxyresorufin dealkylase and BP hydroxylase activities were destroyed to a much greater extent in PB- than in 3MC-treated rats.

We have observed a differential recovery as well as a loss of monooxygenase activity after AIA administration [186]. In mice, AIA produced maximal losses of cytochrome P-450, ethylmorphine, aminopyrine, and para-nitrophenetole dealkylase and aniline hydroxylase activities of 55, 80, 70, 58, and 68%, respectively, within 2 to 6 hr after its administration (Fig. 3). All values were restored to normal levels within 12-18 hr. Aniline hydroxylase and para-nitrophenetole deethylase activities remained at about the normal level for the remainder of the 48-hr experimental period, but cytochrome P-450 and ethylmorphine and aminopyrine N-demethylase activities reached levels 1.36-, 2.4-, and 2.1-fold greater than normal, respectively. Normal, minimal, and maximal specific activities (nmol substrate metabolized/nmol P-450/min) observed throughout the time course of the experiment were 13.0, 6.0, and 29.8; 15.2, 14.2, and 29.3; 2.8, 2.0, and 4.5; 1.5, 1.2, and 1.6 for ethylmorphine, aminopyrine, para-nitrophenetole, and aniline metabolism, respectively. This study not only demonstrates the multiple nature of cytochrome P-450-linked hepatic monooxygenase systems, but suggests that different species of cytochrome P-450 are synthesized at different rates.

Fluroxene (2,2,2-trifluoroethyl vinyl ether) also destroys hepatic cytochrome P-450 without affecting other microsomal proteins [185,187]. As with AIA, this destruction requires metabolic activation of the agent to a reactive intermediate by a cytochrome P-450-catalyzed reaction [187]. The effect of administered fluroxene on cytochrome P-450 levels in hepatic microsomes was similar to that seen with AIA; i.e., the P-450 induced by

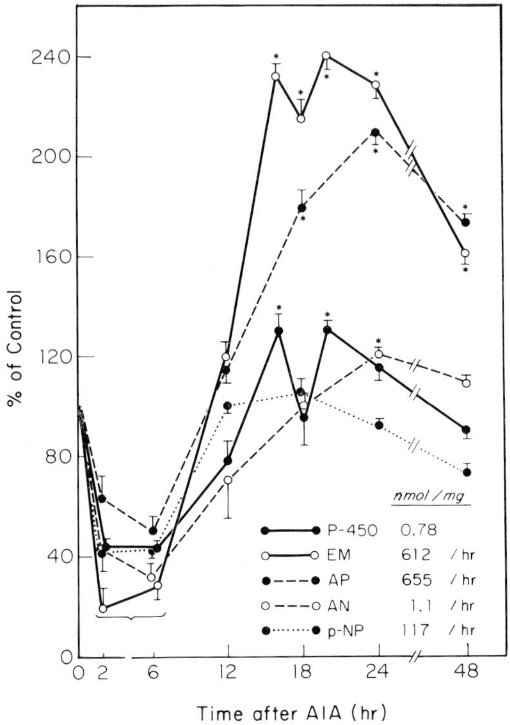

FIGURE 3 Loss and recovery of microsomal cytochrome P-450 and monooxygenase activity after the administration of allylisopropylacetamide (AIA) to mice (400 mg/kg, I.P.). $p < 0.05$ (all 2 and 6 hr except 2-hr p-NP). EM, AP, p-NP = ethylmorphine-, aminopyrine-, and para-nitrophenetole dealkylation, respectively; An = aniline hydroxylation. Values (0.78 etc.) are the 100% control values obtained at 0 time. (From Ref. 186. Reproduced by kind permission of Academic Press.)

PB was more susceptible to destruction than that induced by 3MC. However, the effects of the two agents on monooxygenase activities were quite different, thus emphasizing the multiplicity of cytochrome P-450. Fluroxene had a greater effect on the para-nitroanisole and ethoxyresorufin dealkylase activities of 3MC microsomes than on the same activities of PB microsomes, which was the opposite of what was observed with AIA. Ethylmorphine N-demethylase activity was lowered about 25% in both PB and 3MC microsomes in contrast to the 78 and 50% losses of activity produced by AIA in PB and 3MC microsomes, respectively. Fluroxene greatly depressed BP hydroxylase activity in microsomes, but was without effect on the activity of PB microsomes; AIA had opposite effects on these microsomes.

i. Multiplicity revealed by differences in oxygen binding: Carbon monoxide inhibits monooxygenase reactions by competing for the oxygen binding site of cytochrome P-450. Cooper and associates [25] showed that BP hydroxylase activity of microsomes from untreated rats was inhibited 50% by carbon monoxide when the CO/O_2 ratio was 1:2, but that a 9:12 ratio was required for the same degree of inhibition when microsomes from animals treated with 3MC or 2,3,7,8-tetrachlorodibenzo-para-dioxin (TCDD) were used. It would thus appear that the oxygen binding site of cytochrome P_1-450 may have a lower affinity for CO relative to O_2 than other kinds of cytochrome P-450.

Gray [188] has distinguished three species of cytochrome P-450 in rat PB microsomes by their second-order rate constants of CO binding.

NADH-supported monooxygenase reactions usually proceed at rates which are only 10 to 20% of those supported by NADPH. Recent studies suggest that two rather than one type of cytochrome P-450 may be involved in respective NADH- and NADPH-supported O-dealkylations of certain substrates. Shigematsu and associates [189] showed that the NADH-dependent O-deethylation of para-nitrophenetole by rabbit liver microsomes requires a higher pO_2 for maximum activity than the NADPH-dependent reaction. The NADPH-dependent reaction was inhibited by CO, but the NADH-dependent reaction was not. This led them to conclude that the NADH-dependent reaction was not cytochrome P-450-linked. However, Kamataki and Kitagawa [190] investigated the O-demethylation of para-nitroanisole and provided indirect evidence that the NADH-supported reaction is cytochrome P-450-linked even though it is not inhibited by high concentrations of CO. For example, they showed that para-nitroanisole increased the rate of reduction of microsomal cytochrome P-450 by NADH. Moreover, the increase in the rate was similar to the rate of O-demethylation of para-nitroanisole. This is consistent with the observation that substrate-stimulated increases in rates of reduction of cytochrome P-450 by NADPH are equal to the rates of oxidation of the same substrates by NADPH- and cytochrome P-450-linked systems [191,192]. They also cite unpublished studies which show that antiserum to cytochrome P-450 inhibited the NADH-supported reaction. In an extension of these studies we have obtained evidence that the NADH-supported O-dealkylation of para-nitrophenetole, the O-dealkylation of ethylmorphine and the N-dealkylation of ethylmorphine are catalyzed by different monooxygenase systems [193]. In Fig. 4 it can be seen that the oxygen requirements and CO inhibition of NADPH- and NADH-supported O-deethylations of para-nitrophenetole are quite different. Near maximal activity of the NADPH-supported reaction occurred when the atmosphere contained 5% O_2, but atmospheres of O_2 greater than 20% were required for maximal activity of the NADH-supported reaction. The NADPH-supported reaction was inhibited by CO, but the NADH-supported reaction was not. The effects of CO on the NADPH- and NADH-supported O-deethylation of ethylmorphine were similar, but the NADH-supported O-dealkylation of ethylmorphine

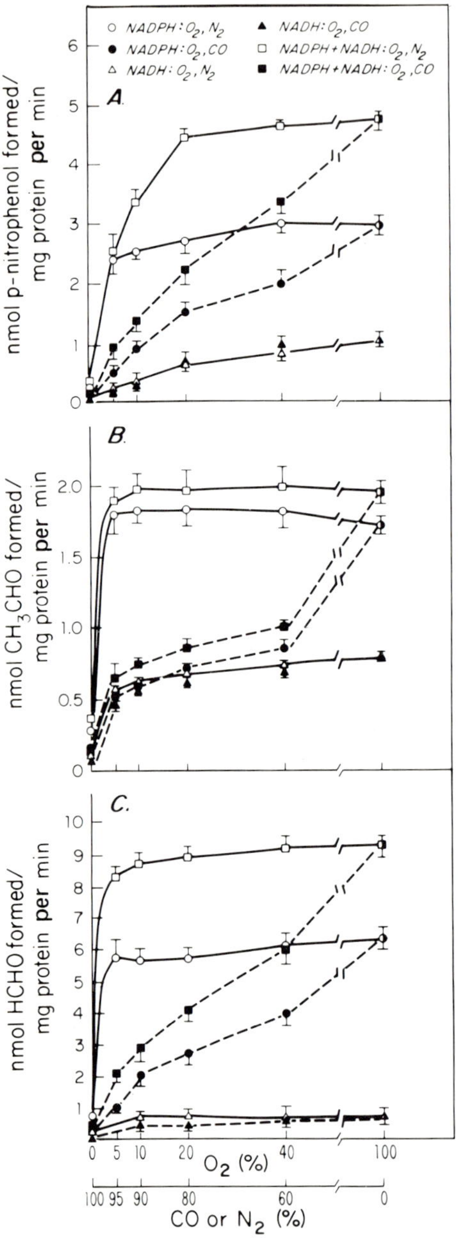

FIGURE 4 Effects of O_2 and CO on NADH- and NADPH-supported O-deethylation of para-nitrophenetole (A), O-deethylation of ethylmorphine (B), and N-demethylation of ethylmorphine (C) by hepatic microsomes from untreated male rats. Each point is the mean ±SE of values obtained in three experiments. (From Ref. 193.)

differed from that of para-nitrophenetole in that it did not require a high pO_2. N-demethylation of ethylmorphine differed from either of the O-dealkylation reactions in that neither the NADPH- nor the NADH-supported reactions required a high pO_2 and both appeared to be inhibited by CO. Differences in NADH synergism of the three dealkylations were also observed. Many hepatic monooxygenase reactions are synergized by NADH; i.e., the velocities of the reactions when both NADPH and NADH are present exceed the sum of the velocities observed when only one or the other nucleotide is present [26,139,194-197]. It is seen in Fig. 4 that the O-deethylation of para-nitrophenetole and the N-demethylation of ethylmorphine were synergized by NADH, but the O-deethylation of ethylmorphine was not. It is also to be noted that no NADH synergism of para-nitrophenetole occurred when atmospheric O_2 was lowered to 5%. These results not only suggest that different cytochrome P-450s are involved in the O-dealkylation of para-nitrophenetole, the O-dealkylation of ethylmorphine and the N-dealkylation of ethylmorphine, but that in the case of para-nitrophenetole, different cytochrome P-450s are involved in the NADPH- and NADH-supported reactions.

j. Multiplicity revealed by ESR and optical substrate binding spectra: The ferric ion of cytochrome P-450 has five d electrons in its outer shell which can be either paired or unpaired depending upon the state of the enzyme and the nature of the ligands bound to it (See Refs. 156 and 198 for reviews). In the low-spin state (single d electron unpaired), the iron atom has two axial ligands and lies in the plane of the porphyrin ring. In the high-spin state (five d electrons unpaired), the iron has a single axial ligand and is out of the plane of the porphyrin ring. Both high- and low-spin forms of cytochrome P-450 are found in control microsomes. The high-spin signal is intensified in microsomes from animals treated with 3MC, BP, TCDD, and other agents known to induce cytochrome P_1-450. High-spin measurements are therefore used to evaluate the induction of cytochrome P_1-450 [199,200]. As will be discussed later (Sec. II.A.3.a), this increase in the high-spin state of microsomes induced by 3MC does not necessarily mean that cytochrome P_1-450 is predominantly a high-spin hemoprotein.

The addition of certain substrates to microsomes shifts the spin equilibrium of cytochrome P-450 toward the high-spin state. This is reflected in a blue shift of the optical spectrum (type I spectrum). Other compounds cause a shift to the low-spin state and produce a red shift in the optical spectrum (type II spectrum). Both the nature of the compound and the kind of cytochrome P-450 with which it reacts determine whether one or the other spectrum will be produced. The binding spectrum observed with any given microsomal preparation is therefore the sum of the binding spectra produced with each of the species of cytochrome P-450 present in the microsomes. Grasdalen and associates [201] used the type I compound SKF-525A and the type II compound metyrapone to reveal the multiplicity of cytochrome P-450 hemoproteins. They concluded from kinetic studies that SKF-525A and metyrapone react selectively with different kinds of microsomal cytochrome P-450; the enzyme induced by PB reacted with metyrapone, but not with SKF-525A. Ullrich and associates [125,202] used 7-ethoxycoumarin to demonstrate differences in the populations of cytochrome P-450s in microsomes from different sources. 7-Ethoxycoumarin gave no binding spectrum with control microsomes, elicited a typical type I spectrum with 3MC microsomes, and produced an unusual type I-like spectrum with PB microsomes. The magnitude of the binding spectra reflected the monooxygenase activities of these microsomes.

k. Multiplicity revealed by the isolation and reconstitution of the components of monooxygenase systems: The opportunity for direct verification of multiple molecular species of cytochrome P-450 was delayed because the usual methods which had been used to solubilize membrane-bound enzymes in their native states proved unsuitable for the isolation of cytochrome P-450. Soon after Ichikawa and Yamano [39] discovered the stabilizing effect of glycerol and other glycols on solubilized cytochrome P-450, Lu and Coon [58] reconstituted the first solubilized cytochrome P-450-linked hepatic monooxygenase system. They used column chromatography to resolve detergent-solubilized microsomes into three components, which in combination, catalyzed the (ω-1)-hydroxylation of laurate. The three components were identified as cytochrome P-450, NADPH-cytochrome c reductase, and a lipid fraction which was later shown to be replaceable by phosphatidylcholine [203,204]. There has been a great deal of interest in reconstituted systems since this work was published over a decade ago (see Refs. 59 and 60 for reviews). Lu and West [60] list 39 drugs, steroids and bile acids, carcinogens, insecticides, anaesthetics, fatty acids, alkanes, and miscellaneous compounds which have been metabolized by reconstituted systems. In many of these studies the cytochrome P-450 was resolved into two or more components which exhibited different catalytic activities and physical characteristics. It was established early that when substrate selectivities of reconstituted systems differed, they did so because their cytochrome P-450 components differed, not because of differences in the reductase or lipid components [205].

Comai and Gaylor [41] were the first to physically separate different forms of cytochrome P-450 from a single source of microsomes. Column chromatography of detergent-solubilized microsomes yielded three cytochrome P-450s with different cyanide binding affinities. Each could be induced selectively by PB, 3MC, or ethanol. Gel electrophoresis of column-fractionated microsomal preparations has been used to great advantage in the isolation and characterization of a variety of different forms of cytochrome P-450 obtained from the livers of several species of untreated and chemically induced animals. Isolated cytochromes have been characterized by their electrophoretic migration patterns, visible absorption spectra, substrate selectivities, and immunological reactivities.

Because of the abundance of indirect evidence that inducing agents cause the synthesis of new forms of cytochrome P-450 or a disproportionate increased synthesis of existing forms, there has been much interest in the isolation of cytochrome P-450 from animals treated with PB, 3MC, and some other inducing agents. Fujita and associates [206] demonstrated qualitative differences in partially purified P-450 cytochromes from MC- and PB-treated rats. Ryan and associates [207] showed that purified cytochrome P-450 from rat 3MC microsomes exhibited different substrate selectivities than that from rat PB microsomes. Moreover, the substrate selectivities of the purified cytochromes were very similar to those of the microsomes from which they were derived. The cytochrome P-450 hemoproteins from 3MC and PB microsomes elicited different redcued CO spectra (λ_{max} 448 nm and λ_{max} 450 nm, respectively), reduced ethyl isocyanide spectra and molecular weights (53,000 and 48,000, respectively). Antibodies produced against the purified cytochromes reacted well with their homologous antigens, but cross-reacted poorly with their heterologous antigens [47]. More recent immunological studies indicate that the purified cytochrome P-450 preparation from PB microsomes contains at least four distinct cytochrome P-450s, and that from 3MC microsomes at least two forms. Welton and Aust [43] showed that cytochrome P-450s with molecular weights of 44,000, 53,000, and 50,000 predominated in PB, 3MC, and control microsomes from rats, respectively. Somewhat similar results were obtained by Alvares and Siekevitz [208] with microsomes from control-, PB-, 3MC-, and polychlorinated biphenyl-induced rats. Bell and Hodgson [209] identified three kinds of cytochrome P-450 in control, PB, and 3MC microsomes; two were selectively induced by PB, one by 3MC.

Coon and associates [50,57,210-212] isolated several species of cytochrome P-450 from rabbits treated with PB or βNF. Two of these, designated cytochromes P-450LM$_2$ and P-450LM$_4$, have been purified to apparent homogeneity. Cytochrome P-450LM$_2$ has a reduced CO spectrum with a λ_{max} at 450 nm, an oxidized spectrum characteristic of a low-spin cytochrome P-450 (λ_{max}: 418 nm), a molecular weight of 48,700, and it hydroxylates benzphetamine, ethylmorphine, and para-nitroanisole preferentially. Cytochrome P-450LM$_4$ has a reduced CO spectrum with a λ_{max} at 448 nm, an oxidized spectrum characteristic of a high-spin cytochrome P-450 (λ_{max}: 394 nm), a molecular weight of 53,300, a high substrate selectivity for BP, but a low substrate selectivity for the substrates hydroxylated preferentially by cytochrome P-450LM$_2$. Cytochrome P-450LM$_1$ and P-450LM$_7$, which are not induced by either PB or β-naphthoflavone (βNF), have molecular weights of 47,000 and 60,000, respectively. Biphenyl was hydroxylated in positions 2 and 4 by all four of these enzymes, but position 4 was preferentially hydroxylated by cytochrome P-450LM$_2$. Testosterone was hydroxylated primarily in position 16α by cytochrome P-450LM$_2$, but in position 6β by a mixture of cytochrome P-450LM$_1$ and P-450LM$_7$. Gustafsson and Ingelman-Sundberg [213] have also concluded from reconstitution studies of fractionated control microsomes from male and female rats that mulple cytochrome P-450s are involved in the hydroxylation of steroids. One form catalyzes the hydroxylation of 5α-androsterone-3α,17β-diol in the 2β and 18 positions, another species the 12β-, 15α-, and 16α-hydroxylations of the same steroid, and a third cytochrome P-450, the 15β-hydroxylation of 5α-androstane-3α,17β-diol 3,17-disulfate.

Haugen and colleagues [48] obtained four major electrophoretic bands of cytochrome P-450 from genetically responsive and nonresponsive control- and PB-, βNF-, PCN-, or TCDD-treated mice. Increased intensities of certain bands were correlated with the induction state of the microsomes as determined by enzymatic and spectral methods. The intensity of band 4 (55,000 daltons; λ_{max} of reduced CO spectrum: 448 nm) was increased by TCDD in both responsive and nonresponsive strains of mice, but βNF induced this cytochrome P-450 only in responsive mice. The other three bands, all of which had a λ_{max} of 450 nm, were not affected by these two inducing agents. Band 4 was associated with the induction of 10 different microsomal monooxygenase activities. Administration of PCN caused an increase in band 3 (54,000); PB increased band 3 (51,000 daltons) primarily, but it also caused smaller increases in band 1 (49,000 daltons) and band 4.

Johnson and Müller-Eberhard [51,214,215] isolated two forms of cytochrome P-450 from hepatic microsomes of rabbits treated with TCDD. Antibody against the major form (54,000 daltons) inhibited microsomal acetanilide hydroxylation, but did not affect BP or coumarin hydroxylation or the dealkylation of aminopyrine or 7-ethoxycoumarin.

Ryan and associates [216] purified a form of cytochrome P-450 from Arochlor 1254-treated rats to apparent homogeneity. It could not be distinguished from a mixture of cytochrome P-450s from PB and 3MC microsomes by its electrophoretic mobility or by its spectral and catalytic properties. However, the effects of antibody to cytochrome P-450 on the metablism of 7-ethoxycoumarin and BP suggested that the species induced by Arochlor 1254 may differ from the mixture of the cytochrome P-450s obtained from PB and 3MC microsomes.

Huang and colleagues [49] obtained four purified cytochrome P-450s (A_1, A_2, C_1, and C_2) from PB microsomes from hybrid mice. They differed in their molecular weights, reduced CO difference spectra, and catalytic properties. Benzphetamine was metabolized preferentially by C_1, BP by A_1 and A_2, and 7-ethoxycoumarin and coumarin by A_1. Testosterone was hydroxylated preferentially in the 6β position by C_1 and C_2, in the 7α position by A_2, and in the 16α position by C_1.

Cytochrome P-450s induced by PB usually give a reduced spectrum with a λ_{max} at about 450 nm, whereas cytochrome P-450s induced by 3MC are associated with a λ_{max} of about 448 nm; their respective molecular weights are about 53,000 and 48,000 to 50,000. However, Philpot and Arinc [46] have obtained two purified cytochrome P-450s from rabbit PB microsomes, one of which had a λ_{max} at 448 nm and the other at 450 nm, yet both appeared to have the same molecular weight (51,500).

Guengerich [217] identified six cytochrome P-450s in control, 3MC, and PB microsomes from the rat and an equal number in control, 3MC, and PB microsomes from the rabbit. The cytochrome P-450s were distinguished by their behaviors in the fractionation systems, their spectral properties, their molecular weights, and the profiles of their substrate selectivities when incorporated into reconstituted systems involving 12 substrates.

Most partially purified preparations of cytochrome P-450 represent only 15% or less of the cytochrome P-450 contained in the microsomes from which they were isolated, although Imai [218] reported a recovery of 50%. Warner and coworkers [219] have recently reported recovery of 70-80% of the cytochrome P-450 from rat microsomes that had been solubilized with a mixture of Emulgen 911, cholate, glycerol, and ethylenediaminetetraacetic acid (EDTA) and resolved into four fractions by anion-exchange chromatography. The four fractions were further resolved by electrofocusing in polyacrylamide into more than eight bands which stained for heme and retained the spectral characteristics of cytochrome P-450 after extraction from the gel.

The separation of multiple forms of cytochrome P-450 and their reconstitution into monooxygenase systems has led to a reassessment of some earlier appraisals of cytochrome P-450 systems. Lu and West [60] summarized some of the current views that take these reassessments into account: (1) The catalytic activity of a particular species of cytochrome P-450 cannot be predicted solely from the λ_{max} of its reduced CO spectrum. As an example of this generalization they point out that rat cytochrome P-448 is 20 times more active than rabbit cytochrome P-448 in supporting BP metabolism. (2) Species of cytochrome P-450 cannot be classified according to the types of reactions they catalyze. Two or more different reactions may be catalyzed by a single species, or a substrate may be hydroxylated at several positions by one or several species of cytochrome P-450. (3) The substrate selectivities of various species of cytochrome P-450 appear to be broad and overlapping.

1. Summary comments: The conclusion that species-, sex-, and age-dependent differences in patterns of drug metabolism reflect the heterogeneity of cytochrome P-450 is based on the principle that when a single enzyme reacts with more than one substrate, substrate selectivities will remain proportionate regardless of the amount or the source of the enzyme; when disproportion occurs, more than one enzyme is involved in the reactions. This principle may not always apply to membrane-bound enzyme systems. In microsomes, the catalytic properties of cytochrome P-450 systems are determined in part by the membrane. The composition of the membrane is certain to differ among mammalian species and with the age, sex, and environment of the same species; the substrate selectivity of a given species of cytochrome P-450 may be altered accordingly. Chemically

induced changes in the membrane might modify specific oxygenase systems in a similar manner. Another possibility to be considered is that a given species of cytochrome P-450 may be located in more than one environment of the membrane and that the degree of reactivity with one substrate or another will depend upon the peculiarities of each environment. Differences or changes in the distribution of a species of cytochrome P-450 among different membrane environments could then account for differences or changes in the proportionality of specific activities. This is not a remote possibility in view of the evidence that microsomal cytochrome P-450 is not uniformly distributed throughout the microsomal membrane [220-223].

The possibility exists that certain of the apparent species differences in substrate selectivity may be due to the lipid peroxidation that occurs when microsomes are incubated with NADPH. Lipid peroxidase activities vary greatly among microsomes from different species; e.g., activities are higher in rat than in rabbit microsomes [170,224]. Lipid peroxidation can alter monooxygenase activity in several ways: (1) The environment of the monooxygenase system can be altered because membrane phospholipids are the substrates for lipid peroxidase. (2) Cytochrome P-450 is denatured by the hydroperoxides formed by lipid peroxidation [169,171,173,224-229]; certain species of membrane-bound cytochrome P-450 are more resistant to lipid peroxidation than others [172]. (3) The lipid peroxidation and cytochrome P-450 systems compete for NADPH-cytochrome P-450 reductase. Discrepancies due to lipid peroxidation can be avoided if EDTA or desferrioxamine is included in the incubation medium to chelate the iron that is required for the reaction [229].

Much of the data that has been used to implicate the multiplicity of cytochrome P-450 systems has depended on evaluations of substrate selectivities. Because of the great complexity of the kinetics of hepatic monooxygenase reactions [230] these data must be interpreted with caution.

Ullrich and Kremers [116] have suggested an evolutionary role of multiple cytochrome P-450 systems. A single-enzyme system with a broad substrate selectivity would necessarily exhibit low substrate affinity and would therefore be of limited value in the detoxification of the many potent toxins in the environment which reach only very low concentrations in the tissues. A limited number of more selective enzymes with relatively high substrate affinities would remove low concentrations of environmental toxins from the tissues more effectively than a single, relatively nonselective enzyme. The economy of the detoxification process is greatly improved when the toxic agent induces an enzyme which is more or less specific for its own metabolism, as is the case when polycyclic aromatic hydrocarbons induce the synthesis of cytochrome P_1-450.

During the last decade great progress has been made in the solubilization, purification, and reconstitution of hepatic cytochrome P-450-linked monooxygenase systems. It can be predicted that when a sufficient number of individual species of purified cytochrome P-450 have been fully characterized, many will be identified with species-, sex-, age-, and environment-related differences that have been associated with membrane-bound monooxygenase systems. However, it may not be possible in all cases to devise reconstituted systems which faithfully duplicate physical and catalytic properties of membrane-bound systems. Thus some of the reasons for observed differences in the behavior of microsomal systems may remain undetermined long after amino acid sequences of every molecular species of cytochrome P-450 have been determined.

The number of species of isolated hepatic cytochrome P-450 hemoproteins appears to be directly proportional to the degree of sophistication of the isolation procedure used. It remains to be seen how many of these newly isolated cytochromes are subunits of their native counterparts and how many are artifacts produced by the solubilization and fractionation procedures.

2. Chemical Composition

Imai and Sato [56] and van der Hoeven et al. [57] were the first to purify cytochrome P-450 to electrophoretic homogeneity. The specific content of their cytochromes, obtained from livers of PB-treated rabbits, was about 17 nmol/mg of protein. "Homogeneous" cytochrome P-450s have since been isolated from PB-treated rats [47,205,232], mice [49], and rabbits [50,56,57], 3MC-treated rats [47,205,232] and rabbits [233,234], Arochlor 1254-treated rats [216], βNF-treated rabbits [50], and TCDD-treated rabbits [215].

Immunological evidence suggests that highly purified preparations of cytochrome P-450 are not always homogeneous, but may consist of two or more closely related species. Highly purified cytochromes P-450 from PB-treated rats and P-448 from 3MC-treated rats contained four and two immunologically distinct forms of cytochrome P-450 hemoprotein, respectively [47,52]. On the other hand, immunological studies did not reveal multiple species of cytochrome P-450 in the most highly purified preparations of cytochrome P-450LM_2 or P-450LM_4 isolated in Coon's laboratory [52,212]. It is to be noted, however, that multiple amino-terminal residues were detected for cytochrome P-450LM_4, which suggests the presence of other proteins, the presence of several highly similar forms of cytochrome P-450, or that the cytochrome had undergone partial proteolysis in vivo or during isolation [235]. In view of the electrophoretic and immunological evidence for homogeneity, the finding of a single carboxyl terminal residue (lysine) [50,52], and other considerations involving the amino-terminal residues, the authors concluded that the cytochrome P-450LM_4 preparation was a mixture of cytochromes which differed only in the degree to which a hydrophobic amino-terminal segment had been degraded by proteolysis. Guengerich [232] has expressed the opinion that "the only enzyme preparation for which rigorous evidence for homogeneity has been presented is the major PB-inducible cytochrome P-450 of rabbit liver microsomes, P-450LM_2."

Each molecule of the purest cytochrome P-450LM_2 and P-450LM_4 isolated in Coon's laboratory contained one molecule of heme and three carbohydrate residues (glucosamine: 0.7 and 0.8; mannose: 1.7 and 2.0; and glucose: 0.2 and 0.9 nmol/nmol of protein for P-450LM_2 and P-450LM_4, respectively). The phospholipid content was only about 0.4 molecule/molecule of protein, which is near the limit of detection [211].

a. Molecular weights: The molecular weights of electrophoretically homogeneous hemoproteins obtained from livers of untreated and induced rabbits, rats, and mice are given in Table 2. Species of cytochrome P-450 are seen to fall roughly into two groups—those with molecular weights approximating 48,000 and those approximating 54,000. The higher-molecular-weight cytochrome P-450s are usually obtained from animals which have received agents that induce cytochrome P_1-450 (3MC, TCDD, βNF), whereas the lower-molecular-weight hemoproteins are obtained from untreated or PB-treated animals. However, there are exceptions to this generalization; e.g., cytochrome P-450LM_4, which has a molecular weight of about 54,000, was isolated from both PB- and βNF-treated rabbits, and cytochromes P-450B and P-450D, which have molecular weights of 53,000 and 54,000, respectively, were isolated from PB-treated rats.

The molecular weight of purified cytochrome P-450LM_2 in the absence of detergents was determined by gel-exclusion chromatography and sucrose-density gradient centrifugation to be about 280,000 daltons [237]. It is assumed that this aggregation of subunits is due to the location of hydrophobic residues in certain parts of the molecule and that the molecular size of the aggregate will vary with conditions. The aggregation of purified membrane proteins is a well-known phenomenon; e.g., it occurs with the microsomal enzymes, NADH-cytochrome c reductase [238], and cytochrome b_5 [239], and with adrenal mitochondrial cytochrome P-450 [240,241].

b. Amino acid composition: The amino acid compositions of seven cytochrome P-450s from the rabbit, rat, and bacteria listed in Table 3 are quite similar. All contain six or seven half-cystine residues except the cytochrome P-450 from R. japonicum, which contains two. Cytochromes P-450LM_2 and PB-450D and both bacterial cytochrome P-450s contain one tryptophan residue, but cytochromes P-450LM_4, PB-450B, and MC-450B contain seven, two, and six tryptophan residues, respectively. The leucine and phenylalanine contents of the cytochromes are relatively high. About 55% of the amino acid residues of the rabbit cytochrome P-450s are nonpolar [178]. This would account for their strong binding to the endoplasmic reticulum and their tendency to aggregate in detergent-free aqueous media. It is of interest that both the membrane-bound mammalian cytochromes and the soluble bacterial cytochromes contain high percentages of nonpolar amino acids.

The amino acids attached to the heme are of particular interest because of concepts that have developed regarding the liganding of the heme iron.

TABLE 2

Specific Content, Molecular Weight, and λ_{max} (Soret Region) of Cytochrome P-450 from the Rabbit, Rat, and Mouse Purified to Apparent Electrophoretic Homogeneity

Designation	Animal source	Inducing agent	Specific content[a]	Mol wt[b] (in thousands)	λ_{max} Fe^{3+}	λ_{max} Fe^{2+}	λ_{max} Fe^{2+} + CO	Reference
P-450LM_2	Rabbit	PB	(20)	47.8 (47.6)	418	413	451	50
P-450LM_4	Rabbit	PB, βNF	(17)	53.0 (54.2)	394	411	448	50
P-450	Rabbit	PB	17	45.0	418	414	450	56
P-450	Rabbit	3MC	17.7	54.0	393	411	448	234
P-450	Rabbit	3MC	(24) 17.2	51.0	416	410	447	233 234
P-450c	Rabbit	TCDD	17.8	54.5	393	412	447	215
P-450	Rat	PB	17	48.0	418	414	450	205
P-450	Rat	PB	16.4	48.5	—	—	—	231
P-450B	Rat	PB	18	53.1	—	—	—	232
P-450D	Rat	PB	14.1	54.25	—	—	—	232
P-450B	Rat	3MC	17.1	55.85	—	—	—	232
P-448	Rat	3MC	17	53.0	417	411	448	205
P-450A2	Mouse	PB	(16.5) 11.7	50.0	417	415	451	49
P-450C2	Mouse	PB	(17.5) 14.7	56.0	417	419	450	49

[a] nmol P-450/mg of protein; values in parentheses were obtained by amino acid rather than by protein analysis.
[b] Values were obtained electrophoretically by the standard Laemmli system [236] except for those in parentheses, which were calculated from amino acid analyses; values may be as much as 15% lower when certain other electrophoretic systems are used [232].

TABLE 3
Amino Acid Composition of Cytochrome P-450 from the Rabbit, Rat, and Bacteria

Amino acid	Rabbit [50,242,243]		Rat [232]			*P. putida* [242,243]	*R. japonicum* [244]
	P-450LM$_2$	P-450LM$_4$	PB-450B	PB-450D	3MC-450B	P-450$_{cam}$	
HaH cystine	6	7	7	7	6	6	2
Asx	36	38	42	41	43	36	33
Met	7	10	11	15	10	9	8
Thr	23	24	29	25	29	19	14
Ser	30	31	30	34	38	21	20
Glx	42	46	52	52	43	55	54
Pro	24	28	27	30	37	27	25
Gly	32	38	33	54	32	26	33
Ala	23	29	29	17	26	34	54
Val	26	32	27	20	28	24	25
Ile	19	22	27	25	24	24	14
Leu	54	58	59	40	54	40	46
Tyr	9	11	14	14	14	9	6
Phe	31	28	32	27	28	17	17
His	11	11	13	10	13	12	12
Lys	19	26	27	38	31	13	14
Trp	1	7	2	1	6	1	1
Arg	29	30	25	22	25	24	29
Totals:	424	482	486	483	487	397	407
NH_2-terminal	Met [235]	Multiple [235]	Asx-Glx-Asx [232]	His [232]	His-Ala-Asx-Tyr [232]	Thr [245]	
COOH-terminal	Arg [50]	Lys [50]	Gly-Ala [232]	—	Val [232]	Val [244,246]	

[a] Numbers in brackets are reference numbers.

Partial degradation of cytochromes $P\text{-}450_{cam}$, $P\text{-}450LM_2$, and $P\text{-}450LM_4$ by BrCN yielded hemopeptides that could be purified without loss of heme [242,243]. The smallest peptides were generally quite similar and each contained single residues of histidine and cysteine. Histidine and a thiolate anion have been implicated as ligands for the iron of cytochrome P-450 (Sec. II.A.2.e).

c. Heme: The alkaline pyridine-hemochromogen spectrum shows that protoheme is the only heme present in hepatic microsomes [15,247]. It has therefore generally been accepted that the heme of hepatic cytochrome P-450 is ferriprotoporphyrin IX. Any doubt that this is the case was removed by Maines and Anders [248], who used a combination of gas chromatography and mass spectroscopy to show that the reductive degradation products of heme derived from microsomal cytochrome P-450 were identical to those obtained from hemoglobin ferriprotoporphyrin IX.

d. Oxidation-reduction potentials: Waterman and Mason [249] examined the redox potential of cytochrome P-450 in hepatic microsomes from PB-treated rabbits under anaerobic conditions, using redox indicator dyes and ESR spectroscopy. The titration curve had an anomalous shape with an apparent midpoint potential of about -410 mV. About 40% of the cytochrome P-450 remained oxidized at about -440 mV at pH 7.0, whereas complete reduction was observed in the presence of CO at more positive potentials. It was concluded that more than one cytochrome P-450 redox couple exists in hepatic microsomes and that about 60% of the dye reducible cytochrome P-450 represents a species with a midpoint potential of -340 mV. This interpretation of the anomalous curve should be evaluated with the usual reservations taken when potentiometric measurements of impure preparations are made and with the understanding that it is not possible to remove all of the oxygen from microsomes by ordinary procedures [250].

The redox potential of pure cytochrome $P\text{-}450LM_2$ was determined by Guengerich and associates [251] to be about -333 mV at pH 7.0. Addition of substrate (benzphetamine), phospholipid, or both substrate and phospholipid did not alter the potential. This was somewhat unexpected in view of the elevation of the potential from -270 to -170 mV that occurs when substrate (camphor) is added to cytochrome $P\text{-}450_{cam}$ [252]. The addition of CO to cytochrome $P\text{-}450LM_2$ raised the potential to -150 mV.

The redox potential of hepatic cytochrome P-450 is the lowest reported for any cytochrome in its native environment [178].

e. Ligands: The spectral, magnetic, chemical, and functional characteristics of individual protoporphyrin hemoproteins result from the specific protein-imposed liganding of the heme iron. The unusual physical and functional properties of cytochrome P-450 which led to its discovery also suggested that the liganding of its iron might be quite different from that of other cytochromes. The ligand field of a hemoprotein that can function both as an electron transferase and as an oxidase would be expected to undergo a series of changes during the sequence of stepwise events that constitute the overall monooxygenase reaction. An understanding of these changes is central to the elucidation of the mechanism of cytochrome P-450-linked monooxygenase reactions.

Four of the six ligands of the iron of cytochrome P-450 are coordinated with pyrrole nitrogens. On the basis of the observation that mercurial sulfhydryl reagents convert cytochrome P-450 to cytochrome P-420, Mason and associates [253, 254] proposed as early as 1965 that a thiolate anion was involved as one of the remaining two ligands. Waterman and Mason [249] also suggested that the low redox potential of cytochrome P-450 is indicative of the presence of a thiolate ligand. The unique optical and ESR spectra of cytochrome P-450 have been largely attributed to the presence of this mercaptide ligand [255-259]. Analytical results showing the presence of cysteine close to the heme of pure cytochrome P-450_{cam} and P-450LM_2 [243, 244] and evaluation of optical and ESR parameters of chemical models [259-268] have provided convincing evidence of the reality of the sulfur ligand (fifth ligand).

The exact nature of the sixth ligand has not been determined. In the absence of its substrate, camphor, ferricytochrome P-450_{cam} exists almost entirely in the low-spin state. The addition of camphor converts it almost completely to the high-spin form [269]. The high-spin cytochrome P-450_{cam} reverts to the low-spin form when the inhibitor, phenylimidazole, is added, putatively because it becomes the sixth ligand. This observation and certain analogies with other known oxygen carriers led Dus and associates [246, 270] to suggest that histidyl imidazole is the sixth ligand. The similarity of IR spectra of the CO adducts of cytochrome P-450_{cam}, hemoglobin, and myoglobin was considered by Dus and Albin [271] to be supportive of the view that the ligand could be a nitrogen histidyl imidazole group. In this context, it is of interest that the smallest heme peptides obtained from degraded cytochromes P-450_{cam} and P-450LM_2 contain one residue each of histidine, cysteine, and heme [242, 243]. However, Gunsalus and colleagues [272] used results from Mössbauer emission spectroscopic studies of model heme complexes to argue against a histidyl ligand.

The water molecule or a hydroxyl group associated with the histidyl imidazole has also been proposed as the sixth ligand [268, 273-276]. Peterson and Griffin [273] concluded from proton-relaxation data for camphor-free cytochrome P-450_{cam} that a molecule of water is present in the first coordination sphere of the ferric ion. Since the low-spin metyrapone and phenylimidazole complexes of ferricytochrome P-450_{cam} do not have exchangeable protons in this coordination sphere, they concluded that the sixth ligand is probably not the imidazole group of a histidine residue. However, Dus [270] points out that the absorbance of cytochrome P-450_{cam} does not change with the pH, as would be expected if water was the ligand, and that the N-3 position of imidazole can change protons quickly with water. Another seeming contradiction that must be addressed when water is proposed as the candidate sixth ligand is that water is a high-spin ligand [277] and would therefore not be expected to form the predominantly low-spin state of the heme complex of cytochrome P-450 that exists in the absence of substrate. Rein and Ristau [278] have suggested a mechanism that would seem to resolve these inconsistencies. If a water molecule and a histidine residue are bridged by a hydrogen bond, water could exist as a weak low-spin ligand. Different protein conformations would produce different states of polarized water. This would account for the differences in spin equilibrium exhibited by individual species of cytochrome P-450.

Cytochrome P-450 exists in temperature-dependent equilibrated high- and low-spin forms both in the presence and absence of substrate [269,279-281]. At any given instant, the iron of a single molecule of cytochrome P-450 is either entirely in the low-spin state ($S = 1/2$) or entirely in the high-spin state ($S = 5/2$). The time spent in each state determines the equilibrium and this is established by the conformation of the protein associated with the heme. Perturbations of the protein may alter the spin state equilibrium. Type I substrates perturb the protein by combining with a substrate binding site located on a hydrophobic region of the protein near the iron; this causes a shift of the equilibrium toward the high-spin state. Type II compounds combine with the iron and cause a shift in the equilibrium toward the low-spin state. The degree of perturbation caused by a type I substrate and the resulting shift in the spin equilibrium depend on both the nature of the substrate and its concentration.

Sligar [269] used optical spectroscopic data at different temperatures to calculate equilibrium constants and thermodynamic parameters of the spin states of cytochrome $P\text{-}450_{cam}$. In the absence of substrate, 92% of the hemoprotein was calculated to be in the low-spin state at room temperature; when complexed with camphor, 94% of the cytochrome was shown to be in the high-spin form.

The substrate binding site of cytochrome P-450 is located on a hydrophobic portion of the protein near the sixth ligand. When the substrate combines with its binding site, the weak sixth ligand of ferricytochrome P-450 is displaced and the 6-coordinated iron (low-spin, 418 nm Soret maximum) shifts to the 5-coordinated iron (high-spin, 393 nm Soret maximum). These substrates are referred to as type I substrates. Other compounds combine with the iron and form a strong ligand that maintains the iron in the low-spin, 6-coordinated state (type II substrates). Still other compounds combine with both the substrate binding site and the iron. The changes in the optical spectra that occur when these compounds are combined with ferricytochrome P-450 will be discussed in the next section.

The generally accepted view that the equilibrium between high- and low-spin states is represented by an equilibrium between 5 and 6-coordinated iron is not uncontested. Rein and Ristau [278] use thermodynamic considerations to argue that the axial low-spin ligand of the heme iron is not split off during transition from the low- to the high-spin state, but rather that the

6-coordinated heme complex is maintained and the spin shift is caused by cooperative breaking of van der Waals contacts between the porphyrin and the protein. They support this concept by citing the results of Iizuka and colleagues [282] and Yonetani and colleagues [283] which show that the spin equilibria of hemoproteins are determined more by specific protein-heme interactions than by the sixth axial ligand of the iron.

3. Optical Properties

The optical properties of hepatic cytochrome P-450 were established with reasonable accuracy long before the cytochromes were solubilized and purified. The molecular extinction coefficient of 91 cm^{-1} mM^{-1} determined in 1962 by Omura and Sato [15] for the reduced CO difference spectrum of cytochrome P-450 between 450 and 490 nm is still considered an accurate index of the cytochrome P-450 content of microsomes and other crude preparations. Absolute spectra of cytochrome P-450 derived by difference spectroscopy of microsomal particles from which cytochrome b_5 had been removed [284,285], or by "offset" difference spectroscopy [286], yielded absolute spectra which compare favorably with those obtained from highly purified preparations of the cytochrome. These early studies revealed several unusual optical properties of cytochrome P-450: (1) CO produces an atypical shift of the Soret peak of the reduced cytochrome to a higher wavelength with almost no change in the visible region. (2) Reduction elicits only a small spectral change. (3) Ethyl isocyanide causes an unusual splitting of the Soret peak into peaks at 430 nm and 455 nm. (4) Blue (type I) and red (type II) shifts of the Soret peak are produced by many substrates and some other compounds. Most of these "anomalous" optical properties can now be explained by recently developed concepts of the nature of the ligand field of the iron of cytochrome P-450 (see preceding section).

Optical properties of cytochrome P-450 are remarkably similar despite their widely different sources and substrate selectivities. Obviously, many major differences in the functions of different species of cytochrome P-450 are not revealed by their spectra.

a. Spectra of purified hepatic cytochrome P-450: The oxidized, reduced, and reduced CO absolute spectra of cytochrome P-450LM$_2$ and P-450LM$_4$ isolated by Haugen and coworkers [210] from rabbit liver are typical of those obtained from the livers of other species (Table 4). Spectra and molecular extinction coefficients of pertinent spectral maxima are given in Fig. 5 and Table 4. Oxidized cytochrome P-450LM$_2$ shows a ferric low-spin-type spectrum. The reduced form shows a ferrous high-spin-type spectrum like that of hemoglobin or peroxidases. Oxidized cytochrome P-450LM$_4$ is of particular interest because it has a typically high-spin spectrum (Soret maximum: 394 nm). Because certain substrates produce a high-spin (type I) spectrum when added to ferricytochrome P-450, the question is raised as to whether the high-spin character of cytochrome

TABLE 4
Absorption Maxima and Molar Extinction Coefficients of Purified Rabbit Liver Cytochrome P-450 (P-450LM$_2$), Membrane-Bound Rat Liver Cytochrome P-450 (Microsomal P-450), and Purified Bacterial Cytochrome P-450 (P-450$_{cam}$)

	P-450LM$_2$[a]		Microsomal P-450[b]		P-450$_{cam}$[c]	
	λ_{max} (nm)	ϵ (mM^{-1} cm^{-1})	λ_{max} (nm)	ϵ (mM^{-1} cm^{-1})	λ_{max} (nm)	ϵ (mM^{-1} cm^{-1})
Oxidized	418	110	417	92	417	115
	535	10.4	535	13	535	11.6
	568	11.2	570	11	569	11.9
Reduced	413	78	411	78	408	76.7
	544	15.1	550	18	540	15.1
Reduced + CO	451	110	449	122	447	121
	552	13.4	555	17	550	14.3

[a] P-450LM$_2$ from rabbit PB microsomes; values are from Ref. 50.
[b] Rat PB microsomes; the linoleic acid hydroperoxide deletion method (Sec. II.A.1.g) was used to derive calculated values [104].
[c] Values are from Ref. 317.

P-450LM$_4$ is due to inherent properties of the hemoprotein or whether it is due to a small molecule that can complex with a low-spin form of the hemoprotein and convert it to a high-spin form. The molecular weight of cytochrome P-450LM$_4$ is about 6000 daltons larger than that of cytochrome P-450LM$_2$ (Table 2); thus, cytochrome P-450LM$_4$ cannot be cytochrome P-450LM$_2$-complexed with a small organic molecule. However, the possibility might be considered that cytochrome P-450LM$_4$ may result from the combination of a lower-molecular-weight low-spin cytochrome P-450 with a hydrophobic peptide of about 6000 daltons which is capable of converting the hemoprotein to the high-spin form. Purified cytochrome P-450s with a Soret maximum at about 393 nm have been isolated from rabbit liver by Johnson and Müller-Eberhard [214] and by Hashimoto and Imai [234]. It is of interest in this context that the high-spin spectrum of purified cytochrome P-450LM$_4$ can be converted to the low-spin spectrum by adding back Renox 690, the detergent that had been used to solubilize the cytochrome. A similar effect of detergent was observed by Hashimoto and Imai. The spectrum reverts to the high-spin form when the detergent is removed [287]. This would suggest that some detergent-dissociable substance may be present in cytochrome P-450LM$_4$ which is capable of shifting the spin equilibrium to the high-spin state.

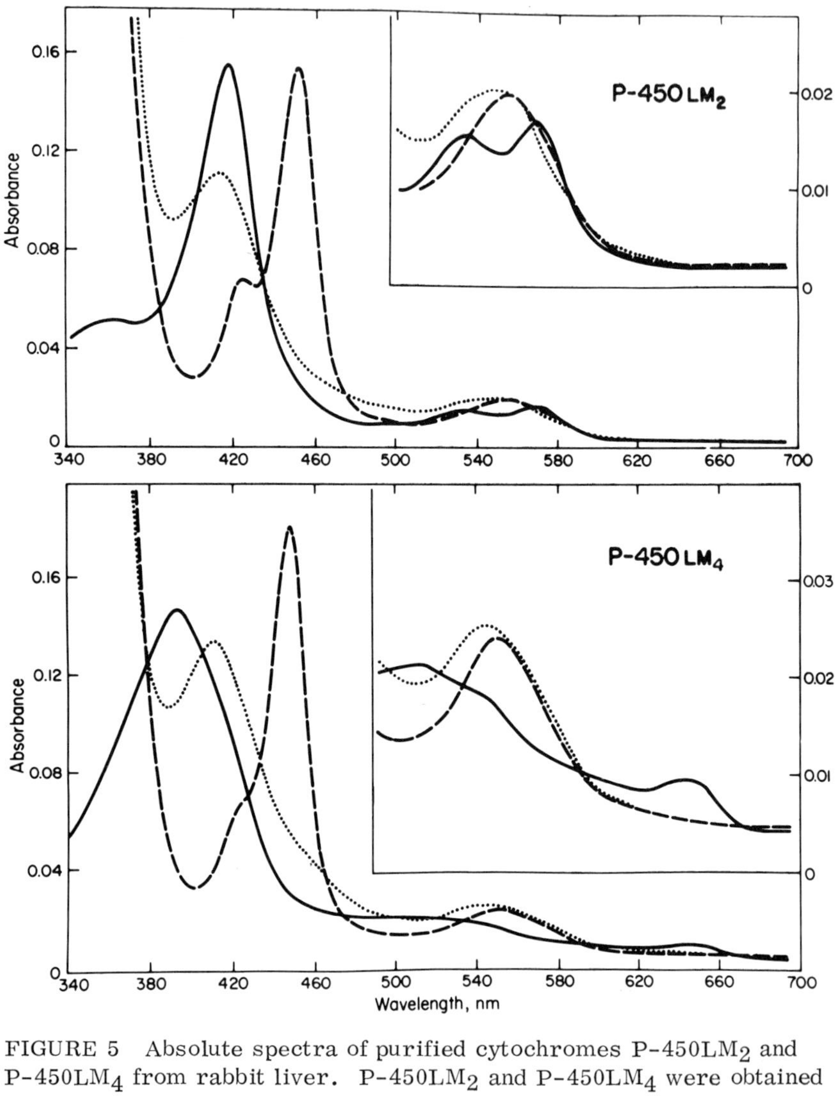

FIGURE 5 Absolute spectra of purified cytochromes P-450LM$_2$ and P-450LM$_4$ from rabbit liver. P-450LM$_2$ and P-450LM$_4$ were obtained from PB and βNF microsomes, respectively. The spectra of the oxidized forms, reduced forms, and reduced CO complexes are represented by the solid, dotted, and dashed curves, respectively. (From Ref. 50. Reproduced by kind permission of Dr. M. J. Coon and the American Society of Biological Chemists.)

Cytochrome P_1-450, the cytochrome or family of cytochromes induced by 3MC and certain other aromatic polycyclic hydrocarbons, was once believed to be a high-spin hemoprotein; the "other" microsomal cytochrome P-450 was thought to be low-spin hemoprotein. Some credence was also given to the possibility that cytochrome P_1-450 represented the high-spin form of a single cytochrome in equilibrium with its own low-spin form. The concept of two cytochrome P-450s, one predominantly high-spin and the other predominantly low-spin, led to several attempts to measure the quantities of each in microsomes by evaluation of electron paramagnetic resonance (EPR) signals or optical spectra [288-290]. These measurements led to the conclusion that cytochrome P_1-450 is a normal component of hepatic microsomes and that its presence in microsomes is increased not only by aromatic polycyclic hydrocarbons, but also by inducing agents such as PB. By this definition, cytochrome P-450LM_4 would seem to satisfy the requirements of cytochrome P_1-450; it is a predominantly high-spin hemoprotein and it has been isolated from the livers of both PB- and 3NF-treated rabbits [50]. However, there is reason to believe that cytochrome P_1-450 per se may not be a predominantly high-spin hemoprotein. It has already been pointed out that detergent converts the high-spin cytochrome P-450LM_4 to a low-spin form [50]. Moreover, a cytochrome P-448 with low-spin optical and ESR characteristics has been isolated from livers of 3MC-treated rats [47]. This highly purified low-spin cytochrome exhibited the substrate selectivity and the ethyl isocyanide spectral characteristics of cytochrome P_1-450. Hashimoto and Imai [234] isolated a high-spin cytochrome P-450 (393-nm Soret maximum absorption) from livers of 3MC-treated rats which they identified as a cytochrome P-450-3MC complex comprised of equal parts of 3MC (or a 3MC metabolite) and cytochrome P-450. These observations suggest the possibility that the increase in the high-spin signals observed in microsomes after the administration of 3MC may be due to the complexing of cytochrome P_1-450 with 3MC or a metabolite of it. Conceivably, cytochrome P_1-450 might have a greater ability to combine with 3MC than the cytochrome P-450s of control or PB microsomes. Preferential, strong binding of an inducing agent to the enzyme that metabolizes it is exactly what would be desired of a detoxifying enzyme, particularly one that must react with an agent that is normally found only in minute concentrations in the environment and the tissues. Another possibility to be considered is that part of the high-spin character of control microsomes is due to the complexing of the enzyme with unidentified endogenous substrates or membrane components and that cytochrome P_1-450 is better able to combine with these substances than are other kinds of cytochrome P-450.

b. Spectra of membrane-bound hepatic cytochrome P-450: A comparison of the spectral data obtained from soluble and membrane-bound cytochrome P-450 (Table 4) shows that the molecular extinction coefficients of the absolute reduced and reduced CO spectra of soluble and membrane-bound cytochrome P-450 are very similar, but that the extinction coefficient of the absolute oxidized spectrum of the microsomal enzyme is lower than that of the soluble one. The reduced and reduced CO spectra are in agreement because reduced cytochrome P-450 is entirely in the high-spin state and reduced CO-complexed cytochrome P-450 is entirely in the low-spin state in both soluble and membrane-bound preparations. However, whereas the oxidized soluble cytochrome P-450 is almost entirely in the low-spin state, an appreciable amount of the membrane-bound cytochrome P-450 exists in the high-spin state. Under aerobic conditions, microsomal cytochrome P-450s exist in both high- and low-spin states and the observed absolute oxidized spectrum reflects this mixture of the two. As has been discussed in the preceding section, high- and low-spin forms of the enzyme have Soret maxima at about 393 and 418 nm, respectively. The observed optical densities of the absolute oxidized spectrum at 393 and 418 nm vary with differences in the relative amounts of high- and low-spin cytochrome P-450 in microsomes. If the molecular extinction coefficients of the absolute oxidized high- and low-spin forms are known, the fraction of the cytochrome P-450 existing in the high-spin state can be calculated from the optical densities observed at 393 and 418 nm [269,291] (Sec. II.A.3.c). We have calculated from the absolute oxidized spectrum obtained by the LAHP deletion technique (Sec. II.A.3.c) that as much as 30% of the total cytochrome P-450 of some preparations of control microsomes was in the high-spin state [292] (Sec. II.A.3.c). Cinti and associates [293] have recently determined the temperature-dependent spin equilibria of microsomal and solubilized rat hepatic cytochrome P-450 from which they calculated that greater than 48% of the membrane-bound enzyme was in the high-spin state, whereas almost all of the soluble enzyme was in the low-spin state. The spin equilibrium of membrane-bound cytochrome P-450 would appear to be largely determined by its lipid environment, by unidentified endogenous substrates, or both.

c. Substrate binding spectra: In 1963, Narasimhulu and coworkers [294,295] observed a difference spectrum with a peak at 390 nm and a trough at 420 nm when 17-hydroxyprogesterone was added to adrenocortical microsomes. The spectrum disappeared when dithionite was added, but reappeared when the microsomes were aerated. NADPH caused a transient disappearance of the spectrum. The spectrum was assumed to be due to a reaction between the steroid and a component of the microsomal 21-hydroxylation system. Shortly after this seminal observation, Remmer and associates [296] and Imai and Sato [297] reported almost simultaneously that a difference spectrum similar to that observed by Narasimhulu and coworkers was obtained when certain substrates were added to hepatic microsomes. This spectrum was designated the type I spectrum. Other compounds produced a second spectrum, designated the type II spectrum, which was roughly the mirror image of the type I spectrum. Still another spectrum, designated the modified type II or reverse type I spectrum, was seen with other compounds.

As was discussed in the preceding section, the type I and II spectra can now be interpreted in light of the changes induced in the ligand field of the heme iron by type I and II compounds: The type I spectrum is associated with a shift of the spin equilibrium of the hemoprotein iron to the high-spin state and the type II spectrum with a shift to the low-spin state. The reverse type I spectrum was originally believed to be due to displacement of an endogenous type I substrate from its binding site. In accordance with this concept, when a reverse type I compound such as 1-butanol is added to the sample cuvette, an unidentified endogenous type I substrate is displaced and the type I binding spectrum produced by this endogenous substrate in the reference cuvette is revealed as the mirror image of a typical type I spectrum. Recent evidence favors the view that the reverse type I spectrum is due to a distinct type of spectrum produced when certain compounds occupy the sixth ligand. Ullrich and associates [176,202,268,298-301] used ESR and optical spectra to demonstrate that phosphines, thiols, thioethers, and nitrogen compounds (e.g., metyrapone) can undergo ligand exchange reactions with the heteroatom occupying the sixth ligand position of cytochrome P-450 and model mercaptide-hemin ligand complexes. Ligands and substrates compete for the active site and can displace each other. That certain compounds can elicit the reverse type I spectrum by forming a ligand does not exclude the possibility that other compounds may produce this spectrum by displacing an endogenous substrate.

Kumaki and Nebert [276] have classified type I, type II, and reverse type I compounds in accordance with their structures. Type I substrates (peak at about 385-390 nm, trough at about 420 nm; examples: cyclohexane, chloroform, n-hexane, carbon tetrachloride, carbon disulfide) are distinctly hydrophobic, which allows them to interact with a hydrophobic portion of the protein moiety of the hemoprotein. Type II compounds (peak at 425-430 nm, trough at 390-410 nm; examples: octylamine, pyridine) are amines which can form a nitrogen ligand with the heme iron. Reverse type I compounds (peak at 420 nm and trough at 385-390 nm; examples: ethanol, 1-butanol, acetone, N,N-dimethylformamide, cyclohexane oxide, dimethylsulfoxide, tetrahydrofuran) form an oxygen ligand with heme iron because they contain lone-pair electrons on sterically accessible oxygen atoms. Ethyl acetate, which is representative of a fourth group of compounds, does not elicit a definitive difference spectrum because it lacks sufficient hydrophobicity and its oxygen is sterically less accessible to the heme iron. A modification of a model by Kumaki and Nebert [276] showing the interaction of type I, type II, and reverse type I compounds with cytochrome P-450 is presented in Fig. 6.

Ullrich and associates [300] have recommended that since the molecular basis for binding spectra is now understood, the operational terms "type I binding" and "type II binding" should be replaced by "substrate binding" and "ligand binding," respectively.

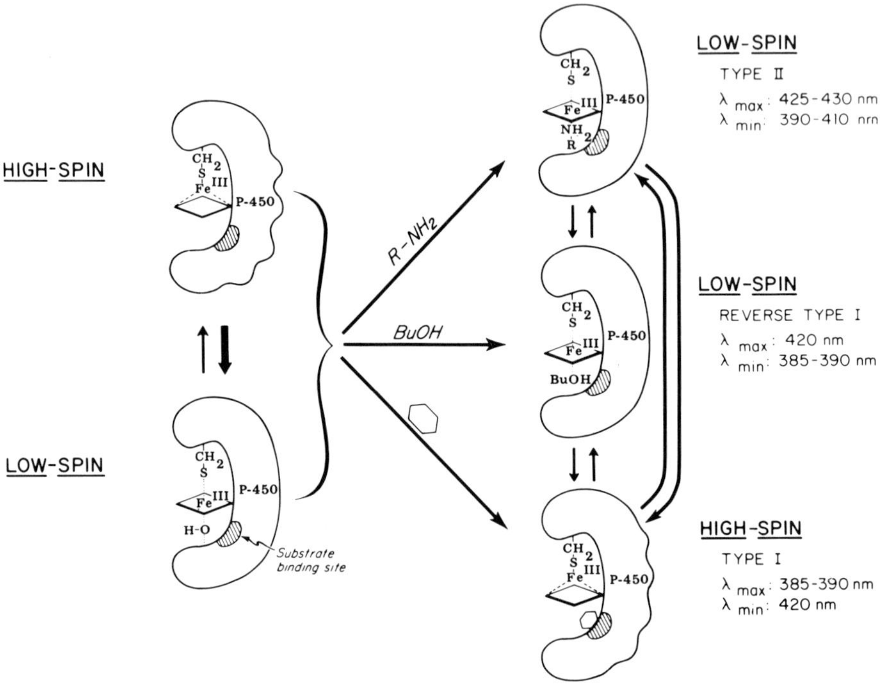

FIGURE 6 Interaction of type I, type II, and reverse type I compounds with cytochrome P-450. (Modification of a drawing published by Kumaki and Nebert [276].

Some compounds can bind both as substrates and as ligands and produce a spectrum that is a mixture of the type I and type II spectra. This was first demonstrated by Schenkman and coworkers [302], who showed that the asymmetrical type II difference spectrum elicited by aniline could be symmetrized by adding a type I substrate (hexobarbital) to the reference cuvette, thereby canceling the type I component of the aniline type II spectrum. The lipophilicity of a compound may determine whether it will bind as a ligand or as a substrate. Thus butylmethyl and pentamethylene sulfides produce the typical low-spin ligand binding spectrum whereas the more lipophilic dibutyl and phenylmethyl sulfides elicit the high-spin type I spectrum [176].

Complex molecules such as phenacetin, piperonyl butoxide, aminoglutethimide, PB, and metyrapone may bind their hydrophobic moieties to the substrate binding site and also form the sixth ligand with their lone-pair electron moieties [276]. Moreover, when more than one molecular species of cytochrome P-450 is present, as is the case in microsomes, these compounds may bind predominantly as a substrate with one species of the enzyme, but also as a ligand with another species. The binding spectra observed when complex drugs are added to microsomes therefore represent composites of type I, type II, and reverse type I spectra. This would explain many of the paradoxical spectra that reflect differences in species [303], strains [304], age [305], tissues [306-308], treatment of the animals with drugs [289,290,302], and techniques used in the preparation of the microsomes [50,309].

Estimates of the magnitude of the substrate-induced shift in the spin equilibrium from optical spectra have not always been consistent with those obtained from ESR measurements. Cyclohexane, a substrate that gives a very large type I spectrum, was estimated by Ullrich [196] to bind 12 and 32% of the cytochrome P-450 of control and PB microsomes, respectively. Using 68 mM^{-1} cm^{-1} as the extinction coefficient ($\Delta\epsilon_{420}$-$\Delta\epsilon_{490}$ mM^{-1} cm^{-1}) for the cytochrome P-450-cyclohexane complex [310], Watterman et al. [311] calculated that cyclohexane converted 27% of the cytochrome P-450 of PB microsomes to the high-spin state. ESR measurements showed that in the absence of substrate, 61% of the hemoprotein was in the low-spin state. The other 39% was presumed to be in the high-spin form due to complex formation with "endogenous substrate." According to ESR measurements, the cytochrome P-450-cyclohexane complex represented 28% of the total cytochrome P-450. This excellent agreement of optical measurements, obtained at room temperature, with ESR measurements obtained at liquid nitrogen temperature, led these investigators to conclude that the spin states of hepatic cytochrome P-450 are not temperature-dependent over this range. Stern and associates [312] calculated from ESR measurements that cytochrome P-450 in control, PCN, and 3MC microsomes from immature rats was 5.7, 2.4, and 13.1% in the high-spin state. Purified rat cytochrome P-450 was determined to be 1.9% and 5.7% in the high-spin state in the absence and presence of benzphetamine, respectively. Corresponding values of 6.3% and 11.4% were obtained with purified cytochrome P-448. Grasdalen and associates [201] used the extinction coefficient for the conversion of purified cytochrome P-450_{cam} ($\Delta\epsilon_{390}$-$\Delta\epsilon_{420}$ = 130 mM^{-1} cm^{-1}) to calculate the increase in the spin state of control and PB microsomes elicited by the type I compound SKF-525A. Of the total cytochrome P-450 of control and PB microsomes 20-25% and 5-15% was converted to the high-spin state by SKF-525A, respectively. Using ESR measurements, they observed that the addition of SKF-525A to control and PB microsomes increased the high-spin component from 11 to 30% and from 7 to 20%, respectively. Thus, while the results obtained by ESR were not completely consistent with those obtained by optical spectroscopy, both methods showed that the cytochrome P-450 induced by PB was less able to bind SKF-525A than that of control microsomes.

Kumaki et al. [313] used the ratio of the high-spin signal (g = 8) at 9.6 K to the low-spin signal (g = 2.24) at 77 K, to calculate the high-spin content of cytochrome P-450 in microsomes from several species of laboratory animals that were untreated or treated with inducing agents. In control microsomes, values ranged from as low as 10% high-spin for the rat to 40% for the rabbit. The effects of administered inducing agents also varied greatly among the different species; e.g., PB greatly decreased the high-spin fraction of guinea pig cytochrome P-450, but did not alter that of the rabbit. The addition of cyclohexane increased high-spin, but the extent depended upon the animal species and the inducing agents they received. Werringloer and associates [314] have recently used the "charge transfer" band at 645 nm, which is indicative of the high-spin state of hemin iron, to estimate the endogenous and substrate-induced spin state of microsomal cytochrome P-450 at room temperature. The endogenous level of high-spin cytochrome P-450 was calculated to be about 55, 40, and 65% in microsomes from untreated, PB-treated, and βNF-treated rats, respectively. Using a variety of substrates, up to 90% of the total cytochrome P-450 could be shifted to the high-spin form.

Rein and coworkers [315] observed that the spin equilibrium of soluble "cytochrome P-450LM" of unspecified purity showed only a small temperature dependency but that the substrate-induced spin state was highly temperature-dependent. Pierson and Cinti [316] also showed that substrate-induced type I and type II spectral changes were affected by temperature. Rein and associates calculated from temperature difference spectra that their cytochrome P-450 preparation was 8% high-spin without substrate and 16% in the presence of benzphetamine. Electrophoretically homogeneous cytochrome P-450LM_2 was calculated to be 7% in the high-spin state at room temperature; benzphetamine produced a shift to 28% [317]. Rein and Ristau [278] pointed out that two spin equilibria determine the spin state of the hemoprotein, namely, the equilibrium in the absence of substrate (K_1 = P-450_H/P-450_L) and the equilibrium in the presence of substrate (K_2 = P-450_H·S/P-450_L·S). They proposed the following reaction scheme:

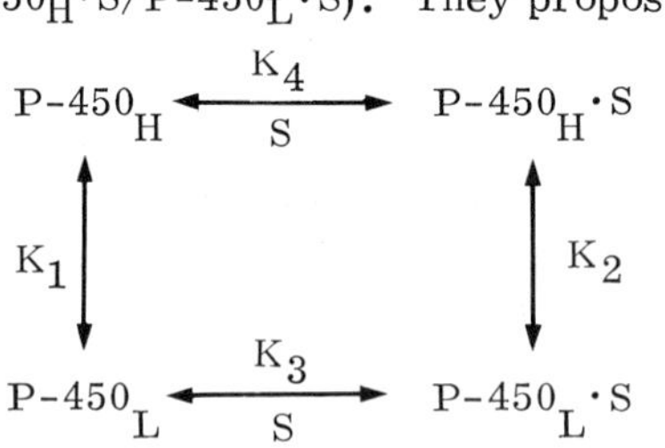

Pierson and Cinti [316] showed that a type I spectrum can be elicited by microsomes in the absence of substrate simply by recording a difference spectrum with the microsomes at different temperatures. This was interpreted to mean that endogenous substrate or the microenvironment of the cytochrome P-450 shifts the spin equilibrium toward the high-spin state and that this equilibrium is temperature-dependent. Thus it would appear that the type I spectrum is temperature-dependent regardless of whether it is induced by exogenous or endogenous substrate. In a more recent study, Cinti and associates [293] used temperature-induced spectral changes of rat hepatic microsomes to derive the thermodynamic parameters of the spin equilibrium, the molar extinction coefficients of the high- and low-spin forms of cytochrome P-450, and the absolute content of the high-spin form in microsomes in the absence of substrate. They concluded that at least 48% of the microsomal enzyme existed in the high spin form. ESR measurements supported this conclusion. In contrast, a soluble preparation of hepatic cytochrome P-450 was found to exist almost entirely in the low-spin form.

The LAHP deletion technique (Sec. II.A.1.g) provides a relatively direct means of determining the absolute and substrate-induced content of high-spin cytochrome P-450 in microsomes. As discussed previously (Sec. II.A.3.b) the absolute oxidized spectrum of microsomal cytochrome P-450 is a composite of the optical spectra produced by high- and low-spin forms of the cytochrome. Figure 7 shows the absolute spectra of oxidized microsomal cytochrome P-450 obtained by the LAHP deletion method in the absence of substrate and in the presence of the type I substrates, cyclohexane, benzphetamine, and hexobarbital. The slight shoulder seen at about 395 nm in the spectrum obtained in the absence of substrate indicates the presence of a high-spin form. The shoulder becomes more prominent when hexobarbital is added and dominates the spectrum when either benzphetamine or cyclohexane is present. The decrease in the optical density at 418 nm concomitant with the substrate-induced increase in the optical density at about 395 nm is indicative of a shift of the spin equilibrium to the high-spin state.

If it is assumed that the absolute spectra of the high- and low-spin forms of hepatic cytochrome P-450 are essentially the same as those that have been determined for pure cytochrome P-450$_{cam}$ [319], one can use the molar extinctions of high-spin P-450$_{cam}$ at 393 and 418 nm, the corresponding molar extinctions of low-spin P-450$_{cam}$ and the observed optical densities of the oxidized absolute spectrum of microsomal P-450 at 393 and 418 nm to calculate the fraction of high-spin cytochrome P-450 in a mixture of the two spin forms as described by Lipscomb [291]:

$$\text{fr x} = \frac{OD_{\lambda x}\,\epsilon^{y}_{\lambda y} - OD_{\lambda y}\,\epsilon^{y}_{\lambda x}}{OD_{\lambda x}\left(\epsilon^{y}_{\lambda y} - \epsilon^{x}_{\lambda y}\right) - OD_{\lambda y}\left(\epsilon^{y}_{\lambda x} - \epsilon^{x}_{\lambda x}\right)}$$

where

fr = fraction of total cytochrome P-450 in the high-spin state

$OD_{\lambda x}$ = observed OD at 393 nm

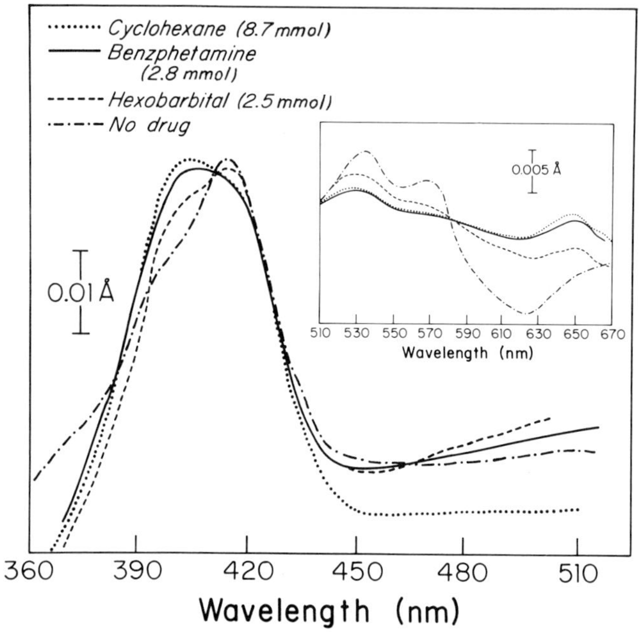

FIGURE 7 Effect of type I substrates on the absolute oxidized spectrum of hepatic microsomal cytochrome P-450. The linoleic acid hydroperoxide deletion method (Sec. II.A.1.g) was used with control microsomes (rat) to obtain the spectra. (From Ref. 292. Reproduced by kind permission of Academic Press.)

$OD_{\lambda y}$ = observed OD at 418 nm

$\epsilon^{y}_{\lambda y}$ = ϵ of low-spin cytochrome P-450 at 418 nm

$\epsilon^{y}_{\lambda x}$ = ϵ of low-spin cytochrome P-450 at 393 nm

$\epsilon^{x}_{\lambda y}$ = ϵ of high-spin cytochrome P-450 at 418 nm

$\epsilon^{x}_{\lambda x}$ = ϵ of high-spin cytochrome P-450 at 393 nm

This formula was used to calculate the percentage of high-spin cytochrome P-450 in microsomes which had been treated with increasing concentrations of LAHP (Fig. 8). The percentage of high-spin cytochrome P-450 in the absence of added substrate is seen to remain at about 30% at each of the concentrations of the enzyme, whereas the levels of substrate-induced high-spin cytochrome P-450 are seen to decrease linearly with successive deletions of cytochrome P-450. An extrapolation of this curve intercepts the endogenous high-spin P-450 curve at the point where no cytochrome P-450 remains. Extrapolation of the curve to the point where none of the cytochrome P-450 has been deleted provides an estimate of the substrate induced high-spin cytochrome P-450 that would have existed in the microsomes before the addition of LAHP. In the example shown in Fig. 8, the high-spin content of microsomal cytochrome P-450 was determined to be 29% in the absence of substrates and 93, 88, and 73% in the presence of cyclohexane, benzphetamine, and hexobarbital, respectively. One interpretation of these results is that microsomes contain two families of P-450 cytochromes. One exists almost entirely in the high-spin state because it is tightly associated with endogenous "substrate." It does not interact with exogenous substrates. The other exists almost entirely in the low-spin state and interacts with exogenous substrates.

The percentage of the microsomal cytochrome P-450 in the high-spin state varied greatly among preparations of microsomes. Untreated rats with the same specifications with respect to age, sex, weight, and source yielded microsomal cytochrome P-450 that varied in high-spin content between 7 and 50%. This suggests that endogenous substrate may be a highly variable component of microsomes. How much this contributes to the considerable day-by-day variation that most investigators encounter in

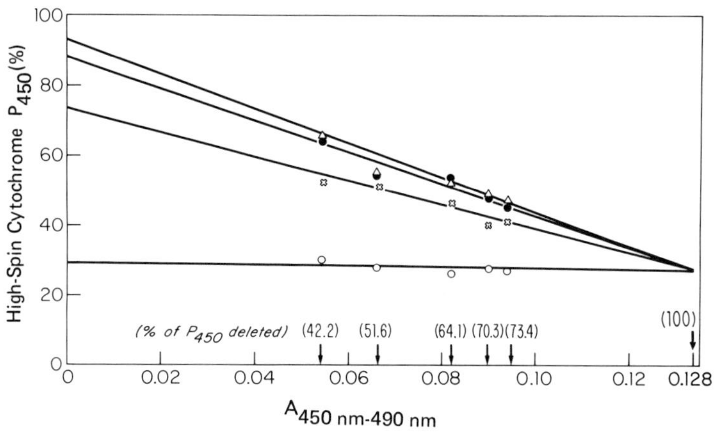

FIGURE 8 Percentage of high-spin cytochrome P-450 in microsomes with and without the addition of type I substrates. The amount of high-spin cytochrome P-450 was calculated from the absolute oxidized spectrum of microsomes from the rat which had been treated with successive increasing concentrations of linoleic acid hydroperoxide to remove cytochrome P-450 [292]. ○ = no added substrate; ✿ = plus hexobarbital (2.5 mM); ● = plus benzphetamine (2.8 mM); Δ = plus cyclohexane (8.7 mM). (From Ref. 292. Reproduced with kind permission of Academic Press.)

the monooxygenase activities of their microsomal preparations remains to be determined.

Most compounds that react with cytochrome P-450 are lipophilic or partly nonpolar at the pH of the reaction. It has therefore been assumed that the ability of a substrate to bind to microsomal cytochrome P-450 is related to the lipophilicity of the substrate [320-324]. The membrane has been assumed to be necessary for the binding of lipophilic substrates, or at least to play a facilitative role [325-328]. However, purified cytochrome P-450 from the rat, which was essentially free of lipid and detergent, gave both type I and type II spectra when appropriate substrates were added [329]. The requirement of phospholipid in reconstituted systems would thus appear to be related more to the interaction of the reductase with the cytochrome P-450-substrate complex than with the formation of the complex. Nevertheless, lipid may facilitate the binding of substrates to the purified enzyme. For example, Coon and associates [330] showed that dilauroyl phosphatidylcholine lowered the K_s for the binding of benzphetamine to cytochrome P-450LM$_2$ from 0.62 mM to 0.1 mM. Substrates that are unavailable to solubilized cytochrome P-450 because of their insolubility in aqueous media may become available after they are solubilized by lipid. Ebel and associates [328] showed that the membrane plays a similar role in microsomal reactions. In an attempt to determine why many investigators failed to obtain good correlation between room temperature optical spectra and ESR spectra, they studied the effects of temperature and the role of the membrane on substrate binding. The magnitude of the type I binding spectra of androstanedione and hexobarbital decreased as the temperature decreased from 36 to 6°C, but spectral binding constants (K_s^{app}) remained unchanged. The temperature effect was more pronounced with hexobarbital than with the steroid. These effects were considered to be due to a function of the microsomal membrane and the lipophilicity of the substrates. Analysis of their data led to the conclusion that the binding of a given substrate to cytochrome P-450 is related to its solubility in the microsomal membrane. Binding therefore appears to be facilitated by the lipids of the membrane. The 20% of the total cytochrome P-450 that were estimated to be bound to "endogenous substrate" underwent a reversible conversion from high- to low-spin as the temperature was lowered from 37 to 4°C. As measured by ESR, this conversion could be prevented by rapid freeze-quenching, which was interpreted to mean that the conversion was not due to a temperature-induced shift in the spin equilibrium. They concluded that endogenous substrates are released from cytochrome P-450 as the membrane cools and becomes less fluid. Their data also indicated that at least 40% of the microsomal cytochrome P-450 of PB microsomes was in the high-spin state in the absence of substrate and that exogenous substrates compete with each other in converting an additional 35% of the cytochrome to the high-spin form.

d. Ethyl isocyanide binding spectrum: The difference spectrum observed when ethyl isocyanide is added to reduced hepatic microsomes is of particular interest because it led to the identification of P-450 hemoproteins as cytochromes [15] and to the recognition of cytochrome P_1-450 as a distinct molecular entity [29]. Omura and Sato [15] used ethyl isocyanide in their early studies because it is known to produce a band in the Soret region with hemoglobin. When they added ethyl isocyanide to reduced hepatic microsomes, they observed a difference spectrum with a peak at 430 nm, which is characteristic of the absorption peak formed with hemoproteins, but they also observed an anomalous peak at 455 nm. The relative heights of the two peaks were found to be pH-dependent [331]. The height of the 455-nm peak increases with an increase in pH, and the height of the 430-nm peak decreases correspondingly, from which it was concluded that cytochrome P-450 exists in two pH-dependent, interconvertible forms. The equilibrium is affected by ionic strength [332] and by certain alcohols at concentrations lower than those required to produce spectral changes with oxidized microsomes [333]. The ratio of the 455-nm/430-nm peaks increases with the concentration and the chain length of the alcohols. The effects of pH and ion strength are seen with partially purified cytochrome P-450 and are therefore not due to changes produced in the membrane [334]. Methyl, tert-butyl, and phenyl isocyanide also elicit pH-dependent peaks at 430 and 455 nm [159]. The 455-nm peak increases and the 430-nm peak decreases with increasing carbon number of the isocyanides. These observations suggest that the equilibrium of the two forms of the hemoprotein is shifted toward the state represented by the 455-nm peak as the hydrophobicity of the environment of the heme is increased. The high 455-nm/430-nm ratio of the ethyl isocyanide spectrum seen with 3MC microsomes [29] and purified cytochrome P-448 prepared from 3MC microsomes [161] can be attributed to the greater hydrophobicity of cytochrome P_1-450 relative to other hepatic cytochrome P-450 hemoproteins. Stern and coworkers [312] have suggested that the 2-nm difference in the Soret maximum of the reduced CO spectra of cytochromes P-448 (e.g., P_1-450) and P-450 is due to a slight difference in the dielectric environments of the hemes produced by their different protein moieties. The maxima produced by ethyl isocyanide are at 430 nm and 455 nm in control and PB microsomes, but at 430 nm and 453 nm in 3MC microsomes [31].

4. Nomenclature

In 1962, when Omura and Sato [14] published their conclusion that Garfinkel's [13] "microsomal carbon monoxide-binding pigment" was a new b-type cytochrome, they proposed that it be named <u>cytochrome P-450</u> "provisionally." At the time, Omura and Sato probably assumed that cytochrome P-450 would be classified and given a permanent name when more was learned about its properties and functions. However, the more that has been learned about this enzyme—or more properly, family of enzymes—the more difficult it has become to fit it into the conventional enzyme classification system. In fact, the question has even been raised [268] as to whether it should be classified as a cytochrome since it is only as the denatured cytochrome P-420 form that it exhibits the spectral features of a cytochrome. Ullrich and associates [268] have proposed that since the sulfur ligand of the iron of cytochrome P-450 is required for the activation of oxygen by this enzyme, the term "heme-sulfur monooxygenase" should be substituted for the "misleading" term "cytochrome P-450." Heme-sulfur proteins would then join the group of electron transfer proteins comprised of iron-sulfur proteins, flavoproteins, and cytochromes.

"Cytochrome P-450" can be defined as any hemoprotein that shows a peak absorbance at about 450 nm when it is reduced and complexed with carbon monoxide. The term is commonly used to designate either a single molecular species or a mixture of cytochromes. The observation that the administration of certain inducing agents caused microsomes to exhibit an absorption maximum at 448 nm rather than at 450 nm [31] led to the term "cytochrome P-448," which was intended to mean that after induction two kinds of P-450 exist in hepatic microsomes, namely, cytochromes P-450 and P-448. The concept of a specific cytochrome P-448 became obsolete when hepatic cytochrome P-450s were purified and several were shown to have absorption peaks at 448 nm rather than at 450 nm. In fact, none of these purified cytochromes have a peak at exactly 450 nm and more have peaks that are closer to 448 than to 450 nm. The practice of classifying cytochrome P-450s in accordance with their "exact" maximum absorbance has lost whatever appropriateness it had originally and should be discouraged.

The substrate method of classifying enzymes is not feasible because all of the hepatic cytochrome P-450s that have been isolated show a broad spectrum of activities.

The designation of purified cytochrome P-450s by gel electrophoresis offers an unorthodox but pragmatic method of classification. The proteins are submitted to discontinuous polyacrylamide gel electrophoresis in the presence of SDS. The resolution of the proteins is reproducible and cytochromes purified in different laboratories give the same electrophoretic patterns [212]. The method has the additional advantage of classifying the cytochromes according to their molecular weights. The electrophoretic method has its discrepancies (e.g., electrophoretically homogeneous preparations of cytochrome P-450 have been shown to contain more than one immunologically distinct species of cytochrome), but it should eliminate some of the multiple naming of cytochrome P-450s. A nomenclature has been proposed which would specify the species, tissue, subcellular fraction, and electrophoretically determined subunit molecular weight of the cytochrome P-450 [335]; for example, rabbit liver microsomal cytochrome P-450 with a molecular weight of 54,000 daltons would be designated RbLvMc $P\text{-}450_{54}$, and rat adrenal mitochondrial cytochrome P-450 with a molecular weight of 52,000 daltons would be RtAdMt $P\text{-}450_{52}$.

The term "cytochrome P_1-450" presents special problems. Cytochrome P_1-450 was originally described as a specific type of cytochrome P-450 induced in rats by the administration of 3MC and certain other aromatic polycyclic hydrocarbons, as exhibiting substrate selectivities different from those of the cytochrome P-450 found in control or PB microsomes, as being resistant to the inhibitory effect of SKF-525A and as eliciting an ethyl isocyanide difference spectrum in the Soret region with an exaggerated 455-nm peak relative to its 430-nm peak at pH 7.4 (see Ref. 30 for review). Metyrapone and αNF are potent inhibitors of cytochrome P_1-450, but not of other cytochrome P-450s [126]. We have repeatedly expressed the opinion that cytochrome P_1-450 appears in the liver only when it is induced by exogenous substrates such as 3MC [30]. Cytochrome P_1-450 has a high specific activity for BP; other cytochrome P-450s have a relatively low specific activity for this substrate. αNF is a potent inhibitor of BP hydroxylation in 3MC microsomes, but has very little inhibitory effect on BP hydroxylation in control or PB microsomes. We consider this to be strong support for the view that appreciable amounts of cytochrome P_1-450 do not exist in control or PB microsomes. Small amounts of cytochrome P_1-450 may occur in control microsomes because animals do not live in an environment that is totally free of agents that induce it. Cytochrome P-450s that do not satisfy all of these criteria are not P_1-450.

From time to time a number of pseudonyms for cytochrome P_1-450 have appeared in the literature: P-448, P-446, high-spin P-450. After it was observed that the reduced CO spectrum of 3MC microsomes yielded a Soret maximum at 448 nm rather than at 450 nm, many investigators substituted the term "cytochrome P-448" for "cytochrome P_1-450." It is now known that several purified hepatic cytochrome P-450s isolated from both control and PB microsomes show a maximum at 448 nm. Most of these cytochrome P-448s do not exhibit the substrate selectivity of cytochrome P_1-450. Thus, not all cytochrome P-450s with a maximum at 448 nm are P_1-450 and the term "cytochrome P-448" should not be used to describe P_1-450.

A difference spectrum with a maximum at 446 nm is observed [288] when control microsomes are balanced against 3MC microsomes by the "offset" spectrophotometric method [286], which eliminates interference due to cytochrome b_5. Because the reduced CO spectra of cytochrome P-450s in the Soret region are not exactly symmetrical, a spectrum with a peak at 446 nm results when the spectrum produced by 3MC microsomes (λ_{max}: 448 nm) is superimposed on the inverse spectrum produced by control microsomes (λ_{min}: 450 nm); in other words, the peak absorbance at 446 nm is an optical artifact.

The term "high-spin cytochrome P-450" was equated with "P_1-450" when it was observed that the high-spin component of microsomes was increased after 3MC administration. The term is inappropriate because all cytochrome P-450s are now believed to exist in high-spin/low-spin equilibria (Sec. II.A.2.e). Moreover, evidence that cytochrome P_1-450 per se is predominantly a high-spin cytochrome is not convincing (Sec. II.A.3.a).

Guenthner and Nebert [55] have redefined cytochrome P_1-450 in accordance with its substrate selectivity. Cytochrome P_1-450 becomes a "polycyclic aromatic-inducible form of cytochrome P-450 associated with induced aryl hydrocarbon hydroxylase activity," and cytochrome P-448 "refers to a polycyclic aromatic-inducible form of cytochrome P-450, having a Soret peak shifted 2-3 nm to the blue when reduced and combined with CO, associated with induced acetanilide 4-hydroxylase activity." This definition is not only arbitrary, but it implies that only two species or classes of cytochrome P-450 are induced by aromatic polycyclic hydrocarbons, one identifiable with aryl hydrocarbon hydroxylase activity and the other with acetanilide hydroxylase activity. The definition does not anticipate the probable contingency that aromatic polycyclic hydrocarbons induce several species of cytochrome P_1-450 with different and overlapping substrate selectivities.

B. Cytochrome b_5

Sanborn and Williams [336] reported in 1950 that Cecropia silkwork larvae contained a cytochrome with a broad spectrum extending between 551 and 562 nm with a maximum at about 557 nm. The pigment, which they termed cytochrome x, was later renamed cytochrome b_5 [337]. Chance and Williams [338] examined the kinetics of the reduction of a hepatic microsomal pigment, which they referred to as cytochrome b_5 because the reduced minus oxidized difference spectrum of the pigment resembled the silkworm cytochrome that Williams had studied earlier. By this time the microsomal hepatic cytochrome had been named cytochrome m by Strittmatter and Ball [339], who reported that it was reduced by both NADH and NADPH and that it was distinct from mitochondrial cytochromes. The pigment was determined to be a b-type cytochrome with iron protoporphyrin IX as its prosthetic group and to function in univalent oxidation-reduction reactions [340]. Microsomal fractions from a variety of extrahepatic tissues have been shown to contain cytochrome b_5; e.g., it is present in the adrenal, pancreas, mammary gland, and intestinal mucosa.

The spectrum of oxidized cytochrome b_5 at neutral pH shows a peak at 413 nm in the Soret region and α- and β-bands at 560 and 530 nm, respectively; the spectrum is characteristic of a low-spin ferric hemoprotein [341]. Corresponding peaks of reduced cytochrome b_5 are 423, 556, and 526 nm.

The heme of cytochrome b_5 is not bound covalently and can be removed from the protein by acid acetone extraction. Cytochrome b_5 is reconstituted when stoichiometric amounts of apocytochrome b_5 and protohematin are mixed. Circular dichroic studies show that the addition of heme stabilizes the ternary structure of the protein. NADH reductase-reducible complexes of apocytochrome b_5 are formed with other iron porphyrins (mesoheme, deuteroheme, pyrroheme, and hematoheme).

Cytochrome b_5 is bound tightly to the microsomal membrane by a hydrophobic portion of the molecule. The hydrophilic portion of the cytochrome is solubilized when microsomes are treated with proteolytic enzymes. The hydrophilic portion, obtained in crystalline form by Raw and Colli in 1959 [342], retains the catalytic and spectral properties of the intact cytochrome. Amino acid sequences have been established for cytochrome b_5 isolated from the calf [343-345], rabbit [343], chicken [346,347], pig [347], horse [348], monkey [347], and man [346,347,349]. The first detailed X-ray crystallographic studies revealing the tertiary structure of cytochrome b_5 were performed by Matthews and Strittmatter [350], who used a crystalline preparation from isolated calf liver microsomes which contained 93 amino acid residues. The molecule has a cylindrical shape with a diameter of approximately 43 Å and a height of about 37 Å. Its heme is buried in a hydrophobic pocket which extends about 40% into the molecule. The iron atom is coordinated by His-39 and His-63 which extend from the walls of the crevice. The nitrogens of these two histidines are in the NH tautomeric form and are hydrogen-bonded to the main chain carbonyl oxygens of Gly-40 and Phe-58, respectively. The first two and the last six residues are disordered and coincide with the two regions that show species variability; they can be removed with trypsin without loss of activity.

The intact cytochrome b_5 can be solubilized if microsomes are treated with detergent rather than with proteolytic enzymes. Using Triton X-100, Ito and Sato [351] were the first to isolate and purify the whole molecule. It forms an octamer in the absence of added detergents. The purified detergent-solubilized cytochrome b_5 yields the hydrophilic and hydrophobic fragments when treated with trypsin [352,353]. The amino acid composition of the whole molecule, the hydrophilic fraction, and the hydrophobic fraction are given in Table 5. The hydrophobic fraction is seen to be rich in hydrophobic amino acids such as alanine, valine, leucine, and isoleucine. No cysteine is present in the whole molecule; membrane proteins are characterized by their low cysteine contents. The primary structure of the nonpolar segment of bovine cytochrome b_5 has been determined recently by Fleming et al. [354].

In hepatic microsomes, cytochrome b_5 is reduced by NADH-cytochrome b_5 reductase (NADH-cytochrome c reductase) or by NADPH-cytochrome P-450 reductase (NADPH-cytochrome c reductase). Cytochrome b_5 does not react readily with molecular oxygen or ligands such as CO or cyanide, although in microsomes the reduced cytochrome is oxidized very slowly by oxygen either directly or indirectly through the autooxidation of other components.

Cytochrome b_5 is a one-electron carrier with an E_0' of +20 mV at pH 7 [340]. It is partially or fully reduced by potassium borohydrate, sodium hydrosulfite, cysteine, and ascorbate and oxidized by potassium ferricyanide, ferric chloride, cytochrome c, and menadione. Strittmatter and Velich [5] isolated an NADH-reductase from hepatic microsomes which reduced cytochrome b_5, but not cytochrome c unless cytochrome b_5 was present.

TABLE 5
Amino Acid Composition of Rabbit Liver Cytochrome b_5

	(A) Heme fragment	(B) Detergent b_5	B - A	Hydrophobic peptide
Lys	10	11	1	1
His	7	7	0	0
Arg	3	4	1	1
Asp	10	16	6	4
Thr	7	10	3	3
Ser	7	10	3	3
Glu	14	15	1	1
Pro	3	5	2	2
Gly	6	7	1	1
Ala	5	10	5	4
Cys	0	0	0	0
Val	4	7	3	3
Met	1	3	2	2
Ile	4	8	4	4
Leu	9	15	6	5
Tyr	3	5	2	2
Phe	3	4	1	1
Trp	1	4	3	3
Totals:	97	141	44	40

Source: From Ref. 341. Reproduced with kind permission of Pharmacological Therapeutics, Series A, and Drs. B. Hagihara and E. Furuya.

Using a reconstituted system, they demonstrated the transfer of electrons from NADH to cytochrome c via the reductase and cytochrome b_5. However, cytochrome c is not a component of the endoplasmic reticulum and the physiological function of cytochrome b_5 remained unknown until the late 1960s when its role in the desaturation of acyl CoA was demonstrated in Sato's laboratory [351,355]. The discovery was stimulated indirectly by Sato's interest in cytochrome P-450 systems. The microsomal enzyme catalyzing the Δ^9-desaturation of long-chain acyl CoA was considered to be an NADPH-linked monooxygenase system [356-358]. The similarity of the cofactor requirement of this system and that of the cytochrome P-450-catalyzed hydroxylation of aniline led to comparisons of the two systems. The observation that ascorbate could substitute for NADH or NADPH as a weak donor of electrons to the desaturase system led to the conjecture that cytochrome b_5 might be involved in the reaction since it is the only microsomal component known to be reducible by all three electron donors. A reconstituted system consisting of NADH, NADH-cytochrome b_5 reductase, cytochrome b_5, and a cyanide-sensitive factor established the participation of cytochrome b_5 in the desaturase reaction. Cytochrome b_5 has been shown to provide reducing equivalents from NADH and NADH-cytochrome b_5 reductase to acyl CoA Δ^5-, Δ^6-, and Δ^9-desaturases, 1-alkyl-2-acyl-sn-glycero-3-phosphoryl ethanolamine desaturase, and possibly 4-methyl sterol oxidase (see Ref. 359 for review). Cytochrome b_5 also transfers electrons to cytochrome P-450, which is the reason for its inclusion in this chapter.

This has been a summary description of cytochrome b_5; for a thorough treatment of the nature and functions of hepatic microsomal cytochrome b_5, the reader is referred to the recent reviews by Strittmatter [360], Strittmatter [361], Oshino [359], and Hagihara and Furuya [341].

C. NADPH-cytochrome P-450 Reductase

An NADPH-linked reductase capable of reducing cytochrome c was discovered in liver in 1950 by Horecker [4]. The enzyme, which became known as NADPH-cytochrome c reductase, was purified by several investigators [5-7] who recognized its microsomal origin. It was shown to be capable of reducing ferric ions, ferricyanide, tetrazolium compounds, menadione, FAD, and azo compounds. It is one of the few flavoproteins which can oxidize cytochrome c directly in vitro. Cytochrome c was known not to be involved in the physiological function of the enzyme because it is not a component of the endoplasmic reticulum. As more was learned about cytochrome P-450-linked monooxygenase systems it became apparent that cytochrome P-450 is the natural acceptor of electrons from the reductase. While the term NADPH-cytochrome c reductase is still used frequently, the more appropriate name for the enzyme is NADPH-cytochrome P-450 reductase.

The reductase was believed at one time to contain two molecules of FAD per molecule of protein [362], but Iyanagi and Mason [363] showed that the prosthetic group consists of one molecule each of FMN and FAD. The reductase from rat liver has been purified to electrophoretic homogeneity by Yasukochi and Masters [364], Knapp and colleagues [365], and Vermilion and Coon [366]. Each of these preparations was determined to have equimolar amounts of FAD, FMN, and protein. Electrophoretically determined molecular weights of 76,000, 79,000, and 76,500 daltons were reported by Yasukochi and Masters, Knapp and colleagues, and Vermilion and Coon,

TABLE 6
Amino Acid Composition of Rat NADPH-cytochrome P-450 Reductase

Amino acid	Knapp et al. [365]	Vermilion and Coon [366]
Val	46	44
Met	24	16
Ile	26	27
Leu	66	62
Tyr	27	32
Phe	33	29
Trp	1	10
Asp	73	62
Glu	91	82
Lys	41	36
His	20	21
Arg	36	35
Thr	45	36
Ser	39	45
Pro	36	31
Gly	52	48
Ala	49	50
Cys	6	7
Totals:	711	673

respectively, which are in relatively good agreement with the estimate made earlier by Welton and associates [367]. The amino acid compositions of the reductase isolated by Knapp and associates and by Vermilion and Coon were quite similar except that the reductase prepared by the first group of investigators had only one tryptophan residue whereas that prepared by Vermilion and Coon had ten (Table 6). The apparently homogeneous reductase prepared in Coon's laboratory could be resolved into two bands by a modification of the electrophoretic procedure [366,368]. The second component, which comprised about 15-25% of the protein, had a minimal molecular weight of 78,000. This second component was considered to be a different form of the reductase, not an impurity.

Vermilion and Coon [366] and Iyanagi [369] showed that under anaerobic conditions the initial addition of NADPH reduced the purified reductase to an air-stable semiquinone form $R—F_1H\cdot—F_2$ (see Sec. III.C for definition of symbols). Additional NADPH produced the $R—F_1H_2—F_2H\cdot$ form of the enzyme and both flavins were fully reduced by an NADPH-regenerating system. The midpoint redox potentials of the reduced and partially reduced forms of the two flavins were determined [366]:

Redox pair	E'/mV
$F_1 \rightleftarrows F_1H\cdot$	-110
$F_1H\cdot \rightleftarrows F_1H_2$	-270
$F_2 \rightleftarrows F_2H\cdot$	-290
$F_2H\cdot \rightleftarrows F_2H_2$	-365

In a more recent publication, Vermilion and Coon [370] showed that F_1 is flavin-adenine dinucleotide (FAD). The similarity of the redox potentials of the redox pairs $F_1H\cdot—F_1H_2$ and $F_2—F_2H\cdot$ suggests that an intramolecular transfer of an electron from F_1 to F_2 occurs with the formation of a species of reductase containing $F_1H\cdot$ and $F_2H\cdot$. $F_1H\cdot$ is stable in air, but $F_2H\cdot$ is not. The difference in the midpoint potentials of NADPH/$NADP^+$ and $F_1/F_1H\cdot$ (250 mV) favors the transfer of electrons from NADPH even when NADPH/$NADP^+$ ratios are quite unfavorable. The implications of this mixture of fully and partially reduced flavins in the transfer of electrons to ferri- and oxyanionferri-P-450 substrate complexes will be discussed later (Sec. III.C).

The reductases associated with bacterial and mitochondrial cytochrome P-450 systems differ from microsomal NADPH-cytochrome P-450 reductase in that they contain only FAD and can only transfer electrons to cytochrome P-450 via intermediate iron-sulfur proteins (putidaredoxin, adrenodoxin). This similarity of the electron-transfer mechanism in both bacteria and mitochondria is of special interest in relation to the symbiotic hypothesis for the bacterial origin of mitochondria [371].

D. Cytochrome b_5 Reductase

Cytochrome c is readily reduced in microsomes by both NADPH and NADH [338,339,372-374]. Electrons from NADPH are transferred directly to cytochrome c by NADPH-cytochrome P-450 reductase. However, electrons from NADH are not transferred directly to cytochrome c by a flavoprotein. Strittmatter and Velick [5] isolated an NADH-specific reductase from pancreatic lipase-treated rabbit microsomes and found that it reduced cytochrome c only when cytochrome b_5 was present; i.e., the reaction required a cytochrome-to-cytochrome electron transfer. The intermediate cytochrome transfer component was recognized as cytochrome b_5 and the enzyme became known as "cytochrome b_5 reductase." Highly purified enzyme-solubilized cytochrome b_5 reductase from calf liver was shown to contain one molecule of FAD per enzyme molecule [375].

Takesue and Omura [376] found that cytochrome b_5 reductase was removed efficiently from hepatic rat microsomes when they were incubated with a lysosomal fraction from the same livers. They obtained a highly purified cytochrome b_5 reductase [377] with properties essentially identical to those of the reductase isolated by Strittmatter and Velick [375] from calf liver. They also provided convincing evidence that the snake venom used to solubilize calf enzyme was not in fact serving that purpose; solubilization had occurred because the hepatic calf microsomes were contaminated with lysosomes [376]. Cytochrome b_5 and NADPH-cytochrome c reductase are solubilized by trypsin and other proteolytic enzymes [6,378-380] but not by lysosomes. On the other hand, proteolytic enzymes do not solubilize NADH-cytochrome b_5 reductase [376].

Like the native forms of NADPH-cytochrome P-450 reductase and cytochrome b_5, native NADH-cytochrome b_5 reductase is comprised of a hydrophilic segment, which contains the catalytic site, and a hydrophobic segment, which anchors the enzyme to the membrane. The whole enzyme is released from the membrane by detergents. Spatz and Strittmatter [238] used Triton X-100 to solubilize calf liver cytochrome b_5 reductase, which they purified to apparent homogeneity. The molecular weight of the native reductase was estimated from its amino acid analysis (Table 7) to be about 43,000. The molecule binds to several membrane structures, including microsomes [238], mitochondria [381], erythrocytes [381], and phospholipid liposomes [382,383], but loses this property after proteolytic conversion to its hydrophilic segment [238,381]. The hydrophilic segment had an estimated molecular weight of 33,000. Fifty-five percent of the amino acids in this segment are hydrophobic, whereas 65% of the amino acids of the smaller segment are hydrophobic. This may seem too small a difference to account for the observed differences in the behavior of the two portions of the reductase, but Spatz and Strittmatter [238] point out that with a suitable molecular configuration of the protein a 10% increase in the content of hydrophobic residues could reduce the number of polar groups available to the surface of the membrane by as much as 20-25%.

Mihara and Sato [381] purified detergent-solubilized cytochrome b_5 reductase from rabbit liver to apparent homogeneity. Its properties were very similar to those of the reductase isolated by Spatz and Strittmatter [238], but its molecular weight was estimated to be 33,000 rather than 43,000. This discrepancy seems too large to be accepted as a species difference; it can be more readily explained on the basis of the different procedures used in the two laboratories to estimate the molecular weights.

TABLE 7
Amino Acid Composition of Lysosomal-extracted Reductase, Detergent-extracted Reductase, and Chymotrypsin-resistant Core of Detergent-extracted Reductase

Amino acid	(A) Detergent-extracted cytochrome b_5 reductase	(B) Lysosomal-extracted cytochrome b_5 reductase	A − B	(C) Chymotryptic core of detergent reductase
Lys	25	20	5	20
His	12	9	3	9
Arg	20	16	4	16
Asp	34	28	6	28
Thr	16	14	2	11
Ser	19	13	6	12
Glu	38	29	9	26
Pro	33	29	4	28
Gly	27	20	7	19
Ala	21	15	6	14
Cys	7	6	1	
Val	28	16	12	19
Met	10	8	2	8
Ile	24	19	5	19
Leu	40	27	13	29
Tyr	13	8	5	9
Phe	18	13	5	13
Trp	6	2	4	2
Totals:	391	292	99	
Molecular weight:	43,320	33,000	10,140	

Source: From Ref. 239. Reproduced with kind permission of Drs. L. Spatz and P. Strittmatter.

The reactivity of the intact reductase with either intact cytochrome b_5 or its hydrophilic segment was greatly enhanced by the addition of Triton X-100 or microsomal phospholipid. The detergent and phospholipid probably simulate a role played by the membrane in the transfer of electrons from the reductase to cytochrome b_5.

E. Microsomal Membrane

Current models [384,385] of membrane structure show a matrix of phospholipids arranged in a bilayer into which proteins are intercalated. The structures are stabilized by hydrophobic interactions among the hydrocarbon moieties of the lipids. Proteins that are integral to the membrane are presumed to possess both hydrophobic and hydrophilic segments. The hydrophobic segment anchors the protein molecule to the apolar hydrocarbon interior of the membrane and the hydrophilic segment extends to the membrane surface where it interacts with the polar head groups of the phospholipids and the aqueous environment. This is certainly true of the proteins that comprise the cytochrome P-450-linked monooxygenase systems of hepatic microsomes. NADPH-cytochrome P-450 reductase, NADPH-cytochrome b_5 reductase, and cytochrome b_5 have hydrophilic moieties which can be cleaved from the membrane enzymatically leaving their hydrophobic moieties embedded in the membrane. The high hydrophobic amino acid content of cytochrome P-450 is in keeping with the view that these cytochromes are deeply embedded in the membrane. The catalytic sites of cytochrome b_5 and the two reductases are known to be located on the hydrophilic segments of these enzymes (Secs. II.B, II.C, and II.D). Immunological studies [47] show that at least a small portion of the cytochrome P-450 protrudes outside the membrane. Each of the enzyme components of the system penetrates the membrane to a depth that allows its catalytic site to assume functional proximity to the catalytic sites of the other components of the system with which it reacts. These sites are on or near the surface of the membrane where they can react readily with cofactors and substrates. A cytochrome P-450 molecule would remain dormant if it were too distant from a reductase molecule, or if it were embedded so deeply in the membrane that it could not react with the reductase. This might explain in part the apparent inability of all cytochrome P-450 molecules to participate in monooxygenase reactions.

Hepatic microsomes contain as many as 20 to 30 times more molecules of cytochrome P-450 than molecules of NADPH-cytochrome P-450 reductase [386]. At first glance this may seem an amomalous situation, but kinetically, the efficiency of the overall reaction is improved when the ratio of cytochrome P-450 to reductase is increased. As will be discussed later (Sec. III.H), the substrate for the reductase is the ferricytochrome P-450-substrate complex, not the substrate per se. Thus, even with a ratio of cytochrome P-450 to reductase of 30:1, the substrate concentration for the reduction reaction is extremely low, which of course explains why these reactions have such low velocities. Should the concentration of cytochrome P-450 in the membrane be lowered to that of the reductase, the velocity of the oxidation of the reductase by ferricytochrome P-450 would be even slower. A kinetically efficient model would show the cytochrome P-450 molecules clustered around the scarce reductase molecules. Moreover, a homogeneous cluster of cytochrome P-450 molecules would be more efficient than a cluster comprised of different species of the enzyme. A cytochrome P-450 molecule is dormant until it binds to a substrate. In a heterogeneous cluster, some of the cytochrome P-450 molecules would remain dormant because they could not form a type I complex with a given substrate and the number of cytochrome P-450-substrate molecules that could react with the reductase would be lowered accordingly. In a homogeneous cluster, all of the cytochrome P-450 molecules would be activated by the substrate and could react with the reductase.

Microsomal particles enriched in cytochrome P-450, cytochrome b_5, NADPH-cytochrome P-450 reductase, and NADH-cytochrome b_5 reductase can be obtained by subfractionation of microsomes [220,221]. This suggests that components of the hepatic monooxygenase systems are in fact arranged in special assemblies within the membranes. Moreover, different subfractions of microsomes were shown to contain different kinds of cytochrome P-450 [222], which suggests that homogenous clusters of cytochrome P-450 may be located in different parts of the endoplasmic reticulum. The activities of microsomal enzymes are correlated with membrane structure, which in turn depends upon lipid-protein interactions [387]. Molecules of protein and phospholipid are bound by relatively weak forces and can therefore form membrane subregions or "patches." This could mean that certain species of cytochrome P-450 could only exist as homogeneous clusters in specific membrane patches.

For several molecules of cytochrome P-450 to react with a single molecule of reductase, one or both of the molecules must migrate in the membrane. The velocity of the movement of a protein in a membrane is an inverse function to its size; thus cytochrome P-450 with a molecular weight of about 50,000 might be expected to move somewhat faster than the reductase, which has a molecular weight of about 80,000. However, almost all of the cytochrome P-450 is embedded in the membrane, whereas only a small hydrophobic segment of the reductase with a molecular weight of about 8000 is buried in the membrane (Sec. II.C). The movement of the reductase is therefore relative to a molecular weight of 8000, not 80,000, and should be considerably more rapid than that of cytochrome P-450.

The properties of the microsomal monooxygenase system are dictated in part by the properties of the lipids and proteins in the membrane. Microsomal membranes are comprised of a mixture of phospholipids with a large portion of unsaturated fatty acyl residues [388]. Cholesterol, which accounts for about 8% of the lipid, undoubtedly plays an important role in determining the packing of phospholipids in the membrane. The importance of relatively small differences in quantities of glycerides, phospholipids, and cholesterol in the membrane awaits a clearer understanding of the location of the components of the monooxygenase systems in the membrane as well as a better evaluation of each reaction in the system. Many of the "animal variations" that plague investigators in this field may find an explanation in the more or less subtle changes that occur in the membrane in response to changes in the environment of the animal.

Amphiphilic substances of membranes exist in the mesomorphic state (liquid-crystalline state), which has properties intermediate between those of the liquid and crystalline states. The properties of a particular mesomorphic state are determined by the mole-fraction composition of the membrane and the temperature. Lipids in bilayers may undergo a temperature-dependent phase separation which produces patches of membranes of different composition [389-391]. Stier and Sackman [392] have shown that the bulk lipid of rabbit microsomal membrane is in a fluid state at 30°C with a lateral diffusion coefficient of 11×10^{-8} cm^2/s. Their spin label studies using tetramethylpiperidine nitroxide-phosphate and the N-oxyl-4,4-dimethyloxazolidine derivative of stearic acid provide evidence for a heterogeneous distribution of lipids located in patches in the membrane. The fluidity of these patches differs from that of the phospholipid of the bulk phase. They propose that cytochrome P-450 and its reductase are embedded in a phospholipid matrix which differs from that of the bulk of the membrane. Their studies indicate that at temperatures below 32°C the enzyme system is enclosed by phospholipid in a quasi-crystalline state. Using nuclear magnetic resonance spectroscopy, Stier and associates [393] showed that the mesomorphic state was converted to the fluid state at 35°C. Thus the two methods gave essentially the same results. It seems likely from the investigations of Stier and associates, and of others who have presented evidence that a tightly bound lipid anulus surrounds some membrane proteins or complexes of proteins [394-398], that boundary lipid is firmly associated with cytochrome P-450 and that phospholipid orients the binding of the latter to NADPH-cytochrome P-450 reductase in the surface of the microsomal membrane.

The lipid in the bulk phase of the membrane is probably in a liquid phase at temperatures above 5°C due to the large percentage of unsaturated fatty acids in liver microsomes [388] and to the cholesterol which decreases and broadens the temperature ranges of the phase transitions [399]. The rapid diffusion rate, even at low temperatures [400], also shows that the bulk phase has considerable fluidity.

The role of lipid in reconstituted systems is not well understood. In the absence of lipid, the rate and extent of reduction of cytochrome P-450 by NADPH-cytochrome P-450 reductase is very low. It seems likely that lipids, which can be replaced with phosphatidylcholine or certain nonionic detergents, may function in several ways: (1) by facilitating the binding of NADPH-cytochrome P-450 reductase to cytochrome P-450; (2) by facilitating the binding of substrate to cytochrome P-450; and (3) by increasing the effective concentration of cytochrome P-450 molecules relative to reductase molecules.

Trypsin-solubilized NADPH-cytochrome P-450 reductase contains the catalytic site of the enzyme but not the hydrophobic portion. It will not react with cytochrome P-450 in reconstituted systems either in the presence or the absence of lipid [366]. Detergent solubilized NADPH-cytochrome P-450 reductase retains both the hydrophilic and the hydrophobic portions of the enzyme. It will react with cytochrome P-450 in reconstituted systems only when lipid is present. This suggests that the hydrophobic portion of the reductase and the lipid act in concert to facilitate binding of the reductase to cytochrome P-450. Coon and associates [330] showed that the binding constant for the binding of reductase to cytochrome P-450 decreased from 0.48 μM to 0.12 μM in the presence of dilauroyl phosphatidylcholine.

While it appears from substrate binding spectra that phospholipids are not absolutely essential for the binding of substrate to cytochrome P-450, they undoubtedly facilitate substrate binding, particularly of highly water-insoluble substrates. Coon and collaborators [330] reported that the apparent K_s for the binding of benzphetamine to cytochrome P-450LM$_2$ decreased from 0.62 to 0.1 mM in the presence of dilauroyl phosphatidylcholine.

A study conducted in our laboratory about a decade ago [401] suggested that lipid may function in reconstituted systems by aggregating cytochrome P-450. Hepatic microsomes from the rabbit were solubilized and resolved into fractions containing cytochrome P-450, NADPH-cytochrome P-450 reductase, or lipid by the procedure described by Lu and Coon [402]. When lipid was excluded from the reconstituted systems, benzphetamine demethylase activity varied greatly from preparation to preparation, which suggested that different amounts of lipid had been retained by the cytochrome P-450 or the reductase fraction during its preparation. Addition of lipid increased the activity of all of these reconstituted systems. After incubation with benzphetamine, part of the mixture was analyzed for its formaldehyde content and another part was centrifuged at 4°C for 1 hr. The cytochrome P-450 contents of the pellet and supernatant fractions were determined. Variations in the activities of the reconstituted systems related directly ($r = 0.87$) to the particulate cytochrome P-450 recovered from the incubation mixture, but bore no relationship ($r = 0.44$) to the total cytochrome P-450 content of the mixture (Fig. 9). While this study is not conclusive, it suggests that cytochrome P-450 functions in reconstituted systems only when it is particulate and that lipid activates the system by aggregating the cytochrome.

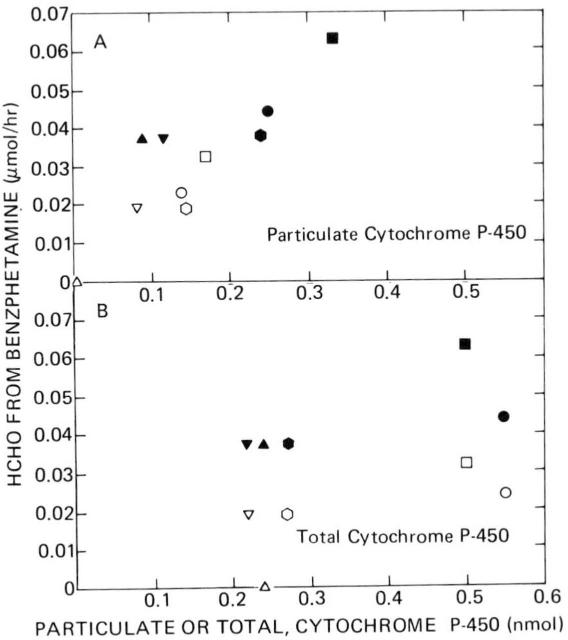

FIGURE 9 Effect of lipid (fraction B) on the aggregation of the cytochrome P-450 and the benzphetamine N-demethylase activity of a reconstituted hepatic monooxygenase system. The benzphetamine N-demethylase activity of the combined microsomal fractions was determined by measuring the amount of formaldehyde formed when the following mixture (total volume 1.5 ml) was incubated for 20 min in air with and without the addition of 0.07 mg of fraction B: 0.4 ml of cytochrome P-450 fraction containing 0.2 to 0.05 nmol of the hemoprotein; 0.3 ml of the NADPH reductase fraction; an NADPH-generating system consisting of 0.5 μmol of NADPH, 2 units of glucose 6-phosphate dehydrogenase, and 1.2 μmol of glucose 6-phosphate; 10 μmol of $MgCl_2$; 5 μmol of semicarbazide; 150 μmol of phosphate buffer, pH 7.4. After 10 min of incubation replicates of these mixtures were centrifuged at 100,000 g for 1 hr; the pellets and supernatant fractions thus obtained were assayed for their cytochrome P-450 contents. Each point is the mean of at least two determinations. In A the rate of HCHO formation is plotted against particulate cytochrome P-450; in B, against total (soluble + particulate) cytochrome P-450. Each of the reconstituted preparations in A and B is represented by a different symbol where either fraction B (solid symbols) or no fraction B (open symbbls) was added. (From Ref. 401. This is a previously unpublished figure presented at the Federation of American Societies for Experimental Biology Meeting in Atlantic City, New Jersey, April 1970.)

III. INTERACTIONS OF THE COMPONENTS OF THE SYSTEMS

Monooxygenase reactions are necessarily very complex because they involve both the transfer of electrons and the activation of oxygen. They are difficult to evaluate because the substrate for one step becomes the catalyst for a subsequent step. The transfer of electrons is intricate. Because NADPH-cytochrome P-450 reductase contains both FAD and FMN and each flavin exists in fully reduced and partially reduced forms, electrons are exchanged between the various forms and it is not known which forms transfer electrons to ferricytochrome P-450 and the oxyanionferricytochrome P-450-substrate complexes. Spontaneous transformations of oxygenated forms of cytochrome P-450 are difficult to identify. Uncoupling may occur when certain substrates are metabolized. The use of reconstituted systems to evaluate individual components of the reaction sequence are difficult to interpret because there is little assurance that solubilized systems function exactly like membrane-bound systems.

Despite these seemingly insurmountable complications, considerable progress has been made toward an understanding of the reaction mechanism. Section III is a brief review of some of the current concepts of how the components of the system are believed to interact.

A. Stoichiometry

By definition, a cytochrome P-450- and NADPH-linked monooxygenase reaction requires equimolar consumption of NADPH, molecular oxygen, and substrate. When rat hepatic microsomes have been used, considerably more NADPH has been oxidized than can be accounted for by product formation [139,197,403-406] although in at least one case [407], the discrepancy in stoichiometry was reversed. The determination of the stoichiometry of NADPH utilization and product formation by microsomes is complicated by endogenous NADPH oxidation. Endogenous enzyme activity (NADPH oxidase activity) may consume as much or more NADPH than is required for the oxidation of added substrate. A stoichiometry of NADPH utilization to product formation of less than one might be explained if endogenous NADPH oxidation is suppressed by the presence of substrate. Recent studies in our laboratory showed [405] that a stoichiometry of greater than one can be explained by the presence of nucleotide pyrophosphatase in microsomes. Earlier studies [406] had demonstrated that when the concentration of EDTA in the medium was high enough to inhibit pyrophosphatase activity, equimolar amounts of NADPH and product formation were observed. A 1:1 relationship of O_2 utilization and product formation was observed by Buening and Franklin [404] when they inhibited pyrophosphatase activity with 5'-AMP. The mechanism by which nucleotide pyrophosphatase distorts stoichiometry remained obscure, however, until it was recognized that the source of the problem is the 2',5'-ADP produced from NADPH through the action of the pyrophosphatase. 2',5'-ADP is formed when exogenous substrate is present; thus substrate appears to stimulate endogenous NADPH oxidation when in reality it permits the reaction to proceed at a less inhibited rate. The K_m for NADPH utilization by the monooxygenase reaction is very low (<1 μM) compared to that for the pyrophosphatase reaction (150 μM). At the initial concentration of NADPH used in these experiments (100 μM), the monooxygenase reaction is of zero order, whereas the pyrophosphatase reaction is of first order. When exogenous substrate is present, the concentration of NADPH is lowered more rapidly as the reaction proceeds than when substrate is absent, and NADPH becomes increasingly more rate-limiting for the pyrophosphatase reaction as the monooxygenase reaction proceeds. This explains why less 2',5'-ADP is formed in the presence of exogenous substrate. When microsomal nucleotide pyrophosphatase was inhibited by EDTA or 5'-AMP, the disparity in NADPH oxidation due to different rates of formation of 2',5'-ADP in the presence and absence of added substrate was eliminated and a 1:1 relationship of NADPH utilization and product formation was observed when aminopyrine, benzphetamine, codeine, or ethylmorphine was the substrate.

The significance of these observations will become more evident when uncoupling is discussed (Sec. III.G).

B. Binding of Substrate to Ferricytochrome P-450

The reaction begins when substrate binds to cytochrome P-450. As has been discussed previously in some detail (Sec. II.A.2.e), substrate binding causes a dissociation or weakening of the sixth ligand of the heme iron and this shifts the spin equilibrium toward the high-spin state. According to Rein and Ristau [278], the transition from the ferric high-spin state to the ferrous high-spin state is favored over the transition of the ferric low-spin state to the ferrous high-spin state:

$$Fe^{III}\ (S = 1/2) + e^{-}\ (S = \pm 1/2) \not\rightarrow Fe^{II}\ (S = 2)$$

$$Fe^{III}\ (S = 5/2) + e^{-}\ (S = -1/2) \rightarrow Fe^{II}\ (S = 2)$$

This concept is supported by studies of the reduction of models of heme complexes [408,409]. The high-spin state of the hemoprotein can be thought of as the "activated" state.

The extent of substrate activation of cytochrome P-450 will depend upon the species of cytochrome P-450 and the absolute and relative substrate and ligand binding constants of the substrate. Not only may substrate binding (type I) constants for a given substrate differ among species of cytochrome

P-450, but ligand binding (type II) constants may also differ. Moreover, the proportion of substrate to ligand binding for a given substrate may be expected to differ for different species of cytochrome P-450. The resultant spin state, and therefore the extent of substrate activation, will be the net effect of the substrate binding (high-spin) and the ligand binding (low-spin) produced by any given substrate with any given species of cytochrome P-450. Thus optical binding constants are not reliable indices of kinetic constants. The K_s and K_m of some substrates are similar (see Ref. 410 for review), but there is little reason to expect that this relationship should exist for all, or even most, substrates.

The ability of the substrate to combine with the binding site relates to its physical characteristics. Hydrophobic substrates generally bind avidly to cytochrome P-450 and the membrane facilitates their binding (Secs. II.A.3.c and II.E).

C. Reduction of Ferricytochrome P-450-substrate Complex

Early studies by Waterman and Mason [411] showed that under anaerobic conditions the cytochrome P-450 of hepatic microsomal preparations is a one-electron acceptor. The cytochrome P-450 of adrenocortical mitochondria [412,413] and purified cytochrome $P\text{-}450_{cam}$ [414] have also been shown to be one-electron acceptors. In 1975, Guengerich and associates [251] in Coon's laboratory reported that the titration of purified cytochrome $P\text{-}450LM_2$ with dithionite revealed the transfer of two electrons rather than one from NADPH. This unexpected finding led briefly to some confusion among investigators in the field and to some new theories describing the mechanism of action of hepatic cytochrome P-450 systems. To the relief of many, a second publication of a collaborative study performed in Coon and Peterson's laboratories [415] showed that purified cytochromes $P\text{-}450LM_2$ and $P\text{-}450LM_4$ are indeed one-electron acceptors and that the reoxidation of the reduced heme is accompanied by the transfer of one electron to oxidizing agents such as cytochrome c, cytochrome b_5, and potassium ferricyanide. In a publication that appeared during the same month, Cooper and colleagues [250] reported that only one electron is required for the formation of membrane-bound ferrocytochrome P-450·CO. They emphasized the essentiality of maintaining strictly anaerobic conditions during electron titration.

Several investigators [311,416-419] had observed that the reduction of ferricytochrome P-450 under anaerobic conditions follows a biphasic time course. Peterson and associates [419] accommodated their data to two first-order reactions occurring simultaneously, with one reaction about 20 times more rapid than the other. They suggested that some molecules of cytochrome P-450 are located in the membrane in clusters associated with the reductase, that others are located outside these clusters and that the slow phase of the reduction is due to the exchange of cytochrome P-450 molecules between the two locations. Gander and Mannering [230] cast doubt on the plausibility of this explanation by pointing out that the lateral diffusion rate of proteins in membranes based on data provided by Cherry [420] is between 0.1 and 0.01 nm/sec, which is too rapid to account for the slow phase. From this and some thermodynamic considerations, they argue that the relocation of cytochrome P-450 molecules in the membrane cannot explain the slow reaction and have proposed a model based on the assumption that the slow and fast reductions of ferricytochrome P-450-substrate complex represent the transfer of electrons from two forms of the NADPH-cytochrome P-450 reductase. Using the designations F_1 for FAD and F_2 for FMN (Sec. II.C), the fast phase would represent the reaction with the fully reduced reductase ($R—F_1H_2—F_2H_2$), and the slow phase, the reaction with a partially reduced reductase ($R—F_1H_2—F_2H$). The model considers the interactions of oxidized, partially reduced and fully reduced species of NADPH-cytochrome P-450 reductase (Sec. II.C) partitioned as follows:

$$[R_t] = [R—F_1—F_2] + [R—F_1H\cdot—F_2] + [R—F_2H_2—F_2] + [R—F_1H\cdot—F_2H\cdot] + [R—F_1H_2—F_2H\cdot] + [R—F_1H_2—F_2H_2]$$

where R_t = total reductase. The concentration of each species of reductase is determined by the K_s for NADPH and by the rate of transfer of electrons to the cytochrome P-450-substrate (XH) complexes. Species of reductase compete with each other when forming complexes with ferri- and oxyanion-ferricytochrome P-450-XH. The concentrations of the reductase P-450-XH complexes depends on the relative affinities of each species of reductase for the oxidized and oxygenated cytochrome P-450 complexes. Electrons from NADPH are transferred only to FAD [366] and ferricytochrome P-450-XH accepts electrons only from FMN [370].

The simplest model consistent with available data suggests that (1) $R—F_1H_2—F_2H_2$ and $F—F_1H_2—F_2H\cdot$ bind to both ferricytochrome P-450-XH and oxyanionferricytochrome P-450-XH; (2) $R—F_1H_2—F_2$ binds to oxyferrocytochrome P-450-XH; (3) $R—F_1H\cdot—F_2H\cdot$ binds to ferricytochrome P-450-XH; (4) $R—F_1H\cdot—F_2$ and $F—F_1H\cdot—F_2H\cdot$ bind to NADPH; and (5) $R—F_1H_2—F_2H_2$ and $R—F_1H_2—F_2H\cdot$ bind to $NADP^+$. $NADP^+$ could be an important "dead-end" inhibitor; that is, it might form an unreactive complex with the species of reductase to which NADPH binds.

The midpoint redox potential ($E^{o'}$) of the F_2H_2 moiety at pH 7.0 (-365 mV) is 75 mV more negative than that of the $F_2H\cdot$ moiety (-290 mV). The $E^{o'}$ of P-450LM is -330 mV [251]. Thus, F_2H_2 should be a better donor of electrons to ferricytochrome P-450-XH than $F_2H\cdot$. Because the concentrations of $R—F_1H_2—F_2H\cdot$ and $R—F_1H_2—F_2H_2$ are determined by the $[NADP^+]/[NADPH]$ ratio, NADPH is the driving force for the reduction of ferricytochrome P-450-XH. Figure 10 shows how these two species of

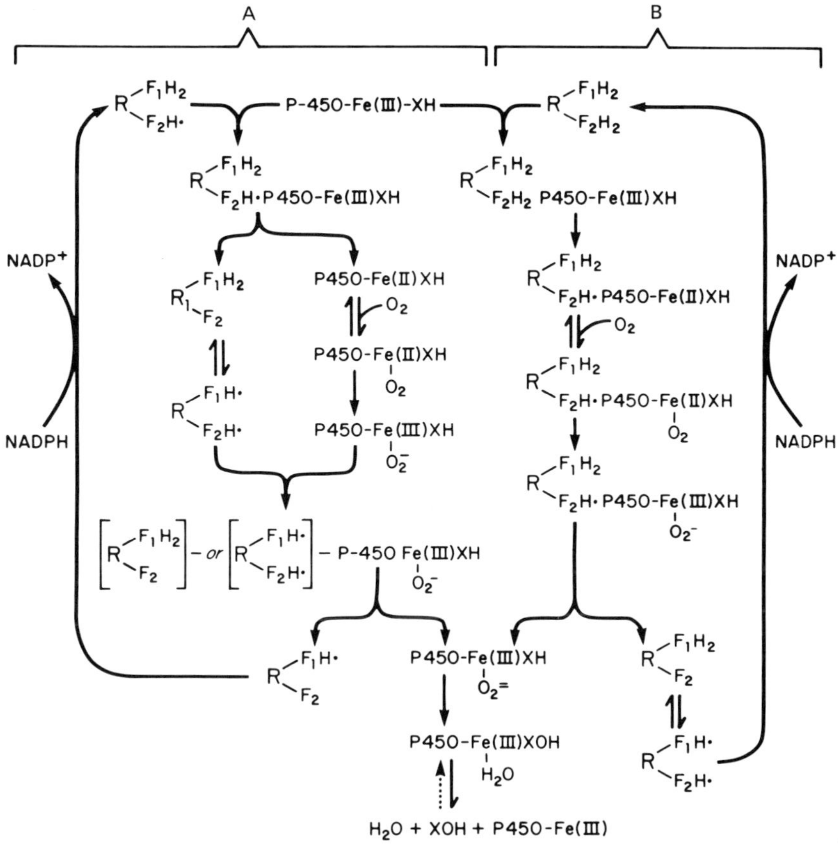

FIGURE 10 Model showing interactions of fully and partially reduced NADPH-cytochrome P-450 reductase with cytochrome P-450 substrate complexes. Parts A and B refer to the slow and fast phases of reduction of cytochrome P-450, respectively. Parts A and B are equivalent to cycle II and cycle I of Fig. 11, respectively. Symbols are defined in Fig. 1. (From Ref. 230. Reproduced by kind permission of Pharmacological Therapeutics, Series A.)

NADPH-cytochrome P-450 reductase are formed by NADPH. Using the Nernst equation to calculate the ratio of the four species of reductase and assuming an $[NADP^+]/[NADPH]$ ratio of 0.1, the ratio of $[R{-}F_1H_2{-}F_2]/[R{-}F_1H_2{-}F_2H_2]$ and $[R{-}F_1H\cdot{-}F_2]/[R{-}F_1H_2{-}F_2H\cdot]$ at equilibrium are 1:7.9 and 1:316, respectively. Both ratios will shift toward a greater percentage of the oxidized species during drug metabolism.

Figure 10 shows the two simultaneous series of reactions. The pathway shown on side B of the figure predominates when the concentration of NADPH is high and the [NADP]/[NADPH] ratio is unity or less. The model predicts that under truly anaerobic conditions and high concentrations of NADPH, one-half of the ferricytochrome P-450-XH will be reduced by the fast reaction (side B) and the other half by the slow reaction (side A) because regeneration of $R-F_1H_2-F_2H_2$ is coupled to NADPH oxidation; i.e., two electrons are transferred to $R-F_1H_2-F_2$ or to $R-F_1H\cdot-F_2H\cdot$. The reduction of $R-F_1H_2-F_2$ to $R-F_1H_2-F_2H_2$ is the slow reaction. Thus, under anaerobic conditions the pathway on side B is coupled to side A through $R-F_1H_2-F_2H\cdot$, and $R-F_1H_2-F_2H_2$ is regenerated by a two-electron reduction. More than 50% of the reduction of ferricytochrome P-450-XH should occur via the fast reaction. The amount of reduction in excess of 50% will depend on the molar ratio of $[R-F_1H_2-F_2H_2]$/[ferricytochrome P-450] at the beginning of the reaction and the relative affinities of $R-F_1H_2-F_2H_2$ and $R-F_1H_2-F_2H\cdot$ for ferricytochrome P-450-XH. Imai and Sato [421] found that about 58% of the ferricytochrome P-450 was reduced by the fast reaction when benzphetamine was the substrate. Matsubara and colleagues [422] also found that about 50% or more of the ferricytochrome P-450 was reduced by the fast reaction when the substrates were hexobarbital (58%), ethylmorphine (46%), cyclohexane (64%), testosterone (46%), and aniline (48%). In the absence of added substrate, 48% of the reduction of ferricytochrome P-450 occurred via the fast reaction. However, the proportion of fast reaction relative to the slow reaction has sometimes been observed to be higher than predicted by the model, e.g., 70% with hexobarbital [419] and 80% with benzphetamine [422].

The reactions shown in Fig. 11 illustrate the role of NADPH in the regeneration of the various species of reductase. The cycle which generates $R-F_1H_2-F_2H_2$ from $R-F_1H\cdot-F_2H\cdot$ (cycle I) is coupled with the cycle which generates $R-F_1H_2-F_2H\cdot$ from $R-F_1H\cdot-F_2$ (cycle II). The relative activities of cycles I and II should depend on both the ratio of $[NADP^+]/[NADPH]$ and the concentration of NADPH. Cycle I is essentially absent when the $[NADP^+]/[NADPH]$ ratio is greater than unity or when the concentration of NADPH is low [10 μM or less). As the ratio of $[NADP^+]/[NADPH]$ increases above unity the redox potential of the system will increase to a level where very little $R-F_1H_2-F_2H_2$ will be regenerated; $R-F_1H\cdot-F_2H\cdot$ formed from $R-F_1H_1-F_2$ will then become the major reductant of ferricytochrome P-450-XH. If the K_m (NADPH) for $R-F_1H\cdot-F_2H\cdot$ and $R-F_1H\cdot-F_2$ are not the same, the Lineweaver-Burk plot of the overall rate of drug metabolism should be nonlinear when NADPH is the variable substrate. At a concentration of 1 mM NADPH the rate of reduction of ferricytochrome P-450 in an anaerobic system occurred via two simultaneous reactions during the first 25 sec, but at a concentration of 10 μM NADPH, only the slow reaction was observed [423]. A rate constant of 0.15/min was obtained for the slow reaction at both concentrations of NADPH. The rates of N-demethylation of ethylmorphine by microsomes were determined at concentrations of NADPH between 0.5 and 400 μM. These data yielded a biphasic Lineweaver-Burk plot with a break at about 25 μM NADPH. These results are consistent with the model shown in Fig. 10. This would mean that at

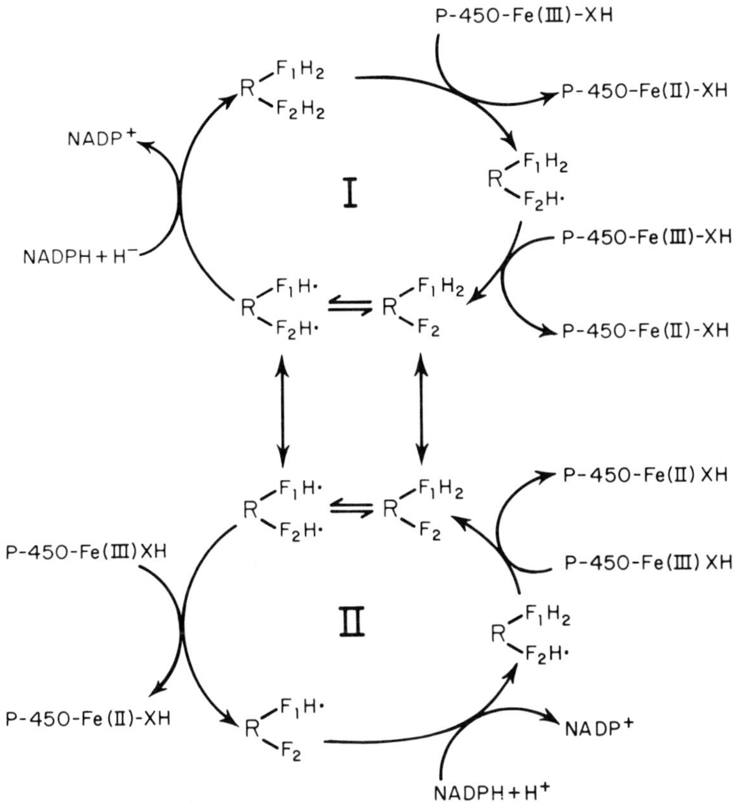

FIGURE 11 Model showing coupling of fast (cycle I) and slow (cycle II) reduction of cytochrome P-450-substrate complex to NADPH reduction of oxidized NADPH-cytochrome P-450 reductase. Symbols are defined in Fig. 1. (From Ref. 230. Reproduced by kind permission of Pharmacological Therapeutics, Series A.)

concentrations of NADPH below 10 μM, ferricytochrome P-450-XH is metabolized primarily by the reactions shown in side A of Fig. 10, and at concentration of NADPH above 10 μM by those on side B.

The model predicts that O_2 should be a potent inhibitor of the reduction of ferricytochrome P-450-XH complex because the addition of O_2 to ferrocytochrome P-450-XH forms a new species which will compete for the reductase. Preliminary evidence shows that O_2 is not a potent inhibitor during the first 1 or 2 sec of ferricytochrome P-450 reduction [423]. This suggests that oxyanionferricytochrome P-450 competes for $R—F_1H_2—F_2H\cdot$ more effectively than it does for $R—F_1H_2—F_2H_2$. A system with competing components would seem unnecessarily disadvantaged. However, in the cell where both NADPH and NADH are present, competition of ferricytochrome P-450-XH and oxyanionferricytochrome P-450-XH for NADPH is minimized or eliminated because oxyanionferricytochrome P-450-XH accepts electrons from NADH via cytochrome b_5. This mechanism is sometimes referred to as "NADH synergism" (Sec. III.F).

D. Oxygenation of Ferricytochrome P-450-substrate Complex and the Activation of Oxygen

When molecular oxygen is added to ferrous cytochrome P-450_{cam} in the presence of its substrate, D-camphor, a new spectral species is formed with absorption maxima at 418 and 555 nm and shoulders at 360 and 580 nm [424-427]. A very similar spectral species has also been observed with rat hepatic microsomes during the aerobic steady state of substrate hydroxylation [428-430]. An oxygen complex forms with ferrous cytochrome P-450_{cam} in the absence of its substrate, but it is 100 times less stable than the complex formed in the presence of substrate [318]. Taken with the spectral and ESR characteristics of the more stable oxygenated species, this observation has led to the conclusion that oxyferrocytochrome P-450 is not a simple adduct of molecular oxygen to the cytochrome, but that it is a tertiary complex of oxygen, substrate, and P-450.

The addition of oxygen to cytochrome P-450 is reversible and oxygen can be displaced with CO to form the characteristic spectrum from which the cytochrome derived its name. Monooxygenase reactions are inhibited by CO because CO competes for the oxygen binding site. Hydroxylation of some drugs is inhibited to a greater extent by CO than others. This may be due to (1) the multiplicity of cytochrome P-450s; (2) substrate-induced differences in the steady-state levels of reduced cytochrome P-450 available for reaction with CO; and (3) differences in the extents of ligand (type II) binding by the substrates.

Evidence that different cytochrome P-450s may have different affinities for oxygen has been presented in Sec. II.A.1.i. Estabrook and collaborators [431] observed that decreasing the concentration of NADPH decreased the CO sensitivity of ethylmorphine N-demethylase without changing the K_m for demethylation and concluded that the steady-state concentration of reduced cytochrome P-450 determines the degree of CO inhibition. Metyrapone and other strong ligand binders interfere with the binding of CO to cytochrome P-450; both metyrapone and CO convert reduced cytochrome P-450 to the low-spin state. Aniline, a type II substrate, decreases both NADPH oxidation and oxygen consumption [432,433].

The rate of binding of oxygen to cytochrome P-450 is about 20 times more rapid than the rate-limiting step of the cytochrome P-450_{cam} reaction [252] and one or two orders of magnitude faster than the rate of product formation by microsomes [434].

Molecular oxygen exists in three states: the ground (triplet) state and two excited (singlet-oxygen) states. In the ground state, the spins of the two unpaired electrons in the two outermost orbitals of the oxygen molecule are parallel. Singlet oxygen is produced when the electrons are rearranged so that they have antiparallel spins in either the same or different orbitals. The energy state is highest when the electrons are in different orbitals. Each of the two outermost orbitals of the oxygen molecule can accommodate another electron. The addition of one electron produces the superoxide anion radical ($O_2^{\bar{\cdot}}$):

$$O_2 + 1e \longrightarrow O_2^{\bar{\cdot}}$$

The addition of two electrons produces the peroxy anion (O_2^{2-}):

$$O_2^{\bar{\cdot}} + 1e \longrightarrow O_2^{2-}$$

The oxygen of oxyferrocytochrome P-450-substrate complex must be activated before it can be added to the substrate. This occurs when an electron from the ferrous iron of the heme is transferred to the oxygen to form the oxyanionferricytochrome P-450-substrate complex (Fig. 1):

$$\underset{\displaystyle O_2}{\overset{|}{\text{P-450-Fe(II)}}}\cdot XH \rightleftarrows \underset{\displaystyle O_2^{\bar{\cdot}}}{\overset{|}{\text{P-450-Fe(III)}}}\cdot XH$$

For cytochrome P-450 and other oxygenases with a transition metal ion, the reactive oxygen species could be a metal ion-complexed O atom (oxene), a peroxy complex, or a hydroxyl radical. As discussed in a recent review by O'Brien [435], several candidates have been nominated only to be rejected, including singlet oxygen, superoxide anion, hydroxyl radical, and hydrogen peroxide. Current thinking favors an oxene intermediate, which is simply atomic oxygen bound to the ferric hemoprotein; as such, it is highly electron-deficient and therefore a potent oxidizing agent. Hamilton [436] noted the similarity of reactions catalyzed by microsomes and and the reactions of carbenes and nitrenes. Carbenes, nitrenes, and oxenes are isoelectronic; all have six electrons in their outer shells and are therefore very reactive by virtue of their electron deficiency. The reactions of carbenes with unactivated carbon-hydrogen bonds to give alkanes, their additions to alkenes to give cyclopropanes, and their reactions with aromatic compounds to give alkyl benzenes and norcaradienes [437] correspond to reactions with oxene which yield alcohols, epoxides, and arene oxides—all known products or intermediates of microsomal oxidations [438]. Jerina and associates [439] tested this analogy by studying the formation of arene oxides from aromatic compounds. They demonstrated the formation of intermediate arene oxides which rearranged to the keto tautomer of the phenol. During this tautomerization, a hydrogen atom shifts from the position to be hydroxylated to the adjacent carbon position. They concluded that this shift (the NIH shift) is mediated by arene oxides. Further support for an oxene intermediate in microsomal reactions comes from the observation that CO and ethyl isocyanide, two potent inhibitors of these reactions, are isoelectronic with oxene [435].

Three species of activated enzyme are possible: (1) an enzyme $\cdot Fe^{+} \cdot O_2$ complex; (2) an enzyme $\cdot Fe^{3+} \cdot$ peroxide complex; and (3) an enzyme $\cdot Fe^{3+} \cdot O$ complex [158]. Hamilton [437] originally favored the peroxide compound as the most probable species, but recent evidence suggests that the enzyme $\cdot Fe^{3+} \cdot O$ complex is the active form of oxygen in cytochrome P-450 reactions. Rahimtula and O'Brien [440] made the important observation that the hydroxylation of a variety of compounds by microsomes is supported by cumene hydroperoxide in the absence of NADPH and O_2. One mole of hydroperoxide was consumed for each mole of substrate hydroxylated. Moreover, the addition of hydroperoxide to hepatic microsomes produced the appropriate transient spectral change and ESR signals [441]. They concluded that the Fe^{3+} O complex is involved in cytochrome P-450-linked monooxygenase reactions. Lichtenberger and colleagues [442] provided evidence that the active oxygen species involves a ferricytochrome containing a single oxygen atom rather than an $Fe^{3+} \cdot$ peroxide by demonstrating that iodosobenzene supported the O-dealkylation of 7-ethoxycoumarin by 3MC microsomes; in fact, the rate of this reaction was 7 times faster than that of the reaction supported by NADPH and O_2. Thus the latest evidence suggests that cytochrome P-450-linked monooxygenase reactions are oxene transfer reactions in which a single oxygen atom bonded to cytochrome P-450 is transferred to the substrate.

For more complete and detailed discussions of activated forms of oxygen and their involvement in biological systems, readers are referred to reviews by Fridovich [443,444], Foote [445], Hamilton [437], O'Brien [435], Paine [446], and Trager [158].

E. Reduction of Oxyanionferricytochrome P-450-substrate Complex and Product Formation

Oxyanionferricytochrome P-450-substrate complex accepts an electron from reduced NADPH-cytochrome P-450 reductase, or preferably, from ferrocytochrome b_5. The oxygen atom is transferred to the substrate, product is released from the enzyme complex, and cytochrome P-450 is restored to its uncomplexed, low-spin ferric state (Fig. 1). The mechanism of dissociation of the hydroxylated product and the restoration of low-spin ferricytochrome P-450 are the least understood steps of the overall reaction. The mechanism is obviously adaptable to the great variety of molecular configurations presented by the diversity of substrates which are known to react with the system. In some cases, epoxide intermediates are formed, as when aromatic polycyclic hydrocarbons are metabolized (see Ref. 447 for review); in other cases, stable product adducts are formed which impede further function of the cytochrome P-450 (see Ref. 448 for review). A consideration of the oxidation of individual substrates or classes of substrates is not only beyond the scope of this review, but this subject has been reviewed by Trager in Chapter 3, Part A, of these two volumes [158].

F. Reduction of Ferri- and Oxyanionferricytochrome P-450-substrate Complexes by Ferrocytochrome b_5; NADH Synergism

Studies which have been attempted to assess the role of the NADH-cytochrome b_5 electron-transfer system (Fig. 1) in cytochrome P-450-linked hepatic monooxygenase reactions have addressed three questions: (1) Is cytochrome b_5 an obligatory component of NADPH-supported reactions? (2) Is cytochrome b_5 a facilitative component of NADPH-supported reactions? (3) Is cytochrome b_5 involved directly or indirectly in the so-called NADH synergism of NADPH-supported reactions? Several experimental approaches have been used: (1) kinetic studies of the effects of substrate on the utilization of NADH and the steady state of reduction of cytochrome b_5 [26]; (2) activation and inhibition of the cytochrome b_5-dependent stearoyl-CoA-desaturase systems to shunt electrons toward or away from the monooxygenase system [139,197]; (3) immunological studies [27,28]; (4) use of reconstituted systems devoid of cytochrome b_5 [57,421,449-452]; (5) addition of homogeneous cytochrome b_5 to microsomes or reconstituted systems [453]; (6) an evaluation of rates of reoxidation of ferrocytochrome P-450 and ferrocytochrome b_5 in the presence of CO [454]. Investigators have generally agreed that cytochrome b_5 is somehow involved in cytochrome P-450-linked monooxygenase reactions, but have frequently disagreed as to the mechanism involved (see Refs. 455 and 456 for reviews).

Most hepatic monooxygenase systems are supported by NADH at only 10-20% of the rate obtained with NADPH. This is usually interpreted to mean that cytochrome P-450 hemoproteins in general are much less able to accept electrons from NADH than from NADPH. The possibility should be considered that certain species of cytochrome P-450 may be more reactive with NADH than others; the observed activity would then represent the mean rate of the reactivity of NADH with several cytochrome P-450s. Certain substrates are metabolized at a relatively high rate when NADH is the only source of electrons. For example, the rate of NADH supported O-deethylation of para-nitrophenetole (5.1 nmol/nmol of cytochrome P-450 per min) by 3MC microsomes is greater than the rate of the NADPH-supported reaction by control microsomes (2.8 nmol/nmol of cytochrome P-450 per min) [193].

As will be discussed in the following paragraphs, there are compelling reasons to believe that when both NADPH and NADH are present, an electron from NADH is donated to oxyanionferricytochrome P-450-substrate complex via NADH-cytochrome b_5 reductase and ferrocytochrome b_5, as shown in Fig. 1. There remains the question of whether ferricytochrome P-450 is reduced directly by NADH-cytochrome b_5 reductase when NADH is the only source of electrons. Since both cytochrome c and stearoyl CoA-desaturase are reduced by ferrocytochrome b_5, but not by NADH-cytochrome b_5 reductase [5,351,355], it seems reasonable to assume that ferricytochrome P-450 is also reduced by ferrocytochrome b_5 that has received an electron from NADH-cytochrome b_5 reductase. Support for this assumption was obtained recently in our laboratory when we showed that antibody to cytochrome b_5 inhibited microsomal O-deethylation of para-nitrophenetole almost completely when NADH was the only source of electrons [193]. Fujita and Peisach [454] used the observation that cytochrome P-450 is the sole microsomal azo reductase engaged in the reduction of amaranth to demonstrate the transfer of electrons from cytochrome b_5 to ferricytochrome P-450. They showed spectrophotometrically that the gradual oxidation of cytochrome P-450 by amaranth in the presence of CO is followed by the oxidation of ferrocytochrome b_5 at essentially the same rate.

Estabrook and associates [26,457] were the first to provide evidence that NADH-dependent cytochrome b_5 systems and NADPH-dependent cytochrome P-450 systems interact in microsomes. They showed that the rate of NADH oxidation by microsomes was increased when NADPH was present and that this increase was related to the rate of oxidation of the substrate. They further implicated cytochrome b_5 in monooxygenase reactions by demonstrating that the steady state of reduced cytochrome b_5 in the presence of both NADPH and NADH was decreased by the addition of substrate (ethylmorphine). An ethylmorphine-enhanced rate of oxygen utilization and product formation linked the oxidation of ethylmorphine to the alteration in the steady-state reduction of cytochrome b_5. The substrate-induced reoxidation of cytochrome b_5 was believed to be due to the reduction of ferricytochrome P-450-substrate complex. Schenkman and associates [453,456] visualize an entirely different role of cytochrome b_5 in NADH synergism whereby cytochrome b_5 shunts electrons away from cytochrome P-450 rather than toward it. They propose that cytochrome b_5 acts as a "drain" for electrons from NADPH-cytochrome P-450 reductase. This deprives ferricytochrome P-450-substrate complex of its full share of electrons from NADPH. An apparent synergism is observed when electrons from NADH are substituted for the electrons from NADPH which were being lost to the cytochrome b_5 "drain." This analysis of NADH synergism assumes that the reduction of ferricytochrome P-450 is rate-limiting in the absence of NADH and that at least part of this rate limitation is due to a competition of ferricytochrome P-450-substrate complex and ferricytochrome b_5 for electrons from NADPH-cytochrome P-450 reductase.

Cytochrome b_5 is involved in the transfer of electrons from NADH to stearoyl CoA-reductase [351,355]. Correia and Mannering [139,197] showed that stearoyl CoA inhibited NADH synergism and that this inhibition was reversed by concentrations of cyanide which were high enough to inhibit stearoyl CoA-desaturase almost completely, but not high enough to inhibit cytochrome P-450. This was interpreted to mean that when NADH is present, second electrons are donated to cytochrome P-450 via cytochrome b_5 and that activation of the cytochrome b_5-dependent desaturase system diverts these electrons from the cytochrome P-450 system. They also studied the role of type I binding in NADH synergism by employing microsomes which varied in their abilities to produce a type I binding spectrum with ethylmorphine. This was accomplished by selecting microsomes from different animal sources (male rats of different ages, female rats, 3MC-treated rats) and by subjecting microsomes from a single source to treatments known to diminish type I binding (treatment with SKF-525A or with phospholipase C or cold storage). Using ethylmorphine as the substrate, type I binding was shown to be directly correlated with NADH synergism and NADH utilization.

Sasame [27] and Mannering [28] and their collaborators observed that antibody against cytochrome b_5 completely inhibited NADH synergism, but reactions supported solely by NADPH were inhibited by only 20-30%. These studies definitely established a role of cytochrome b_5 in NADH synergism, but did not distinguish between the mechanism proposed by Hildebrandt and Estabrook and Schenkman and coworkers. These studies also suggested that when NADPH is the only electron donor, the reduction of oxyanionferricytochrome P-450-substrate complex is not mediated primarily by cytochrome b_5 as had been suggested by Hildebrandt and Estabrook [26]. The 20-30% inhibition of the NADPH-supported reaction by antibody against cytochrome b_5 could mean that 20-30% of second electrons from NADPH are transferred to cytochrome P-450 by cytochrome b_5, that the latter acts as an "effector" in microsomes in a manner similar to that proposed for putidaredoxin in the cytochrome P-450_{cam} system [272,426], or that the reaction of antibody with cytochrome b_5 perturbs the monooxygenase system adversely in a manner not directly related to the transfer of electrons through cytochrome b_5.

Cytochrome b_5 appears to play a larger role in NADPH-supported reactions in the kidney and lung than in the liver. Antibody against cytochrome b_5 inhibited laureate hydroxylation in kidney cortex microsomes by 55% [458] and the metabolism of 4-ipomeanol in lung microsomes by 60-70% [459] when NADPH was the only electron source.

Purified cytochrome b_5 from detergent-solubilized hepatic microsomes can be incorporated into the microsomal membrane where it functions in the NADH-cytochrome c reductase and fatty acyl CoA-desaturase systems [382,453,460,461]. Jansson and Schenkman [453] showed a progressive inhibition of NADPH-supported aminopyrine demethylation with increasing concentrations of incorporated cytochrome b_5. This observation was used to support their hypothesis that cytochrome b_5 does not participate directly in the transport of the second electron from cytochrome P-450, but diverts electrons from NADPH away from the latter. If this is the mechanism of NADH synergism, the endogenous cytochrome b_5 of microsomes which have not been enriched with exogenous cytochrome b_5 should exert an inhibitory effect on monooxygenase activity when NADPH is the only source of electrons and antibody against cytochrome b_5 should relieve this inhibition; i.e., antibody against b_5 should stimulate monooxygenase activity in microsomes that have not been enriched with cytochrome b_5, not inhibit it slightly, as is the case [27,462]. The antibody studies argue strongly against the mechanism of NADH synergism proposed by Schenkman and associates.

A number of factors might explain why exogenous cytochrome b_5 inhibits monooxygenase activity while endogenous cytochrome b_5 does not: (1) It cannot be assumed that exogenous cytochrome b_5 should necessarily interact with cytochrome P-450 like endogenous cytochrome b_5 even though both may function in a like manner with stearoyl CoA-desaturase. Endogenous cytochrome b_5 appears to be distributed uniformly throughout the membrane [463,464] where it may function in the maintenance of the membrane as a component of the desaturase system. Unlike cytochrome b_5, cytochrome P-450 appears to be located in patches throughout the membrane [220-223]. This may suggest that the cytochrome P-450 systems are complexes which function most efficiently when their components form structured units. The addition of exogenous cytochrome b_5 might not disturb a randomly distributed desaturase system, but might disrupt a structured cytochrome P-450 unit by displacing phopholipids or by interfering with the movements of other components of the system. Although cytochrome b_5 may be randomly distributed throughout the membrane, it may not function uniformly. Archakov and coworkers [465-467] presented kinetic evidence for the existence of two pools of cytochrome b_5 in hepatic microsomes and suggested that only about one-fifth to one-third of the cytochrome b_5 participates in the transfer of electrons to cytochrome P-450. Muna and Smuckler [468] observed that while all of the exogenous cytochrome b_5 bound to microsomes was reducible with dithionite, only about 25% of that in excess of endogenous cytochrome b_5 was reducible by NADH. They concluded that only a small fraction of the added cytochrome b_5 was combined with specific binding sites in the membrane. (2) Exogenous cytochrome b_5 might act as an electron sink, in which case its effect could be likened to the inhibition of monooxygenase activity that occurs when cytochrome c is added to microsomes. Cytochrome c inhibits the monooxygenase reaction by competing with ferricytochrome P-450-substrate complex for electrons from NADPH-cytochrome P-450 reductase. (3) Added cytochrome b_5 might participate more actively than endogenous cytochrome b_5 in reactions not directly coupled to the monooxygenase system and thereby divert electrons from cytochrome P-450 that would not normally have been diverted in this fashion by endogenous cytochrome b_5. (4) The possibility that the inhibitory effect of the detergent-solubilized cytochrome b_5 used by Jansson and Schenkman was due to contaminating detergent must also be considered. Small concentrations of detergent are very difficult to detect by conventional methods. A small amount of detergent attached to the hydrophobic region of cytochrome b_5 would have excellent access to the hydrophobic region of cytochrome P-450 where it could exert a greater effect than detergent distributed randomly throughout the membrane. Studies by Cinti and Ozols [469] strongly implicate detergent as the source of inhibition. They repeated the study of Jansson and Schenkman using highly purified detergent-solubilized cytochrome b_5 and observed that it functioned in the desaturase system and inhibited monooxygenase activity. When they used cytochrome b_5 which had been reconstituted from purified apocytochrome b_5 and heme, they found that it functioned in the desaturase system, but did not inhibit monooxygenase activity. They concluded that detergent-free cytochrome b_5 does not inhibit monooxygenase activity when added to microsomes.

Staudt and associates [470] postulated a role of cytochrome b_5 in uncoupled monooxygenase reactions. Certain compounds (e.g., perfluoro-n-hexane) bind to cytochrome P-450 but are not oxidized; the active oxygen is reduced to water rather than incorporated into the compound. The phenomenon is termed uncoupling (see Sec. III.G). These investigators postulated that when uncoupling occurs and both NADH and NADPH are present, active oxygen is reduced to water preferentially by the NADH-cytochrome b_5 system. Electrons from NADPH are thus made more available for the reduction of ferricytochrome P-450-substrate complex and this accounts for NADH synergism. Since NADH synergism is observed with the majority of substrates that have been tested, this interpretation of the mechanism of NADH synergism requires that the majority of substrates be uncoupling agents to some extent. This in turn means that a stoichiometry of NADPH to product formation of greater than unity be observed with the majority of substrates. However, as has been discussed previously (Sec. III.A), this does not appear to be the case. Thus, while the mechanism proposed by Staudt and associates may explain NADH synergism when substrates are uncoupling agents, it does not explain NADH synergism for the most commonly used substrates [405].

Correia and Mannering [139,197] explained NADH synergism on the basis of relative rate limitations imposed by the introduction of the first and second electrons. Their observation that NADH synergism occurs with type I substrates, but not with type II substrates, suggested that when NADPH is the only source of electrons, the rate of entry of the second electron is rate-limiting relative to the rate of entry of the first electron and that the rate of introduction of the first electron becomes rate-limiting only when both NADPH and NADH are present. In accordance with this concept, the introduction of type I substrates creates an increased demand for both first and second electrons. NADPH can satisfy the demand for first electrons, but not for second electrons; i.e., the second electron is rate-limiting. NADH is a more efficient donor of second electrons than NADPH because NADH can provide second electrons to the monooxygenase system via cytochrome b_5, whereas NADPH cannot, or at least not very well. After addition of NADH to the NADPH-supported reaction, second electrons are now more available to the system than first electrons, or at least as available; i.e., the second electron is no longer rate-limiting. However, the rate-limiting step is now functioning at a higher level of electron flux than when NADPH was the sole electron donor. The result is "NADH synergism." NADH synergism is not seen with type II substrates because the first electron is rate-limiting regardless of whether or not NADH is present. The rate of hydroxylation of type II compounds is so slow that the demand for second electrons from NADPH are able to keep pace with the input of first electrons and therefore no benefit is derived from the addition of NADH. Fujita and Peisach [454] have drawn attention to data of Sasame and associates [462] which showed that antibodies to cytochrome b_5 had a greater inhibitory effect on the faster NADPH-supported reactions. They believe this implies that the introduction of the first electron becomes rate-limiting as the rate of reaction increases and the electron transport from cytochrome b_5 becomes more important.

In their recent review, Gander and Mannering [230] point out the precaution that must be taken before assigning a rate-limiting role to a single step of a multistep reaction. The term "rate limitation" can be avoided if one simply recognizes that the monooxygenase reaction is an "internally impeded" reaction when NADPH is the only source of electrons because ferricytochrome P-450-substrate complex and oxyanionferricytochrome P-450-substrate complex complete for electrons from NADPH-cytochrome P-450 reductase. This competitive inhibition is relieved when another source of second electrons replaces those supplied by NADPH. This occurs when electrons from NADH are transferred to oxyanionferricytochrome P-450 via ferrocytochrome b_5. Not only is a better term than "NADH synergism" needed for the phenomenon, but we should discontinue thinking of the NADPH-supported reaction as a "normal" or "physiological" reaction. The complete monooxygenase system as it functions in the hepatocyte consists of cytochrome P-450, cytochrome b_5, NADPH-cytochrome P-450 reductase, NADH-cytochrome b_5 reductase, NADPH, NADH, O_2, and substrate.

The two microsomal electron-transfer systems are designed so that they do not compete with each other for electrons; i.e., NADPH is specific for NADPH-cytochrome P-450 reductase and NADH is specific for NADH-cytochrome b_5 reductase. Bacterial and mitochondrial cytochrome P-450s systems are comprised of a single-electron-transport system consisting of a reductase and an iron-sulfur protein. The dual-electron-transport system of the monooxygenase systems of the hepatic endoplasmic reticulum may represent an evolutionary refinement of the mechanism.

The failure of anti-cytochrome b_5 immunoglobin to inhibit NADPH-supported drug metabolism appreciably [27, 28, 462] suggests that cytochrome b_5 is not a necessary component of cytochrome P-450-dependent systems. Reconstituted cytochrome P-450 systems free of cytochrome b_5 metabolized benzphetamine, cyclohexane, aniline, laurate, chlorobenzene, benzo[a]-pyrene, and N,N-dimethylaniline [57, 421, 449-452]. Depending on the substrate and the species of cytochrome P-450, cytochrome b_5 may enhance, inhibit, or have no effect on the rate of product formation by reconstituted systems. Lu and associates [450] observed an inhibition of benzphetamine demethylation when cytochrome b_5 was added to a system consisting of cytochrome P-450, NADPH, NADPH-cytochrome P-450 reductase and lipid. The addition of NADH and NADH-cytochrome b_5 reductase relieved the inhibition. They suggested that the observed synergistic effect of NADH on the demethylation of benzphetamine by microsomes may be due to a prevention of the inhibition of the reaction by cytochrome b_5. This seems unlikely in view of the failure of anti-cytochrome b_5 immunoglobin to enhance NADPH-supported drug demethylation by microsomes [27, 28, 462]. The hydroxylation of BP by a reconstituted system consisting of cytochrome P-448, NADPH-cytochrome P-450 reductase, NADPH, and lipid was not inhibited by cytochrome b_5. When NADH, NADH-cytochrome b_5 reductase, and cytochrome b_5 were added to this system, BP hydroxylation was increased by an amount that could be accounted for by the NADH-dependent hydroxylation pathway via NADH-cytochrome b_5 reductase and cytochrome b_5; i.e., no NADH synergism was observed.

The hydroxylation of chlorobenzene by a reconstituted system containing cytochrome P-450, NADPH, NADPH-cytochrome P-450 reductase, and lipid was doubled when cytochrome b_5 was added, even though NADH and NADH-cytochrome b_5 reductase were not present [449]. No cytochrome b_5-induced increase in chlorobenzene hydroxylation occurred when cytochrome P-448 was substituted for cytochrome P-450 in the system.

Imai and Sato [421] observed a stimulation rather than an inhibition of benzphetamine demethylation when they added cytochrome b_5 to a reconstituted system containing cytochrome P-450, NADPH, NADPH-cytochrome b_5 reductase, and sodium cholate. A similar result was obtained when N,N-dimethylaniline was the substrate. The increased amount of formaldehyde formed from benzphetamine or N,N-dimethylaniline in this system was considerably less than the amount of NADPH oxidized, but the stoichiometry approached unity when cytochrome b_5 was added. Thus, cytochrome b_5 improved the coupling of NADPH oxidation to demethylation. When cytochrome b_5, NADH, and NADH-cytochrome b_5 reductase were added to the system, benzphetamine demethylation was synergized and the oxidation of NADH accounted for all of the second electrons required for the reaction.

They concluded that cytochrome b_5 functioned in their reconstituted system both by improving coupling and by supplying second electrons.

The membrane both restricts and directs the activity of its enzymes; the absence of these restraints in reconstituted systems may account for those effects of cytochrome b_5 observed with reconstituted systems which differ from those observed with microsomes.

G. Uncoupling

Certain compounds bind to cytochrome P-450 and stimulate oxygen uptake without incorporating active oxygen. The phenomenon is called "uncoupling" [471-473]; compounds that produce the effect are called "uncoupling agents." Some compounds (e.g., perfluoro-n-hexane) are complete uncoupling agents, whereas others (n-hexane, hexobarbital, benzphetamine) are partial uncouplers, i.e., they incorporate part of the generated active oxygen. With regard to cytochrome P-450 systems, two kinds of uncoupling agents have been described: (1) compounds which produce increased formation of water; and (2) compounds which cause the formation of hydrogen peroxide. With uncoupling agents of the first type, two moles of NADPH are used per mole of oxygen; with the second type, the increased rate of oxygen utilization is accompanied by an equivalent increase in the rate of NADPH oxidation. In either case, if uncoupling is complete, no product is formed. Of the known uncoupling agents of the first type (perfluoro-n-hexane, n-hexane) none was also an uncoupling agent of the second type [470,472]. It is not known why compounds uncouple reactions by different mechanisms.

Possible mechanisms by which cytochrome P-450 systems are believed to form hydrogen peroxide are shown in Fig. 12. $Fe^{3+} \cdot O_2^- \cdot R$ dissociates to give ferricytochrome P-450-substrate complex and the superoxide anion, which forms hydrogen peroxide by dismutation ($2O_2 + 2H^+ \rightleftarrows H_2O_2 + O_2$). $Fe^{3+} \cdot O_2 \cdot R$ may undergo further reduction (introduction of the second electron) to form the peroxide anion derivative, P-450-$Fe^{3+} \cdot O_2^-$, which is protonated and dissociated to H_2O_2. Which of these two mechanisms accounts for hydrogen peroxide generation is still a matter of speculation. However, the observation that NADH does not synergize endogenous hydrogen peroxide formation by PB microsomes favors the dismutation mechanism. NADH synergism is believed to be due to facilitation of the introduction of the second electron (Sec. III.F); the lack of NADH synergism suggests that H_2O formation occurs before the peroxide anion is formed. We have observed that NADH synergizes benzphetamine-induced hydrogen peroxide generation in control microsomes, but not in PB microsomes [423]. This might suggest not only that both mechanisms of hydrogen peroxide formation can occur, but also that the species of cytochrome P-450 may determine which mechanism prevails.

Gillette and associates [474] observed as early as 1957 that hydrogen peroxide is generated when microsomes are incubated with NADPH. Hydrogen

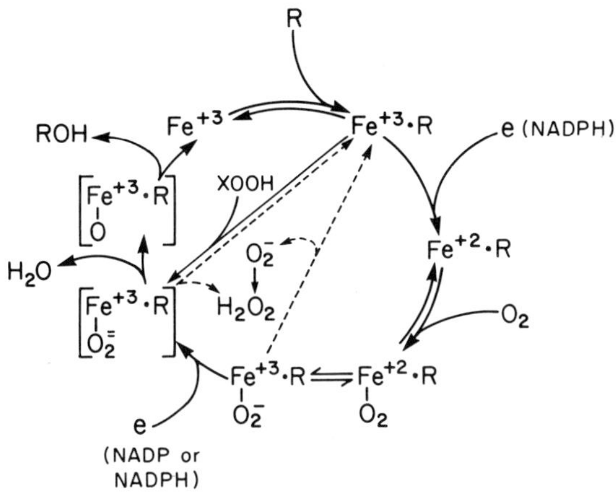

FIGURE 12 Proposed mechanisms of hydrogen peroxide generation by cytochrome P-450 systems. (Modification of a figure from Ref. 476.)

peroxide is converted to water in microsomal preparations by adventitious catalase that adheres to the microsomes during their preparation. This conversion can be avoided by adding a catalase inhibitor such as azide or by introducing methanol and catalase to form the catalase $\cdot H_2O_2\cdot$ methanol complex which dissociates to form formaldehyde, a readily assayable product. The latter method is preferred because accumulated hydrogen peroxide is lost, at least in part through the peroxidative action of cytochrome P-450 [475]. The apparent involvement of cytochrome P-450 in the formation of hydrogen peroxide by microsomes was demonstrated through the use of cytochrome P-450 inhibitors. Carbon monoxide inhibits H_2O_2 formation. Moreover, the extent of the inhibition of H_2O_2 generation caused by various mixtures of O_2 and CO was almost identical to the inhibition of ethylmorphine N-demethylation observed with the same gas mixtures [476]. On the other hand, a concentration of metyrapone that caused a 90% inhibition of ethylmorphine N-demethylation inhibited H_2O_2 production by only 50%. This was interpreted "to imply that all forms of cytochrome P-450 present in liver microsomes can participate in hydrogen peroxide formation whereas a unique metyrapone binding form functions in ethylmorphine N-demethylation reactions." Alternatively, it might be concluded that essentially all of whatever percentage of the cytochrome P-450 that is responsible for ethylmorphine N-demethylation is inhibited by metyrapone, whereas only 50% of whatever percentage of the cytochrome P-450 that is capable of producing hydrogen peroxide is inhibited by metyrapone. The observations that the K_m (NADPH), activation energy, and effect of pH were the same for hydrogen peroxide formation and ethylmorphine N-demethylation further strengthened the view that cytochrome P-450 is involved in both reactions [476].

The mechanism by which NADPH causes the formation of hydrogen peroxide in microsomes in the absence of exogenous substrate is not understood. If the hydrogen peroxide is produced by one or both of the mechanism shown in Fig. 12, active oxygen must be preceded by the binding to cytochrome P-450 of endogenous substrates or membrane components that are uncoupling agents. The mechanism by which exogenous substrates induce hydrogen peroxide formation is also not well understood, but it seems likely that most if not all of these substrates will be found to produce uncoupling by forming intermediate metabolites which bind strongly to cytochrome P-450 thereby producing a "defective" cytochrome P-450 that can no longer transfer active oxygen to the substrate efficiently. Benzphetamine, the most studied inducer of hydrogen peroxide formation in microsomes, undergoes several sequential oxidations [477]:

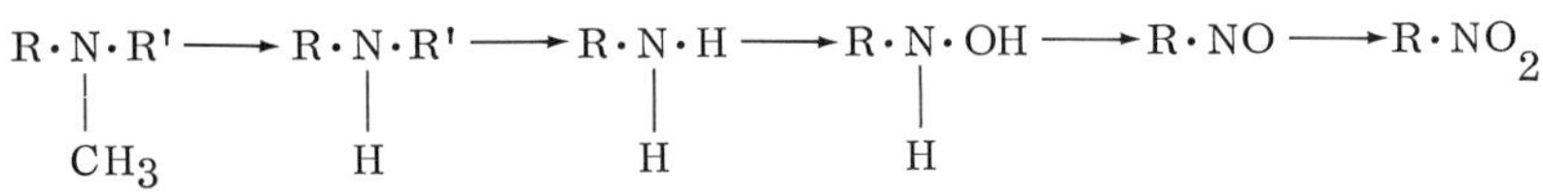

R·NO forms a complex with P-450 that elicits an absorption peak at 455 nm (see Ref. 448 for review). Hexobarbital, which is also known to induce hydrogen peroxide formation, does not produce an absorption peak indicative of a metabolite adduct. However, we have recently obtained indirect evidence that it may in fact form a stable cytochrome P-450 adduct when incubated with microsomes [423]. SKF-525A forms a stable adduct with cytochrome P-450 which has an absorption maximum at 452 nm. These adducts impair CO binding. The addition of ferricyanide removes the adduct and restores CO binding [478]. CO binding is also decreased in microsomes that have been incubated with hexobarbital, and this is restored by ferricyanide; thus it would appear that like SKF-525A and benzphetamine, hexobarbital forms an adduct that inhibits CO binding.

Our recent observation [423] that benzphetamine induces hydrogen peroxide formation in PB microsomes, but not in control microsomes, suggests that substrate induced hydrogen peroxide generation may relate to the species of cytochrome P-450 involved as well as to the substrate. We also observed that benzphetamine does not induce hydrogen peroxide production in 3MC microsomes. A concentration of benzphetamine that produced the adduct with the absorption maximum at 455 nm in PB microsomes did not cause the peak to appear in control microsomes. When PB microsomes are used, hydrogen peroxide production is increased when the concentration of benzphetamine is increased from 0.05 mM to 1 mM, but the formation of the 455-nm absorption peak is decreased. This suggests that the intermediate metabolite responsible for hydrogen peroxide generation is not the nitroso derivative.

Eventually it may be possible to identify substrates that stimulate hydrogen peroxide generation by their chemical structures. We have observed that with the exception of barbital, which is not metabolized by microsomes, all of the barbiturates we have tested induce hydrogen peroxide formation in both control and PB microsomes, including hexobarbital, PB, amobarbital, pentobarbital, and secobarbital [423]. No induction of hydrogen peroxide generation was seen in either control or PB microsomes when ethylmorphine, codeine, or aminopyrine was the substrate.

Although the evidence for direct involvement of cytochrome P-450 in H_2O_2 formation seems quite convincing, an alternative mechanism can be postulated which implicates flavoprotein as the primary site. The possibility that hydrogen peroxide is produced by the donation of electrons from NADPH-cytochrome P-450 reductase has been generally dismissed on the basis that hydrogen peroxide production is inhibited by CO, which inhibits cytochrome P-450, but not the reductase. However, my colleague Elizabeth Jeffery has pointed out that the semiquinone forms of the flavoprotein are unstable and might readily reduce O_2 to superoxide, which would condense to form hydrogen peroxide. Hydrogen peroxide production would then depend upon the concentration of the two semiquinones, which in turn may be controlled by the NADP-NADPH couple and the rate at which cytochrome P-450 accepts electrons from $RF_1H_2F_2H_2$ to form $RF_1H_2F_2H\cdot$ (Sec. III.C). Thus hydrogen peroxide formation may be controlled rather than formed by cytochrome P-450.

An observation of Mason and Holtzman [479] suggests still another mechanism for the formation of hydrogen peroxide. Nitroreduction of a variety of compounds is mediated by NADPH-cytochrome P-450 reductase under anaerobic conditions. Mason and Holtzman observed that nitroreduction does not occur in an atmosphere of oxygen, but uptake of O_2 is increased by the substrate. They suggest that under these conditions the flavoprotein transfers an electron to the substrate and the substrate forms superoxide by donating an electron to O_2. Superoxide, and subsequently hydrogen peroxide, could be produced in the manner suggested by the studies of Mason and Holtzman if cytochrome P-450 were to convert a substrate to a metabolite that could undergo nitroreduction under anaerobic conditions. In fact, benzphetamine is metabolized to 2-nitro-1-phenylpropane, a suitable substrate for nitroreduction.

Because uncoupling aborts electrons and active oxygen, the question may be raised as to its physiological significance. Is the generation of toxic oxygen radicals and hydrogen peroxide a price that must be paid for the benefits derived from monooxygenase systems, or is hydrogen peroxide formation by microsomes an artifact? The possibility should be considered that the conversion of the endoplasmic reticulum to microsomes may alter the membrane in such a way that previously unavailble endogenous substrates or membrane components may become available to cytochrome P-450 where they can act as uncoupling agents. Reconstituted systems comprised of purified components produce hydrogen peroxide in amounts equimolar to O_2 and NADPH utilization [480], which may suggest that endogenous substrates are not required for hydrogen peroxide generation. However, the possibility should not be overlooked that impurities or the dilauroyl-GPC used in this study as a required component of the reconstituted system may have acted as an uncoupling agent. The dilauroyl-GPC probably functions by facilitating the binding of the reductase to cytochrome P-450, but it might also uncouple the reaction. As mentioned previously, benzphetamine stimulates hydrogen peroxide production in PB microsomes, but not in control microsomes. The most likely explanation for this is that PB induces species of cytochrome P-450 that can be uncoupled readily by a benzphetamine metabolite and that control microsomes do not contain the kinds of cytochrome P-450 induced by PB. Alternatively, the de novo cytochrome P-450 may be "crowding" the membrane in such a way that it is not "constrained" in the normal manner and is thus more vulnerable to uncoupling. Similar disturbances of the binding of cytochrome P-450 systems to membrane components may occur when microsomes are prepared; thus it cannot be assumed that either endogenous or substrate-induced hydrogen peroxide generation by cytochrome P-450 systems occurs in vivo.

H. The Rate-limiting Step

Many attempts have been made to locate a rate-limiting step in the overall microsomal cytochrome P-450-linked monooxygenase reaction. This section will not summarize the many studies that have led to the claim that one step or another is rate-limiting, a subject that has been discussed thoroughly in Bjorkhem's recent review [481], but will deal with some of the factors that may affect reaction rates of individual steps and with the question of how much significance should be attached to the designation of a rate-limiting step derived from kinetic evaluations of individual steps.

The turnover numbers of several well-known enzymes and the velocities of some commonly studied hepatic monooxygenase reactions obtained under optimal experimental conditions are listed in Table 8. The velocities of the monooxygenase reactions are at least two orders of magnitude lower than the slowest of the other reactions. Monooxygenase reactions are slow because they have very few substrate molecules to react with. In soluble systems, the ratio of substrate to enzyme is usually in the order of 10,000:1 and a velocity approaching the V_{max} can be achieved when high concentrations of substrate are used. However, the substrate for NADPH-cytochrome P-450 reductase is not the exogenous substrate per se, as has so frequently been assumed, but the ferricytochrome P-450-substrate complex. Thus, regardless of the amount of exogenous "substrate" that is made available to the system, the ratio of the true substrate to the reductase cannot exceed the ratio of the number of cytochrome P-450 molecules to reductase molecules. This can only be as high as 10:1 to 30:1 if all of the cytochrome P-450 molecules in the microsomes combine with the added drug-substrate and react with the reductase. The ratio is considerably less than 10:1 to

TABLE 8
Comparison of Reaction Rates of Some Hepatic Cytochrome P-450-linked Monooxygenase Reactions with the Turnover Numbers of Some Common Enzymes

Monooxygenase reactions[a] (nmol substrate transformed/nmol P-450 per min)	
Aminopyrine N-demethylase	13
Ethylmorphine N-demethylase	10
p-Nitrophenetole O-deethylase	3
Hexobarbital hydroxylase	2.5
Aniline hydroxylase	1.2
Other reactions[b] (nmol substrate transformed/nmol of enzyme per min)	
Carbonic anhydrase c	36,000,000
Δ^3-ketosteroid isomerase	17,100,000
Catalase	5,600,000
β-amylase	1,100,000
β-glactosidase	12,500
Phosphoglucomutase	1,240
Succinate dehydrogenase	1,150

[a] Typical rates observed in our laboratory with rat control microsomes.
[b] From Ref. 482.

30:1 because not all species of cytochrome P-450 bind to all added substrates. Michaelis-Menten kinetics is based on the assumption that the concentration of the substrate is greatly in excess of the enzyme, even at the lowest concentrations of substrate. When the ratios of substrate to enzyme become as low as 10 or 30 to 1, the applicability of Michaelis-Menten kinetics can be questioned. It is to be noted that curves usually satisfy criteria of Michaelis-Menten kinetics when reaction rates are plotted against concentrations of added substrate, which means that a first-order substrate-saturable reaction is taking place. However, it is the ferrocytochrome P-450 that is saturable, not the reductase. The mobilities of the components of the system in the membrane impose additional restrictions on the velocity of the reaction. The mobility of the reductase may in fact control the rate of the reaction.

The ability of NADPH-cytochrome P-450 reductase to accept electrons from NADPH is not rate-limiting. When the reductase can be supplied with an abundance of substrate, as is the case when cytochrome c is the electron acceptor, the reaction rate greatly exceeds that of the overall monooxygenase reaction. The turnover number for the reductase when cytochrome c is the electron acceptor is about 4000 but less than 100 when the acceptor is ferricytochrome P-450 [366, 419].

The concentrations of enzyme and substrate, the temperature, and the magnitude of one or more rate constants all contribute to the observed rate of the overall reaction. When any of these factors is altered, an apparent rate limitation may shift from one step to another. For example, ferricytochrome P-450-substrate complex and oxyanionferricytochrome P-450-substrate complex compete for NADPH-cytochrome P-450 reductase, and the ratio of the concentrations of reduced and partially reduced species of reductase depends on the ratio of the concentrations of $NADP^+$ and NADPH at constant pH. A change in the ratio of reductase bound to ferri- and oxyanionferricytochrome P-450-substrate complexes from 80:20 to 20:80 would result in a 16-fold change in the relative rate of the two reductions without changing the observed overall rate of product formation [230]. Thus a reciprocal relationship in the activities of the fiest and second reductions would occur with this change in conditions. The relative concentrations of (1) NADPH-cytochrome P-450 reductase-ferricytochrome P-450-substrate complex, (2) NADPH-cytochrome P-450 reductase-oxyanionferricytochrome P-450-substrate complex, and (3) oxyanionferricytochrome P-450-substrate complex (Fig. 1) will determine the rates at three potentially rate-limiting steps. Thus, any condition which alters the concentration of any species of cytochrome P-450 in a microsomal preparation, the ratio of cytochrome P-450 to NADPH-cytochrome P-450 reductase, or the $NADP^+$/NADPH ratio may result in a shift of the apparent rate-limiting step from one site in the reaction sequence to another site.

Estabrook and coworkers [427, 483] showed that a spectral intermediate appears when ethylmorphine and other type I substrates are metabolized. This intermediate is thought to represent the oxyanionferricytochrome P-450-substrate complex. The addition of NADH to the reaction mixture caused a decrease of the spectral intermediate. This shows an increase in the rate of the second reduction, but does not necessarily locate the rate-limiting step at this site because it does not exclude the possibility that the rate of disappearance of the spectral intermediate is rate-limiting. The proposed intermediate species was detected in PB microsomes but not in control microsomes but not in control microsomes; this illustrates how a change in conditions may change the flux of electrons through the system.

Miwa and associates [484] conclude that the apparent rate-limiting step is determined by a number of factors including the substrate, the kinds of agents used to induce the cytochrome P-450 system, the species and age of the laboratory animal, and other experimental conditions. The fact that there can be an apparent change in the rate-limiting step when experimental conditions change suggests a reciprocal relationship between some of the slower reactions in the system.

If a reaction sequence has a rate-limiting step, then the energy of activation (E_a) of the overall reaction should be neither higher nor lower than that of the rate-limiting step. The E_a of aminopyrine demethylation (12.8 kcal/mol) is about the same as that for cytochrome P-450 reductase (11.2 kcal/mol) [432,417], which suggests that reduction of the ferricytochrome P-450-substrate complex is rate-limiting [481]. However, if the rate-limiting step and some other step have the same E_a, it is not possible to determine which step is rate-limiting on the basis of the E_a of the reaction. An E_a of 16.8 kcal/mol was observed for ethylmorphine N-demethylation [417,433]. Thus, if a rate-limiting step exists in ethylmorphine metabolism, it is not the reduction of the ferricytochrome P-450 substrate complex.

The rate of cleavage of the $C—^2H$ and of the $C—^3H$ bonds are often about two- and threefold slower, respectively, than that of the $C—^1H$ bond. Thompson and Holtzman [485] showed that [$^3H—CH_3$] ethylmorphine was dealkylated 2.5 times more slowly than [$^1H—CH_3$] ethylmorphine, but Miwa and associates [484] found no isotope effect on the demethylation of [$^2H—CH_3$] phentermines. The absence of an isotope effect cannot be used as evidence that a given step in a reaction sequence is not rate-limiting [486]. Thompson and Holtzman used control microsomes, but Miwa and colleagues used PB microsomes. The difference in results obtained by these authors may be another example of how the rate limitation can be changed by conditions.

The studies of Matsubara and coworkers [422] and Guengerich and coworkers [429] suggest that the slowest step occurs after the formation of the oxyferrocytochrome P-450-substrate complex. Guengerich and associates used a reconstituted system composed of photoreduced (methylviologen and light) cytochrome P-450LM, dilauroyl-phosphatidylcholine and benzphetamine to determine the rate constants for the formation of complex I, complex II, and P-450Fe(III) after the addition of O_2:

$$\text{P-450-Fe(II)XH} \xrightarrow[k_1]{O_2} \text{complex I} \xrightarrow{k_2} \text{complex II} \xrightarrow{k_3} \text{P-450-Fe(III)}$$

Addition of NADPH-cytochrome P-450 reductase and NADPH to this system increased the k_3 to 23/min, which corresponds with a k_3 of 24/min for benzphetamine demethylation by the system. While k_3 appears to be the rate-limiting constant in this reconstituted system, it remains to be seen if this is the case in microsomal systems where the membrane imposes restraints that are not readily duplicated outside the microsome.

When the rate constants of the individual steps of a multistep reaction are quite similar, the velocity of the overall reaction will be determined by the combined velocities of all the steps, not by a single step that may be slightly slower than any of the others. This is a principle that has been consistently overlooked by investigators who have attempted to assign a rate-limiting step to a hepatic monooxygenase reaction on the basis that one step is slower than certain other steps and not faster than the overall reaction. The reciprocal of the observed velocity (v_{obs}) of the overall reaction is equal to the sum of the reciprocals of the velocities of each of the steps of the overall reaction [487]:

$$\frac{1}{v_{obs}} = \frac{1}{v_1} + \frac{1}{v_2} + \cdots + \frac{1}{v_n} = \sum_{i=1}^{N} \frac{1}{v_i}$$

where v_1 represents the velocity of each of N steps of the reaction. The hepatic cytochrome P-450-linked monooxygenase system is comprised of at least seven steps (Fig. 1). Therefore, the concept of a rate-limiting step can only be meaningful if the second slowest step is at least 30 times faster than the next slowest step [230]. A difference in velocities of the two slowest steps of this magnitude has not been demonstrated.

When isotopes are employed in attempts to ascertain the rate-limiting step, the maximum isotope effect is observed when the isotope is involved in the rate-limiting step. When this is not the case, the observed isotope effect decreases as the rate of the reaction involving the isotope exceeds that of the rate-limiting step. If the velocity of the step involving the isotope is 30 or more times greater than that of the rate-limiting step, the isotope effect will not be observed [230].

Gander and Mannering [230] conclude that "the concept of a single rate-limiting step for drug metabolism by microsomal systems has many limitations."

IV. CONCLUSIONS

The hepatic cytochrome P-450-linked monooxygenase system consists of an undetermined number of species of cytochrome P-450 associated with NADPH-cytochrome P-450 reductase. When NADH is present as well as NADPH, cytochrome b_5 may donate the second of the two electrons required by monooxygenase reactions. When this is the case, NADH-cytochrome b_5 reductase and cytochrome b_5 should be included as components of the system. It is conceivable that cytochrome b_5 may be a facilitative component of certain P-450 systems, an obligate component of others, nonparticipative in certain systems, and in still other systems the obligate source of both electrons. Whether or not cytochrome b_5 participates or not in a given system may also depend on the substrate, the $NADP^+$/NADPH redox couple, as well as the species of cytochrome P-450.

Many studies which used intact animals and hepatic microsomes provided indirect evidence for the multiplicity of hepatic P-450 cytochromes. More recently, isolation and purification studies have provided direct evidence for at least six molecular species of hepatic cytochrome P-450 which exhibit distinctive patterns of substrate selectivity, electrophoretic mobilities, and immunological reactivities. That several more cytochrome P-450s will be isolated can be predicted from preliminary studies that have been published; the number may be astronomical if a concept recently suggested by Nebert proves to be correct. Nebert [488] has hypothesized that as many species of cytochrome P-450 may exist as there are chemicals capable of inducing this enzyme system. According to his concept, specific cytochrome P-450s are formed by individual hepatocytes in the same manner that immunoglobulins are formed by individual B-lymphocytes. Each immunoglobulin is composed principally of one chain of variable light (V_L), variable heavy (V_H), constant light (C_L), and constant heavy (C_H) chains. B-lymphocytes are differentiated so that each is restricted to synthesizing immunoglobulin with only a single V_L and V_H region. Many thousands of different V_L-V_H paired combinations may develop in one host organism and thus many thousands of antibodies can be formed in response to as many antigens. In theory, hepatocytes would possess a similar system for the formation of specific species of cytochrome P-450 in response to specific chemicals. Each of these cytochrome P-450s would have a high specific activity for the biotransformation of the chemical that induced it, but some other species of the enzyme would also react with that chemical to a lesser extent. This is an intriguing hypothesis that would not only account for the broad substrate selectivity of cytochrome P-450 systems, but would also explain how the liver could "anticipate" the metabolism of a chemical before it had come into existence. Hepatic cytochrome P-450 systems are depressed by agents that modulate immune systems [489-496] and immune systems are depressed by agents that induce hepatic cytochrome P-450 systems [497-499]. This is not only supports Nebert's hypothesis, but suggests that the two systems may interact.

Excellent progress has been made in the past decade on the isolation and purification of P-450 cytochromes; however, the elucidation of molecular structures has just begun. With only about 5% of the amino acid sequence of any purified species of hepatic cytochrome P-450 having been determined, it is too early to predict how closely the molecular structures of individual P-450 cytochromes will resemble one another. Conceivably, it may develop that although individual cytochrome P-450s may differ quite markedly in their structures, they will be classifiable into a small number of groups that categorize these differences. Individual species within each of these groups would then exhibit minor differences which would impart substrate selectivity. In any event, elucidation of the structures of cytochrome P-450s, particularly with reference to the substrate binding site and the liganding of the heme iron, will be essential for a thorough understanding of the monooxygenase reaction. After the molecular properties of the cytochrome P-450s are thoroughly understood, it will be necessary to return to the intact microsomes in order to discover how these enzymatic systems function in their natural environment.

NADPH-cytochrome P-450 reductase, the other major component of the hepatic monooxygenase system, appears to be a single enzyme, but the existence of more than one similar reductase in hepatic microsomes has not been excluded. An interesting feature of this enzyme is that it possesses an FAD and an FMN, which transfer electrons between their partially and fully reduced forms. This offers a variety of possible mechanisms for the transfer of first and second electrons to cytochrome P-450-substrate complexes. The predominance or pattern of electron transfer mechanisms that will exist under a given set of steady-state conditions will depend on the NADPH-$NADP^+$ redox couple, the species of cytochrome P-450, the substrate, and the availability of second electrons from cytochrome b_5. The mechanism of transfer of electrons from the reductase to cytochrome P-450-substrate complexes is not well understood. It is known that FAD is the acceptor of electrons from NADPH and that ferricytochrome P-450-substrate complex is the acceptor of an electron from FAD, but it is now known whether oxyanionferricytochrome P-450 accepts its electron from FAD, from FMN, or from both flavins.

Monooxygenase reactions take place on or near the outer surface of the membrane. Cytochrome P-450 is deeply embedded in the membrane but a small portion is exposed to the surface. The exposed region contains the catalytic and substrate binding sites. NADPH-cytochrome P-450 reductase is comprised of a hydrophilic and a hydrophobic region. The catalytic site resides in the hydrophilic portion. The hydrophobic region, which accounts for about one-tenth of the molecule, is embedded in the membrane to the extent that the catalytic site of the reductase is in juxtaposition with the catalytic site of the cytochrome P-450. Similar hydrophobic regions of NADH-cytochrome b_5 reductase and cytochrome b_5 also provide the opportunity for their interaction at the catalytic site of cytochrome P-450. These cytochrome P-450 molecules are believed to form a rosette around a single molecule of the reductase such that the reductase can react first with one and then with another of the cytochrome P-450 molecules. The suggestion has also been made that the reductase may meander among cytochrome P-450 molecules distributed more or less randomly throughout the membrane [488]. In either event, the kinetics of the overall reaction will depend in part on the rate at which the reductase displaces lipid molecules as it crosses the membrane from one cytochrome P-450 molecule to the other. The membrane both facilitates and restricts monooxygenase reactions in ways that may be difficult, if not impossible, to duplicate exactly in reconstituted systems.

Kinetics of hepatic microsomal monooxygenase systems are extremely complicated because (1) they are membrane-bound systems and thus do not always follow the rules that have been formulated for soluble systems; (2) the overall reaction is comprised of several sequential steps; (3) the membrane contains multiple cytochrome P-450-cytochromes; and (4) the concentration of the substrate binding to the reductase (namely, the ferricytochrome P-450-substrate complex) is limited to the concentration of cytochrome P-450 in the membrane. This last factor accounts for the very slow velocities of the overall reactions. Attempts that have been made to assign a rate-limiting step to microsomal monooxygenase systems have not always taken into account the complexity of these reactions.

ABBREVIATIONS

BP, benzo[a]pyrene; MC, 3-methylcholanthrene; 3MMAB, 3-methyl-4-methylaminoazobenzene; βNF, β napthoflavone; PB, phenobarbital; SKF 525-A, 2-diethylaminoethyl 2,2-diphenylvalerate; TCDD, tetrachlorodibenzo-p-dioxin; control-microsomes, MC-microsomes and PB-microsomes are microsomes obtained from untreated, MC-treated and PB-treated animals, respectively.

REFERENCES

1. G. C. Mueller and J. A. Miller, J. Biol. Chem. 180:1125 (1949).
2. G. C. Mueller and J. A. Miller, J. Biol. Chem. 202:579 (1953).
3. B. B. Brodie, J. Axelrod, J. R. Cooper, L. Gaudette, B. N. La Du, C. Mitoma, and S. Udenfriend, Science 121:603 (1955).
4. B. L. Horecker, J. Biol. Chem. 183:593 (1950).
5. P. Strittmatter and S. F. Velick, J. Biol. Chem. 221:277 (1956).
6. A. H. Phillips and R. G. Langdon, J. Biol. Chem. 237:2652 (1962).
7. C. H. Williams, Jr. and H. Kamin, J. Biol. Chem. 237:587 (1962).
8. H. S. Mason, W. L. Fowlks, and E. Peterson, J. Amer. Chem. Soc. 77:2914 (1955).
9. O. Hayaishi, M. Katagiri, and S. Rothberg, J. Amer. Chem. Soc. 77:5450 (1955).
10. H. S. Mason, Science 125:1185 (1957).
11. O. Hayaishi, in Oxygenases (O. Hayaishi, Ed.). Academic, New York, 1962, pp. 1-29.
12. M. Klingenberg, Arch. Biochem. Biophys. 75:376 (1958).
13. D. Garfinkel, Arch. Biochem. Biophys. 77:493 (1958).
14. T. Omura and R. Sato, J. Biol. Chem. 237:1375 (1962).
15. T. Omura and R. Sato, J. Biol. Chem. 239:2379 (1964).
16. Y. Hashimoto, T. Yamano, and H. S. Mason, J. Biol. Chem. 237:3843 (1962).
17. Y. Ichikawa, B. Hagihara, and T. Yamano, Arch. Biochem. Biophys. 120:204 (1967).
18. Y. Ichikawa and T. Yamano, Arch. Biochem. Biophys. 121:742 (1967).
19. D. Y. Cooper, Life Sci. 13:1151 (1973).
20. K. Ryan and L. Engel, J. Biol. Chem. 225:103 (1957).
21. O. Warburg, Biochem. Z. 177:471 (1926).
22. R. W. Estabrook, D. Y. Cooper, and O. Rosenthal, Biochem. Z. 338:741 (1963).
23. O. Warburg, in Heavy Metal Prosthetic Groups and Enzyme Action. Clarendon Press, Oxford, 1949, Chap. IX, pp. 73-89.
24. D. Y. Cooper, S. Levin, S. Narasimhulu, O. Rosenthal, and R. W. Estabrook, Science 147:400 (1965).

25. D. Y. Cooper, H. Schleyer, O. Rosenthal, W. Levin, A. Y. H. Lu, R. Kuntzman, and A. H. Conney, Eur. J. Biochem. 74:69 (1977).
26. A. Hildebrandt and R. W. Estabrook, Arch. Biochem. Biophys. 143:66 (1971).
27. H. A. Sasame, J. R. Mitchell, S. Thorgeirsson, and J. R. Gillette, Drug Metab. Disp. 1:150 (1973).
28. G. J. Mannering, S. Kuwahara, and T. Omura, Biochem. Biophys. Res. Comm. 57:476 (1974).
29. N. E. Sladek and G. J. Mannering, Biochem. Biophys. Res. Comm. 24:668 (1966).
30. G. J. Mannering, Metabolism 20:228 (1971).
31. A. P. Alvares, G. Schilling, W. Levin, and R. Kuntzman, Biochem. Biophys. Res. Comm. 29:521 (1967).
32. A. G. Hildebrandt, H. Remmer, and R. W. Estabrook, Biochem. Biophys. Res. Comm. 30:607 (1968).
33. J. B. Schenkman, H. Greim, M. Zauge, and H. Remmer, Biochim. Biophys. Acta 171:23 (1969).
34. Y. Imai and P. Siekevitz, Arch. Biochem. Biophys. 144:143 (1971).
35. A. Y. H. Lu and W. Levin, Biochem. Biophys. Res. Comm. 46:1334 (1972).
36. A. Y. H. Lu, R. Kuntzman, S. West, M. Jacobson, and A. H. Conney, J. Biol. Chem. 247:1727 (1972).
37. T. Fujita, D. W. Shoeman, and G. J. Mannering, J. Biol. Chem. 248:2192 (1973).
38. D. W. Nebert, J. K. Heidema, H. W. Strobel, and M. J. Coon, J. Biol. Chem. 248:7631 (1973).
39. Y. Ichikawa and T. Yamano, Biochim. Biophys. Acta 131:490 (1967).
40. Y. Miyake, J. L. Gaylor, and H. S. Mason, J. Biol. Chem. 243:5788 (1968).
41. K. Comai and J. L. Gaylor, J. Biol. Chem. 248:4947 (1973).
42. A. P. Alvares and P. Siekevitz, Biochem. Biophys. Res. Comm. 54:923 (1973).
43. A. F. Welton and S. D. Aust, Biochem. Biophys. Res. Comm. 56:898 (1974).
44. P. E. Thomas, A. Y. H. Lu, D. Ryan, S. West, and W. Levin, Life Sci. 15:1475 (1974).
45. D. Ryan, A. Y. H. Lu, S. West, and W. Levin, J. Biol. Chem. 250:2157 (1975).
46. R. M. Philpot and E. Arinc, Mol. Pharmacol. 12:483 (1976).
47. P. E. Thomas, A. Y. H. Lu, D. Ryan, S. B. West, J. Kawalek, and W. Levin, J. Biol. Chem. 251:1385 (1976).
48. D. A. Haugen, M. J. Coon, and D. W. Nebert, J. Biol. Chem. 251:1817 (1976).
49. M.-T. Huang, S. B. West, and A. Y. H. Lu, J. Biol. Chem. 251:4659 (1976).
50. D. A. Haugen and M. J. Coon, J. Biol. Chem. 251:7929 (1976).

51. E. F. Johnson and U. Müller-Eberhard, J. Biol. Chem. 252:2839 (1977).
52. W. L. Dean and M. J. Coon, J. Biol. Chem. 252:3255 (1977).
53. D. Y. Bell and E. Hodgson, Gen. Pharmac. 8:121 (1977).
54. J. Deutsch, J. C. Leutz, S. K. Yang, H. V. Gelboin, Y. L. Chiang, K. P. Vatsis, and M. J. Coon, Proc. Nat. Acad. Sci. USA 75:3123 (1978).
55. T. M. Guenthner and D. W. Nebert, Eur. J. Biochem. 91:449 (1978).
56. Y. Imai and R. Sato, Biochem. Biophys. Res. Comm. 60:8 (1974).
57. T. A. van der Hoeven, D. A. Haugen, and M. J. Coon, Biochem. Biophys. Res. Comm. 60:569 (1974).
58. A. Y. H. Lu and M. J. Coon, J. Biol. Chem. 243:1331 (1968).
59. A. Y. H. Lu and W. Levin, Biochim. Biophys. Acta 344:205 (1974).
60. A. Y. H. Lu and S. B. West, Pharmacol. Ther., (A) 2:337 (1978).
61. A. Ellin, S. Jakobson, J. B. Schenkman, and S. Orrenius, Arch. Biochem. Biophys. 150:64 (1972).
62. Y. Takesue and R. Sato, J. Biochem. 64:885 (1968).
63. A. P. Poland, E. Glover, J. R. Robinson, and D. W. Nebert, J. Biol. Chem. 249:5599 (1974).
64. G. Betz, P. Tsai, and R. Weakley, J. Biol. Chem. 251:2839 (1976).
65. R. A. Meigs and K. J. Ryan, Biochim. Biophys. Acta 165:470 (1968).
66. J. A. Cohn, A. P. Alvares, and A. Kappas, J. Exp. Med. 145:1607 (1977).
67. B. W. Harding, S. H. Wong, and D. H. Nelson, Biochim. Biophys. Acta 92:415 (1964).
68. J. L. Purvis, J. A. Canick, J. H. Rosenbaum, J. Hologgitas, and S. A. Lafif, Arch. Biochem. Biophys. 159:32 (1973).
69. T. Yohro and S. Horie, J. Biochem. 61:515 (1967).
70. H. L. Henry and A. W. Norman, J. Biol. Chem. 249:7529 (1974).
71. J. G. Ghazarian, C. R. Jefcoate, J. C. Knutson, W. H. Orme-Johnson, and H. F. DeLuca, J. Biol. Chem. 249:3026 (1974).
72. S. Taniguchi, N. Hoshita, and K. Okuda, Eur. J. Biochem. 40:607 (1973).
73. R. Sato, Y. Atsuta, Y. Imai, S. Taniguchi, and K. Okuda, Proc. Nat. Acad. Sci. USA 74:5477 (1977).
74. A. S. Khandwala and C. P. Kasper, Biochem. Biophys. Res. Comm. 54:1241 (1973).
75. D. Garfinkel, Comp. Biochem. Physiol. 8:367 (1963).
76. C. F. Strittmatter and F. T. Umberger, Biochim. Biophys. Acta 180: 18 (1969).
77. A. Morello, W. Bleecka, and M. Agosin, Biochem. J. 124:199 (1971).
78. F. W. Plapp and J. E. Casida, J. Econ. Entomol. 63:1091 (1970).
79. J. Capdevila, N. Ahmad, and M. Agosin, J. Biol. Chem. 250:1048 (1975).
80. P. J. Murphy and C. A. West, Arch. Biochem. Biophys. 133:395 (1969).

81. J. R. M. Potts, R. Weklych, and E. E. Conn, J. Biol. Chem. 249: 5019 (1974).
82. P. R. Rich and D. S. Bendall, Eur. J. Biochem. 55:333 (1975).
83. O. Young and H. Beevers, Phytochemistry 15:372 (1976).
84. K. M. Madyastha, T. D. Meehan, and C. J. Coscia, Biochemistry 15:1097 (1976).
85. K. M. Madyastha, J. E. Ridgeway, J. G. Dwyer, and C. J. Coscia, J. Cell. Biol. 72:302 (1977).
86. A. Lindenmayer and L. Smith, Biochim. Biophys. Acta 93:445 (1964).
87. C. A. Appleby, Biochim. Biophys. Acta 147:399 (1967).
88. M. Katagiri, B. N. Ganguli, and I. C. Gunsalus, J. Biol. Chem. 243:3543 (1968).
89. S. H. Ambike, R. M. Baxter, and N. D. Zahid, Phytochemistry 9: 1959 (1970).
90. G. Cardini and P. Jurtshuk, J. Biol. Chem. 245:2789 (1970).
91. W. Duppel, J.-M. Lebeault, and M. J. Coon, Eur. J. Biochem. 36: 583 (1973).
92. Y. Yoshida, H. Kumaoka, and R. Sato, J. Biochem. 75:1201 (1974).
93. G. Murphy, G. Vogel, G. Krippahl, and F. Lynen, Eur. J. Biochem. 49:443 (1974).
94. A. M. Vygantas and J. M. Corcoran, Fed. Proc. 33:1233 (1974).
95. A. Berg, J.-A. Gustafsson, M. Ingelman-Sundberg, and K. Carlström, J. Biol. Chem. 251:2831 (1976).
96. K. T. W. Alexander, K. A. Mitropoulos, and G. F. Gibbons, Biochem. Biophys. Res. Comm. 60:460 (1974).
97. G. F. Gibbons and K. A. Mitropoulos, Eur. J. Biochem. 40:269 (1973).
98. G. S. Boyd, A. M. Grimwade, and M. E. Lawson, Eur. J. Biochem. 37:334 (1973).
99. E. R. Simpson and G. S. Boyd, Biochem. Biophys. Res. Comm. 24: 110 (1966).
100. R. A. Meigs and K. J. Ryan, J. Biol. Chem. 246:83 (1971).
101. E. A. Thompson, Jr. and P. K. Siiteri, J. Biol. Chem. 249:5373 (1974).
102. M. H. Bhattacharyya and H. F. DeLuca, Arch. Biochem. Biophys. 160:58 (1974).
103. D. E. Nerland and G. J. Mannering, Drug Metab. Disp. 6:150 (1978).
104. D. E. Nerland and G. J. Mannering, unpublished data.
105. S. el Defrawy el Masry, G. M. Cohen, and G. J. Mannering, Drug Metab. Disp. 2:267 (1974).
106. H. L. Richardson and L. Cunningham, Cancer Res. 11:274 (1951).
107. A. H. Conney, E. C. Miller, and J. A. Miller, Cancer Res. 16:450 (1956).
108. H. Remmer, Naturwissenschaften 45:189 (1958).
109. A. H. Conney, Pharmacol. Rev. 19:317 (1967).

110. G. J. Mannering, in Selected Pharmacological Testing Methods (A. Burger, Ed.). Marcel Dekker, New York, 1968, pp. 51-119.
111. R. Kuntzman, Ann. Rev. Pharmacol. 9:21 (1969).
112. G. J. Mannering, in Handbook of Experimental Pharmacology, Vol. 28, Part 2 (B. B. Brodie and J. R. Gillette, Eds.). Springer-Verlag, Berlin, 1971, pp. 452-476.
113. M. W. Anders, Ann. Rev. Pharmacol. 11:37 (1971).
114. N. E. Sladek and G. J. Mannering, Mol. Pharmacol. 5:186 (1969).
115. M. W. Anders and G. J. Mannering, Mol. Pharmacol. 2:319 (1966).
116. V. Ullrich and P. Kremers, Arch. Toxicol. 39:41 (1977).
117. U. Frommer, V. Ullrich, and S. Orrenius, FEBS Lett. 41:14 (1974).
118. V. Ullrich, J. Schadelin, and H. Staudinger, FEBS Symp. 16:261 (1969).
119. V. Ullrich, P. Weber, and P. Wollenberg, Biochem. Biophys. Res. Comm. 64:808 (1975).
120. U. Frommer, V. Ullrich, and H. Staudinger, Hoppe-Seyler's Z. Physiol. Chem. 351:903 (1970).
121. M. D. Burke and R. T. Mayer, Drug Metab. Disp. 3:245 (1975).
122. T. Fischbach and W. Lenk, in Microsomes and Drug Oxidations (V. Ullrich, I. Roots, A. Hildebrandt, R. Estabrook, and A. H. Conney, Eds.). Pergamon, New York, 1977, pp. 39-46.
123. H. G. Selander, D. M. Jerina, and J. W. Daly, Arch. Biochem. Biophys. 168:309 (1975).
124. M. D. Burke and J. W. Bridges, Xenobiotica 5:357 (1975).
125. V. Ullrich, U. Frommer, and P. Weber, Hoppe-Seyler's Z. Physiol. Chem. 354:514 (1973).
126. D. W. Nebert, J. R. Robinson, A. Niwa, K. Kumaki, and A. P. Poland, J. Cell. Physiol. 85:393 (1975).
127. D. W. Nebert and A. R. Boobis, in Biological Reactive Intermediates (D. J. Jallow, J. J. Kocsis, R. Snyder, and H. Vainio, Eds.). Plenum, New York, 1977, pp. 125-145.
128. S. S. Thorgeirsson and D. W. Nebert, Advan. Cancer Res. 25:149 (1977).
129. A. R. Boobis and D. W. Nebert, in Advances in Enzyme Regulation, Vol. 15 (G. Weber, Ed.). Pergamon, New York, 1977, pp. 339-362.
130. D. W. Nebert, Biochimie, 60:1019 (1978).
131. D. W. Nebert, in Pharmacological Intervention in the Aging Process (J. Roberts, R. C. Adelman, and V. J. Cristofalo, Eds.). Plenum, New York, 1978, pp. 55-79.
132. D. W. Nebert and N. M. Nelson, CRC Critical Rev. Biochem. 6:401 (1979).
133. A. R. Boobis, D. W. Nebert, and O. Pelkonen, Biochem. Pharmacol. 28:111 (1979).
134. G. Powis, R. E. Talcott, and J. B. Schenkman, in Microsomes and Drug Oxidations (V. Ullrich, I. Roots, A. Hildebrandt, R. Estabrook, and A. H. Conney, Eds.). Pergamon, New York, 1977, pp. 127-135.

135. S. Cha, Mol. Pharmacol. 4:621 (1968).
136. N. E. Sladek and G. J. Mannering, Mol. Pharmacol. 5:174 (1969).
137. A. P. Alvares and G. J. Mannering, Mol. Pharmacol. 6:206 (1970).
138. G. J. Mannering, unpublished observation.
139. M. A. Correia and G. J. Mannering, Mol. Pharmacol. 9:455 (1973).
140. A. Rubin, T. R. Tephly, and G. J. Mannering, Biochem. Pharmacol. 13:1007 (1964).
141. J. F. Henderson and P. Mazel, Biochem. Pharmacol. 13:1471 (1964).
142. N. E. Sladek, Studies on the stimulation of drug metabolism by phenobarbital and polycyclic hydrocarbons. Ph.D. Thesis, University of Minnesota, 1966.
143. A. P. Alvares, G. R. Schilling, and R. Kuntzman, Biochem. Biophys. Res. Comm. 30:588 (1968).
144. H. L. Gurtoo, T. C. Campbell, R. E. Webb, and K. M. Plowman, Biochem. Biophys. Res. Comm. 31:588 (1968).
145. N. G. Zampaglione and G. J. Mannering, J. Pharmacol. Exp. Ther. 185:676 (1973).
146. D. S. Davies, P. L. Gigon, and J. R. Gillette, Biochem. Pharmacol. 17:1865 (1968).
147. J. A. Castro and J. R. Gillette, Biochem. Biophys. Res. Comm. 28:426 (1967).
148. J. B. Schenkman, I. Frey, H. Remmer, and R. W. Estabrook, Mol. Pharmacol. 3:516 (1967).
149. T. C. Pederson and S. D. Aust, Biochem. Pharmacol. 19:2221 (1970).
150. F. Wada, H. Shimakawa, M. Takasugi, T. Kotake, and Y. Sakamoto, J. Biochem. 64:109 (1968).
151. S. E. Lewis, C. F. Wilkinson, and J. W. Ray, Biochem. Pharmacol. 16:1195 (1967).
152. P. Jenner and B. Testa, in Drug Metabolism Reviews, Vol. 2 (F. J. DiCarlo, Ed.). Marcel Dekker, New York, 1974, pp. 117-184.
153. L. K. Low and N. Castagnoli, Jr., in Annual Reports in Medicinal Chemistry (F. H. Clarke, Ed.). Academic, New York, 1978, pp. 304-315.
154. L. R. Pohl, S. D. Nelson, W. A. Garland, and W. F. Trager, Biomed. Mass Spect. 2:23 (1975).
155. L. R. Pohl, S. D. Nelson, W. R. Porter, W. F. Trager, M. J. Fasco, F. D. Baker, and J. W. Fenton II, Biochem. Pharmacol. 25:2153 (1976).
156. W. F. Trager, in Drug Metabolism Concepts (D. M. Jerina, Ed.). Amer. Chem. Soc. Symposium Series 44, Washington, D.C., 1977, pp. 81-98.
157. L. R. Pohl, W. R. Porter, W. F. Trager, M. J. Fasco, and J. W. Fenton II, Biochem. Pharmacol. 26:109 (1977).
158. W. F. Trager, in Concepts in Drug Metabolism, Part A (P. Jenner and B. Testa, Eds.). Marcel Dekker, New York, 1979, pp. 177-209.

159. Y. Ichikawa and T. Yamano, Biochim. Biophys. Acta 153:753 (1968).
160. C. Hashimoto, Y. Imai, and R. Sato, Seikagaku 48:508 (1976).
161. W. Levin and R. Kuntzman, J. Biol. Chem. 244:3671 (1969).
162. W. Levin and R. Kuntzman, Mol. Pharmacol. 5:499 (1969).
163. W. Levin, D. Ryan, R. Kuntzman, and A. H. Conney, Mol. Pharmacol. 11:190 (1975).
164. U. A. Meyer and H. S. Marver, Science 171:64 (1971).
165. D. P. Tschudy and H. L. Bonkowsky, Fed. Proc. 31:147 (1972).
166. R. Schmid, Drug Metab. Disp. 1:256 (1973).
167. F. De Matteis, Drug Metab. Disp. 1:267 (1973).
168. S. Granick, P. Sinclair, S. Sassa, and G. Grieninger, J. Biol. Chem. 250:9215 (1975).
169. D. M. Bissell and L. E. Hammaker, Arch. Biochem. Biophys. 176: 103 (1976).
170. W. Levin, A. Y. H. Lu, M. Jacobson, R. Kuntzman, J. L. Poyer, and P. B. McCay, Arch. Biochem. Biophys. 158:842 (1973).
171. T. C. Pederson, J. A. Buege, and S. D. Aust, J. Biol. Chem. 248: 7134 (1973).
172. E. Jeffery, A. Kotake, R. el Azhary, and G. J. Mannering, in Microsomes and Drug Oxidations (V. Ullrich, I. Roots, A. Hildebrandt, R. W. Estabrook, and A. H. Conney, Eds.). Pergamon, New York, 1976, pp. 323-330.
173. E. Jeffery, A. Kotake, R. el Azhary, and G. J. Mannering, Mol. Pharmacol. 13:415 (1977).
174. M. M. Iba and G. J. Mannering, unpublished data.
175. P. J. O'Brien and J. Rahimtula, J. Agric. Food Chem., 23:154 (1975).
176. W. Nastainzcyk, H. R. Ruf, and V. Ullrich, Eur. J. Biochem. 60: 615 (1975).
177. T. Yamano and Y. Ichikawa, Pharmacol. Ther., (A) 2:673 (1978).
178. Y. Imai, in Cytochrome P-450 (R. Sato and T. Omura, Eds.). Academic, New York, 1978, pp. 37-72.
179. M. R. Franklin, Mol. Pharmacol. 8:711 (1972).
180. M. R. Franklin, Mol. Pharmacol. 8:722 (1972).
181. J. W. DePierre and L. Ernster, FEBS Lett. 55:18 (1975).
182. M. D. Chaplin and G. J. Mannering, Mol. Pharmacol. 6:631 (1970).
183. K. Takeshige, A. Ito, and S. Minakami, J. Biochem. 72:1361 (1972).
184. F. DeMatteis, in Heme and Hemoproteins (F. De Matteis and W. N. Aldridge, Eds.). Springer-Verlag, New York, 1978, pp. 95-127.
185. J. J. Bradshaw, M. R. Ziman, and K. M. Ivanetich, Biochem. Biophys. Res. Comm. 85:859 (1978).
186. L. Deloria, J. Low, and G. J. Mannering, in Microsomes, Drug Oxidations, and Chemical Carcinogenesis, Vol. II (M. J. Coon, A. H. Conney, R. W. Estabrook, H. V. Gelboin, J. R. Gillette, and P. J. O'Brien, Eds.). Academic, New York, 1980, pp. 861-864.

187. K. M. Ivanetich, J. A. Marsh, J. J. Bradshaw, and L. S. Kaminsky, in Microsomes and Drug Oxidations (V. Ullrich, I. Roots, A. Hildebrandt, R. Estabrook, and A. H. Conney, Eds.). Pergamon, New York, 1977, pp. 76-81.
188. R. D. Gray, J. Biol. Chem. 253:4364 (1978).
189. H. Shigematsu, S. Yamano, and H. Yoshimura, Arch. Biochem. Biophys. 173:178 (1976).
190. T. Kamataki and H. Kitagawa, Biochem. Biophys. Res. Comm. 76: 1007 (1977).
191. P. L. Gigon, T. E. Gram, and J. R. Gillette, Mol. Pharmacol. 5: 109 (1969).
192. J. L. Holtzman and M. L. Carr, Mol. Pharmacol. 8:481 (1972).
193. S. Kuwahara and G. J. Mannering, in Microsomes, Drug Oxidations, and Chemical Carcinogenesis, Vol. II (M. J. Coon, A. H. Conney, R. W. Estabrook, H. V. Gelboin, J. R. Gillette, and P. J. O'Brien, Eds.). Academic, New York, 1980, pp. 973-976.
194. A. H. Conney, R. R. Brown, J. A. Miller, and E. C. Miller, Cancer Res. 17:628 (1957).
195. A. Nilsson and B. C. Johnson, Arch. Biochem. Biophys. 101:494 (1963).
196. V. Ullrich, Hoppe-Seyler's Z. Physiol. Chem. 350:357 (1969).
197. M. A. Correia and G. J. Mannering, Mol. Pharmacol. 9:470 (1973).
198. T. Yamano and T. Iizuka, in Cytochrome P-450 (R. Sato and T. Omura, Eds.). Academic, New York, 1978, pp. 106-126.
199. D. W. Nebert and H. Kon, J. Biol. Chem. 248:169 (1973).
200. D. W. Nebert and J. R. Robinson, J. Biol. Chem. 248:7637 (1973).
201. H. Grasdalen, D. Backström, L. E. G. Ericksson, A. Ehrenberg, P. Moldeus, C. Von Bahr, and S. Orrenius, FEBS Lett. 60:294 (1975).
202. V. Ullrich and W. Duppel, in The Enzymes, Vol. 12 (P. Boyer, Ed.). Academic, New York, 1975, pp. 253-297.
203. A. Y. H. Lu, K. W. Junk, and M. J. Coon, J. Biol. Chem. 244:3714 (1969).
204. H. W. Strobel, A. Y. H. Lu, J. Heidema, and M. J. Coon, J. Biol. Chem. 245:4851 (1970).
205. A. Y. H. Lu, R. Kuntzman, S. West, and A. H. Conney, Biochem. Biophys. Res. Comm. 42:1200 (1971).
206. T. Fujita, D. W. Shoeman, and G. J. Mannering, J. Biol. Chem. 248:2192 (1973).
207. D. Ryan, A. Y. H. Lu, J. Kawalek, S. B. West, and W. Levin, Biochem. Biophys. Res. Comm. 64:1134 (1975).
208. A. P. Alvares and P. Siekevitz, Biochem. Biophys. Res. Comm. 54: 923 (1973).
209. D. Y. Bell and E. Hodgson, Gen. Pharmacol. 8:121 (1977).
210. D. A. Haugen, T. A. van de Hoeven, and M. J. Coon, J. Biol. Chem. 250:3567 (1975).
211. M. J. Coon, D. P. Ballou, D. A. Haugen, S. O. Krezoski, G. D. Nordblom, and R. E. White, in Microsomes and Drug Oxidations

(V. Ullrich, I. Roots, A. Hildebrandt, R. Estabrook, and A. H. Conney, Eds.). Pergamon, New York, 1977, pp. 82-94.
212. M. J. Coon, R. E. White, G. D. Nordblom, D. P. Ballou, and F. P. Guengerich, Croatica Chem. Acta 49:163 (1977).
213. J. A. Gustaffsson and M. Ingelman-Sundberg, Eur. J. Biochem. 64: 35 (1976).
214. E. F. Johnson and U. Müller-Eberhard, Biochem. Biophys. Res. Comm. 76:644 (1977).
215. E. F. Johnson and U. Müller-Eberhard, Biochem. Biophys. Res. Comm. 76:652 (1977).
216. D. E. Ryan, P. E. Thomas, and W. Levin, Mol. Pharmacol. 13:521 (1977).
217. F. P. Guengerich, J. Biol. Chem. 252:3970 (1977).
218. Y. Imai, J. Biochem. 80:267 (1976).
219. M. Warner, M. V. LaMarca, and A. H. Neims, Drug Metab. Disp. 6:353 (1978).
220. H. U. Schulze and H. Staudinger, Hoppe-Seyler's Z. Physiol. Chem. 352:1659 (1971).
221. A. Amar-Costesec, H. Beaufay, M. Wibo, D. Thines-Sempoux, E. Feytmans, M. Robbi, and J. Berthet, J. Cell Biol. 61:201 (1974).
222. R. B. Mailman, L. G. Tate, K. E. Muse, L. B. Coons, and E. Hodgson, Chem.-Biol. Interact. 10:215 (1975).
223. R. B. Mailman, G. T. Barthalmus, K. Muse, and E. Hodgson, Gen. Pharmacol. 8:275 (1977).
224. F. De Matteis, in Proc. 5th Int. Congr. Pharmacol., San Francisco 2:89 (1972).
225. F. De Matteis, FEBS Lett. 6:343 (1970).
226. F. De Matteis, Biochem. J. 124:767 (1971).
227. B. A. Schacter, H. S. Marver, and U. A. Meyer, Biochim. Biophys. Acta 279:221 (1972).
228. B. A. Schacter, H. S. Marver, and U. A. Meyer, Drug Metab. Disp. 1:286 (1973).
229. F. De Matteis and R. G. Sparks, FEBS Lett. 29:141 (1973).
230. J. E. Gander and G. J. Mannering, Pharmacol. Ther. 10:191 (1980).
231. T. Kamataki, D. H. Belcher, and R. A. Neal, Mol. Pharmacol. 12: 921 (1976).
232. F. P. Guengerich, J. Biol. Chem. 253:7931 (1978).
233. J. C. Kawalek, W. Levin, D. Ryan, P. E. Thomas, and A. Y. H. Lu, Mol. Pharmacol. 11:874 (1975).
234. C. Hashimoto and Y. Imai, Biochem. Biophys. Res. Comm. 68:821 (1976).
235. D. A. Haugen, L. G. Armes, K. T. Yasunobu, and M. J. Coon, Biochem. Biophys. Res. Comm. 77:967 (1977).
236. U. K. Laemmli, Nature 227:680 (1970).

237. T. A. van der Hoeven and M. J. Coon, J. Biol. Chem. 249:6302 (1974).
238. L. Spatz and P. Strittmatter, J. Biol. Chem. 248:793 (1973).
239. L. Spatz and P. Strittmatter, Proc. Nat. Acad. Sci. USA 68:1042 (1971).
240. M. Shikita and P. F. Hall, J. Biol. Chem. 248:5598 (1973).
241. M. Shikita and P. F. Hall, J. Biol. Chem. 248:5605 (1973).
242. K. Dus, W. J. Litchfield, A. G. Miguel, T. A. van der Hoeven, D. A. Haugen, W. L. Dean, and M. J. Coon, Biochem. Biophys. Res. Comm. 60:15 (1974).
243. K. Dus, D. Carey, R. Goewert, and R. A. Swanson, in Microsomes and Drug Oxidations (V. Ullrich, I. Roots, A. Hildebrandt, R. Estabrook, and A. H. Conney, Eds.). Pergamon, New York, 1977, pp. 95-102.
244. K. Dus, R. Goewert, C. C. Weaver, D. Carey, and C. A. Appleby, Biochem. Biophys. Res. Comm. 69:437 (1976).
245. M. Tanaka, S. Zeitlin, K. T. Yasunobu, and I. C. Gunsalus, in Iron and Copper Proteins (K. T. Yasunobu, H. F. Mower, and O. Hayaishi, Eds.). Plenum, New York, 1976, pp. 263-269.
246. K. Dus, M. Katagiri, C.-A. Yu, D. L. Erbes, and I. C. Gunsalus, Biochem. Biophys. Res. Comm. 40:1423 (1970).
247. T. Omura and R. Sato, J. Biol. Chem. 239:2370 (1964).
248. M. D. Maines and M. W. Anders, Arch. Biochem. Biophys. 159:201 (1973).
249. M. R. Waterman and H. S. Mason, Arch. Biochem. Biophys. 150:57 (1972).
250. D. Y. Cooper, M. D. Cannon, H. Schleyer, and O. Rosenthal, J. Biol. Chem. 252:4755 (1977).
251. F. P. Guengerich, D. P. Ballou, and M. J. Coon, J. Biol. Chem. 250:7405 (1975).
252. I. C. Gunsalus and J. D. Lipscomb, in The Molecular Basis of Electron Transport (J. Schultz and B. F. Cameron, Eds.). Academic, New York, 1972, pp. 179-192.
253. H. S. Mason, Ann. Rev. Biochem. 34:595 (1965).
254. H. S. Mason, J. C. North, and M. Vanneste, Biochem. Biophys. Res. Comm. 24:1072 (1965).
255. K. Murakami and H. S. Mason, J. Biol. Chem. 242:1102 (1967).
256. C. R. Jefcoate and J. L. Gaylor, Biochemistry 8:3464 (1969).
257. A. Röder and E. Bayer, Eur. J. Biochem. 11:89 (1969).
258. D. W. Smith and R. J. Williams, Struct. Bonding (Berlin) 7:1 (1970).
259. R. Tsai, C. A. Yu, I. C. Gunsalus, J. Peisach, W. E. Blumberg, W. H. Orme-Johnson, and H. Beinert, Proc. Nat. Acad. Sci. USA 66:1157 (1970).
260. H. A. O. Hill, A. Roeder, and R. J. Williams, Naturwissenschaften 57:69 (1970).

261. J. O. Stern and J. Peisach, J. Biol. Chem. 249:7495 (1974).
262. S. Koch, S. C. Tang, R. H. Holm, and R. B. Frankel, J. Amer. Chem. Soc. 97:914 (1975).
263. S. Koch, S. C. Tang, R. H. Holm, R. B. Frankel, and J. A. Ibers, J. Amer. Chem. Soc. 97:916 (1975).
264. J. P. Collman and T. N. Sorrell, J. Amer. Chem. Soc. 97:4133 (1975).
265. T. Watanabe and S. Horie, J. Biochem. 79:829 (1976).
266. C. K. Chang and D. Dolphin, J. Amer. Chem. Soc. 98:1607 (1976).
267. M. Sato, H. Kon, K. Kumaki, and D. W. Nebert, Biochim. Biophys. Acta 498:403 (1977).
268. V. Ullrich, H. H. Ruf, and P. Wende, Croatica Chem. Acta 49:213 (1977).
269. S. G. Sliger, Biochemistry 15:5399 (1976).
270. K. Dus, in The Enzymes of Biological Membranes, Vol. 4 (A. Martinosi, Ed.). Plenum, New York, 1976, p. 213.
271. K. Dus and J. Albin, unpublished results cited by Dus [270].
272. I. C. Gunsalus, J. R. Meeks, J. D. Lipscomb, P. Debrunner, and E. Munck, in Molecular Mechanisms of Oxygen Activation (D. Hayaishi, Ed.). Academic, New York, 1974, p. 559.
273. J. A. Peterson and B. W. Griffin, Drug Metab. Disp. 1:14 (1973).
274. B. W. Griffin and J. A. Peterson, J. Biol. Chem. 250:6445 (1975).
275. S. Maricic, S. Vuk-Parlovic, B. Benko, J. Porok, H. Rein, G. G. Jänig, and K. Ruckpaul, Croatica Chem. Acta 49:323 (1977).
276. K. Kumaki and D. W. Nebert, Pharmacology 17:262 (1978).
277. J. C. Schäffer and C. K. Jörgensen, J. Inorg. Nucl. Chem. 8;143 (1958).
278. H. Rein and O. Ristau, Pharmazie 33:325 (1978).
279. P. George, J. Beelestone, and J. S. Griffith, Rev. Med. Phys. 36:44 (1964).
280. J. Blanck and W. Scheler, Acta Biol. Med. Ger. 25:29 (1970).
281. M. Sharrock, E. Münck, P. G. Debrunner, V. Marshall, J. D. Lipscomb, and I. C. Gunsalus, Biochemistry 12:258 (1973).
282. T. Iizuka, M. Kotani, and T. Yonetani, J. Biol. Chem. 246:4731 (1971).
283. T. Yonetani, T. Iizuka, T. Asakura, J. Otsuka, and M. Kotani, J. Biol. Chem. 247:863 (1972).
284. H. Nishibayashi and R. Sato, J. Biochem. 63:766 (1968).
285. H. Nishibayashi, T. Omura, R. Sato, and R. W. Estabrook, in Structure and Function of Cytochromes (K. Okunuki, M. D. Kamen, and I. Sekuzu, Eds.). University of Tokyo Press, Tokyo, 1968, p. 658.
286. T. Kinoshita and S. Horie, J. Biochem. 61:26 (1967).
287. M. J. Coon, personal communication.

288. A. G. Hildebrandt and R. W. Estabrook, in Microsomes and Drug Metabolism (J. R. Gillette, A. H. Conney, G. J. Cosmides, R. W. Estabrook, J. R. Fouts, and G. J. Mannering, Eds.). Academic, New York, 1969, pp. 331-347.
289. C. R. E. Jefcoate, J. L. Gaylor, and R. L. Calabrese, Biochemistry 8:3455 (1969).
290. C. R. E. Jefcoate, R. L. Calabrese, and J. L. Gaylor, Mol. Pharmacol. 6:391 (1970).
291. J. D. Lipscomb, Ph.D. Thesis. University of Illinois, Urbana, 1974.
292. M. M. Iba, D. E. Nerland, and G. J. Mannering, in Microsomes, Drug Oxidations, and Chemical Carcinogenesis, 4th Int. Symp. Microsomes and Drug Oxidation, Vol. I (M. J. Coon, A. H. Conney, R. W. Estabrook, H. V. Gelboin, J. R. Gillette, and P. J. O'Brien, Eds.). Academic, New York, pp. 151-154.
293. D. L. Cinti, S. G. Sligar, G. G. Gibson, and J. B. Schenkman, Biochemistry 18:36 (1979).
294. S. Narasimhulu, Fed. Proc. 22:530 (1963).
295. S. Narasimhulu, D. Y. Cooper, and O. Rosenthal, Life Sci. 4:2101 (1965).
296. H. Remmer, J. Schenkman, R. W. Estabrook, H. Sasame, J. Gillette, S. Narasimhulu, D. Y. Cooper, and O. Rosenthal, Mol. Pharmacol. 2:187 (1966).
297. Y. Imai and R. Sato, Biochem. Biophys. Res. Comm. 22:620 (1966).
298. J. A. Peterson, V. Ullrich, and A. G. Hildebrandt, Arch. Biochem. Biophys. 145:531 (1971).
299. D. Mansuy, W. Duppel, H. H. Ruf, and V. Ullrich, Hoppe-Seyler's Z. Physiol. Chem. 355:1341 (1974).
300. V. Ullrich, W. Nastainczyk, and H. H. Ruf, Biochem. Soc. Transactions 3:803 (1975).
301. W. Nastainczyk, H. H. Ruf, and V. Ullrich, Chem.-Biol. Interact. 14:251 (1976).
302. J. B. Schenkman, Biochemistry 9:2081 (1970).
303. J. B. Schenkman, D. L. Cinti, S. Orrenius, P. Moldeus, and R. Kraschnitz, Biochemistry 11:4243 (1972).
304. F. M. Coujon, D. W. Nebert, and J. E. Gielen, Mol. Pharmacol. 8:667 (1972).
305. G. M. Cohen and G. J. Mannering, Drug Metab. Disp. 2:285 (1974).
306. D. Kupfer and S. Orrenius, Mol. Pharmacol. 6:221 (1970).
307. S. Orrenius, D. Kupfer, and L. Ernster, FEBS Lett. 6:249 (1970).
308. A. Ellin, S. Orrenius, A. Pilotti, and C. G. Swahn, Arch. Biochem. Biophys. 158:597 (1973).
309. S. Burstein, N. Co, M. Gut, H. Schleyer, D. Y. Cooper, and O. Rosenthal, Biochemistry 11:573 (1972).
310. H. Diehl, J. Schadelin, and V. Ullrich, Hoppe-Seyler's Z. Physiol. Chem. 351:1359 (1970).

311. M. R. Waterman, V. Ullrich, and R. W. Estabrook, Arch. Biochem. Biophys. 155:355 (1973).
312. J. O. Stern, J. Peisach, W. E. Blumberg, A. Y. H. Lu, and W. Levin, Arch. Biochem. Biophys. 156:404 (1973).
313. K. Kumaki, M. Sato, H. Kon, and D. W. Nebert, J. Biol. Chem. 253:1048 (1978).
314. J. Werringloer, S. Kawano, and R. W. Estabrook, Pharmacologist 20:170 (1978).
315. H. Rein, O. Ristau, J. Friedrich, G.-R. Jänig, and K. Ruckpaul, FEBS Lett. 75:19 (1977).
316. W. C. Pierson and D. L. Cinti, Biochem. Biophys. Res. Comm. 78: 1139 (1977).
317. O. Ristau, H. Rein, G.-R. Jänig, and K. Ruckpaul, cited by Rein and Ristau [278], 1978.
318. I. C. Gunsalus, J. R. Meeks, J. D. Lipscomb, D. Debrunner, and E. Munck, in Molecular Mechanisms of Oxygen Activation (O. Hayaishi, Ed.). Academic, New York, 1974, pp. 559-613.
319. I. C. Gunsalus and G. C. Wagner, in Methods of Enzymology, Vol. 52 (S. Fleischer and L. Packer, Eds.). Academic, New York, 1978, pp. 166-188.
320. J. R. Gillette in Drugs and Enzymes, Proceedings of the Second International Pharmacological Meeting. Pergamon, Oxford, 1965, pp. 9-22.
321. S. Orrenius, B. J. Wilson, C. von Bahr, J. B. Schenkman, in Biological Hydroxylation Mechanisms (G. S. Body and R. M. Smellie, Eds.). Academic, New York, 1972, pp. 55-77.
322. I. Jansson, S. Orrenius, L. Ernster, and J. B. Schenkman, Arch. Biochem. Biophys. 151:391 (1972).
323. M. H. Bickel and J. W. Steele, Chem.-Biol. Interact. 8:151 (1974).
324. D. S. Sitar and G. J. Mannering, Biochem. Pharmacol. 26:988 (1977).
325. A. L. Ibbetson and R. B. Freedman, Biochem. Soc. Trans. 2:343 (1974).
326. G. Parry, D. N. Palmer, and D. J. Williams, FEBS Lett. 67:123 (1976).
327. J. W. DePierre and L. Ernster, Ann. Rev. Biochem. 46:201 (1977).
328. R. E. Ebel, D. H. O'Keeffe, and J. A. Peterson, J. Biol. Chem. 253:3888 (1978).
329. W. Levin, D. Ryan, S. West, and A. Y. H. Lu, J. Biol. Chem. 249: 1747 (1974).
330. M. J. Coon, D. A. Haugen, F. P. Guengerich, J. L. Vermilion, and W. L. Dean, in The Structural Basis of Membrane Function (Y. Hatefi and L. Djavadi-Ohaniance, Eds.). Academic, New York, 1976, pp. 409-427.
331. Y. Imai and R. Sato, J. Biochem. 62:464 (1967).
332. Y. Imai and R. Sato, J. Biochem. 63:270 (1968).

333. Y. Imai and H. S. Mason, unpublished data cited by Y. Imai, in Cytochrome P-450 (R. Sato and T. Omura, Eds.). Academic, New York, 1978, p. 63.
334. Y. Imai and R. Sato, J. Biochem. 75:689 (1974).
335. S. A. Atlas, A. R. Boobis, J. S. Felton, S. S. Thorgiersson, and D. W. Nebert, J. Biol. Chem. 252:4712 (1977).
336. R. C. Sanborn and C. M. Williams, J. Gen. Physiol. 33:579 (1950).
337. A. M. Pappenheimer, Jr., and C. M. Williams, J. Biol. Chem. 209:915 (1954).
338. B. Chance and G. R. Williams, J. Biol. Chem. 209:945 (1954).
339. C. F. Strittmatter and E. G. Ball, Proc. Nat. Acad. Sci. USA 38: 19 (1952).
340. S. F. Velick and P. Strittmatter, J. Biol. Chem. 221:265 (1956).
341. B. Hagihara and E. Furuya, Pharmacol. Ther., (A) 2:537 (1978).
342. I. Raw and W. Colli, Nature 184:1798 (1959).
343. A. Tsugita, M. Kobayashi, T. Kajihara, and B. Hagihara, J. Biochem. 64:727 (1968).
344. J. Ozols and P. Strittmatter, J. Biol. Chem. 243:3367 (1968).
345. J. Ozols and P. Strittmatter, J. Biol. Chem. 243:3376 (1968).
346. A. Tsugita, M. Kobayashi, S. Tani, S. Kyo, M. A. Rashid, Y. Yushida, T. Kajihara, and B. Hagihara, Proc. Nat. Acad. Sci. USA 67:442 (1970).
347. F. G. Nobrega and J. Ozols, J. Biol. Chem. 246:1706 (1971).
348. J. Ozols, C. Gerard, and F. G. Nobrega, J. Biol. Chem. 251:6767 (1976).
349. M. A. Rashid, B. Hagihara, M. Kobayashi, S. Tani, and A. Tsugita, J. Biochem. 74:985 (1973).
350. F. S. Mathews and P. Strittmatter, J. Molec. Biol. 41:295 (1969).
351. A. Ito and R. Sato, J. Biol. Chem. 243:4922 (1968).
352. L. Spatz and P. Strittmatter, Proc. Nat. Acad. Sci. USA 68:1042 (1971).
353. L. Visser, C. Neal, N. C. Robinson, and C. Tanford, Biochemistry 14:1194 (1975).
354. P. J. Fleming, H. A. Dailey, D. Corcoran, and P. Strittmatter, J. Biol. Chem. 253:5369 (1978).
355. N. Oshino, Y. Imai, and R. Sato, 7th International Congress of Biochemistry. Tokyo, 1967, p. 725 (abstract).
356. D. K. Bloomfield and K. Bloch, J. Biol. Chem. 235:337 (1960).
357. W. Stoffel, Biochem. Biophys. Res. Comm. 6:270 (1961).
358. J. B. Marsh and A. T. James, Biochim. Biophys. Acta 60:320 (1962).
359. N. Oshino, Pharmacol. Ther., (A) 2:477 (1978).
360. C. F. Strittmatter, in Haematin Enzymes, Vol. 2 (J. E. Folk, R. Lemberg, and R. K. Morton, Eds.). Pergamon, New York, 1961, pp. 461-473.

361. P. Strittmatter, in The Enzymes (P. D. Boyer, H. A. Lardy, and K. Myrbäck, Eds.). Academic, New York, 1963, pp. 113-145.
362. B. S. S. Masters, H. Kamin, Q. H. Gibson, and C. H. Williams, Jr., J. Biol. Chem. 240:921 (1965).
363. T. Iyanagi and H. S. Mason, Biochemistry 12:2297 (1973).
364. Y. Yasukochi and B. S. S. Masters, J. Biol. Chem. 251:5337 (1976).
365. J. A. Knapp, J. D. Dignam, and H. W. Strobel, J. Biol. Chem. 252: 437:(1977).
366. J. L. Vermilion and M. J. Coon, J. Biol. Chem. 253:2694 (1978).
367. A. F. Welton, T. C. Pederson, J. A. Buege, and S. D. Aust, Biochem. Biophys. Res. Comm. 54:161 (1973).
368. M. J. Coon, J. L. Vermilion, K. P. Vatsis, J. S. French, W. L. Dean, and D. A. Haugen, in Drug Metabolism Concepts (D. M. Jerina, Ed.). American Chemical Society Symposium Series, No. 44, American Chemical Society, Washington, D.C., 1977, pp. 46-71.
369. T. Iyanagi, Biochemistry 16:2725 (1977).
370. J. L. Vermilion and M. J. Coon, J. Biol. Chem. 253:8812 (1978).
371. L. Sagan, J. Theoret. Biol. 14:225 (1967).
372. V. R. Potter, J. Biol. Chem. 165:311 (1946).
373. G. H. Hogeboom, J. Biol. Chem. 177:847 (1949).
374. M. Bailie and R. K. Morton, Nature 176:111 (1955).
375. P. Strittmatter and S. F. Velick, J. Biol. Chem. 228:785 (1957).
376. S. Takesue and T. Omura, J. Biochem. 67:259 (1970).
377. S. Takesue and T. Omura, J. Biochem. 67:267 (1970).
378. T. Omura, P. Siekevitz, and G. E. Palade, J. Biol. Chem. 242:2389 (1967).
379. T. Kajihara and B. Hagihara, J. Biochem. 63:453 (1968).
380. A. Ito and R. Sato, J. Cell Biol. 40:179 (1969).
381. K. Mihara and R. Sato, J. Biochem. 78:1057 (1975).
382. M. J. Rogers and P. Strittmatter, J. Biol. Chem. 248:800 (1973).
383. M. J. Rogers and P. Strittmatter, J. Biol. Chem. 250:5713 (1975).
384. D. F. H. Wallach and P. H. Zahler, Proc. Nat. Acad. Sci. USA 56: 1552 (1966).
385. S. J. Singer and G. L. Nicolson, Science 175:720 (1972).
386. R. W. Estabrook, J. Werringloer, B. S. S. Masters, H. Jonen, T. Matsubara, R. Ebel, D. O'Keefe, and J. A. Peterson, in The Structural Basis of Membrane Function (Y. Hatefi and L. Djavadi-Ohaniance, Eds.). Academic, New York, 1976, pp. 429-445.
387. B. F. Trump, S. M. Duttera, W. L. Byrne, and A. V. Arstila, Proc. Soc. Nat. Acad. Sci. USA 66:433 (1970).
388. G. Dallner and L. Ernster, J. Histochem. Cytochem. 16:611 (1968).
389. C. J. Scandella, P. Devaux, and H. M. McConnell, Proc. Nat. Acad. Sci. USA 69:2056 (1972).
390. S. Wu and H. M. McConnell, Biochemistry 14:847 (1975).

391. E. J. Luna and H. M. McConnell, Biochim. Biophys. Acta 470:303 (1977).
392. A. Stier and E. Sackman, Biochim. Biophys. Acta 331:400 (1973).
393. A. Stier, W. Kühnle, and R. Rösen, Hoppe-Seyler's Z. Physiol. Chem. 357:1057 (1976).
394. P. C. Jost, O. H. Griffith, R. A. Capaldi, and G. Vanderkooi, Proc. Nat. Acad. Sci. USA 70:480 (1973).
395. G. B. Warren, P. A. Toon, M. J. M. Birdsall, A. G. Lee, and J. C. Metcalfe, Proc. Nat. Acad. Sci. USA 71:622 (1974).
396. M. Nakamura and S. Ohnishi, J. Biochem. 78:1039 (1975).
397. J. J. Baldassare, K. B. Rhinehart, and D. F. Silbert, Biochemistry 15:2986 (1976).
398. J. J. Baldassare, G. M. Brenckle, M. Hoffman, and D. F. Silbert, J. Biol. Chem. 252:8797 (1977).
399. M. C. Phillips, R. M. Williams, and D. Chapman, Chem. Phys. Lipids 3:234 (1969).
400. H. Träuble and E. Sackmann, J. Am. Chem. Soc. 94:4499 (1972).
401. D. W. Shoeman, J. G. White, and G. J. Mannering, Pharmacologist 12:260 (1970).
402. A. Y. H. Lu and M. J. Coon, J. Biol. Chem. 243:1331 (1968).
403. B. S. Cohen and R. W. Estabrook, Arch. Biochem. Biophys. 143:46 (1971).
404. M. K. Buening and M. R. Franklin, Mol. Pharmacol. 10:999 (1974).
405. E. H. Jeffery and G. J. Mannering, Mol. Pharmacol. 15:396 (1979).
406. E. H. Jeffery and G. J. Mannering, Mol. Pharmacol. 10:1004 (1974).
407. B. Stripp, N. Zampaglione, M. Hamrick, and J. R. Gillette, Mol. Pharmacol. 8:189 (1972).
408. K. M. Kadish and D. G. Davis, Ann. New York Acad. Sci. 206:495 (1973).
409. P. M. Champion, E. Münck, P. G. Debrunner, T. H. Moss, J. D. Lipscomb, and I. C. Gunsalus, Biochim. Biophys. Acta 376:579 (1975).
410. G. J. Mannering, in Drugs and Cell Regulation: Organizational and Pharmacological Aspects on the Molecular Level (E. Mihich, Ed.). Academic, New York, 1971, pp. 197-225.
411. M. R. Waterman and H. S. Mason, Biochem. Biophys. Res. Comm. 39:450 (1970).
412. D. Y. Cooper, H. Schleyer, and O. Rosenthal, Hoppe-Seyler's Z. Physiol. Chem. 349:1592 (1968).
413. H. Schleyer, D. Y. Cooper, and O. Rosenthal, in Magnetic Resonances in Biological Research (C. Franconi, Ed.). Gordon and Breach, New York, 1971, pp. 247-265.
414. I. C. Gunsalus, J. D. Lipscomb, V. Marshall, H. Frauenfelder, E. Greenbaum, and E. Münck, in Biological Hydroxylation Mechanisms, Biochemical Society Symposia 34 (G. S. Boyd and R. M. S. Smellie, Eds.). Academic, New York, 1972, pp. 135-157.

415. J. A. Peterson, R. E. White, Y. Yasukochi, M. L. Coomes, D. H. O'Keeffe, R. E. Ebel, B. S. S. Masters, D. P. Ballou, and M. J. Coon, J. Biol. Chem. 252:4431 (1977).
416. P. L. Gigon, T. E. Gram, and J. R. Gillette, Biochem. Biophys. Res. Comm. 31:558 (1968).
417. J. L. Holtzman and M. L. Carr, Arch. Biochem. Biophys. 150:227 (1972).
418. C. S. Yang and F. S. Strickhart, J. Biol. Chem. 250:7968 (1975).
419. J. A. Peterson, R. E. Ebel, D. H. O'Keeffe, T. Matsubara, and R. W. Estabrook, J. Biol. Chem. 251:4010 (1976).
420. J. R. Cherry, FEBS Lett. 55:1 (1975).
421. Y. Imai and R. Sato, Biochem. Biophys. Res. Comm. 75:420 (1977).
422. T. Matsubara, J. Baron, L. L. Peterson, and J. A. Peterson, Arch. Biochem. Biophys. 172:463 (1976).
423. E. H. Jeffery and G. J. Mannering, unpublished data.
424. Y. Ishimura, V. Ullrich, and J. A. Peterson, Biochem. Biophys. Res. Comm. 42:140 (1971).
425. J. A. Peterson, Y. Ishimura, and B. W. Griffin, Arch. Biochem. Biophys. 149:197 (1972).
426. C. A. Tyson, J. D. Lipscomb, and I. C. Gunsalus, J. Biol. Chem. 247:5777 (1972).
427. R. W. Estabrook, A. G. Hildebrandt, J. Baron, K. J. Netter, and K. Leibman, Biochem. Biophys. Res. Comm. 42:132 (1971).
428. I. C. Gunsalus, C. A. Tyson, R. Tsai, and J. D. Lipscomb, Chem. Biol. Interactions 4:75 (1971).
429. P. Rösen and A. Stier, Biochem. Biophys. Res. Comm. 51:603 (1973).
430. F. P. Guengerich, D. P. Ballou, and M. J. Coon, Biochem. Biophys. Res. Comm. 70:951 (1976).
431. R. W. Estabrook, M. R. Franklin, and A. Hildebrandt, Ann. N.Y. Acad. Sci. 174:218 (1970).
432. J. B. Schenkman, Chem.-Biol. Interact. 3:306 (1971).
433. J. B. Schenkman, Mol. Pharmacol. 8:178 (1972).
434. J. Blanck, G. Smettan, G.-R. Jänig, and K. Ruckpaul, Acta Biol. Med. Ger. 35:1455 (1976).
435. P. J. O'Brien, Pharmacol. Ther., (A) 2:517 (1978).
436. G. A. Hamilton, J. Am. Chem. Soc. 86:3391 (1964).
437. G. A. Hamilton, in Molecular Mechanisms of Oxygen Activation (O. Hayaishi, Ed.). Academic, New York, 1974, pp. 405-451.
438. D. M. Jerina, H. Yagi, and J. W. Daly, Heterocycles 1:267 (1973).
439. D. M. Jerina, J. W. Daly, and B. Wilcop, Biochemistry 10:366 (1971).
440. A. D. Rahimtula and P. J. O'Brien, Biochem. Biophys. Res. Comm. 60:440 (1974).
441. A. D. Rahimtula, P. J. O'Brien, E. G. Hrycay, J. A. Peterson, and R. W. Estabrook, Biochem. Biophys. Res. Comm. 60:695 (1974).

442. F. Lichtenberger, W. Nastainczyk, and V. Ullrich, Biochem. Biophys. Res. Comm. 70:939 (1976).
443. I. Fridovich, Advan. Enzymol. 41:35 (1974).
444. I. Fridovich, Ann. Rev. Biochem. 44:147 (1975).
445. C. S. Foote, in Free Radicals in Biology, Vol. 2 (W. A. Pryor, Ed.). Academic, London, 1976, pp. 85-133.
446. A. J. Paine, Biochem. Pharmacol. 27:1805 (1978).
447. C. Heidelberger, Ann. Rev. Biochemistry 44:79 (1975).
448. M. R. Franklin, Pharmacol. Ther., (A) 2:227 (1977).
449. A. Y. H. Lu, W. Levin, H. Selander, and D. M. Jerina, Biochem. Biophys. Res. Comm. 61:1348 (1974).
450. A. Y. H. Lu, S. B. West, M. Vore, D. Ryan, and W. Levin, J. Biol. Chem. 249:6701 (1974).
451. A. Y. H. Lu, W. Levin, S. B. West, M. Vore, D. Ryan, R. Kuntzman, and A. H. Conney, Advan. Exp. Med. Biol. 58:447 (1975).
452. M. J. Coon, T. A. Haugen, D. A. van der Hoeven, F. P. Guengerich, J. L. Vermilion, and D. P. Ballou, Advan. Exp. Med. Biol. 58:26 (1975).
453. I. Jansson and J. B. Schenkman, Mol. Pharmacol. 9:840 (1973).
454. S. Fujita and J. Peisach, Biochem. Biophys. Res. Comm. 78:328 (1977).
455. G. J. Mannering, Advan. Exp. Med. Biol. 58:405 (1975).
456. J. B. Schenkman, I. Jansson, and K. M. Robie-Suh, Life Sci. 19:611 (1976).
457. R. W. Estabrook, M. Franklin, J. Baron, A. Shigematsu, and A. Hildebrandt, in Drugs and Cell Regulation: Organizational and Pharmacological Aspects on the Molecular Level (E. Mihich, Ed.). Academic, New York, 1971, pp. 227-257.
458. H. A. Sasame, S. S. Thorgeirsson, J. R. Mitchell, and J. R. Gillette, Life Sci. 14:35 (1974).
459. H. A. Sasame, J. R. Gillette, and M. R. Boyd, Biochem. Biophys. Res. Comm. 84:389 (1978).
460. P. Strittmatter, M. J. Rogers, and L. Spatz, J. Biol. Chem. 247:7188 (1972).
461. K. Enomoto and R. Sato, Biochem. Biophys. Res. Comm. 51:1 (1973).
462. H. A. Sasame, S. S. Thorgeirsson, J. R. Mitchell, and J. R. Gillette, Advan. Exp. Med. Biol. 58:435 (1975).
463. M. J. Rogers and P. Strittmatter, J. Biol. Chem. 249:895 (1974).
464. J. Remacle, S. Fowler, H. Beaufay, and J. Berthet, J. Cell Biol. 61:237 (1974).
465. A. I. Archakov, V. M. Devichensky, and A. V. Karjakin, Arch. Biochem. Biophys. 166:295 (1975).
466. A. I. Archakov, V. M. Devichensky, I. I. Karvzina, and A. V. Karjakin, Arch. Biochem. Biophys. 166:308 (1975).

467. A. I. Archakov and V. M. Devichensky, Arch. Biochem. Biophys. 166:313 (1975).
468. W. F. Muna and E. A. Smuckler, Res. Commun. Chem. Path. Pharmacol. 14:287 (1976).
469. D. L. Cinti and J. Ozols, Advan. Exp. Med. Biol. 58:467 (1975).
470. H. Staudt, F. Lichtenberger, and V. Ullrich, Eur. J. Biochem. 46 99 (1974).
471. R. H. White-Stevens and H. Kamin, Biochem. Biophys. Res. Comm. 38:882 (1970).
472. V. Ullrich and H. Diehl, Eur. J. Biochem. 30:509 (1971).
473. S. Narasimhulu, Arch. Biochem. Biophys. 147:384 (1971).
474. J. R. Gillette, B. B. Brodie, and B. N. LaDu, J. Pharmacol. Exp. Ther. 119:532 (1957).
475. A. G. Hildebrandt, M. Speck, and I. Roots, Biochem. Biophys. Res. Comm. 54:968 (1973).
476. R. W. Estabrook and J. Werringloer, in Drug Metabolism Concepts (D. M. Jerina, Ed.). American Chemical Society Symposium Series 44, Washington, D.C., 1977, pp. 1-26.
477. A. H. Beckett and G. G. Gibson, J. Pharm. Pharmacol. 29:756 (1977).
478. M. K. Buening and M. R. Franklin, Drug Metab. Disp. 4:244 (1976).
479. R. P. Mason and J. L. Holtzman, Biochem. Biophys. Res. Comm. 67:1267 (1975).
480. G. D. Nordblom and M. J. Coon, Arch. Biochem. Biophys. 180:343 (1977).
481. I. Björkhem, Pharmacol. Ther. (A) 1:327 (1977).
482. A. H. Leninger, in Biochemistry, 2nd ed. Worth, New York, 1975, p. 208.
483. R. W. Estabrook, J. Baron, and A. Hildebrandt, Chem.-Biol. Interact. 3:260 (1971).
484. G. T. Miwa, S. B. West, and A. Y. H. Lu, J. Biol. Chem. 253: 1921 (1978).
485. J. A. Thompson and J. L. Holtzman, Drug Metab. Disp. 2:577 (1974).
486. D. B. Northrup, Biochemistry 14:2644 (1975).
487. G. Yagil and H. D. Hoberman, Biochemistry 8:352 (1969).
488. D. W. Nebert, Mol. Cell. Biochem. 27:27 (1979).
489. K. W. Renton and G. J. Mannering, Drug. Metab. Disp. 4:223 (1976).
490. K. W. Renton and G. J. Mannering, Biochem. Biophys. Res. Comm. 73:343 (1976).
491. J. F. Williams and A. Szentivanyi, Europ. J. Pharmacol. 43:281 (1977).
492. K. W. Renton, J. Pharmacol. Exp. Ther. 208:267 (1979).

493. K. W. Renton, D. E. Keyler, and G. J. Mannering, Biochem. Biophys. Res. Comm. 88:1017 (1979).
494. R. El Azhary and G. J. Mannering, Mol. Pharmacol. 15:698 (1979).
495. K. W. Renton, L. B. Deloria, and G. J. Mannering, Mol. Pharmacol. 14:672 (1978).
496. L. F. Soyka, W. G. Hunt, S. E. Knight, and R. S. Foster, Jr., Canc. Res. 35:4425 (1976).
497. R. L. Levy, M. H. Barrington, R. A. Lerner, G. J. Griffin, and C. E. Whitmire, Cancer Res. 37:3892 (1977).
498. J. G. Vos and J. A. Moore, Int. Arch. Allergy Appl. Immunol. 47:777 (1974).
499. S. K. Park and J. Brody II, Nature New Biol. 233:181 (1971).

Chapter 3

TOXIFICATION AND DETOXIFICATION AS A RESULT OF XENOBIOTIC METABOLISM

Brian G. Lake and Sharat D. Gangolli

The British Industrial Biological Research Association
Carshalton, Surrey, England

People are exposed to a multitude of foreign compounds (xenobiotics) of both natural and synthetic origin. The majority of xenobiotics which enter our bodies are subjected to metabolic transformations mediated by numerous enzymes present in the liver and in other tissues. While metabolism often results in the conversion of xenobiotics to less toxic polar products, some metabolites may be more toxic than the parent compound resulting in tissue damage and even the initiation of carcinogenesis. In this chapter we briefly review the range of hepatic and extrahepatic xenobiotic-metabolizing enzymes and the various factors which may modify these enzyme activities. We illustrate the principle of xenobiotic metabolism resulting in either detoxification and/or toxification by considering the metabolism of paracetamol, phenacetin, benzo[a]pyrene, 2-acetylaminofluorene, and allyl alcohol in detail. Finally, the various methods available for studying the metabolism of xenobiotics are discussed.

I. INTRODUCTION

An inevitable result of modern scientific and technological progress has been the inexorable increase in the numbers of new compounds in the environment. As a consequence human exposure to such chemicals, either deliberate or inadvertent, has correspondingly multiplied. Drugs, food additives, and cosmetic products are the major sources of human contact with chemicals and this group has been vastly augmented in recent times. For example, over 3000 drugs were listed in the Extra Pharmacopoeia in 1967 [1], and this number was increased to over 4000 compounds in the 1977 edition [2]. As regards chemicals used as food additives, over 200 compounds are permitted in the United Kingdom, and the Food Chemical Codex [3] mentions over 600 compounds. Additionally, many substances of natural origin and often of complex chemical composition are employed as flavoring and dispersing agents in foods. Cosmetic products also contain a wide variety of both synthetic and naturally occurring compounds [4].

One additional and important source of human exposure to foreign compounds or xenobiotics is from pesticides, agrochemicals, and compounds used in industrial processes. Apart from accidental direct human contact, many of these compounds in the absence of stringent preventative measures gain access to the environment, enter the food chain, and hence eventually the human diet as contaminants (Fig. 1).

There is a growing awareness of the toxic hazards in the human chemical environment and a general recognition that dire and irrevocable consequences may follow if the widespread pollution of the biosphere is allowed to proceed unchecked. Support for this view is derived from the accumulating body of evidence relating human and animal illnesses to deliberate or adventitious chemical exposure. New therapeutic drugs, despite extensive animal studies, have been found to produce toxic effects in humans [5], and even drugs long established in official pharmacopoeias such as paracetamol (acetaminophen), phenacetin (acetophenetidine), and aspirin (acetylsalicylic acid), have since been shown to cause serious injury in humans [6-8]. Environmental chemical pollutants have presented far more insidious and sinister problems in terms of human and animal toxicity. Episodes of acute and chronic poisoning have been associated with exposure to air, water, and foods contaminated by mercury [9], cadmium [10], lead [11], organophosphorus pesticides [12], and various halogenated chemicals including aldrin and dieldrin [13], polychlorinated polycyclic compounds [14], and polybrominated biphenyls [15]. Furthermore, in the etiology of human cancers it has been postulated that 80 to 90% of incidences may be attributed to environmental chemicals [16-18].

Thus the importance of relevant information of toxic hazards posed by chemicals and the urgent need for adequate statutory controls on the production, usage, and disposal of toxic substances is widely accepted.

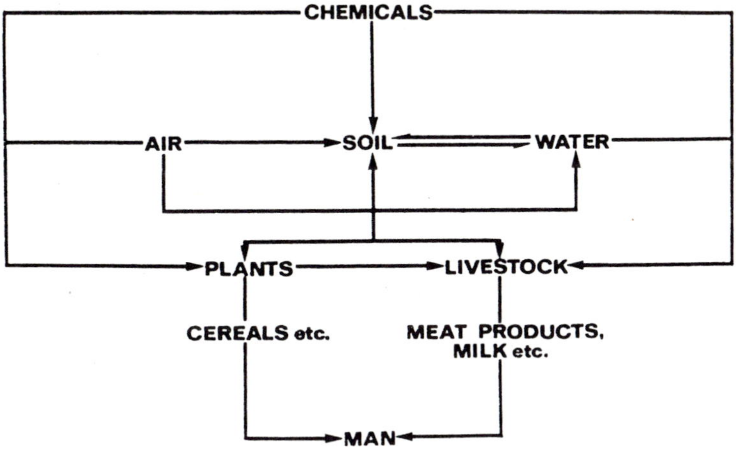

FIGURE 1 Schematic representation of routes whereby chemical contaminants enter the human diet.

Toward this end toxicity studies on a wide variety of compounds in experimental animals are actively pursued. The information generated forms the basis on which regulatory controls are made. However, toxicity data per se are insufficient for the extrapolation of animal findings to humans and for the meaningful toxicological assessment of a chemical hazard in terms of human exposure, account must be taken of the suitability and sensitivity of the experimental animal model used and the pharmacokinetics and metabolism of the compound in the experimental animals and in humans. Other relevant factors meriting consideration are the influence of the dosage, route, and mode of administration on the absorption, metabolism, and disposition of a compound on the eventual toxicological sequelae in the animal. Equally germane in this context is the need for an understanding and elucidation of biochemical mechanisms involved in bioactivation and detoxification processes determining the manifestation of toxic effects in the animal.

This chapter attempts to review the salient features of the enzymic systems mediating the activation and/or deactivation of xenobiotics present in our environment, and the influence of various modifying factors—e.g., nutritional state, genetic variation—on these processes.

II. HEPATIC AND EXTRAHEPATIC XENOBIOTIC METABOLISM

Xenobiotic-metabolizing enzyme activity exists in many tissues, the liver, however, being the principal organ responsible for the activation (for example isoniazid or acetylisoniazid, see Ref. 19-21) and/or deactivation of foreign compounds by functionalization and conjugation reactions [22,23].

The microsomal monooxygenase complex with its requirement for both NADPH and molecular oxygen [24-27] consists of two electron-transport chains of which the cytochrome P-450 hemoproteins are the terminal oxygenases [28,29] catalyzing a variety of functionalization reactions [30-47]. Any particular xenobiotic may of course be metabolized by more than one pathway, as exemplified by the carcinogen 2-acetylaminofluorene which undergoes N-hydroxylation, aromatic C-hydroxylation, and deacetylation, as well as subsequent conjugation with D-glucuronic acid and sulfate [35,48,49]. Recent work has demonstrated that microsomal cytochrome P-450 consists of a number of distinct hemoproteins [50-52] which have been shown to exhibit marked differences in both the qualitative and quantitative metabolism of xenobiotics [53-55]. Furthermore, the relative amounts of these different hemoproteins are altered when the xenobiotic-metabolizing enzyme system is stimulated by the administration of inducing agents such as barbiturates, polychlorinated biphenyls, polycyclic hydrocarbons, etc. (see Sec. IV).

In addition to the microsomal monooxygenase-catalyzed biotransformations, xenobiotics may also be metabolized by a variety of other enzyme systems distributed throughout all subcellular compartments of the hepatocyte (Table 1). For example, amines, depending on their structure, may be metabolized by a number of non-cytochrome P-450-dependent amine

TABLE 1
Subcellular Localization of Various Hepatic Xenobiotic-metabolizing Enzymes

Subcellular fraction	Enzymic pathway	Reference(s)
Nuclei	Cytochrome P-450s and associated xenobiotic-metabolizing enzyme activities	56, 57
	Epoxide hydrase	58, 59
Mitochrondria	Cytochrome P-450s involved in cholesterol catabolism and other biotrans formations?	60, 61
	Aldehyde dehydrogenase	62
	Monoamine oxidase	63, 64
	Nonspecific esterases	65, 66
	Superoxide dismutase	67
	Conjugation with amino acids	23, 68

TABLE 1 (continued)

Subcellular fraction	Enzymic pathway	Reference(s)
Lysosomes	Acid hydrolases, including nonspecific esterases	66,69,70
Peroxisomes (microbodies)	Peroxidative enzymes, including catalase	64
Microsomes	Cytochrome P-450-dependent monooxygenase complex incorporating associated electron-transport chain components (e.g., cytochrome b_5, NADPH- and NADH-cytochrome c reductases) catalyzing both xenobiotic oxidation and reduction transformations	25-29, 46,47
	Aldehyde dehydrogenase	62
	Epoxide hydrase	71,72
	Monoamine oxidase	64,73
	Non-cytochrome P-450-dependent N-oxidation and N-hydroxylation enzymes, including the Ziegler mixed-function amine oxidase	74,75
	Nonspecific esterases	65,69,70
	Nonspecific N- and O-methyltransferases	76,77
	Conjugation with D-glucuronic acid	78,79
Cytosol (soluble fraction)	Alcohol dehydrogenase	80
	Aldehyde dehydrogenase	62
	Azo and nitro group reductions	44,45
	Catechol O-methyltransferase	81
	Superoxide dismutase	67
	Conjugation with acetate	82,83
	Conjugation with glutathione	84,85
	Conjugation with sulfate	86,87

Recent work by Ota and Hammock [72a] has demonstrated the existence of an epoxide hydrase enzyme with different specificities in the cytosolic fraction of rodent liver.

oxidases [64,73-75,88] localized in several subcellular fractions. The intracellular distribution of enzymes capable of metabolizing xenobiotics may result in the exposure of the hepatocyte to substances which are activated at one site, but are deactivated by either further functionalization or conjugation at other site(s). For example, the cytochrome P-450-dependent monooxygenases present in the nuclear and microsomal fractions have been shown to metabolize the carcinogen benzo[a]pyrene to reactive intermediates [57,89], whereas additional detoxifying enzymes such as glutathione S-transferases and sulfotransferases are located in the soluble fraction (see Sec. III).

Although the majority of studies on hepatic xenobiotic metabolism have been performed on tissues obtained from experimental animals, a few studies have been conducted on human liver. Various xenobiotic-metabolizing enzyme activities have been demonstrated in either human biopsy or autopsy liver tissues, e.g., monooxygenase components [90-96], epoxide hydrase [97], uridine diphosphate (UDP)-glucuronyltransferase [94], and glycine conjugation [98]. Thus human liver xenobiotic-metabolizing enzymes would appear to be qualitatively similar to those of other mammals although the liver-to-body weight ratio exhibits a marked species difference [92,99]. Xenobiotics are capable of being metabolized by extrahepatic tissues from both experimental animals and humans. Although the levels of xenobiotic-metabolizing enzymes are generally lower than the corresponding hepatic enzyme activities, extrahepatic xenobiotic metabolism may be of great importance especially when the xenobiotic passes through the tissue, e.g., lung, gut, skin, before reaching the liver. The range of xenobiotic transformations appears to be similar to that of the liver with both functionalization enzymes including cytochrome P-450 and associated components of the microsomal electron-transport chain, together with other enzymes such as epoxide hydrase, UDP-glucuronyltransferase and glutathione S-transferase (Table 2). As with the liver (see Sec. IIE) xenobiotic-metabolizing enzyme activities may not be uniformly distributed throughout the extrahepatic tissue. For example, the activities of cytochrome P-450s [101], benzo[a]-pyrene hydroxylase [127], and UDP-glucuronyltransferase [128] are highest in the proximal portion of the rat small intestine and activity exhibits a differential distribution in various regions of the rat kidney [129] and testes [110]. In the lung, xenobiotic-metabolizing enzyme activities have been detected by biochemical, histochemical, and autoradiographic techniques in a number of distinct cell types including alveolar macrophages [130], Clara cells [131], and the cells of the alveolar [132,133] and bronchiolar epithelium [133]. As with the activities of hepatic xenobiotic-metabolizing enzymes, extrahepatic enzyme levels may also be influenced as the result of administration of various foreign compounds (see Sec. IV).

In addition to the hepatic and extrahepatic xenobiotic-metabolizing enzymes of the animal, the gastrointestinal flora are also known to contribute to the activation and/or deactivation of ingested xenobiotics. The gut

TABLE 2

Xenobiotic-Metabolizing Enzyme Activities Detected in Extrahepatic Tissues of Rodents (References)

	Enzymic activity							
				Monooxygenase substrate metabolism				
Tissue	Cytochrome P-450	Cytochrome b_5	NADPH-cytochrome c reductase	Benzo[a]pyrene[a]	7-Ethoxycoumarin	Epoxide hydrase[b]	Glutathione S-transferase[c]	UDP-Glucuronyl-transferase[d]
Small intestine	100,101	101,111	100	101,109,113, 114	118	118,119	118,120	118,122
Kidney	102,103	111	103	104,113,114	118	118,119	118,120, 121	118,121, 122
Lung	103	111	103	109,113,114	118	118,119	118,121	118,121, 122
Skin	104,105	105	112	104,105,115	112	119		123
Adrenal	106,107	111		113,114		107,119	107,108	122
Mammary				116,117				
Ovary	107,108	108	103	108		107,108 119	107,108	
Placenta	109		103	109				109,122
Spleen			103	109,113		119		122
Testis	103,110	111	103	109,110,114	118	110,118, 119	110,118	118

[a] Benzo[a]pyrene hydroxylase is also known as aryl hydrocarbon hydroxylase. In most studies a fluorescence assay is used which measures predominantly 3-hydroxybenzo[a]pyrene [124], but in some instances several benzo[a]pyrene metabolites have been determined in studies with extrahepatic tissues [115, 125, 126].

[b] Measured employing either styrene 7,8-oxide or benzo[a]pyrene 4,5-oxide as the substrate.

[c] Measured employing either sytrene 7,8-oxide, benzo[a]pyrene 4,5-oxide, or 3,4-dichloronitrobenzene as the substrate.

[d] Measured employing either 4-nitrophenol, 2-aminophenol, or 4-methylumbelliferone as the aglycone.

bacteria are extremely versatile and can carry out various enzymic reactions including the hydrolysis of glucuronides and other conjugates, dehydroxylations, decarboxylations, dealkylations, dehalogenations, deaminations, aromatization reactions, ring fission reactions, the reduction of nitro and azo groups, etc. [134-136].

III. EXAMPLES OF TOXIFICATION AND DETOXIFICATION

The role of xenobiotic-metabolizing enzyme systems is to increase the polarity of the xenobiotic and thus favor its elimination from the organism. In the case of drugs the pharmacological effectiveness may be either diminished (deactivation) or enhanced (activation) as a consequence of metabolism. For example, the hypnotic drug phenobarbital is inactivated by metabolism to 4-hydroxyphenobarbital, whereas acetanilide is converted to the active analgesic agent paracetamol [137]. However, xenobiotic metabolism does not always lead to beneficial effects for the organism and many instances are known where the metabolite(s) of a xenobiotic are more toxic than the parent compound. For example, the hepatotoxin carbon tetrachloride is activated to reactive products by the cytochrome P-450-dependent monooxygenase system [138]. As would be expected the compound is more toxic in animals with induced levels of monooxygenase activity than in animals with depressed levels of xenobiotic-metabolizing enzymes [139].

In recent years many examples have been recorded where the activation and/or deactivation of a xenobiotic may be markedly affected by manipulation of the various enzyme systems involved in the metabolism of the compound. By considering the metabolism of paracetamol, phenacetin, benzo[a]pyrene, 2-acetylaminofluorene, and allyl alcohol, it is intended in this section to illustrate and to interrelate the basic pathways responsible for the activation and/or deactivation of xenobiotics in mammals.

A. Paracetamol

Paracetamol (acetaminophen, N-acetyl-4-aminophenol) is a widely used non-narcotic analgesic drug. However, when administered in large doses paracetamol causes both hepatic and renal necrosis in humans [7, 8] and in experimental animals [140-142]. Studies on the metabolism of paracetamol in vivo [143-147] and with both liver and kidney cell suspensions in vitro [148-150] have indicated that paracetamol is excreted unchanged and as glucuronide, sulfate, and thiol conjugates. However, the studies of Mitchell and coworkers [140-142, 145, 151-155] have demonstrated that while the sulfate and glucuronide conjugates of paracetamol represent the products of detoxification, the thiol conjugates (particularly with reduced glutathione) represent detoxified products of metabolically activated paracetamol. Indeed, the investigations of Mitchell and coworkers have demonstrated that the metabolic activation of paracetamol involves an initial N-hydroxylation reaction catalyzed by enzymes of the cytochrome P-450-dependent monooxygenase complex. N-Hydroxyparacetamol then rearranges to N-acetylbenzoquinonimine (also termed acetamidoquinone), a highly reactive electrophilic arylating intermediate which can bind covalently to tissue macromolecules (Fig. 2).* However, these activated intermediates may be detoxified by reacting either enzymatically [156] or nonenzymatically [145, 155] with intracellular reduced glutathione. The formation of N-hydroxyparacetamol as the toxic intermediate has recently been confirmed by the observations that N-methylparacetamol (where the methyl substituent blocks N-hydroxylation) does not produce either hepatic or renal necrosis [157], whereas N-hydroxyparacetamol produces both liver and kidney damage in experimental animals [158].

The metabolism of paracetamol and its subsequent hepatotoxicity may be greatly influenced by modifying either the activity of the cytochrome P-450-dependent monooxygenase complex or by altering the intracellular levels of reduced glutathione. Thus the stimulation of monooxygenase activity in mice by treatment with phenobarbital enhances both the covalent binding of reactive paracetamol metabolites and hepatic necrosis, whereas the toxification of the analgesic is depressed in animals with monooxygenase activity reduced by prior treatment with either cobalt chloride, piperonyl butoxide, or metyrapone [151,152,159]. Similarly, the prior depletion of hepatic glutathione levels by treatment with compounds such as diethyl maleate [160] or diisopropylidene acetone (phorone) [161], increases paracetamol hepatotoxicity [153,160] whereas the administration of glutathione [162,163] protects against the toxic effects of the analgesic. Other sulfur-containing compounds such as cysteamine (2-aminoethanethiol) [145,163, 164], L-cysteine [153,163,164], L-methionine [164,165], N-acetylcysteine [166,167], dimercaprol (2,3-dimercapto-1-propanol) [145], dithiocarb (sodium diethyldithiocarbamate) [163,164], and α-mercaptopropionylglycine [168] also protect against paracetamol-induced liver necrosis and subsequent mortality. However, not all of these sulfur-containing compounds appear to act in the same manner as glutathione. For example, while L-cysteine and L-methionine may protect by repleting hepatic glutathione stores [153,

---

*While recent studies [155a] have demonstrated the formation of N-acetylbenzoquinonimine by incubating paracetamol with mouse hepatic microsomes, N-hydroxyparacetamol was not a metabolite of paracetamol incubated with hamster hepatic microsomes although it was formed from the metabolism of N-hydroxyphenacetin [155b]. Thus the possibility exists that the bioactivation of paracetamol does not arise from an initial N-hydroxylation step as indicated in Fig. 2; however, the ultimate reactive metabolite of both paracetamol and phenacetin may still be N-acetylbenzoquinonimine [155, 155b,244,245].

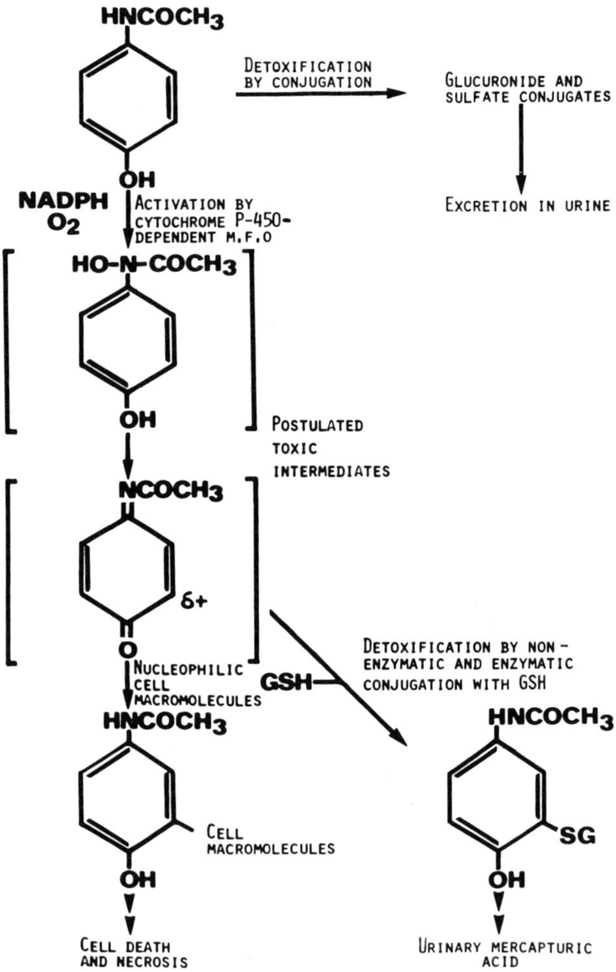

FIGURE 2 Pathways of activation and detoxification of paracetamol.

163,164], compounds such as cysteamine and dithiocarb may at least partially act by inhibiting the activity of the monooxygenase complex [164,169].*
The inhibition of paracetamol hepatotoxicity by sulfhydryl agents such as cysteamine and L-methionine has been successfully employed in recent years as antidotes for the treatment of cases of paracetamol overdosage in humans [170,171].

Paracetamol hepatotoxicity also serves to illustrate the effect of dosage on the subsequent route of xenobiotic metabolism. At low doses paracetamol is largely conjugated and excreted as glucuronide and sulfate conjugates [144,172] with any monooxygenase-derived activated metabolites being conjugated with glutathione and excreted. However, higher doses of the analgesic progressively deplete hepatic glutathione levels and thus result in the extensive covalent binding of reactive metabolites and subsequent hepatic necrosis [153,154]. Furthermore, the dose threshold that exists for paracetamol toxicity following the extensive depletion of tissue glutathione levels is potentiated by the observation that the amount of the analgesic that can be conjugated with either D-glucuronic acid or sulfate in both experimental animals [144,172,173] and humans [174] is saturable at high doses of paracetamol. Thus the reduction in the detoxification pathways of paracetamol glucuronide and sulfate conjugations further enhances the metabolism of the analgesic by the monooxygenase-dependent toxification pathway. Indeed, while the coadministration of sodium sulfate with a hepatotoxic dose of paracetamol substantially reduces subsequent mortality in the mouse [175], the administration of salicylamide—which inhibits both the glucuronidation and sulfation of paracetamol—to hamsters markedly potentiated the hepatotoxicity of the analgesic [176]. Similarly, several compounds, including some drugs, have been shown to inhibit paracetamol glucuronide formation by rat liver microsomal preparations in vitro [177] and the administration of acetylsalicylic acid inhibits the sulfate conjugation of the analgesic in the mouse and hamster [178,179]. A number of human studies have also demonstrated that the metabolism of low (therapeutic) doses of paracetamol may be affected by the coadministration of agents such as L-ascorbic acid and salicylamide [180,181]. These studies would suggest that in certain instances drugs and other compounds which compete for the conjugative pathways of glucuronidation and sulfation may result in increased toxicity of the analgesic in humans. However, in the case of L-ascorbic acid a recent study has shown that vitamin C protects against paracetamol-induced mortality in mice [182]. One possible mechanism of

---

*Indeed, recent studies [169a] employing a high-performance liquid chromatography procedure to separate paracetamol metabolite-nucleophile adducts generated by a mouse hepatic microsomal system have confirmed that covalent binding of paracetamol metabolites can be inhibited by adduct formation and/or inhibition of reactive metabolite generation.

L-ascorbic acid protection may be that the vitamin is acting as a scavenging agent [183] by reacting with the activated paracetamol intermediates.

Another aspect of detoxification and toxification illustrated by paracetamol hepatotoxicity is that of species differences. While the mouse and hamster are highly susceptible to paracetamol induced hepatic necrosis, the rat, guinea pig, and rabbit are relatively resistant [141,144,184]. These differences are directly attributable to the higher rates of reactive metabolite formation via the monooxygenase-mediated N-hydroxylation of paracetamol in the mouse and hamster [141,152,154], hence leading at high doses of the analgesic to hepatic glutathione depletion, macromolecular binding, and subsequent necrosis. However, a species difference does occur with respect to paracetamol toxicity in the mouse and hamster after the induction of hepatic microsomal monooxygenase activity by phenobarbital. While treatment with the barbiturate stimulates the covalent binding of reactive paracetamol metabolites in vitro and in vivo and thus potentiates liver necrosis, phenobarbital decreases paracetamol hepatotoxicity in the hamster [184]. This apparent anomaly has been explained on the basis that paracetamol glucuronidation, i.e., detoxification, is markedly stimulated in the hamster leading to a shorter half-life of the analgesic and, in addition, phenobarbital only slightly enhances the rate of hepatic monooxygenase-dependent paracetamol activation [154,184]. In contrast, treatment with 3-methylcholanthrene markedly potentiates reactive metabolite formation and tissue necrosis in the hamster [154].

While the above discussion has been devoted to the mechanism of and modification of paracetamol-induced hepatoxicity, recent studies have demonstrated that the renal toxicity of the analgesic is also due to the generation of a chemically reactive species from the metabolism of paracetamol [142,185]. Paracetamol depletes glutathione levels in both the liver and kidney of rats and mice, and the inhibition of monooxygenase enzyme activity by cobalt chloride reduces covalent binding and subsequent necrosis in both tissues. However, while 3-methylcholanthrene treatment stimulates hepatic covalent binding and necrosis in the rat and mouse, there was no significant effect on renal macromolecular binding and necrosis. This finding may indicate a tissue difference in the response of hepatic and renal monooxygenases to stimulation by 3-methylcholanthrene.

The investigations into the metabolism and toxicity of paracetamol have demonstrated that tissue necrosis is associated with the covalent binding of reactive paracetamol metabolites to intracellular macromolecular components. However, many other xenobiotics including certain drugs, carcinogens, steroids, and industrial chemicals have been shown to be metabolized by mammalian hepatic microsomal fractions to reactive intermediates which may subsequently become bound to tissue macromolecules such as lipids, proteins, and nucleic acids (Table 3). While not all xenobiotics have been as exhaustively studied as paracetamol, most workers assume that nonextractable radioactively labeled xenobiotic residues are

TABLE 3
The Metabolic Activation of Xenobiotics to Reactive Intermediates Catalyzed by Hepatic Microsomal Fractions In Vitro

Compound[a]	Postulated metabolic pathway(s) leading to reactive intermediate(s)[b]	Reference(s)
2-Acetylaminofluorene	N-hydroxylation	152
Acetylhydrazine	N-hydroxylation and subsequent rearrangement	19
Aflatoxin B_1	Epoxidation	186,187,188
Antipyrine	Epoxidation	189
Benzene	Epoxidation and further metabolism	190
Benzo[a]pyrene and related compounds	Epoxidation, and other pathways?	191,192,193
Biphenyl and 4-chlorobiphenyl	Epoxidation?	194
Bromobenzene	Epoxidation	195
4-Bromobiphenyl	Epoxidation	196
Bromotrichloromethane	Free radical formation	197
Carbonyl (1-naphthyl-N-methylcarbamate)	Epoxidation?	198
Carbon disulfide	Oxidation with release of sulfur	199
Carbon tetrachloride	Free radical formation	197
Chloramphenicol	Formation of oxamyl chloride intermediate	200
Chloroform	Free radical formation	197,201
Cyclophosphamide	4-hydroxylation and subsequent rearrangement	202
2,4-Diaminoanisole	N-hydroxylation and ring hydroxylation with subsequent rearrangement?	203

(continued)

TABLE 3 (continued)

Compound[a]	Postulated metabolic pathway(s) leading to reactive intermediate(s)[b]	Reference(s)
2,4-Diaminotoluene	Hydroxylation followed by oxidation of catechol nucleus?	204
Eraldin (practolol)	N-hydroxylation and/or epoxidation	205
Furosemide and related compounds	Epoxidation of furan ring	206,207,208
Halothane	Free radical formation	201
Hexachlorophene	Epoxidation	209
2-Hydroxyestradiol and related compounds	Ring hydroxylation and subsequent oxidation of catechol nucleus	210,211,212, 213
Imipramine	Epoxidation	214
4-Ipomeanol	Oxidation of furan ring	215
Isopropylhydrazine	N-hydroxylation and subsequent rearrangement	19
Methimazole	Oxidation with release of sulfur	216
α-Methyldopa and related compounds	Oxidation of catechol nucleus	217
α-Naphthylisothiocyanate	Epoxidation?	218
Norethindrone	Epoxidation?	219
Paracetamol	N-hydroxylation?	152,155
Parathion	Oxidation with release of sulfur	220
Phenacetin	N-hydroxylation and epoxidation?	155,221
Polychlorinated biphenyls	Epoxidation and ring hydroxylation with subsequent oxidation of catechol nucleus	222,223
Thioacetamide	S-oxidation and subsequent further metabolism	224

TABLE 3 (continued)

Compound[a]	Postulated metabolic pathway(s) leading to reactive intermediate(s)[b]	Reference(s)
Trichloroethylene	Epoxidation	225
Vinyl chloride	Epoxidation, and other pathways?	226,227

[a] The metabolic activation of these xenobiotics to reactive intermediates was normally demonstrated with hepatic microsomal fractions from rats, mice, or hamsters and an NADPH-generating system.
[b] In most instances the activation of the xenobiotic is considered to be mediated by the cytochrome P-450-dependent monooxygenase complex. Evidence for the particular metabolic pathway(s) involved may be derived from inhibitor studies. For example, an increase in covalent binding after the addition of either 3,3,3-trichloropropylene oxide or cyclohexene oxide (which inhibit microsomal epoxide hydrase [97]) would provide evidence for an epoxide intermediate.

either "irreversibly" or "covalently" bound to tissue macromolecules. Furthermore, although the covalent binding of reactive intermediates may, like paracetamol, represent only a small portion of the metabolism of the xenobiotic, the metabolic pathways leading to the formation of these intermediates are diverse and may involve N-hydroxylation, epoxidation, free radical formation, etc. Studies with human liver microsomal preparations have also demonstrated that compounds such as chloroform, furosemide, imipramine, α-methyldopa, and paracetamol can be metabolized to covalently bound products [214,228,229]. In addition to the hepatic metabolic activation of xenobiotics, many extrahepatic tissues such as the kidney [142,185,208,230], lung [215,230-232], placenta [233], and brain [234] have also been found to catalyze the covalent binding of reactive intermediates in vitro and in vivo.

The presence of small amounts of residual radioactivity in the tissues of experimental animals after the administration of isotopically labeled xenobiotics may present considerable problems in the interpretation of toxicity data. Such radioactivity may be covalently bound and hence indicate possible tissue toxicity due to the generation of reactive metabolites of the xenobiotic. However, the radioactivity may represent the reversible binding of the xenobiotic and/or its metabolite(s) to tissue components or, conversely the radioactivity may represent endogenous compounds which have been synthesized from radioactive metabolites of the xenobiotic that have entered normal metabolic pathways. Gillette [20,235,236] has suggested various procedures for investigating the covalent binding of xenobiotic metabolites to tissue macromolecules and for the determination of the nature of radioactive residues in tissues.

B. Phenacetin

The minor analgesic drug phenacetin (acetophenetidine, 4-ethoxyacetanilide), like paracetamol, produces both hepatic [237-239] and renal necrosis [240] in experimental animals and is metabolized to reactive intermediates which can bind covalently to tissue macromolecules [155, 239]. Although phenacetin is closely related structurally to paracetamol, recent studies have shown that phenacetin may be activated by at least three different mechanisms.

1. Phenacetin is deethylated by a monooxygenase-dependent reaction to paracetamol [155, 239, 241] and subsequently activated to reactive intermediates (see Fig. 2).
2. Phenacetin is metabolized to a 3,4-epoxide intermediate which then rearranges to the reactive intermediate derived from paracetamol (Fig. 2) with the concomitant loss of the 4-ethoxy substituent [155, 238]. Evidence for this pathway is derived from studies with ^{18}O-labeled compounds where approximately 50% of the stable isotope is incorporated into a phenacetin-glutathione conjugate [155]. If phenacetin was solely activated by conversion to paracetamol and then hydroxylated, the incorporated oxygen atom would not be retained in the reactive N-acetylbenzoquinonimine intermediate (Fig. 2) and hence also in the metabolite-glutathione conjugate [155]. Furthermore, the addition of sodium fluoride does not stimulate the covalent binding of reactive phenacetin metabolites to microsomal protein in vitro, whereas fluoride is known to stimulate the N-hydroxylation of other arylamines including paracetamol [152, 242]. Additionally, while the macromolecular binding of reactive paracetamol metabolites is stimulated in hamsters by 3-methylcholanthrene treatment, that of phenacetin is not affected [155]. These studies thus indicate that phenacetin is not solely activated by an enzymic pathway identical with that activating paracetamol.
3. Phenacetin is known to be N-hydroxylated by a monooxygenase-dependent reaction [243, 244]. Although the N-hydroxyphenacetin formed cannot directly react with tissue macromolecules [155, 243], conjugation to yield either N-O-sulfate or N-O-glucuronide products results in the activation of N-hydroxyphenacetin with the subsequent arylation of tissue macromolecules [221, 244, 245]. Studies on the breakdown of the glucuronide of N-hydroxyphenacetin have indicated that the major reactive metabolite is identical with that derived from paracetamol, i.e., N-acetylbenzoquinonimine [245]. Finally, Mulder et al. [245] have suggested that phenacetin N-O-glucuronide may at least in part be responsible for the nephrotoxicity of the

analgesic as the conjugate formed in the liver would become concentrated in the kidney prior to excretion.

The activation of phenacetin serves to illustrate two observations of relevance to the toxification and detoxification of xenobiotics. First, although phenacetin is structurally related to paracetamol, it can be activated by different metabolic pathways; and secondly, the glucuronide and sulfate conjugates are not always detoxification products.* Indeed, conjugation reactions are known to be responsible for the metabolic activation of a range of carcinogenic aromatic amides and amines (see Sec. III.D).

C. Benzo[a]pyrene

Benzo[a]pyrene and certain other polycyclic aromatic hydrocarbons are examples of xenobiotics which require metabolic activation in order to exert their toxic, mutagenic, and carcinogenic effects [246]. The metabolism of these compounds is complex and a variety of phenols, dihydrodiols, quinones, and arene oxide derivatives together with conjugates of sulfate, D-glucuronic acid, and glutathione have been described [246-248]. The initial metabolic activation of these compounds is the formation of arene oxides [249] which can either be further metabolized, bind covalently with tissue macromolecules, or rearrange nonenzymatically to phenols. The enzyme(s) responsible for the metabolism of benzo[a]pyrene and related compounds have been termed "aryl hydrocarbon hydroxylase(s)" and shown to be part of the cytochrome P-450-dependent monooxygenase complex present in both the liver and in extrahepatic tissues (see Sec. II). Recent studies have demonstrated that the principal metabolically activated form of benzo[a]pyrene is the bay region antidiol epoxide, which is formed from the epoxide hydrase-catalyzed conversion of benzo[a]pyrene 7,8-oxide to the corresponding dihydrodiol followed by a second monooxygenase-catalyzed epoxidation reaction [250,251] at the 9,10-position [250,251]. The enantiomers of 7,8-dihydroxy-9,10-epoxy-7,8,9,10-tetrahydrobenzo[a]pyrene so formed have been shown to react with DNA [250,252,253] and to be highly mutagenic [254,255].

Thus the initial monooxygenase-catalyzed step cannot be considered to be wholly a toxification pathway as some phenolic products formed are not mutagenic either directly or following further metabolism [255,256], whereas the epoxide hydrase-catalyzed step is not wholly a detoxification pathway owing to its role in the synthesis of the antidiol epoxide. However,

---

*Although three possible pathways of phenacetin activation have been demonstrated in vitro, the conversion of phenacetin to paracetamol followed by activation of the latter component is considered to be the predominant pathway in the hamster in vivo [244].

like paracetamol, alterations in the levels of the various enzymes involved in the metabolism of benzo[a]pyrene can markedly affect the nature of the products formed. The metabolism of benzo[a]pyrene to either toxic and/or nontoxic products has been investigated by both covalent binding studies and by mutagenicity studies employing detection systems such as the Ames test [257,258]. For example, the stimulation of benzo[a]pyrene arene oxide formation by increased microsomal monooxygenase activity enhances both the covalent binding of benzo[a]pyrene metabolites to DNA [259] and their mutagenicity in the Ames test [260]. However, the degree of induction of aryl hydrocarbon hydroxylase activity is dependent on the particular inducing agent employed and on the nature of the cytochrome P-450 species present after induction (see Sec. IV). Conversely, the inhibition of aryl hydrocarbon hydroxylase activity by α-naphthoflavone (7,8-benzoflavone) [261] decreased the covalent binding of benzo[a]pyrene metabolites to DNA catalyzed either by microsomal fractions [262] or in isolated hepatocytes [263]. Similarly compounds such as harman and norharman or ellipticine, which also inhibit aryl hydrocarbon hydroxylase, markedly reduce the mutagenicity of benzo[a]pyrene in the Ames test [264,265]. Changes in benzo[a]pyrene toxicity may also be elicited by varying the activities of epoxide hydrase and the glutathione, sulfate, and glucuronide conjugation enzymes. Thus the covalent binding of activated benzo[a]pyrene metabolites to DNA in isolated hepatocytes was enhanced [263] by adding 3,3,3-trichloropropylene oxide (an inhibitor of epoxide hydrase [97]), diethyl maleate (which depletes glutathione levels [160]), and salicylamide (which inhibits conjugation with either sulfate or D-glucuronic acid). In mutagenicity studies, while the addition of purified epoxide hydrase to the hepatic microsomal-supernatant "S9 fraction" activating system diminishes mutagenicity [266], the addition of inhibitors such as 3,3,3-trichloropropylene oxide and cyclohexane oxide enhances mutagenicity [267,268].

While enhanced epoxide hydrase activity normally results in the decreased mutagenicity of benzo[a]pyrene metabolites, highly mutagenic products, presumably diol epoxides (see above), were obtained in studies where benzo[a]pyrene 7,8-oxide replaced the parent polycyclic hydrocarbon as the substrate and purified epoxide hydrase was included in the activation system [256]. While epoxide hydrase is involved in both the activation and deactivation of metabolites of benzo[a]pyrene, the enzyme glutathione S-epoxide transferase most probably represents solely a detoxification pathway. Thus benzo[a]pyrene mutagenicity may be enhanced by either depleting glutathione levels in the "S9 fraction" [260] by the addition of diethyl maleate [268] or by using microsomes alone as the activating system [269] where glutathione and the soluble glutathione S-epoxide transferase enzymes are absent (see Sec. II).

The metabolism of polycyclic hydrocarbons and its relationship to cancer has recently been reviewed by DePierre and Ernster [248]. Obviously the interpretation of data derived from in vitro covalent binding studies to DNA and other macromolecules and mutagenicity studies employing the Ames test etc. requires caution when attempting to extrapolate to man. In addition, the different susceptibilities of various tissues to tumor production by polycyclic hydrocarbon administration also requires elucidation. For example, the liver and lung possess both microsomal aryl hydrocarbon hydroxylase and epoxide hydrase enzyme activities. However, although the activities of both enzymes are lower in rat lung the ratio of the levels of the hydrase enzyme to the hydroxylase enzyme is higher in the liver than in the lung [248]. Does this different enzyme ratio make the lung more susceptible than the liver to polycyclic hydrocarbon-induced carcinogenesis, particularly when the carcinogens are inhaled? Attempts have been made to correlate benzo[a]pyrene metabolism with carcinogenicity in in vivo studies. For example, the antioxidant butylated hydroxyanisole has been shown to prevent the induction of forestomach and lung tumors in mice fed the polycyclic hydrocarbon [270,271]. Although benzo[a]pyrene metabolism was not studied in the target organs, the hepatic metabolism of the carcinogen to the detoxification product 3-hydroxybenzo[a]pyrene was enhanced after the antioxidant treatment whereas the formation of epoxides was diminished [272].

D. 2-Acetylaminofluorene

Like benzo[a]pyrene, 2-acetylaminofluorene [2-acetamidofluorene, N-(2-fluorenyl)-acetamide] requires metabolic activation in order to exert its carcinogenic effect. Both the N- and the ring (carbon)-hydroxylations have been shown to be catalyzed by enzymes of the cytochrome P-450-dependent monooxygenase complex [273-277]. While the ring hydroxylations of 2-acetylaminofluorene may be considered to be pathways of detoxification, various investigations have demonstrated that an initial N-hydroxylation reaction is responsible for both the mutagenic and carcinogenic effects of this compound [278-280]. Thus both 2-acetylaminofluorene and N-hydroxy-2-acetylaminofluorene are potent carcinogens in the rat [281-283] whereas ring hydroxylated products such as 7-hydroxy-2-acetylaminofluorene are considered to be either noncarcinogenic or far less carcinogenic than the parent amine [282-285]. Indeed, the administration of 7-hydroxy-2-acetylaminofluorene produced no tumors in rats, while the synthetic compound N-hydroxy-(7-hydroxy)-2-acetylaminofluorene produced a 50% tumor incidence [285]. Further evidence for the relationship between N-hydroxylation and carcinogenesis was provided by the observation that the rate of N-hydroxylation of 2-acetylaminofluorene is some 40-50 times greater than that of its isomer 3-acetylaminofluorene [276], which has only marginal carcinogenicity in the rat [286]. In addition, 3-acetylaminofluorene, but not 2-acetylaminofluorene, is extensively metabolized by oxidation of the carbon atom in position 9 [287]. Finally, mutagenicity studies employing the Ames test have demonstrated that 2-acetylaminofluorene is not converted to toxic epoxide intermediates as the epoxide hydrase inhibitor 3,3,3-trichloropropylene oxide [97], had no effect on 2-acetylaminofluorene mutagenicity while markedly stimulating that of benzo[a]pyrene [268].

Whereas the N-hydroxylation of 2-acetylaminofluorene represents the initial activation step a number of different mechanisms have been postulated for the subsequent conversion of N-hydroxy-2-acetylaminofluorene to reactive mutagenic and carcinogenic products. These may be summarized as follows:

1. N-hydroxy-2-acetylaminofluorene is converted to the highly reactive electrophilic N-O-sulfate ester by a sulfotransferase enzyme present in the soluble fraction. This product then rearranges to yield reactive intermediates which may bind covalently to either protein or nucleic acids [278,288,289]. Indeed, the treatment of rats with sodium sulfate increases the binding of carcinogen metabolites to tissue macromolecules and subsequent toxicity of a dose of N-hydroxy-2-acetylaminofluorene [290].
2. N-hydroxy-2-acetylaminofluorene is converted by microsomal UDP-glucuronyltransferase to the N-O-glucuronide which has been shown to react both in vitro and in vivo with nucleic acids and amino acids [291-294]. Analysis of the adducts formed have demonstrated that covalent binding occurs at the C-8 of guanine and that the N-acetyl group of N-hydroxy-2-acetylaminofluorene is normally retained in binding to RNA, but largely lost in binding to DNA [291, 293]. As the synthetic O-glucuronide of N-hydroxy-2-aminofluorene has been shown to react with GMP [295], there may be more than one mechanism involved in the interaction of conjugated 2-acetylaminofluorene derivatives with nucleic acids.
3. N-hydroxy-2-acetylaminofluorene may also be possibly converted to reactive esters by combination with either acetic acid [296] or phosphoric acid [297].
4. N-hydroxy-2-acetylaminofluorene can be activated by a soluble acetyltransferase enzyme [298,299]. The mechanism of activation thus involves the transfer of the N-acetyl group to the oxygen of the hydroxylamine resulting in the formation of the reactive electrophile N-acetoxy-2-aminofluorene [298].
5. Recent studies on the mutagenicity of N-hydroxy-2-acetylaminofluorene utilizing the Ames test have indicated that while the hepatic soluble sulfotransferase enzyme may even reduce mutagenicity [300,301] a microsomal deacetylase enzyme appears to be responsible for the further activation of N-hydroxy-2-acetylaminofluorene [280,301,302]. Indeed, the compound paraoxon completely inhibits both the microsomal deacetylation [303] and mutagenesis [301,302] of N-hydroxy-2-acetylaminofluorene, whereas the deacetylated product N-hydroxy-2-aminofluorene is highly mutagenic in the Ames test [304,305].

As would be expected, the carcinogenicity of 2-acetylaminofluorene may be greatly influenced by alterations in the levels of hepatic microsomal activating enzymes. For example, 2-acetylaminofluorene is not carcinogenic in the guinea pig [283] as this species is unable to N-hydroxylate the carcinogen unlike the rat, mouse, rabbit, and hamster [278]. Thus the feeding of the carcinogen to guinea pigs does not result in urinary N-hydroxy-2-acetylaminofluorene excretion [48] and guinea pig hepatic microsomal preparations catalyze only the ring hydroxylation of 2-acetylaminofluorene [306]. However, as would be expected, the administration of the activated carcinogen N-hydroxy-2-acetylaminofluorene produces tumors in both the guinea pig and other species [282,283,307]. The metabolism of 2-acetylaminofluorene to both N- and ring (carbon)-hydroxylated products by hepatic microsomal fractions is markedly stimulated in animals treated with monooxygenase-inducing agents such as phenobarbital and 3-methylcholanthrene [273,277,306,308,309,310]. However, the feeding of 2-acetylaminofluorene with 3-methylcholanthrene to rats markedly reduces the subsequent tumor incidence [281,307] whereas the monooxygenase enzyme inducer has no such protective effect on 2-acetylaminofluorene carcinogenesis in the hamster [308]. It would appear that in the rat 3-methylcholanthrene treatment induces both N- and ring-hydroxylations [306,309], thus resulting in a reduction in the levels of and urinary excretion of N-hydroxy-2-acetylaminofluorene [48,306], whereas in the hamster, where 3-methylcholanthrene primarily increased the N-hydroxylation toxification pathway [277,306,308], no significant effect on urinary N-hydroxy-2-acetylaminofluorene excretion was observed [261]. As would be expected, 3-methylcholanthrene administration does not protect against tumor formation by N-hydroxy-2-acetylaminofluorene in the rat [282]; while treatment with the enzyme inducer reduces the amount of radioactivity bound to liver nucleic acids following a dose of labeled 2-acetylaminofluorene, it has no reductive effect after a dose of labeled N-hydroxy-2-acetylaminofluorene [307].

As with certain inducers of hepatic xenobiotic metabolism 2-acetylaminofluorene is known to stimulate its own metabolism to N-hydroxy-2-acetylaminofluorene. Thus 2-acetylaminofluorene treatment enhances rat hepatic microsomal N-hydroxylase activity [311] and stimulates the urinary excretion of N-hydroxy-2-acetylaminofluorene [48,312]. However, the 2-acetylaminofluorene-mediated increase in its toxification pathway does not appear to be the result of a general stimulation of microsomal xenobiotic metabolism as the increase in 2-acetylaminofluorene N-hydroxylase activity occurs without any increases in microsomal monooxygenase electron-transport components such as cytochrome P-450s or NADPH-cytochrome c reductase [311].

In addition to the effects of known inducers of hepatic microsomal monooxygenases, certain other agents including acetanilide, 4-hydroxyacetanilide, and other related compounds have been shown to inhibit tumor production by both 2-acetylaminofluorene [313-315] and N-hydroxy-2-acetylaminofluorene [314,316]. Acetanilide appears to inhibit tumor production by a number of different mechanisms. For example, in the case of 2-acetylaminofluorene, acetanilide appears to inhibit N-hydroxylation resulting in reduced binding of carcinogen metabolites to tissue macromolecules [317]. Indeed, acetanilide and/or its metabolites have been shown to bind to tissue macromolecules [318] and may therefore be blocking carcinogen receptor sites. The inhibition of N-hydroxy-2-acetylaminofluorene carcinogenicity may be due to reduced formation of the activated sulfate ester as the major metabolite of acetanilide, namely, 4-hydroxyacetanilide, is partially excreted as a sulfate conjugate [318,319]. Hence the administration of additional dietary sulfate reverses the acetanilide-mediated protection against N-hydroxy-2-acetylaminofluorene hepatocarcinogenicity but has no effect on the inhibition of 2-acetylaminofluorene tumor production [316].

While the modification of 2-acetylaminofluorene metabolism by acetanilide and related compounds appears to result in detoxification of the carcinogen, not all inhibitors may have such beneficial effects. For example, although the pesticide synergist piperonyl butoxide inhibits the overall rate of 2-acetylaminofluorene metabolism by mouse liver microsomal preparations, only ring hydroxylations are decreased whereas N-hydroxylation is markedly enhanced [320]. The stimulation of 2-acetylaminofluorene toxification in vitro is paralleled in vivo by increased covalent binding of carcinogen metabolites to liver nucleic acids. A similar differential effect on the in vitro rate of 2-acetylaminofluorene metabolism by hepatic microsomal preparations has been observed after treatment of hamsters with 3-amino-1,2,4-triazole [277].

To summarize, the metabolism and toxicity of 2-acetylaminofluorene provides an example of species differences in metabolism, where species unable to N-hydroxylate the xenobiotic are protected from the carcinogenic effects. Furthermore, the metabolism of this xenobiotic to toxic products requires both functionalization and conjugation enzymes.

E. Allyl Alcohol

Allyl alcohol and certain of its esters such as allyl formate have been shown to produce periportal hepatic necrosis [321,322], which is associated with the covalent binding of allyl alcohol metabolites to tissue macromolecules [322]. However, unlike paracetamol, benzo[a]pyrene, and 2-acetylaminofluorene, allyl alcohol is not activated by enzymes of the microsomal cytochrome P-450-dependent monooxygenase complex, but is converted to acrolein (Fig. 3) by cytosolic alcohol dehydrogenase [321-323]. Acrolein is an extremely reactive hepatotoxic agent and has been shown to inhibit both protein synthesis [321] and mitochondrial function [324] in vitro. Additional in vivo studies have demonstrated that acrolein inhibits both hepatic DNA and RNA synthesis [325] whereas the administration of allyl alcohol results in the inhibition of a number of enzyme activities including cytochrome P-450s, monooxygenases, and alcohol dehydrogenase [326,327].

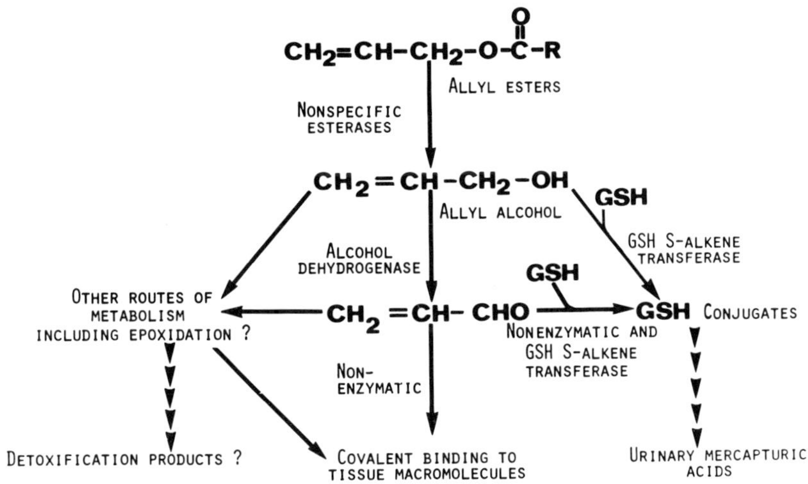

FIGURE 3 Pathways of metabolism of allyl esters and allyl alcohol. The allyl ester side chain is indicated by R.

Evidence for the metabolic pathway shown in Fig. 3 comes from the observations that inhibitors of alcohol dehydrogenase markedly reduce the metabolism of allyl alcohol to acrolein in liver homogenates [323] and prevent the covalent binding of allyl alcohol metabolites and subsequent hepatic necrosis in vivo [322], whereas the induction of monooxygenase activity by pretreatment with phenobarbital has no effect [322]. Furthermore, the hepatotoxicity of allyl alcohol in isolated perfused organ studies is abolished by the prior perfusion of ethanol presumably due to competition between the two alcohols for alcohol dehydrogenase [328]. Similarly, the hepatotoxicity of the esters allyl acetate and allyl cinnamate could be prevented [329] by the treatment of rats with the alcohol dehydrogenase inhibitor pyrazole [330]. In addition, the hydrolysis of these two esters could be prevented by the administration of tri-ortho-tolyl phosphate, which inhibits the nonspecific carboxylesterases catalyzing the hydrolysis of allyl esters in rat liver homogenates [329].

As with paracetamol, the intracellular levels of reduced glutathione are of paramount importance in determining the subsequent toxicity of allyl alcohol. For example, allyl alcohol may serve as a substrate for glutathione S-alkenetransferase [331] whereas acrolein can react both enzymatically [332] and nonenzymatically [333] with reduced glutathione. Indeed, urinary mercapturic acid conjugates have been detected after the administration of acrolein, allyl alcohol, and several allyl esters to rats [334].

As would be expected, the depletion of intracellular glutathione levels by the administration of diethyl maleate potentiates the hepatotoxicity of allyl alcohol [335].

In contrast to hepatotoxins such as paracetamol, carbon tetrachloride, and bromobenzene which give rise to necrosis of the centrilobular areas of the liver lobule [140,336,337], allyl alcohol produces necrosis in the periportal regions [321,322]. These observations may be simply explained on the basis that the enzymes which activate these hepatotoxins have been shown not to be uniformly distributed throughout the parenchymal cells of the liver lobule. Thus the enzymes of the monooxygenase complex including cytochrome P-450 [338,339], cytochrome b_5 [340], aryl hydrocarbon hydroxylase [132], NADPH-cytochrome c reductase [341], and larger amounts of smooth endoplasmic reticulum [342] are concentrated in hepatocytes around the central veins, whereas alcohol dehydrogenase has been shown to be more active in the periportal areas [321,343]. However, it should be noted that not all hepatotoxins believed to be activated by cytochrome P-450-dependent monooxygenases produce centrilobular liver lesions. For example, treatments which either enhance or depress monooxygenase enzyme activity have been shown to shift the site of the lesion produced by the sesquiterpene ngaione in mice [344]. Furthermore, although the highest concentrations of cytochrome P-450 occur in the centrilobular cells, the various forms of this hemoprotein which have different catalytic activities (see Sec. IV) are not uniformly distributed throughout the cells of the liver lobule [339].*

In summary, allyl alcohol is an example of a xenobiotic not activated to toxic products by enzymes of the microsomal monooxygenase complex. Studies with this hepatotoxin also demonstrate that xenobiotic-metabolizing enzyme activities are not uniformly distributed through the cells of the liver.

IV. MODIFYING FACTORS

The detoxification and/or activation of a xenobiotic may be altered as a consequence of the influence on the organism of a variety of factors including

---

*Although previous histochemical studies have indicated that hepatic-reduced glutathione content shows a fairly uniform distribution throughout the cells of the liver lobule [344a], recent studies employing a more quantitative procedure [344b] have demonstrated that periportal cells may contain more than twice as much reduced glutathione as centrilobular hepatocytes. Thus, as many reactive metabolites are detoxified by conjugation with glutathione, this may provide an additional reason for the higher susceptibility of centrilobular cells to hepatotoxins such as bromobenzene and paracetamol.

exposure to other xenobiotics. Furthermore, in addition to environmental changes marked species, strain and sex differences have also been observed. A number of factors known to affect the activities of hepatic xenobiotic-metabolizing enzymes are shown in Table 4. It should also be noted that extrahepatic xenobiotic-metabolizing enzyme activities can be modified by the administration of foreign compounds [109,362] (also see below) and by dietary manipulation including starvation [101,363-365]. As with hepatic xenobiotic-metabolizing enzymes, extrahepatic enzyme activity exhibits circadian rhythms [366], may be affected in disease states [367], and develops with age, being low in fetal and newborn animals [368-370].

In this section a few of the more important variables affecting the metabolism of xenobiotics will be considered.

A. Enzyme Induction and Inhibition

As stated in Sec. II, the enzymes of the hepatic microsomal cytochrome P-450-dependent monooxygenase complex may be stimulated by many foreign compounds, of which the two "model" inducers are phenobarbital and 3-methylcholanthrene [345]. Furthermore, it has been established that hepatic microsomes from both untreated and induced animals contain multiple forms

TABLE 4
Factors Affecting the Activities of Hepatic Xenobiotic-metabolizing Enzymes

Factor	Reference(s)
Enzyme induction	345
Sex differences	346,347
Strain differences	348,349
Species differences	22,184,350
Age differences	351,352
Hormonal status	353
Nutritional status	347,354,355
Pregnancy	356,357
Disease	353,358
Circadian variation	359,360
Stress	361

of cytochrome P-450 which exhibit widely different substrate and catalytic affinities [50-55]. Similarly multiple hemoprotein types have also been detected in extrahepatic tissues [371,372]. While phenobarbital induces many types of hepatic xenobiotic biotransformations, 3-methylcholanthrene stimulates only certain enzyme activities [345]. The major forms of microsomal hemoprotein present after induction by these two compounds are termed cytochrome P-450 and P-448 (or P_1-450) respectively [51,54]. Recent studies with either commercial polychlorinated biphenyl [373] or polybrominated biphenyl [374] mixtures have led to "mixed-type" patterns of induction in that the induced microsomal enzymes have properties of both the drug type, e.g., phenobarbital and the polycyclic hydrocarbon classes of inducers. The duration of and magnitude of induction of hepatic xenobiotic metabolism by the various inducing agents differs greatly, for example, 3-methylcholanthrene and β-naphthoflavone both induce cytochrome P-448 and associated enzymes, but induction by the former compound is more prolonged as β-naphthoflavone is more rapidly excreted by the animal [375]. In addition, the compound 2,3,7,8-tetrachlorodibenzo-para-dioxin is 30,000 times more potent as an inducer of aryl hydrocarbon hydroxylase in the rat than 3-methylcholanthrene [376], with an oral dose as low as 2 ng/kg producing a significant stimulation of enzyme activity [377]. The studies of Nebert and coworkers with strains of inbred mice have demonstrated that the induction of cytochrome P-448 and associated monooxygenase enzyme activities is genetically linked, in that animals may be classified as either genetically "responsive" or "nonresponsive" to the administration of polycyclic hydrocarbon inducers [378-380]. However, the administration of inducing agents other than polycyclic hydrocarbons can stimulate enzyme activities in both categories of mouse strains [381].

In addition to quantitative differences in levels of stimulation of monooxygenases by various inducers, the nature of the different forms of cytochrome P-450 produced may also cause qualitative differences in the metabolism of xenobiotics. For example, the monooxygenase substrates testosterone, bromobenzene, n-hexane, and benzo[a]pyrene are primarily metabolized at different positions by microsomal preparations from animals pretreated with either phenobarbital or 3-methylcholanthrene [379]. In the case of the hepatotoxin bromobenzene, phenobarbital stimulates the monooxygenase-catalyzed formation of reactive epoxide intermediates and subsequent hepatic necrosis in the rat, whereas treatment with 3-methylcholanthrene protects against bromobenzene toxicity [195,382,383]. This protection is due to the stimulation of the conversion of the toxic 3,4-bromobenzene oxide to the corresponding nontoxic dihydrodiol and also to the greatly enhanced formation of 2-bromophenol, another product of detoxification [383]. Studies on the binding of benzo[a]pyrene metabolites to DNA catalyzed by liver microsomal preparations from mice treated with several inducing agents have demonstrated that the various forms of cytochrome P-450 are responsible for large differences in both the magnitude and the nature of the benzo[a]pyrene metabolite-DNA adducts formed [384].

Other aspects of enzyme induction that warrant consideration are the induction of non-monooxygenase-dependent xenobiotic-metabolizing enzymes and both tissue and subcellular differences in response to inducing agents. For example, in addition to their effects on monooxygenases, phenobarbital and 3-methylcholanthrene also induce other xenobiotic-metabolizing enzymes such as UDP-glucuronyltransferase [385,386], epoxide hydrase [71,387], and glutathione S-transferase [120,388,389]. However, the activities of these enzymes toward particular substrates may not be always induced as a result of the administration of monooxygenase-inducing agents. Recent studies have suggested that certain epoxides such as trans-stilbene oxide at low doses may stimulate hepatic microsomal epoxide hydrase activity without affecting either levels of cytochrome P-450s or monooxygenase activity [390-392]. The induction of xenobiotic-metabolizing enzymes other than those of the monooxygenase complex can greatly complicate the interpretation of experiments where induced animals have been employed as tools to study the metabolism of a xenobiotic. Furthermore, the resultant toxicity of a xenobiotic may be greatly influenced by the relative percentage increase in monooxygenase and other xenobiotic-metabolizing enzyme activities, e.g., see benzo[a]pyrene (Sec. II.C). With regard to tissue differences in enzyme induction, extrahepatic tissues are often refractory to the effects of known inducers of hepatic xenobiotic metabolism [109,393,394]. Although 3-methylcholanthrene induces certain xenobiotic-metabolizing enzymes in extrahepatic tissues of the rat, phenobarbital is a poor inducer of extrahepatic enzymes in this species [109,394,395] and even the potent inducer of hepatic xenobiotic metabolism 2,3,7,8-tetrachlorodibenzo-para-dioxin was found to be ineffective in stimulating aryl hydrocarbon hydroxylase in rat testis [118,396]. Recent studies have demonstrated that the nuclear fraction contains cytochrome P-450s, monooxygenases and epoxide hydrase [56,57,58,59,397] and that these enzymes, like their microsomal counterparts, are inducible by certain foreign compounds [57,398]. These nuclear xenobiotic-metabolizing enzymes may be of great importance in chemical carcinogenesis owing to their close proximity to the genetic material of the cell. Indeed, these enzymes have been shown to catalyze the formation of metabolite-DNA adducts from carcinogens such as benzo[a]pyrene and 2-acetylaminofluorene [57,89,399,400].

Finally, it should be noted that enzyme induction is not necessarily sustained by the continued administration of the compound to the animal. For example, while the prolonged administration of either butylated hydroxytoluene or phenobarbital results in sustained enzyme induction [401,402], other compounds such as dieldrin, methyl butter yellow, safrole, and Ponceau MX, which also initially stimulate hepatic xenobiotic-metabolizing enzymes, result in a decline of enzyme activities on prolonged treatment [403,404].

Enzyme induction is important in humans not only with respect to possible effects on the metabolism of xenobiotics, but also for adverse effects on the metabolism of endogenous substrates of the microsomal monooxygenase complex. Indeed, adverse effects on the metabolism of folic acid [405], steroids [406], and vitamin D [407] have been observed in epileptic patients receiving anticonvulsant drugs such as phenobarbital and diphenylhydantoin which are known to stimulate hepatic xenobiotic metabolism in humans [406,408]. Similarly, enzyme induction may be of importance in instances where one drug enhances the metabolism and subsequent pharmacological effectiveness of another drug [409].

The activities of xenobiotic-metabolizing enzymes are often found to be impaired in a number of liver disease states in humans such as hepatitis, cirrhosis, cholestasis, obstructive jaundice, and neoplasia [353,358,410]. Apart from diminished enzyme activities, liver disease may also result in alterations in the biliary excretion of xenobiotics and in their binding to serum proteins [410]. Thus liver disease and certain other abnormal physiological states (see Table 4) may result in the prolonged exposure of the organism to xenobiotics with a possible concomitant increase in toxicity.

B. Nutrition

A number of studies have demonstrated that variation in the amount of nutrients in the diet can markedly affect xenobiotic metabolism in both experimental animals and in humans. For example, low-protein diets [139,165, 411] and fat-free diets [412] are known to decrease hepatic xenobiotic-metabolizing enzymes and cytochrome P-450 content. Similarly, studies in humans have demonstrated that the plasma half-lives of antipyrine and theophylline were shortened (i.e., induced) by the administration of a high-protein/low-carbohydrate diet but prolonged by a low-protein/high-carbohydrate diet [413]. In addition to changes in enzyme activities, nutritionally inadequate diets may affect the metabolism of xenobiotics by altering the levels of essential cofactors and coenzymes. For example, a low-protein diet reduces the hepatic content of reduced glutathione and consequently enhances paracetamol hepatotoxicity, despite the fact that the levels of cytochrome P-450 (which activates the analgesic—see Sec. III.A) are also reduced [165].

Apart from variations in xenobiotic metabolism due to high or low intake of nutrients, dietary anutrients possibly represent the highest source of human exposure to foreign compounds. While certain food additives (e.g., the antioxidant butylated hydroxytoluene [414]) and contaminants (e.g., the pesticide dichlorodiphenyltrichloroethane [415] and polychlorinated biphenyls [373]) are known inducers of xenobiotic metabolism in animals, a number of naturally occurring compounds may also affect the rate of foreign compound metabolism. For example, the natural anutrients β-ionone [416], safrole [401,416], linalol [417], caffeine [418], flavones and related compounds [419], phenothiazine and certain of its derivatives [113], and various indole derivatives [363,413,420] have been found to stimulate either extrahepatic and/or hepatic xenobiotic metabolism in experimental animals. Similarly, the consumption of vegetables such as Brussels sprouts and cabbage, which contain enzyme-inducing indoles [363,413,420], has been shown to induce the metabolism of antipyrine and phenacetin in humans [421]. In addition, levels of both hepatic and extrahepatic xenobiotic-metabolizing enzymes are lower in experimental animals fed purified semisynthetic diets instead of normal stock diets which contain vegetable matter [422-425]. A number of studies have demonstrated that polycyclic hydrocarbons, whether consumed in the diet, e.g., in charcoal-broiled beef, or inhaled in cigarette smoke also stimulate hepatic and extrahepatic xenobiotic metabolism in experimental animals [413,425,426] and in humans [413,425-429]. Indeed, cigarette smoking may have toxicological consequences for the human fetus as certain xenobiotic-metabolizing enzyme activities including aryl hydrocarbon hydroxylase are elevated in the placentas of women who smoked during pregnancy [109,425,427,430].

A number of investigations have demonstrated that the dietary administration of enzyme inducers, including those of natural origin, can reduce the tumor incidence of a number of carcinogens. For example, food antioxidants including butylated hydroxytoluene inhibit the tumorigenesis of benzo[a]pyrene, 2-acetylaminofluorene, and N-hydroxy-2-acetylaminofluorene [271,272,431], whereas certain flavones and phenothiazine reduce the carcinogenicity of benzo[a]pyrene [432] and bracken fern [433], respectively. The carcinogenicity of xenobiotics may be also affected by other components of the diet. For example, the carcinogenicity of 4-dimethylaminoazobenzene is enhanced by feeding riboflavin-deficient diets, as riboflavin was found to be essential for the hepatic metabolism of the carcinogen to nontoxic products by reduction of the axo linkage [434]. Indeed, riboflavin deficiency has been shown to depress a number of xenobiotic-metabolizing enzymes [435,436]. Another important dietary constituent is L-ascorbic acid (vitamin C), which is essential for the maintenance of xenobiotic-metabolizing enzyme activities in the guinea pig [437]. In addition, recent studies have demonstrated that highly carcinogenic nitrosamines may be formed in vivo from sodium nitrite and secondary amines ingested in the diet [438,439]. However, the coadministration of L-ascorbic acid with the nitrosamine precursors blocks the formation of the nitrosamines in the stomachs of rats and mice [440,441]. Thus dietary L-ascorbic acid may serve to protect humans against the toxic effects of nitrosamines synthesized from dietary components.

C. Genetic Factors

A number of studies have demonstrated that genetic differences (including both species and strain differences) can markedly affect the metabolism and subsequent toxicity of xenobiotics. For example, studies with inbred strains of mice have demonstrated genetic differences in aryl hydrocarbon hydroxylase inducibility, benzo[a]pyrene toxicity, 3-methylcholanthrene initiated tumorigenesis, paracetamol-induced hepatotoxicity, etc. [379,380, 442]. Furthermore, in the case of enzyme activities the magnitude of enzyme induction may vary greatly with the tissue, strain, and species, indicating genetic differences in the regulation of enzyme activities with regard to basal levels and in response to stimulation [443].

Studies in man have demonstrated wide interindividual differences in xenobiotic metabolism as assessed both by the in vitro measurement of enzyme activities and the in vivo determination of plasma drug half-lives [96,425,430,444,445]. The wide variations encountered in human xenobiotic metabolism have been attributed to both environmental and to genetic factors [444,446-448] and complicate the assessment of animal studies in terms of possible human hazards.

V. METHODS FOR ASSESSING XENOBIOTIC METABOLISM

Studies in intact experimental animals and in humans are obviously the means for assessing the biological fate of xenobiotics in terms of their absorption, metabolism, disposition, and excretion. In the case of drugs, investigations into pharmacokinetics and bioavailability are essential prerequisites for developing a sound basis for chemotherapy. This experimental approach, equally valid in the context of chemicals used as food additives and in cosmetic preparations, is widely used and the literature is replete with references on the metabolic disposition of xenobiotics in live animals and humans.

However, before investigations in humans are undertaken it is imperative that complete and detailed information generated from animal experiments is available on the metabolic fate and toxicity of a test compound. A fuller understanding of the biochemical mechanisms mediating the bioactivation and detoxification of xenobiotics and of the factors influencing these processes can best be obtained by studies on intact organs or tissue preparations. Equally in the case of toxic chemicals and carcinogens where human exposure is clearly undesirable, assessment of the human hazard can be made more meaningful by data generated in in vitro studies. Three experimental approaches employed in the study of the metabolism of xenobiotics will be considered briefly. These are isolated organ perfusion technique, cell suspension and cell culture systems, and tissue preparations. As the liver is the principal organ involved in xenobiotic metabolism, consideration will be mainly confined to hepatic metabolism. This does not minimize the role of other organs and tissues in the biotransformation of foreign compounds, and techniques developed for studies on the liver are equally applicable to other organs.

The isolated liver perfusion technique, admirably described in detail by Miller [449], can be readily applied to the study of the metabolism of xenobiotics. Examples of such studies include the hepatic metabolism of diazepam [450], procarbazine [451], and nortriptyline [452]; and in isolated rabbit lung, the metabolism of benzo[a]pyrene [453]. The isolated organ perfusion technique offers certain advantages not only by virtue of its ability to mediate the multistep metabolism of substances, thereby providing a system for elucidating the intermediate pathways of biodegradation, but also enables the study of the distribution, storage, and excretion of xenobiotics and their metabolites in tissues. Conversely, the technique requires considerable surgical operative skill, is time-consuming and expensive, and presents problems in maintaining consistent and reproducible viability of the isolated organ during a perfusion study.

The isolated cell suspension and cell culture systems have been extensively used in recent years for the study of xenobiotic metabolism. The methods employed for isolating whole cell preparations from the liver and other organs and cell culture techniques have been fully described by Fry and Bridges [454]. This review also cites numerous examples of the application of these systems for investigating the metabolism of xenobiotics. More recently isolated hepatocyte suspensions have been used for studying the metabolism of biphenyl [455], norbenzphetamine [456], aminopyrine [457], and of drugs metabolized by aromatic and aliphatic hydroxylation, N-demethylation, and glucuronidation [458]. The metabolism of paracetamol by isolated kidney cells has been studied [150], comparative studies carried out on a number of substrates metabolized by the monooxygenase complex in rat hepatocytes and kidney tubule fragments [459], and species differences in benzoic acid metabolism have been investigated [460]. While the isolated cell suspension and cell culture systems have undoubted advantages, there are also problems associated with their use. These problems stem mainly from technical difficulties associated with the handling of cells, the identification and estimation of minute amounts of metabolites formed, and the expression of results.

By far the most extensively used method for investigating xenobiotic metabolism is to employ homogenate preparations of tissues and subcellular fractions obtained by differential centrifugation procedures. The literature on the methodology, kinetics, cofactor requirements, and effects of inhibitors and inducers on enzymic biotransformation of xenobiotics in these in vitro systems is copious and commendable reviews on this subject appear regularly. Useful starting points are either Handbook of Experimental Pharmacology [461] or Methods in Enzymology [462]. Undoubtedly the use of in vitro systems including the many refinements such as the use of purified enzyme preparations has added immeasurably to the understanding of the biochemical mechanisms underlying the biotransformation of xenobiotics. Nevertheless it must be recognized that the in vitro system, a biochemist's artifact, has certain serious drawbacks and limitations. Preparative procedures, ionic strength and pH of the medium, levels of cofactors, and other variables can influence the metabolism of compounds. Furthermore, membrane transport, the interplay of multistep metabolic processes and vectorial factors, all essential features in the biotransformation and disposition of xenobiotics in the intact organ, cannot be studied in homogenate preparations. In addition, the results of enzyme induction and enzyme inhibition studies require careful interpretation. For example, the compounds 3,3,3-trichloropropylene oxide and cyclohexene oxide are often employed as inhibitors of epoxide hydrase activity in vitro [97,463]; however, when administered in vivo both compounds enhance hepatic epoxide hydrase activity while reducing liver reduced glutathione content [463]. Indeed, 3,3,3-trichloropropylene oxide also inhibits monooxygenase activity [464], whereas the monooxygenase inhibitor metyrapone may increase the rate of hydration of certain epoxides [465]. Similarly, in studies where monooxygenase activities are depleted in vivo by treatment with cobalt chloride, the tissue levels of reduced glutathione are enhanced, which may further diminish the toxification of certain xenobiotics [466].

All of the techniques described have an important role in elucidating the metabolism of xenobiotics. Each of the methods has certain advantages and limitations and an intelligent appreciation of these is essential for a sound and meaningful assessment of the biological fate of xenobiotics.

VI. CONCLUSION

The biological fate of xenobiotics in the intact organism is governed by a number of interrelated factors. These include the form, dose, and route of exposure, absorption, metabolism, disposition, and excretion. Each of these factors has an essential role to play in regulating the bioavailability of a xenobiotic, in the processes mediating its activation and detoxification, in the pharmacological effects exerted, and the toxicological sequelae following exposure.

The liver, replete with a variety of processing enzymes, essential cofactors, and endogenous scavengers of reactive metabolites such as reduced glutathione and vitamin E, is undoubtedly the principal organ mediating the biotransformation of xenobiotics. However, other sites in the body have an equally important and, in certain situations even a crucial function to fulfill in the metabolism and disposition of xenobiotics. Thus, depending on the amount and route of exposure, the skin, lung, small intestine, and gastrointestinal microflora may either in part or wholly determine the metabolic fate of a compound.

Equally germane in this context is the influence of modifying factors on enzyme systems involved in biotransformation processes and their effects on enhancing or ameliorating the toxicity of compounds. A wide variety of compounds, including drugs, food additives, pesticides, and environmental chemicals have the ability of inducing or inhibiting the monooxygenase system, thereby altering not only their own metabolic fate and pharmacotoxicological effects but also that of other xenobiotics and endogenous substances. Additionally, other factors such as age, sex, genetic defects, and diet have a profound influence in modifying the activation and detoxification mechanisms involved in the metabolic fate of xenobiotics.

The picture that emerges is one of complex and dynamic systems wherein interrelated and conflicting factors operating either in tandem or in parallel act upon xenobiotics and influence their metabolic fate in the body. The net effect of these interactions on a compound determines its pharmacological activity and toxicity in an organism. Clearly, a reasonable understanding of these biochemical mechanisms of toxification and detoxification and of pharmacokinetics is essential in both the strategy and tactics of the approaches to the toxicological evaluation of xenobiotics present in the human chemical environment.

REFERENCES

1. R. G. Todd (Ed.), Extra Pharmacopoeia Martindale, 25th ed. Pharmaceutical Press, London, 1967.
2. A. Wade (Ed.), Extra Pharmacopoeia Martindale, 27th ed. Pharmaceutical Press, London, 1977.
3. Food Chemical Codex, 2nd ed. National Academy of Sciences, Washington, D.C., 1972.
4. Harry's Cosmeticology, 6th ed. (rev. J. B. H. Wilkinson). Intertext Group, London, 1973.
5. P. Wright, Brit. Med. J. 1:595-598 (1975).
6. J. O. Craig, I. C. Ferguson, and J. Syme, Brit. Med. J. 1:757-761 (1966).
7. J. R. Mitchell, R. J. McMurtry, C. N. Statham, and S. D. Nelson, Amer. J. Med. 62:518-526 (1977).
8. L. F. Prescott, Brit. J. Clin. Pharmacol. 7:453-462 (1979).
9. Environmental Health Criteria, Vol. 1. Mercury. World Health Organization, Geneva, 1976.
10. Cadmium: Criteria (Dose/Effect Relationships) for Commission of the European Communities. Pergamon, London, 1978.
11. Food Additives and Contaminants Committee Review of Lead in Food Regulations, FAC/REP/21. Her Majesty's Stationary Office, London, 1975.
12. R. L. Rodnitzky, H. S. Levin, and D. L. Mick, Arch. Environ. Health 30:98-103 (1975).
13. K. W. Jager, Aldrin, Dieldrin, Endrin, and Telodrin. Elsevier, Amsterdam, 1970.
14. R. D. Kimbrough, Crit. Rev. Toxicol. 2:445-498 (1974).
15. L. J. Carter, Science 192:240-243 (1976).
16. E. Boyland, Proc. Roy. Soc. Med. 60:93-99 (1967).

17. R. Doll, Prevention of Cancer: Pointers from Epidemiology. Whitefriars, London, 1967.
18. J. Higginson, Present trends in cancer epidemiology, Canadian Cancer Conf. 8:40-75 (1969).
19. S. D. Nelson, J. R. Mitchell, J. A. Timbrell, W. R. Snodgrass, and C. B. Corcoran III, Science 193:901-903 (1976).
20. J. R. Gillette and L. R. Pohl, J. Toxicol. Environ. Health 2:849-871 (1977).
21. S. D. Nelson, J. R. Mitchell, W. R. Snodgrass, and J. A. Timbrell, J. Pharmacol. Exp. Ther. 206:574-585 (1978).
22. R. T. Williams, Fed. Proc. Fed. Amer. Soc. Exp. Biol. 26:1029-1039 (1967).
23. D. V. Parke, The Biochemistry of Foreign Compounds. Pergamon, Oxford, 1968.
24. P. Siekevitz, Fed. Proc. Fed. Amer. Soc. Exp. Biol. 24:1153-1154 (1965).
25. B. B. Brodie, J. Axelrod, J. R. Cooper, L. Gaudette, B. N. La Du, C. Mitoma, and S. Udenfriend, Science 121:603-604 (1955).
26. H. S. Mason, Science 125:1185-1188 (1957).
27. H. S. Mason, J. C. North, and M. Vanneste, Fed. Proc. Fed. Amer. Soc. Exp. Biol. 24:1172-1180 (1965).
28. T. Omura, R. Sato, D. Y. Cooper, O. Rosenthal, and R. W. Estabrook, Fed. Proc. Fed. Amer. Soc. Exp. Biol. 24:1181-1189 (1965).
29. A. Hildebrandt and R. W. Estabrook, Arch. Biochem. Biophys. 143:66-79 (1971).
30. C. Mitoma, H. S. Posner, H. C. Reitz, and S. Udenfriend, Arch. Biochem. Biophys. 61:431-444 (1956).
31. A. H. Conney, E. C. Miller, and J. A. Miller, J. Biol. Chem. 228:753-766 (1957).
32. P. J. Creaven, D. V. Parke, and R. T. Williams, Biochem. J. 96:879-885 (1965).
33. U. Frommer, V. Ullrich, H. Staudinger, and S. Orrenius, Biochim. Biophys. Acta 280:487-494 (1971).
34. J. R. Cooper and B. B. Brodie, J. Pharmacol. Exp. Ther. 114:409-417 (1955).
35. C. C. Irving, J. Biol. Chem. 239:1589-1596 (1964).
36. B. N. La Du, L. Gaudette, N. Trousof, and B. B. Brodie, J. Biol. Chem. 214:741-752 (1955).
37. G. C. Mueller and J. A. Miller, J. Biol. Chem. 202:579-587 (1953).
38. V. Ullrich and P. Weber, Hoppe-Seyler's Z. Physiol. Chem. 353:1171-1177 (1972).
39. K. J. Netter and G. Seidel, J. Pharmacol. Exp. Ther. 146:61-65 (1964).

40. P. Mazel, J. F. Henderson, and J. Axelrod, J. Pharmacol. Exp. Ther. 143:1-6 (1964).
41. J. Axelrod, J. Biol. Chem. 214:753-763 (1955).
42. R. A. Van Dyke and M. B. Chenoweth, Biochem. Pharmacol. 14:603-609 (1965).
43. N. P. Salzman and B. B. Brodie, J. Pharmacol. Exp. Ther. 118:46-54 (1956).
44. J. R. Fouts, J. J. Kamm, and B. B. Brodie, J. Pharmacol. Exp. Ther. 120:291-300 (1957).
45. J. R. Fouts and B. B. Brodie, J. Pharmacol. Exp. Ther. 119:197-207 (1957).
46. J. R. Gillette, J. J. Kamm, and H. A. Sasame, Mol. Pharmacol. 4:541-548 (1968).
47. P. H. Hernandez, P. Mazel, and J. R. Gillette, Biochem. Pharmacol. 16:1877-1888 (1967).
48. J. A. Miller, J. W. Cramer, and E. C. Miller, Cancer Res. 20:950-962 (1960).
49. J. H. Peters and H. R. Gutmann, J. Biol. Chem. 216:713-726 (1955).
50. K. Comai and J. L. Gaylor, J. Biol. Chem. 248:4947-4955 (1973).
51. A. P. Alvares and P. Siekvitz, Biochem. Biophys. Res. Commun. 54:923-929 (1973).
52. M. Warner, M. V. LaMarca, and A. H. Neims, Drug Metab. Dispos. 6:353-362 (1978).
53. D. A. Haugen, T. A. van der Hoeven, and M. J. Coon, J. Biol. Chem. 250:3567-3570 (1975).
54. D. Ryan, A. Y. H. Lu, J. Kawalek, S. B. West, and W. Levin, Biochem. Biophys. Res. Commun. 64:1134-1141 (1975).
55. F. P. Guengerich, J. Biol. Chem. 252:3970-3979 (1977).
56. C. B. Kasper, J. Biol. Chem. 246:577-581 (1971).
57. E. G. Rogan, P. Mailander, and E. Cavalieri, Proc. Nat. Acad. Sci. U.S. 73:457-461 (1976).
58. W. A. Bornstein, H. Chuang, E. Bresnick, H. Mukhtar, and J. R. Bend, Chem.-Biol. Interact. 21:343-346 (1978).
59. H. Mukhtar, T. H. Elmanlouk, R. M. Philpot, and J. R. Bend, Mol. Pharmacol. 15:192-196 (1979).
60. R. Sato, Y. Atsuta, Y. Imai, S. Taniguchi, and K. Okuda, Proc. Nat. Acad. Sci. U.S. 74:5477-5481 (1977).
61. I. Raw, Biochem. Biophys. Res. Commun. 81:1294-1297 (1978).
62. T. Koivula and M. Koivusalo, Biochim. Biophys. Acta 397:9-23 (1975).
63. G. C. Cotzias and V. P. Dole, Proc. Soc. Exp. Biol. Med. 78:157-160 (1951).
64. P. Baudhuin, H. Beaufay, Y. Rahman-Li, O. Z. Sellinger, R. Wattiaux, P. Jaques, and C. De Duve, Biochem. J. 92:179-184 (1964).
65. K. Hayase and A. L. Tappel, J. Biol. Chem. 244:2269-2274 (1969).
66. R. E. Talcott, Toxicol. Appl. Pharmacol. 47:145-150 (1979).

67. R. A. Weisiger and I. Fridovich, J. Biol. Chem. 248:3582-3592 (1973).
68. K. Irjala, Ann. Acad. Sci. Fenn., Ser. A 5:154, 40 pp (1972).
69. C. De Duve, B. C. Pressman, R. Gianetto, R. Wattiaux, and F. Appelmans, Biochem. J. 60:604-617 (1955).
70. W. Guder, L. Weiss, and O. Wieland, Biochim. Biophys. Acta 187: 173-185 (1969).
71. F. Oesch, Xenobiotica 3:305-340 (1973).
72. A. Y. H. Lu, D. Ryan, D. M. Jerina, J. W. Daly, and W. Levin, J. Biol. Chem. 250:8283-8288 (1975).
72a. K. Ota and B. D. Hammock, Science 207:1479-1481 (1980).
73. V. G. Erwin and R. A. Deitrich, Mol. Pharmacol. 7:219-228 (1971).
74. D. M. Ziegler and C. H. Mitchell, Arch. Biochem. Biophys. 150: 116-125 (1972).
75. J. W. Gorrod, Chem.-Biol. Interact. 7:289-303 (1973).
76. J. Axelrod, Science 140:499-500 (1963).
77. J. K. Inscoe, J. Daly, and J. Axelrod, Biochem. Pharmacol. 14: 1257-1263 (1965).
78. K. J. Isselbacher and J. Axelrod, J. Amer. Chem. Soc. 77:1070-1071 (1955).
79. G. J. Dutton, Biochem. J. 64:693-701 (1956).
80. A. Nyberg, J. Schuberth, and L. Änggård, Acta Chem. Scand. 7: 1170-1172 (1953).
81. J. Axelrod and R. Tomchick, J. Biol. Chem. 233:702-705 (1958).
82. W. W. Weber and S. N. Cohen, Mol. Pharmacol. 3:266-273 (1967).
83. G. M. Lower, Jr. and G. T. Bryan, Biochem. Pharmacol. 22:1581-1588 (1973).
84. L. F. Chasseaud, Adv. Cancer Res. 29:175-274 (1979).
85. W. H. Habig, M. J. Pabst, and W. B. Jakoby, J. Biol. Chem. 249: 7130-7139 (1974).
86. R. K. Banerjee and A. B. Roy, Mol. Pharmacol. 2:56-66 (1966).
87. F. A. McEvoy and J. Carroll, Biochem. J. 123:901-906 (1971).
88. E. A. Zeller, in The Enzymes: Chemistry and Mechanism of Action, Vol. 2, Part 1 (J. S. Sumner and K. Myrbäck, Eds.). Academic, New York, 1951.
89. J. M. Pezzuto, M. A. Lea, and C. S. Yang, Cancer Res. 37:3427-3433 (1977).
90. A. P. Alvares, G. Schilling, W. Levin, R. Kuntzman, L. Brand, and L. C. Mark, Clin. Pharmacol. Ther. 10:655-659 (1969).
91. E. B. Nelson, P. P. Raj, K. J. Belfi, and B. S. S. Masters, J. Pharmacol. Exp. Ther. 178:580-588 (1971).
92. B. Schoene, R. A. Fleischmann, H. Remmer, and H. F. V. Oldershausen, Eur. J. Clin. Pharmacol. 4:65-73 (1972).
93. O. Pelkonen, E. H. Kaltiala, T. K. I. Larmi, and N. T. Kärki, Chem.-Biol. Interact. 9:205-216 (1974).

94. D. S. Lecamwasam, C. Franklin, and P. Turner, Brit. J. Clin. Pharmacol. 2:257-262 (1975).
95. N. Ahmad and M. Black, J. Pharmacol. Exp. Ther. 203:397-408 (1977).
96. R. Kuntzman, L. C. Mark, L. Brand, M. Jacobson, W. Levin, and A. H. Conney, J. Pharmacol. Exp. Ther. 152:151-156 (1966).
97. F. Oesch, Biochem. J. 139:77-88 (1974).
98. J. Caldwell, J. R. Moffatt, and R. L. Smith, Xenobiotica 6:275-280 (1976).
99. C. L. Litterst, T. E. Gram, E. G. Mimnaugh, P. Leber, D. Emmerling, and R. I. Freudenthal, Drug Metab. Dispos. 4:203-207 (1976).
100. R. J. Chhabra, R. J. Pohl, and J. R. Fouts, Drug Metab. Dispos. 2:443-447 (1974).
101. H. Hoensch, C. H. Woo, and R. Schmid, Biochem. Biophys. Res. Commun. 65:399-406 (1975).
102. S. Jakobsson, H. Thor, and S. Orrenius, Biochem. Biophys. Res. Commun. 39:1073-1080 (1970).
103. M. Del C. Villarruel, E. G. D. De Toranzo, and J. A. Castro, Toxicol. Appl. Pharmacol. 41:337-344 (1977).
104. D. R. Bickers, A. Kappas, and A. P. Alvares, J. Pharmacol. Exp. Ther. 188:300-309 (1974).
105. W. P. Norred and F. J. Akin, Biochem. Pharmacol. 25:732-734 (1976).
106. B. W. Harding, S. H. Wong, and D. H. Nelson, Biochim. Biophys. Acta 92:415-417 (1964).
107. H. Mukhtar, R. M. Philpot, and J. R. Bend, Drug Metab. Dispos. 6:577-583 (1978).
108. H. Mukhtar, R. M. Philpot, and J. R. Bend, Biochem. Biophys. Res. Commun. 81:89-98 (1978).
109. B. G. Lake, R. Hopkins, J. Chakraborty, J. W. Bridges, and D. V. Parke, Drug Metab. Dispos. 1:342-349 (1973).
110. H. Mukhtar, I. P. Lee, G. L. Foureman, and J. R. Bend, Chem.-Biol. Interact. 22:153-165 (1978).
111. D. Garfinkel, Comp. Biochem. Physiol. 8:367-379 (1963).
112. R. J. Pohl, R. M. Philpot, and J. R. Fouts, Drug Metab. Dispos. 4:442-450 (1976).
113. L. W. Wattenberg and J. L. Leong, Cancer Res. 25:365-370 (1965).
114. A. P. Alvares and A. Kappas, J. Biol. Chem. 252:6373-6378 (1977).
115. D. L. Berry, W. R. Bracken, T. J. Slaga, N. M. Wilson, S. G. Butty, and M. R. Juchau, Chem.-Biol. Interact. 18:129-142 (1977).
116. A. H. L. Chuang and E. Bresnick, Cancer Res. 36:4125-4129 (1976).
117. J. M. Fysh and A. B. Okey, Biochem. Pharmacol. 27:2968-2972 (1978).
118. A. Aitio and M. G. Parkki, Toxicol. Appl. Pharmacol. 44:107-114 (1978).

119. F. Oesch, H. Glatt, and H. Schmassmann, Biochem. Pharmacol. 26:603-607 (1977).
120. G. Clifton and N. Kaplowitz, Biochem. Pharmacol. 27:1284-1287 (1978).
121. C. L. Litterst, E. G. Mimnaugh, R. L. Reagan, and T. E. Gram, Drug Metab. Dispos. 3:259-265 (1975).
122. A. Aitio, Int. J. Biochem. 5:325-330 (1974).
123. G. J. Dutton and I. H. Stevenson, Biochim. Biophys. Acta 58:633-634 (1962).
124. G. Holder, H. Yagi, W. Levin, A. Y. H. Lu, and D. M. Jerina, Biochem. Biophys. Res. Commun. 65:1363-1370 (1975).
125. S. J. Stohs, R. C. Grafström, M. D. Burke, and S. Orrenius, Arch. Biochem. Biophys. 179:71-80 (1977).
126. P. Uotila, M. G. Parkki, and A. Aitio, Toxicol. Appl. Pharmacol. 46:671-683 (1978).
127. L. W. Wattenberg, J. L. Leong, and P. J. Strand, Cancer Res. 22:1120-1125 (1962).
128. C. M. Schiller and G. W. Lucier, Chem;-Biol. Interact. 22:199-209 (1978).
129. T. V. Zenser, M. B. Mattammal, and B. B. Davis, J. Pharmacol. Exp. Ther. 207:719-725 (1978).
130. G. E. R. Hook, J. R. Bend, and J. R. Fouts, Biochem. Pharmacol. 21:3267-3277 (1972).
131. M. R. Boyd, Nature 269:713-715 (1977).
132. L. W. Wattenberg and J. L. Leong, J. Histochem. Cytochem. 10:412-420 (1962).
133. P. Grasso, M. Williams, R. Hodgson, M. G. Wright, and S. D. Gangolli, Histochem. J. 3:117-126 (1971).
134. R. Walker, Food Cosmet. Toxicol. 8:659-676 (1970).
135. R. T. Williams, Toxicol. Appl. Pharmacol. 23:769-781 (1972).
136. R. Scheline, Pharmacol. Rev. 25:452-523 (1973).
137. R. T. Williams, FEBS Symp. 16:81-95 (1969).
138. T. F. Slater, Free Radical Mechanisms in Tissue Injury. Pion, London, 1972.
139. A. E. M. McLean and E. K. McLean, Biochem. J. 100:564-571 (1966).
140. J. R. Mitchell, D. J. Jollow, W. Z. Potter, D. C. Davis, J. R. Gillette, and B. B. Brodie, J. Pharmacol. Exp. Ther. 187:185-194 (1973).
141. D. C. Davis, W. Z. Potter, D. J. Jollow, and J. R. Mitchell, Life Sci. 14:2099-2109 (1974).
142. R. J. McMurtry, W. R. Snodgrass, and J. R. Mitchell, Toxicol. Appl. Pharmacol. 46:87-100 (1978).
143. G. Levy and H. Yamada, J. Pharm. Sci. 60:215-221 (1971).

144. D. J. Jollow, S. S. Thorgeirsson, W. Z. Potter, M. Hashimoto, and J. R. Mitchell, Pharmacology 12:251-271 (1974).
145. J. R. Mitchell, S. S. Thorgeirsson, W. Z. Potter, D. J. Jollow, and H. Keiser, Clin. Pharmacol. Ther. 16:676-684 (1974).
146. D. Howie, P. I. Adriaenssens, and L. F. Prescott, J. Pharm. Pharmacol. 29:235-237 (1977).
147. A. Klutch, W. Levin, R. L. Chang, F. Vane, and A. H. Conney, Clin. Pharmacol. Ther. 24:287-293 (1978).
148. P. Moldéus, Biochem. Pharmacol. 27:2859-2863 (1978).
149. P. Moldéus, D. P. Jones, K. Ormstad, and S. Orrenius, Biochem. Biophys. Res. Commun. 83:195-200 (1978).
150. D. P. Jones, G.-B. Sundby, K. Ormstad, and S. Orrenius, Biochem. Pharmacol. 28:929-935 (1979).
151. D. J. Jollow, J. R. Mitchell, W. Z. Potter, D. C. Davis, J. R. Gillette, and B. B. Brodie, J. Pharmacol. Exp. Ther. 187:195-202 (1973).
152. W. Z. Potter, D. C. Davis, J. R. Mitchell, D. J. Jollow, J. R. Gillette, and B. B. Brodie, J. Pharmacol. Exp. Ther. 187:203-210 (1973).
153. J. R. Mitchell, D. J. Jollow, W. Z. Potter, J. R. Gillette, and B. B. Brodie, J. Pharmacol. Exp. Ther. 187:211-217 (1973).
154. W. Z. Potter, S. S. Thorgeirsson, D. J. Jollow, and J. R. Mitchell, Pharmacology 12:129-143 (1974).
155. J. A. Hinson, S. D. Nelson, and J. R. Mitchell, Mol. Pharmacol. 13:625-633 (1977).
155a. D. J. Miner and P. T. Kissinger, Biochem. Pharmacol. 28:3285-3290 (1979).
155b. J. A. Hinson, L. R. Pohl, and J. R. Gillette, Life Sci. 24:2133-2138 (1979).
156. D. E. Rollins and A. R. Buckpitt, Toxicol. Appl. Pharmacol. 47:331-339 (1979).
157. S. D. Nelson, A. J. Forte, and R. J. McMurtry, Res. Commun. Chem. Path. Pharmacol. 22:61-71 (1978).
158. K. Healey, I. C. Calder, A. C. Yong, C. A. Crowe, C. C. Funder, K. N. Ham, and J. D. Tange, Xenobiotica 8:403-411 (1978).
159. M. Goldstein and E. B. Nelson, Res. Commun. Chem. Path. Pharmacol. 23:203-206 (1979).
160. E. Boyland and L. F. Chasseaud, Biochem. Pharmacol. 19:1526-1528 (1970).
161. R. Van Doorn, Ch.-M. Leijdekkers, and P. Th. Henderson, Toxicology 11:225-233 (1978).
162. M. Strolin Benedetti, A. Louis, A. Malnoë, M. Schneider, R. Lam, L. Kreber, and R. L. Smith, J. Pharm. Pharmacol. 27:629-632 (1975).

163. O. Strubelt, C. P. Siegers, and A. Schutt, Arch. Toxicol. 33:55-64 (1974).
164. F. D. Harvey and T. E. Levitt, J. Int. Med. Res. 4:130-137 (1976).
165. A. E. M. McLean and P. A. Day, Biochem. Pharmacol. 24:37-42 (1975).
166. E. Piperno and D. A. Berssenbruegge, Lancet ii:738-739 (1976).
167. J. G. Gerber, J. S. MacDonald, R. D. Harbison, J.-P. Villeneuve, A. J. J. Wood, and A. S. Nies, Lancet i:657-658 (1977).
168. D. Labadarios, M. Davis, B. Portmann, and R. Williams, Biochem. Pharmacol. 26:31-35 (1977).
169. R. Mull, W. Hinkelbein, J. Gertz, and K. Flemming, Biochim. Biophys. Acta 481:407-419 (1977).
169a. A. R. Buckpit, D. E. Rollins, and J. R. Mitchell, Biochem. Pharmacol. 28:2941-2946 (1979).
170. P. Crome, J. A. Vale, G. N. Volans, B. Widdop, and R. Goulding, Lancet ii:829-830 (1976).
171. L. F. Prescott, J. Park, G. R. Sutherland, I. J. Smith, and A. T. Proudfood, Lancet ii:109-113 (1976).
172. H. Büch, W. Rummel, K. Pfleger, Ch. Eschrich, and N. Texter, Naunyn-Schmiedebergs Arch. Pharmacol. Exp. Pathol. 259:276-289 (1968).
173. M. Davis, N. G. Harrison, G. Ideo, B. Portmann, D. Labadarios, and R. Williams, Xenobiotica 6:249-255 (1976).
174. M. Davis, C. J. Simmons, N. G. Harrison, and R. Williams, Quart. J. Med. 45:181-191 (1976).
175. J. T. Slattery and G. Levy, Res. Commun. Chem. Path. Pharmacol. 18:167-170 (1977).
176. D. J. Jollow and C. Smith, in Biological Reactive Intermediates: Formation, Toxicity, and Inactivation (D. J. Jollow, J. J. Kocsis, R. Snyder, and H. Vainio, Eds.). Plenum, New York, 1977, pp. 42-59.
177. W. Bolanowska and T. Gessner, J. Pharmacol. Exp. Ther. 206:233-238 (1978).
178. L. W. Whitehouse, C. J. Paul, and B. H. Thomas, Toxicol. Appl. Pharmacol. 38:571-582 (1976).
179. L. T. Wong, G. Solomonraj, and B. H. Thomas, Xenobiotica 6:575-584 (1976).
180. J. B. Houston and G. Levy, J. Pharm. Sci. 65:1218-1221 (1976).
181. G. Levy and H. Yamada, J. Pharm. Sci. 60:215-221 (1971).
182. T. C. Raghuram, D. Krishnamurthi, and R. Kalamegham, Toxicol. Lett. 2:175-178 (1978).
183. J. A. Edgar, Nature 248:136-137 (1974).
184. J. R. Gillette, in Drug Metabolism from Microbe to Man (D. V. Parke and R. L. Smith, Eds.). Taylor and Francis, London, 1977, pp. 147-168.

185. G. H. Mudge, M. W. Gemborys, and G. G. Duggin, J. Pharmacol. Exp. Ther. 206:218-226 (1978).
186. D. H. Swenson, J. A. Miller, and E. C. Miller, Biochem. Biophys. Res. Commun. 53:1260-1267 (1973).
187. D. H. Swenson, E. C. Miller, and J. A. Miller, Biochem. Biophys. Res. Commun. 60:1036-1043 (1974).
188. H. L. Gurtoo and T. C. Campbell, Mol. Pharmacol. 10:776-789 (1974).
189. S. Tabarelli-Poplawski and H. Uehleke, Naunyn-Schmiedeberg's Arch. Pharmacol. Exp. Pathol. 297:105-110 (1977).
190. A. Tunek, K. L. Platt, P. Bentley, and F. Oesch, Mol. Pharmacol. 14:920-929 (1978).
191. P. L. Grover and P. Sims, Biochem. J. 110:159-160 (1968).
192. J. F. Waterfall and P. Sims, Biochem. Pharmacol. 22:2469-2483 (1973).
193. K. Burki, T. A. Stoming, and E. Bresnick, J. Nat. Cancer Inst. 52: 785-788 (1974).
194. C. Wyndham and S. Safe, Can. J. Biochem. 56:993-997 (1978).
195. D. J. Jollow, J. R. Mitchell, N. Zampaglione, and J. R. Gillette, Pharmacology 11:151-169 (1974).
196. J. Kohli, C. Wyndham, M. Smylie, and S. Safe, Biochem. Pharmacol. 27:1245-1249 (1978).
197. I. G. Sipes, G. Krishna, and J. R. Gillette, Life Sci. 20:1541-1548 (1977).
198. A. Miller III, M. C. Henderson, and D. R. Buhler, Chem.-Biol. Interact. 24:1-17 (1979).
199. R. R. Dalvi, A. L. Hunter, and R. A. Neal, Chem.-Biol. Interact. 10:349-361 (1975).
200. L. R. Pohl, S. D. Nelson, and G. Krishna, Biochem. Pharmacol. 27:491-496 (1978).
201. H. Uehleke and Th. Werner, Arch. Toxicol. 34:289-308 (1975).
202. H. L. Gurtoo, R. Dahms, J. Hipkens, and J. B. Vaught, Life Sci. 22:45-52 (1978).
203. E. Dybing, T. Aune, and S. D. Nelson, Biochem. Pharmacol. 28: 43-50 (1979).
204. T. Aune, S. D. Nelson, and E. Dybing, Chem.-Biol. Interact. 25: 23-33 (1979).
205. T. C. Orton, C. Lowery, and W. E. Lindup, Brit. J. Pharmacol. 60:319 P (1977).
206. P. J. Wirth, C. J. Bettis, and W. L. Nelson, Mol. Pharmacol. 12: 759-768 (1976).
207. J. R. Mitchell, W. L. Nelson, W. Z. Potter, H. A. Sasame, and D. J. Jollow, J. Pharmacol. Exp. Ther. 199:41-52 (1976).
208. R. J. McMurtry and J. R. Mitchell, Toxicol. Appl. Pharmacol. 42: 285-300 (1977).

209. A. Miller III, M. C. Henderson, and D. R. Buhler, Mol. Pharmacol. 14:323-336 (1978).
210. S. D. Nelson, J. R. Mitchell, E. Dybing, and H. A. Sasame, Biochem. Biophys. Res. Commun. 70:1157-1165 (1976).
211. F. Marks and E. Hecker, Biochim. Biophys. Acta 187:250-265 (1969).
212. H. Kappus, H. M. Bolt, and H. Remmer, Steroids 22:203-225 (1973).
213. H. M. Bolt, H. Kappus, and R. Käsbohrer, J. Clin. Endocrinol. Metab. 39:1072-1080 (1974).
214. H. Kappus and H. Remmer, Biochem. Pharmacol. 24:1079-1084 (1975).
215. M. R. Boyd, L. T. Burka, B. J. Wilson, and H. A. Sasame, J. Pharmacol. Exp. Ther. 207:677-686 (1978).
216. P. W. Lee and R. A. Neal, Drug Metab. Dispos. 6:591-600 (1978).
217. E. Dybing, S. D. Nelson, J. R. Mitchell, H. A. Sasame, and J. R. Gillette, Mol. Pharmacol. 12:911-920 (1976).
218. A. M. El-Hawari and G. L. Plaa, Biochem. Pharmacol. 26:1857-1866 (1977).
219. H. Kappus and H. Remmer, Drug Metab. Dispos. 3:338-344 (1975).
220. B. J. Norman, R. E. Poore, and R. A. Neal, Biochem. Pharmacol. 23:1733-1744 (1974).
221. G. J. Mulder, J. A. Hinson, and J. R. Gillette, Biochem. Pharmacol. 26:189-196 (1977).
222. T. Shimada and R. Sato, Biochem. Pharmacol. 27:585-593 (1978).
223. S. Hesse, M. Mezger, and T. Wolff, Chem.-Biol. Interact. 20:355-365 (1978).
224. W. R. Porter and R. A. Neal, Drug Metab. Dispos. 6:379-388 (1978).
225. B. L. Van Duuren and S. Banerjee, Cancer Res. 36:2419-2422 (1976).
226. H. Kappus, H. M. Bolt, A. Buchter, and W. Bolt, Toxicol. Appl. Pharmacol. 37:461-471 (1976).
227. F. P. Guengerich and P. G. Watenabe, Biochem. Pharmacol. 28:589-596 (1979).
228. Th. Cresteil, Ph. Beaune, J. P. Leroux, M. Lange, and D. Mansuy, Chem.-Biol. Interact. 24:153-165 (1979).
229. E. Dybing, Acta Pharmacol. Toxicol. 41:89-93 (1977).
230. P. Uotila, M. G. Parkki and A. Aitio, Toxicol. Appl. Pharmacol. 46:671-683 (1978).
231. M. R. Boyd and L. T. Burka, J. Pharmacol. Exp. Ther. 207:687-697 (1978).
232. E. Dybing, Drug Metab. Dispos. 4:513-516 (1976).
233. F. Martz, C. Failinger III, and D. A. Blake, J. Pharm. Exp. Ther. 203:231-239 (1977).
234. H. A. Sasame, M. M. Ames, and S. D. Nelson, Biochem. Biophys. Res. Commun. 78:919-926 (1977).
235. J. R. Gillette, Biochem. Pharmacol. 23:2785-2794 (1974).

236. J. R. Gillette, Biochem. Pharmacol. 23:2927-2938 (1974).
237. E. M. Boyd, Toxicol. Appl. Pharmacol. 1:240-249 (1959).
238. S. D. Nelson, M. R. Boyd, and J. R. Mitchell, in Drug Metabolism Concepts (D. M. Jerina, Ed.). American Chemical Society Symposium Series 44, Washington, D.C., 1977, pp. 155-185.
239. S. D. Nelson, W. A. Garland, J. R. Mitchell, Y. Vaishnav, C. N. Statham, and A. R. Buckpitt, Drug Metab. Dispos. 6:363-367 (1978).
240. I. C. Calder, M. J. Creek, P. J. Williams, C. C. Funder, C. R. Green, K. N. Ham, and J. D. Tange, J. Med. Chem. 16:499-502 (1973).
241. W. A. Garland, S. D. Nelson, and H. A. Sasame, Biochem. Biophys. Res. Commun. 72:539-545 (1976).
242. J. Booth and E. Boyland, Biochem. J. 91:362-369 (1964).
243. J. A. Hinson and J. R. Mitchell, Drug Metab. Dispos. 4:430-435 (1976).
244. J. A. Hinson, S. D. Nelson, and J. R. Gillette, Mol. Pharmacol. 15:419-427 (1979).
245. G. J. Mulder, J. A. Hinson, and J. R. Gillette, Biochem. Pharmacol. 27:1641-1649 (1978).
246. C. Heidelberger, An. Rev. Biochem. 44:79-121 (1975).
247. P. Sims, Biochem. Pharmacol. 19:795-818 (1970).
248. J. W. DePierre and L. Ernster, Biochim. Biophys. Acta 473:149-186 (1978).
249. D. M. Jerina and J. W. Daly, Science 185:573-582 (1974).
250. P. Sims, P. L. Grover, A. Swaisland, K. Pal, and A. Hewer, Nature 252:326-328 (1974).
251. D. R. Thakker, H. Yagi, A. Y. H. Lu, W. Levin, A. H. Conney, and D. M. Jerina, Proc. Nat. Acad. Sci. U.S. 73:3381-3385 (1976).
252. H. W. S. King, M. R. Osborne, F. A. Beland, R. G. Harvey, and P. Brookes, Proc. Nat. Acad. Sci. U.S. 73:2679-2681 (1976).
253. J. D. Regan, A. A. Francis, W. C. Dunn, O. Hernandez, H. Yagi, and D. M. Jerina, Chem.-Biol. Interact. 20:279-287 (1978).
254. R. F. Newbold and P. Brookes, Nature 261:52-54 (1976).
255. E. Huberman, L. Sachs, S. K. Yang, and H. V. Gelboin, Proc. Nat. Acad. Sci. U.S. 73:607-611 (1976).
256. A. W. Wood, W. Levin, A. Y. H. Lu, H. Yagi, O. Hernandez, D. M. Jerina, and A. H. Conney, J. Biol. Chem. 251:4882-4890 (1976).
257. B. N. Ames, W. E. Durston, E. Yamasaki, and F. D. Lee, Proc. Nat. Acad. Sci. U.S. 70:2281-2285 (1973).
258. J. McCann and B. N. Ames, Proc. Nat. Acad. Sci. U.S. 73:950-954 (1976).
259. H. V. Gelboin, Cancer Res. 29:1272-1276 (1969).
260. B. N. Ames, J. McCann, and E. Yamasaki, Mutation Res. 31:347-364 (1975).

261. F. J. Wiebel, J. C. Leutz, L. Diamond, and H. V. Gelboin, Arch. Biochem. Biophys. 144:78-86 (1971).
262. W.-I. Liu and N. H. Sloane, Xenobiotica 9:165-171 (1979).
263. M. D. Burke, H. Vadi, B. Jernström, and S. Orrenius, J. Biol. Chem. 252:6424-6431 (1977).
264. R. C. Levitt, C. Legraverend, D. W. Nebert, and O. Pelkonen, Biochem. Biophys. Res. Commun. 79:1167-1175 (1977).
265. P. Lesca, P. Lecointe, C. Paoletti, and D. Mansuy, Biochem. Pharmacol. 27:1203-1209 (1978).
266. F. Oesch, P. Bentley, and H. R. Glatt, Int. J. Cancer 18:448-452 (1976).
267. H. R. Glatt, F. Oesch, A. Frigerio, and S. Garattini, Int. J. Cancer 16:787-797 (1975).
268. J. S. Felton and D. W. Nebert, J. Biol. Chem. 250:6769-6778 (1975).
269. J. Ashby and J. A. Styles, Nature 271:452-455 (1978).
270. L. W. Wattenberg, J. Nat. Cancer Inst. 48:1425-1430 (1972).
271. L. W. Wattenberg, J. Nat. Cancer Inst. 50:1541-1544 (1973).
272. L. K. T. Lam and L. W. Wattenberg, J. Nat. Cancer Inst. 58:413-417 (1977).
273. J. W. Cramer, J. A. Miller, and E. C. Miller, J. Biol. Chem. 235:250-256 (1960).
274. P. D. Lotlikar and K. Zaleski, Biochem. J. 150:561-564 (1975).
275. S. S. Thorgeirsson, D. J. Jollow, H. A. Sasame, I. Green, and J. R. Mitchell, Mol. Pharmacol. 9:398-404 (1973).
276. H. R. Gutmann and P. Bell, Biochim. Biophys. Acta 498:229-243 (1977).
277. T. Matsushima and J. H. Weisburger, Xenobiotica 2:423-430 (1972).
278. J. A. Miller, Cancer Res. 30:559-576 (1970).
279. J. H. Weisburger and E. K. Weisburger, Pharmacol. Rev. 25:1-66 (1973).
280. J. S. Felton, D. W. Nebert, and S. S. Thorgeirsson, Mol. Pharmacol. 12:225-233 (1976).
281. E. C. Miller, J. A. Miller, R. R. Brown, and J. C. MacDonald, Cancer Res. 18:469-477 (1958).
282. E. C. Miller, J. A. Miller, and H. A. Hartmann, Cancer Res. 21:815-824 (1961).
283. E. C. Miller, J. A. Miller, and M. Enomoto, Cancer Res. 24:2018-2031 (1964).
284. E. K. Weisburger and J. H. Weisburger, Advan. Cancer Res. 5:331-431 (1958).
285. H. R. Gutmann, S. B. Galitski, and W. A. Foley, Cancer Res. 27:1443-1455 (1967).
286. H. R. Gutmann, D. S. Leaf, Y. Yost, R. E. Rydell, and C. C. Chen Cancer Res. 30:1485-1498 (1970).

287. E. Kaplan, H. R. Gutmann, and T. H. Emory, Biochem. Pharmacol. 27:1581-1589 (1978).
288. J. R. DeBaun, E. C. Miller, and J. A. Miller, Cancer Res. 30:577-595 (1970).
289. L. S. Andrews, J. M. Fysh, J. A. Hinson, and J. R. Gillette, Life Sci. 24:59-64 (1979).
290. J. R. DeBaun, J. Y. R. Smith, E. C. Miller, and J. A. Miller, Science 167:184-186 (1970).
291. E. Kriek, Biochim. Biophys. Acta 161:273-275 (1968).
292. C. C. Irving, R. A. Veazey, and J. T. Hill, Biochim. Biophys. Acta 179:189-198 (1969).
293. C. C. Irving, R. A. Veazey, and L. T. Russell, Chem.-Biol. Interact. 1:19-26 (1969).
294. E. C. Miller, P. D. Lotlikar, J. A. Miller, B. W. Butler, C. C. Irving, and J. T. Hill, Mol. Pharmacol. 4:147-154 (1968).
295. C. C. Irving and L. T. Russell, Biochemistry 9:2471-2476 (1970).
296. P. D. Lotlikar and L. Luha, Mol. Pharmacol. 7:381-388 (1971).
297. P. D. Lotlikar and M. B. Wasserman, Biochem. J. 120:661-665 (1970).
298. H. Bartsch, M. Dworkin, J. A. Miller, and E. C. Miller, Biochim. Biophys. Acta 286:272-298 (1972).
299. C. M. King, Cancer Res. 34:1503-1515 (1974).
300. G. J. Mulder, J. A. Hinson, W. L. Nelson, and S. S. Thorgeirsson, Biochem. Pharmacol. 26:1356-1358 (1977).
301. L. S. Andrews, J. A. Hinson, and J. R. Gillette, Biochem. Pharmacol. 27:2399-2408 (1978).
302. H. A. J. Schut, P. J. Wirth, and S. S. Thorgeirsson, Mol. Pharmacol. 14:682-692 (1978).
303. C. C. Irving, Cancer Res. 26:1390-1396 (1966).
304. B. N. Ames, F. D. Lee, and W. E. Durston, Proc. Nat. Acad. Sci. U.S. 70:782-786 (1973).
305. W. E. Durston and B. N. Ames, Proc. Nat. Acad. Sci. U.S. 71:737-741 (1974).
306. P. D. Lotlikar, M. Enomoto, J. A. Miller, and E. C. Miller, Proc. Soc. Exp. Biol. Med. 125:341-346 (1967).
307. C. C. Irving, T. C. Peeler, R. A. Veazey, and R. Wiseman, Jr., Cancer Res. 31:1468-1472 (1971).
308. M. Enomoto, M. Miyake, and K. Sato, Gann 59:177-186 (1968).
309. P. D. Lotlikar, Biochem. J. 118:513-518 (1970).
310. T. Matsushima, P. H. Grantham, E. K. Weisburger, and J. H. Weisburger, Biochem. Pharmacol. 21:2043-2051 (1972).
311. D. Malejka-Giganti, R. C. McIver, A. L. Glasebrook, and H. R. Gutmann, Biochem. Pharmacol. 27:61-69 (1978).
312. J. W. Cramer, J. A. Miller, and E. C. Miller, J. Biol. Chem. 235:885-888 (1960).

313. R. S. Yamamoto, R. M. Glass, H. H. Frankel, E. K. Weisburger, and J. H. Weisburger, Toxicol. Appl. Pharmacol. 13:108-117 (1968).
314. J. H. Weisburger, E. K. Weisburger, R. M. Madison, M. L. Wenk, and D. S. Klein, J. Nat. Cancer Inst. 51:235-240 (1973).
315. R. S. Yamamoto, H. H. Frankel, and J. H. Weisburger, Toxicol. Appl. Pharmacol. 17:98-106 (1970).
316. R. S. Yamamoto, G. M. Williams, H. L. Richardson, E. K. Weisburger, and J. H. Weisburger, Cancer Res. 33:454-457 (1973).
317. P. H. Grantham, L. Mohan, R. S. Yamamoto, E. K. Weisburger, and J. H. Weisburger, Toxicol. Appl. Pharmacol. 13:118-130 (1968).
318. P. H. Grantham, T. Matsushima, L. Mohan, E. K. Weisburger, and J. H. Weisburger, Xenobiotica 2:551-565 (1972).
319. H. Büch, W. Rummel, K. Pfleger, Ch. Eschrich, and N. Texter, Naunyn-Schmiedebergs Arch. Pharmakol. Exp. Pathol. 259:276-289 (1968).
320. M. A. Friedman and S. Woods, Res. Commun. Chem. Pathol. Pharmacol. 17:623-630 (1977).
321. K. R. Rees and M. J. Tarlow, Biochem. J. 104:757-761 (1967).
322. W. D. Reid, Experientia 28:1058-1061 (1972).
323. F. Serafini-Cessi, Biochem. J. 128:1103-1107 (1972).
324. H. Zollner, Biochem. Pharmacol. 22:1171-1178 (1973).
325. N. Munsch and C. Frayssinet, Biochimie 53:243-248 (1971).
326. S. S. Thorgeirsson, J. R. Mitchell, H. A. Sasame, and W. Z. Potter, Chem.-Biol. Interact. 15:139-147 (1976).
327. B. G. Lake, S. D. Gangolli, M. G. Wright, P. Grasso, F. M. B. Carpanini, and K. R. Butterworth, Biochem. Soc. Trans. 6:145-147 (1978).
328. V. Schwarzmann, R. Infante, A. Raisonnier, and J. Caroli, C. R. Soc. Biol. 161:2425-2439 (1967).
329. E. H. Silver and S. D. Murphy, Toxicol. Appl. Pharmacol. 45:377-389 (1978).
330. H. Theorell, T. Yonetani, and B. Sjöberg, Acta Chem. Scand. 23:255-260 (1969).
331. E. Boyland and L. F. Chasseaud, Biochem. J. 109:651-661 (1968).
332. E. Boyland and L. F. Chasseaud, Biochem. J. 104:95-102 (1967).
333. H. Esterbauer, H. Zollner, and N. Scholz, Z. Naturforsch. 30c:466-473 (1975).
334. C. M. Kaye, Biochem. J. 134:1093-1101 (1973).
335. S. K. Hanson and M. W. Anders, Toxicology Lett. 1:301-305 (1978).
336. G. R. Cameron and W. A. E. Karunaratne, J. Pathol. Bacteriol. 42:1-21 (1936).
337. B. B. Brodie, W. D. Reid, A. K. Cho, G. Sipes, G. Krishna, and J. R. Gillette, Proc. Nat. Acad. Sci. U.S. 68:160-164 (1971).
338. P. E. Gooding, J. Chayen, B. Sawyer, and T. F. Slater, Chem.-Biol. Interact. 20:299-310 (1978).

339. J. Baron, J. A. Redick, and F. P. Guengerich, Life Sci. 23:2627-2632 (1978).
340. M. Tavassoli, J. Ozols, G. Sugimoto, K. H. Cox, and U. Muller-Eberhard, Biochem. Biophys. Res. Commun. 72:281-287 (1976).
341. J. Baron, J. A. Redick, P. Greenspan, and Y. Taira, Life Sci. 22:1097-1102 (1978).
342. E. D. Massey and W. H. Butler, Chem.-Biol. Interact. 24:329-344 (1979).
343. N. J. Greenberger, R. B. Cohen, and K. J. Isselbacher, Lab. Invest. 14:264-271 (1965).
344. A. A. Seawright and J. Hrdlicka, Brit. J. Exp. Pathol. 53:242-252 (1972).
344a. K. Ashgar, B. G. Reddy, and G. Krishna, J. Histochem. Cytochem. 23:774-779 (1975).
344b. M. T. Smith, N. Loveridge, E. D. Wills, and J. Chayen, Biochem. J. 182:103-108 (1979).
345. A. H. Conney, Pharmacol. Rev. 19:317-366 (1967).
346. G. P. Quinn, J. Axelrod, and B. B. Brodie, Biochem. Pharmacol. 1:152-159 (1958).
347. R. Kato and J. R. Gillette, J. Pharmacol. Exp. Ther. 150:279-284 (1965).
348. R. L. Cram, M. R. Juchau, and J. R. Fouts, Proc. Soc. Exp. Biol. Med. 118:872-875 (1965).
349. J. G. Page and E. S. Vesell, Pharmacology 2:321-336 (1969).
350. R. T. Williams, Biochem. Soc. Trans. 2:359-377 (1974).
351. T. K. Basu, J. W. T. Dickerson, and D. V. Parke, Biochem. J. 124:19-24 (1971).
352. C. R. Short, D. A. Kinden, and R. Stith, Drug Metab. Rev. 5:1-42 (1976).
353. R. Kato, Xenobiotica 7:25-92 (1977).
354. W. J. Marshall and A. E. M. McLean, Biochem. Pharmacol. 18:153-157 (1969).
355. A. H. Conney, E. J. Pantuck, R. Kuntzman, A. Kappas, K. E. Anderson, and A. P. Alvares, Clin. Pharmacol. Ther. 22:707-720 (1977).
356. M. R. Juchau and J. R. Fouts, Biochem. Pharmacol. 15:891-898 (1966).
357. M. G. Neale and D. V. Parke, Biochem. Pharmacol. 22:1451-1461 (1973).
358. E. S. Vesell, Drug Metab. Rev. 8:265-291 (1978).
359. F. M. Radzialowski and W. F. Bousquet, J. Pharmacol. Exp. Ther. 163:229-238 (1968).
360. B. G. Lake, J. M. Tredger, M. D. Burke, J. Chakraborty, and J. W. Bridges, Chem.-Biol. Interact. 12:81-90 (1976).

361. R. L. Furner, E. D. Neville, K. S. Talarico, and D. D. Feller, Toxicol. Appl. Pharmacol. 21:569-581 (1972).
362. B. Testa and P. Jenner, in Drug Metabolism: Chemical and Biochemical Aspects. Marcel Dekker, New York, 1976.
363. E. J. Pantuck, K.-C. Hsiao, W. D. Loub, L. W. Wattenberg, R. Kuntzman, and A. H. Conney, J. Pharmacol. Exp. Ther. 198:278-283 (1976).
364. C. L. Litterst, E. G. Mimnaugh, and T. E. Gram, Biochem. Pharmacol. 26:749-755 (1977).
365. E. Hietanen and M. Laitinen, Biochem. Pharmacol. 27:1095-1097 (1978).
366. J. M. Tredger and R. S. Chhabra, Xenobiotica 7:481-489 (1977).
367. S. J. Stohs, L. A. Reinke, J. M. Hassing, and H. Rosenberg, Drug Metab. Dispos. 7:49-51 (1979).
368. J. R. Fouts and T. R. Devereux, J. Pharmacol. Exp. Ther. 183:458-468 (1972).
369. J. M. Tredger, R. S. Chhabra, and J. R. Fouts, Drug Metab. Dispos. 4:17-24 (1976).
370. M. O. James, G. L. Foureman, F. C. Law, and J. R. Bend, Drug Metab. Dispos. 5:19-28 (1977).
371. C. R. Wolf, M. M. Szutowski, L. M. Ball, and R. M. Philpot, Chem.-Biol. Interact. 21:29-43 (1978).
372. F. P. Guengerich and P. S. Mason, Mol. Pharmacol. 15:154-164 (1979).
373. A. P. Alvares and A. Kappas, Clin. Pharmacol. Ther. 22:809-816 (1977).
374. J. G. Dent, K. J. Netter, and J. E. Gibson, Toxicol. Appl. Pharmacol. 38:237-249 (1976).
375. A. R. Boobis, D. W. Nebert, and J. S. Felton, Mol. Pharmacol. 13:259-268 (1977).
376. A. Poland and E. Glover, Mol. Pharmacol. 10:349-359 (1974).
377. K. T. Kitchin and J. S. Woods, Toxicol. Appl. Pharmacol. 47:537-546 (1979).
378. S. A. Atlas and D. W. Nebert, Arch. Biochem. Biophys. 175:495-506 (1976).
379. D. W. Nebert and J. S. Felton, Fed. Proc. Fed. Amer. Soc. Exp. Biol. 35:1133-1141 (1976).
380. D. W. Nebert, R. C. Levitt, M. M. Orlando, and J. S. Felton, Clin. Pharmacol. Ther. 22:640-658 (1977).
381. R. S. Chhabra, J. M. Tredger, R. M. Philpot, and J. R. Fouts, Chem.-Biol. Interact. 15:21-31 (1976).
382. W. D. Reid, B. Christie, M. Eichelbaum, and G. Krishna, Exp. Mol. Pathol. 15:363-372 (1971).
383. N. Zampaglione, D. J. Jollow, J. R. Mitchell, B. Stripp, M. Hamrick, and J. R. Gillette, J. Pharmacol. Exp. Ther. 187:218-227 (1973).

384. A. R. Boobis, D. W. Nebert, and O. Pelkonen, Biochem. Pharmacol. 28:111-121 (1979).
385. K. W. Bock, W. Fröhling, H. Remmer, and B. Rexer, Biochim. Biophys. Acta 327:46-56 (1973).
386. H. Vainio and A. Aitio, Acta Pharmacol. Toxicol. 34:130-140 (1974).
387. D. M. Jerina, P. M. Dansette, A. Y. H. Lu, and W. Levin, Mol. Pharmacol. 13:342-351 (1977).
388. H. Mukhtar and E. Bresnick, Chem-Biol. Interact. 15:59-67 (1976).
389. A. J. Baars, M. Jansen, and D. D. Breimer, Biochem. Pharmacol. 27:2487-2494 (1978).
390. H. Schmassmann and F. Oesch, Mol. Pharmacol. 14:834-847 (1978).
391. H. Schmassmann, A. Sparrow, K. Platt, and F. Oesch, Biochem. Pharmacol. 27:2237-2245 (1978).
392. F. Oesch and H. Schmassmann, Biochem. Pharmacol. 28:171-176 (1979).
393. G. Feuer, J. C. Sosa-Lucero, G. Lumb, and G. Moddel, Toxicol. Appl. Pharmacol. 19:579-589 (1971).
394. S. J. Stohs, R. C. Grafström, M. D. Burke, and S. Orrenius, Drug Metab. Dispos. 4:517-521 (1976).
395. T. Matsubara, R. A. Prough, M. D. Burke, and R. W. Estabrook, Cancer Res. 34:2196-2203 (1974).
396. G. E. R. Hook, J. K. Haseman, and G. W. Lucier, Chem.-Biol. Interact. 10:199-214 (1975).
397. E. Rogan and E. Cavalieri, Mol. Pharmacol. 14:215-219 (1978).
398. A. Viviani, W. K. Lutz, and C. Schlatter, Biochem. Pharmacol. 27:2103-2108 (1978).
399. B. Jernström, H. Vadi, and S. Orrenius, Chem.-Biol. Interact. 20:311-321 (1978).
400. S. Sakai, C. E. Reinhold, P. J. Wirth, and S. S. Thorgeirsson, Cancer Res. 38:2058-2067 (1978).
401. R. F. Crampton, T. J. B. Gray, P. Grasso, and D. V. Parke, Toxicology 7:289-306 (1977).
402. B. G. Lake, R. C. Longland, R. A. Harris, B. J. Severn, and S. D. Gangolli, Biochem. Pharmacol. 27:2357-2361 (1978).
403. F. Hutterer, F. M. Klion, A. Wengraf, F. Schaffner, and H. Popper, Lab. Invest. 20:455-464 (1969).
404. R. F. Crampton, T. J. B. Gray, P. Grasso, and D. V. Parke, Toxicology 7:307-326 (1977).
405. D. Labadarios, J. W. T. Dickerson, D. V. Parke, E. G. Lucas, and G. H. Obuwa, Brit. J. Clin. Pharmacol. 5:167-173 (1978).
406. A. Richens, in Anticonvulsant Drugs and Enzyme Induction (A. Richens and F. P. Woodford, Eds.). Elsevier/North-Holland, Amsterdam, 1976, pp. 3-12.

407. J. Hunter, in Anticonvulsant Drugs and Enzyme Induction (A. Richens and F. P. Woodford, Eds.). Elsevier/North-Holland, Amsterdam, 1976, pp. 77-85.
408. I. H. Stevenson, K. O'Malley, and A. M. M. Shepherd, in Anticonvulsant Drugs and Enzyme Induction (A. Richens and F. P. Woodford, Eds.). Elsevier/North-Holland, Amsterdam, 1976, pp. 37-46.
409. S. P. Sher, Toxicol. Appl. Pharmacol. 18:780-834 (1971).
410. G. R. Wilkinson and S. Schenker, Biochem. Pharmacol. 25:2675-2681 (1976).
411. T. C. Campbell, Clin. Pharmacol. Ther. 22:699-706 (1977).
412. L. Rowe and E. D. Wills, Biochem. Pharmacol. 25:175-179 (1976).
413. A. Kappas, K. G. Anderson, A. H. Conney, and A. P. Alvares, Clin. Pharmacol. Ther. 20:643-643 (1976).
414. D. Gilbert and L. Golberg, Food Cosmet. Toxicol. 3:417-432 (1965).
415. L. G. Hart and J. R. Fouts, Proc. Soc. Exp. Biol. Med. 114:388-392 (1963).
416. D. V. Parke, in Enzyme Induction (D. V. Parke, Ed.). Plenum, London, 1975, pp. 207-271.
417. D. V. Parke, Kh. M. Q. Rahman, and R. Walker, Biochem. Soc. Trans. 2:615-618 (1974).
418. C. Mitoma, L. Lombrozo, S. E. LeValley, and F. Dehn, Arch. Biochem. Biophys. 134:434-441 (1969).
419. L. W. Wattenberg, M. A. Page, and J. L. Leong, Cancer Res. 28:934-937 (1968).
420. W. D. Loub, L. W. Wattenberg, and D. W. Davis, J. Nat. Cancer Inst. 54:985-988 (1975).
421. E. J. Pantuck, C. B. Pantuck, W. A. Garland, B. H. Min, L. W. Wattenberg, K. E. Anderson, A. Kappas, and A. H. Conney, Clin. Pharmacol. Ther. 25:88-95 (1979).
422. R. R. Brown, J. A. Miller, and E. C. Miller, J. Biol. Chem. 209:211-222 (1954).
423. L. W. Wattenberg, Toxicol. Appl. Pharmacol. 23:741-748 (1972).
424. A. E. M. McLean and H. E. Driver, Biochem. Pharmacol. 26:1299-1302 (1977).
425. A. H. Conney, E. J. Pantuck, K.-C. Hsiao, R. Kuntzman, A. P. Alvares, and A. Kappas, Fed. Proc. Fed. Amer. Soc. Exp. Biol. 36:1647-1652 (1977).
426. R. Kuntzman, E. J. Pantuck, S. A. Kaplan, and A. H. Conney, Clin. Pharmacol. Ther. 22:757-764 (1977).
427. M. Jacobson, W. Levin, P. J. Poppers, A. W. Wood, and A. H. Conney, Clin. Pharmacol. Ther. 16:701-710 (1974).
428. R. R. Miller, Clin. Pharmacol. Ther. 22:749-756 (1977).

429. A. Kappas, A. P. Alvares, K. E. Anderson, E. J. Pantuck, G. B. Pantuck, R. Chang, and A. H. Conney, Clin. Pharmacol. Ther. 23: 445-450 (1978).
430. R. M. Welch, Y. E. Harrison, B. W. Gommi, P. J. Poppers, M. Finster, and A. H. Conney, Clin. Pharmacol. Ther. 10:100-109 (1969).
431. B. M. Ullard, J. H. Weisburger, R. S. Yamamoto, and E. K. Weisburger, Food Cosmet. Toxicol. 11:199-207 (1973).
432. L. W. Wattenberg and J. L. Leong, Cancer Res. 30:1922-1925 (1970).
433. A. M. Pamukcu, L. W. Wattenberg, J. M. Price, and G. T. Bryan, J. Nat. Cancer Inst. 47:155-159 (1971).
434. C. J. Kensler, J. Biol. Chem. 179:1079-1084 (1949).
435. C. S. Catz, M. R. Juchau, and S. J. Yaffe, J. Pharm. Exp. Ther. 174:197-205 (1970).
436. J. M. Patel and S. S. Pawar, Biochem. Pharmacol. 23:1467-1477 (1974).
437. V. G. Zannoni, E. J. Flynn, and M. Lynch, Biochem. Pharmacol. 21:1377-1392 (1972).
438. M. Greenblatt, S. Mirvish, and B. T. So, J. Nat. Cancer Inst. 46: 1029-1034 (1971).
439. W. Lijinsky and M. Greenblatt, Nature New Biol. 236:177-178 (1972).
440. M. Greenblatt, J. Nat. Cancer Inst. 50:1055-1056 (1973).
441. J. J. Kamm, T. Dashman, A. H. Conney, and J. J. Burns, Proc. Nat. Acad. Sci. U.S. 70:747-749 (1973).
442. S. S. Thorgeirsson, J. S. Felton, and D. W. Nebert, Mol. Pharmacol. 11:159-165 (1975).
443. D. W. Nebert and H. V. Gelboin, Arch. Biochem. Biophys. 134: 76-89 (1969).
444. E. S. Vesell, G. T. Passananti, F. E. Greene, and J. G. Page, Ann. N.Y. Acad. Sci. 179:752-773 (1971).
445. R. Kalameghan, K. Krishnaswamy, S. Krishnamurthy, and R. N. K. Bhargava, Clin. Pharmacol. Ther. 25:67-73 (1979).
446. E. S. Vesell, Fed. Proc. Fed. Amer. Soc. Exp. Biol. 31:1253-1269 (1972).
447. H. S. Fraser, C. J. Bulpitt, C. Kahn, G. Mould, J. C. Mucklow, and C. T. Dollery, Clin. Pharmacol. Ther. 20:369-376 (1976).
448. R. A. Branch, S. Y. Salih, and M. Homeida, Clin. Pharmacol. Ther. 24:283-286 (1978).
449. L. L. Miller, in Isolated Liver Perfusion and Its Application (I. Bartošek, A. Guaitani, and L. L. Miller, Eds.). Raven, New York, 1973, pp. 11-53.
450. J. Kvetina, A. Guaitani, C. Pugliatti, and E. Veneroni, Pharmacology 2:17-20 (1969).

451. M. Baggiolini, B. Dewald, and H. Aebi, Biochem. Pharmacol. 18: 2187-2196 (1969).
452. C. von Bahr, F. Sjöqvist, and S. Orrenius, Eur. J. Pharmacol. 9: 106-110 (1970).
453. B. R. Smith, R. M. Philpot, and J. R. Bend, Drug Metab. Dispos. 6:425-431 (1978).
454. J. R. Fry and J. W. Bridges, in Progress in Drug Metabolism, Vol. 2 (J. W. Bridges and L. F. Chasseaud, Eds.). Wiley, London, 1977, pp. 71-118.
455. P. Wiebkin, J. R. Fry, C. A. Jones, R. K. Lowing, and J. W. Bridges, Biochem. Pharmacol. 27:1899-1970 (1978).
456. M. Hirata, B. Lindeke, and S. Orrenius, Biochem. Pharmacol. 28: 479-484 (1979).
457. D. J. Stewart and T. Inaba, Biochem. Pharmacol. 28:461-464 (1979).
458. R. E. Billings, R. E. McMahon, J. Ashmore, and S. R. Wagle, Drug Metab. Dispos. 5:518-526 (1977).
459. J. R. Fry, P. Wiebkin, J. Kao, C. A. Jones, J. Gwynn, and J. W. Bridges, Xenobiotica 8:113-120 (1978).
460. J. Kao, C. A. Jones, J. R. Fry, and J. W. Bridges, Life Sci. 23: 1221-1228 (1978).
461. B. B. Brodie and J. R. Gillette (Eds.), Handbook of Experimental Pharmacology, Vol. 28, Concepts in Biochemical Pharmacology Part 2. Springer-Verlag, Berlin, 1971.
462. S. Fleischer and L. Packer (Eds.), Methods in Enzymology, Vol. 3, Biomembranes, Part C. Academic, New York, 1978.
463. F. Oesch, D. M. Jerina, J. W. Daly, and J. M. Rice, Chem.-Biol. Interact. 6:189-202 (1973).
464. T. Shimada and R. Sato, Biochem. Pharmacol. 28:1777-1781 (1979).
465. W. Levin, P. E. Thomas, D. Korzeniowski, H. Seifried, D. M. Jerina, and A. Y. H. Lu, Mol. Pharmacol. 14:1107-1120 (1978).
466. H. A. Sasame and M. R. Boyd, J. Pharmacol. Exp. Ther. 205: 718-724 (1978).

Chapter 4

AN OVERVIEW OF THE PHENOMENA OF ENZYME INDUCTION AND INHIBITION: THEIR RELEVANCE TO DRUG ACTION AND DRUG INTERACTIONS

Helmut A. Greim

Department of Toxicology
Munich Society for Radiation and Environment Research
Neuherberg, Federal Republic of Germany

The present chapter considers enzyme induction and inhibition from a general mechanistic and therapeutic point of view. Although a number of factors, both endogenous and exogenous, affect drug metabolism, many adverse effects result from drug interactions at the metabolic sites.

General features of induction in humans are presented. This allows an evaluation of common properties of inducing agents, and some possibility to predict a microsomal enzyme induction during therapy. A limited number of drugs detectably increase drug-metabolizing enzyme activity when administered over longer periods of time. This may result in dangerous side effects, as illustrated by several examples including barbiturates, tricyclic drugs, rifampicin, and diphenylhydantoin.

In contrast, more drugs compete for the drug-metabolizing enzyme systems, resulting in inhibition phenomena. The general features and characteristics of enzyme inhibition are presented, allowing an understanding of the conditions required for inhibitory drug-drug interactions. The most important clinical consequences of these interactions are illustrated; special attention is drawn to the oral contraceptives.

Various methods used to detect enzyme induction and inhibition are critically evaluated.

I. INTRODUCTION

In 1964, Remmer and Siegert observed a prolonged duration of hexobarbital anesthesia in dogs on the first day of phenobarbital administration (80 mg/kg daily); with increasing time of phenobarbital administration, however, the duration of anesthesia shortened [1]. Such an observation comprises both topics of this contribution, namely, the inhibition of drug metabolism shortly after administration of a modifying compound, and an enhanced drug conversion thereafter. During the following years, evidence accumulated that many drugs and other environmental chemicals including pesticides alter the activities of hepatic microsomal enzymes. As a consequence, the inhibition or stimulation of their own metabolism or that of other drugs, including endogenous compounds such as steroids, has been observed. To the clinical pharmacologist these findings explained several then unexpected adverse drug reactions which occurred when drug combinations were administered. Meanwhile, considerable information on drug-drug interaction in humans due to such effects became available; moreover, environmental chemicals and dietary factors were shown to affect microsomal metabolism [2-6].

In this chapter, I try to summarize this information on the basis of biochemical or pharmacological considerations which may be of assistance in understanding the background involved. It may also explain why the actual number of compounds exhibiting such effects of clinical importance in humans remains relatively small.

II. FACTORS MEDIATING VARIATION OF DRUG METABOLISM

The intensity and duration of effect of many foreign compounds, especially of many drugs, depend on the rate of enzymatic degradation by the host. The enzyme systems involved are located in many tissues including the kidney, gut, brain, and particularly the liver. These versatile xenobiotic-metabolizing systems serve two major functions [7]. First, in many cases, they metabolically inactivate the parent compound by reducing its initial biological activity. Secondly, they convert the usually lipophilic substrates into polar derivatives which are soluble in water and can be eliminated by means of the urinary or biliary systems. Without such a conversion, drugs or other foreign material would remain in the organism for years with the consequence of accumulation and intoxication. Such consequences can be observed in peri- and postnatal periods when conjugation of bilirubin or chloramphenicol is insufficient leading to hyperbilirubinemia and the Gray syndrome, respectively, or in severe liver disease when the metabolism of hexobarbital [8] or many other drugs can be impaired [9-12].

A. Endogenous Variations of Drug Metabolism

It is accepted that the same dose of a drug given by the same route to patients of the same age and sex suffering from the same disease may produce toxicity in some, the desired therapeutic effect in others, and no effect in the rest. The basis for this discrepancy lies in the immense variations that exists between subjects. This biological variation occurs for a number of different reasons, one of which is due to differences in drug-metabolizing activity [13-15]. Since relatively little work on the variation of drug-metabolizing enzymes in humans has been performed for obvious ethical reasons, we are not aware at the present time of the precise manner in which host variations affect the action of drugs. However, a number of studies have been undertaken to evaluate the activity of microsomal monooxygenase systems in samples of human liver taken postmortem. As shown in Table 1, great variation exists in the amount of NADPH-cytochrome c reductase and cytochrome P-450 found [16]. Although it cannot be excluded that the patients had previously been exposed to inducing drugs or environmental chemicals, the large differences in enzyme content may reflect potential endogenous differences in the capacity to metabolize drugs and other toxic agents. Czygan and colleagues [17] reported similar variations in the cytochrome P-450 content of human liver biopsies, whereas other studies [18-21] showed relatively constant cytochrome P-450 levels in the livers of patients suffering from liver disease. Only those patients with severe hepatic disease showed lowered cytochrome P-450 levels and drug-metabolizing enzyme activity in the liver biopsies. Such differences are also reflected in vivo since individual differences in halothane metabolism in the order of magnitude of 2:1 have been reported [22]. Further, an almost tenfold variation in diphenylhydantoin blood levels during administration of the same daily doses has been described by Remmer and associates [23]. This may be partially explained by a genetically determined deficiency in diphenylhydantoin hydroxylase activity since large interindividual differences in the ratio between plasma concentrations of diphenylhydantoin and its para-hydroxylated metabolite have been observed [24].

Of similar clinical importance are differences in the activity of acetyltransferase, the enzyme responsible for the conjugation of isoniazid, dapsone, phenelzine, hydralazine, sulfamethoxine, and other sulfonamides such as sulfamethylazine [25]. The human population can be divided into two groups, namely, slow and fast acetylators. Slow acetylators who are given isoniazid frequently suffer from polyneuropathia unless lower doses of the drug are given. Moreover, Kutt and associates [26] found that 10% of epileptics who have been treated with 300 mg daily of diphenylhydantoin showed symptoms of intoxication with the latter drug when para-aminosalicylic acid or isoniazid had been given. All of the patients were slow acetylators in whom the elevated isoniazid blood levels inhibited microsomal transformation of diphenylhydantoin. When the dose of the latter

TABLE 1
Microsomal Drug-metabolizing Enzymes in Normal Human Livers

Patient age (years) + sex	Autopsy (hr after death)	Aminopyrine demethylation[a]	NADPH-cytochrome c reductase[a]	Cytochrome P-450[b]
44 M	3	N. D.	58	0.4
26 F	1	3.4	91	0.6
16 M	3	0.9	90	0.2
22 M	2	0.14	7	0.2
26 F	1	2.1	24	0.3
26 F	5	N.D.	4	0.2
25 M	6	0.2	10	0.3
45 M	2	1.2	47	0.5
20 M	3	0.7	9	0.2
49 M	4	1.0	10	0.3
31 M	2	1.6	29	0.2
28 M	3	0.7	14	0.1

[a] nmol/min per mg microsomal protein; N.D. = not determined.
[b] nmol/mg microsomal protein.
Source: Modified from Ref. 16. Williams & Wilkins Co., Baltimore.

drug was reduced the symptoms of intoxication disappeared. Further examples of adverse drug reactions having a genetic basis have been reviewed in detail [27-29].

Of great importance has been the finding that aromatic hydrocarbon-responsive mice are more susceptible to 3-methylcholanthrene-initiated tumors and to the toxicity of certain polycyclic hydrocarbons. This suggested the existence of genetic loci that modulate the response to environmental chemicals, in particular carcinogenic compounds. Evidence that similar phenomena occur in man comes from a number of sources. Cigarette smoke, which contains benzo[a]pyrene and other polycyclic aromatic hydrocarbons, induces aryl hydrocarbon hydroxylase (AHH), a multicomponent hydroxylase system utilizing NADPH and molecular oxygen and involving the microsomal electron-transport chain of which cytochrome P_1-450 is a major part [2,30,31]. The activity of this enzyme in human pulmonary alveola macrophages was found to be considerably higher in smokers than in nonsmokers [32]. Furthermore, benzo[a]pyrene hydroxylase activity was very low or nondetectable in human placenta obtained at term from women who were nonsmokers. However, among smokers placental benzo[a]-pyrene hydroxylase activity varied over a 70-fold range [33]. The basis for this variability is unknown but may be related to genetic differences in the inducibility of this enzyme which could be associated with genetic differences in susceptibility to the action of carcinogenic chemicals. There is evidence that AHH inducibility in cultures of human leucocytes correlates well with that in other tissues, such as lung, skin, and colon [34,35]. A study of more than 350 normal white subjects revealed that they could be classified in three distinct groups displaying low, intermediate, and high degrees of AHH inducibility [36]. Phenotype frequency was 53% low, 37% intermediate, and 10% high. A study of leucocyte AHH inducibility in a group of 50 patients with bronchiogenic carcinoma, all having been heavy smokers, revealed striking differences in the proportion of these three phenotypes from the normal population. Only 4% of the patients were in the low-inducibility group, whereas 66% were intermediate and 30% were of the high-inducibility group. Thus, persons showing intermediate and high inducibility of AHH have been calculated to have a 16 to 36 times higher risk for bronchiogenic carcinoma than those with low AHH inducibility [36]. These observations provide a genetic basis for the epidemiologic findings of Tocuhata [37] suggesting hereditary factors in susceptibility to lung cancer. They also strikingly illustrate genetic differences in the susceptibility of man to endogenous agents.

B. Mechanism of Enzyme Induction and Inhibition

1. Enhanced Drug Metabolism Due to Induction

When an animal is given an inducing agent such as phenobarbital over a period of several days, alteration in the drug-metabolizing enzyme system can be readily demonstrated. Morphologically, a proliferation of hepatic endoplasmic reticulum is observable by electron microscopy [38,39]. In addition, there is an apparent increase in microsomal protein per gram of liver concomitant with the development of increased drug tolerance. For example, when rats or dogs are treated with phenobarbital (80 mg/kg daily) for 3 days, both the sleeping time and plasma half-life of pentobarbital are reduced by more than 50% [1,40]. When hepatic microsomes of animals treated with an inducer like phenobarbital are isolated, their drug-metabolizing activity is enhanced for a wide variety of substrates. This enhancement is due to increased enzyme content rather than to increased enzyme activity. Michaelis constant (K_m) and inhibitor constants K_i for the overall reaction of drug metabolism are similar in induced and noninduced microsomal enzyme systems, indicating that a quantitative rather than a qualitative change is produced by the inductive process [41].

There is strong evidence to suggest that the induction phenomenon represents de novo synthesis of enzymatic proteins rather than either activation of preexisting enzyme forms or a decrease in the rate of protein degradation [42]. Ethionine, which is known to block protein synthesis by decreasing hepatic high-energy phosphate levels, prevents phenobarbital-stimulated induction of drug metabolism [43]. Puromycin and actinomycin D, which block RNA translation and transcription, respectively, also prevent enzyme induction [44,45]. Both transcriptional and translational control appear to regulate the synthesis of microsomal cytochrome P-450 enzymes [46,47]. A model system has been proposed by Marshall and McClean [48,49] and Marshall and Naughton [50] in which an exogenous inducer competes with an endogenous substrate (which is also an inducer) at the binding site of the enzyme system reducing the metabolism of the latter inducer and increasing its concentration. This increase derepresses cytochrome P-450 synthesis causing an enhanced enzyme formation until a new steady state is reached. Removal of the exogenous inducer finally results in rapid metabolism of the endogenous inducer leading to a reduced state of enzyme synthesis until the normal steady-state level is reached. Marshall and Naughton [50] suggest that the putative endogenous inducer might be identical with, or at least closely related to, lipid peroxides. This is based on the observation that phenobarbital induces hepatic lipid peroxidation. Recent work on the mechanism of induction suggests that lipid peroxidation of a specific membrane site by singlet oxygen released from cytochrome P-450 may be the common key by which a wide variety of molecules induce the cytochrome P-450 system [50-53]. However, the findings of Poland and coworkers [54], Guenthner and Nebert [55], and Nebert [56] contradict the concept of a common inducer. Thus, even excess concentrations of inducing agents like phenobarbital, pregnenolone-16α-carbonitrile, and other steroids do not displace active inducers from the cytosolic receptor of the locus regulating cytochrome P_1-450 enzyme synthesis. It is unlikely, however, that each inducing agent interacts specifically with a separate receptor controlling a specific form of cytochrome P-450. This would imply that thousands of receptors must exist to respond to the inducing capability of thousands of environmental chemicals. One possibility by which the genetic material could respond to the diverse range of inducing agents might be the phenomenon of intervening sequences which has been recently reviewed by Leder [57]. Genes for several proteins contain two or more discontinuous segments separated from each other by intervening sequences. Following transcription of the entire genome these sequences are removed and the assembled RNA can be translated into the polypeptide. To explain formation of the multiple forms of cytochrome P-450 system, Nebert [56] postulates that the various inducers interact with a "sensor system" which induces formation of a specific receptor by removing intervening sequences from the precursor in RNA. Subsequently, the inducer is able to interact with newly formed cytosolic receptors. These inducer-receptor complexes again remove specific intervening sequences from the precursor RNA synthesized by the structural genes of cytochrome P-450 resulting in the assembly of specific amino acid sequences of a specific cytochrome P-450. This newly induced form then represents a large portion of the total cytochrome P-450 content of the cell. In newborn rabbits treated with 3-methylcholanthrene, cytochrome P_1-450 comprises more than 80% of hepatic cytochrome P-450 content [58]. This would explain the overlapping substrate or inhibitor selectivities observed. It further implies the existence of a great variety of inducer-specific cytochrome P-450 forms which may only differ in certain variable regions of the cytochromal polypeptide explaining the increasing number of isolated cytochrome P-450 forms reported. The clinical consequence of the existence and inducibility of the different cytochrome P-450 forms is not clear. Since they seem to differ in their K_m values, it is extremely difficult to predict the consequences of enhanced formation of a particular cytochrome due to an inducing agent on the metabolism of other drugs.

Regardless of which mechanisms are involved in the induction process, there seem to be several pharmacological properties which are correlated with the inducing capability of a xenobiotic. From animal studies and investigations in humans the following properties are apparent [2]:

1. The inducing compound is sufficiently lipid-soluble to enter hepatocytes.
2. The inducer accumulates or at least maintains a certain intracellular level on repeated administration.
3. The inducer is a substrate of the microsomal enzyme system.

2. Enhanced Drug Metabolism Due to Factors Other than Induction

Enhanced drug metabolism is not necessarily due to an induction of drug-metabolizing enzymes. It can also occur when the free concentration of a drug in plasma and in liver increases. In severe liver and kidney disease (for review, see Refs. 9,11) and in nephrotic syndromes, when the level of albumin and other plasma proteins is diminished, the amount of drug bound to circulating proteins may be altered. If the drug is highly bound to proteins (90% or more), any decrease in the binding capacity of proteins will significantly increase the free concentration of the drug. Since liver monooxygenase enzymes are never saturated under normal in vivo conditions, increased free drug concentrations in plasma increase the drug concentration in the enzyme compartment with the consequence of accelerated metabolism. This explains why the oxidation rate of tolbutamide and phenylbutazone [59], which are highly bound to plasma proteins, are found to be increased during liver cirrhosis and kidney disease when the serum albumin concentration is decreased [60]. By contrast, the elimination of the weakly bound antipyrine and aminopyrine is decreased under such conditions due to diminished metabolism [61]. Moreover, when conjugation reactions are involved in the metabolic fate of a drug, elimination may be increased during severe liver disease. The glucuronyltransferase which is located in the endoplasmic reticulum of the liver is easily activated tenfold by detergents such as bile acids in vitro [62]. Since the concentration of bile acids is greatly increased in pathologically altered livers [12,63], increased glucuronidation of drugs may occur.

3. Impaired Drug Metabolism

An early clue to the mechanism of action of enzyme inhibitors was provided by McMahon [64] who studied the nature of inhibition of microsomal demethylation by 2,4-dichloro-6-phenylphenoxyethylamine, observing that this compound competitively inhibited the N-demethylation of butynamine and meperidine. In addition, the demethylation of a variety of other substrates was inhibited. SKF-525A, Lilly-18947, and desmethylmeperidine were also shown to be competitive inhibitors of butynamine demethylation. From these studies, McMahon [64] concluded that substrates and inhibitors compete for the same enzymatic site.

Due to the wide substrate range of the microsomal enzyme system resulting from a low substrate selectivity of cytochrome P-450, almost all compounds that are metabolized by this enzyme may a priori inhibit the metabolism of other substrates. In vivo, piperonyl butoxide and many other methylenedioxyphenyl derivatives prolong the sleeping time of barbiturates and the paralysis time of zoxazolamine [65-70]. Similarly, the acute toxicity of Freons, griseofulvine, and benzo[a]pyrene is increased by piperonyl butoxide in infant mice [71,72]. However, careful in vitro studies revealed that piperonyl butoxide produced competitive inhibition, but that the degree of inhibition increased with time [73,74]. Spectral studies of the microsomal system revealed two major perturbations. Firstly, and similarly to most of the compounds that are metabolized by cytochrome P-450 [75-77], addition of piperonyl butoxide resulted in a type I spectrum [78]. Secondly, after prolonged incubation in the presence of NADPH and oxygen an absorbance at 455 nm appeared [79]. Electron paramagnetic resonance spectra indicated this peak to be due to a newly formed drug-cytochrome P-450 complex. At the same time, the competitive inhibition of ethylmorphine demethylation became noncompetitive. Further studies revealed the ligandlike nature of the complex, and also that the extent of its formation was well correlated with the degree of inhibition [73]. From this it can be concluded that drug-metabolizing enzyme activity cannot be inhibited only by drugs acting as alternate substrates but also by the formation of metabolites which generate stable cytochrome P-450 complexes.

Similar inhibitory effects of hydroxylated metabolites have been demonstrated in vitro with 5-(para-hydroxyphenyl)-5-phenylhydantoin and 2-hydroxydesmethylimipramine [80,81]. In vivo studies similarly inducate the inhibitory effects of hydroxyphenylhydantoin and oxyphenylbutazone on the elimination of the parent compounds [82,83]. Moreover, drug metabolites can also inhibit the biotransformation of other drugs. Such cross-inhibition was observed in vitro for the combination of hydroxyphenylhydantoin with phenylbutazone [84], hexobarbital and ethylmorphine [85], zoxazolamine and aniline [86], and oxyphenylbutazone and diphenylhydantoin [84]. Hydroxyphenylhydantoin prolonged the hexobarbital sleeping time in mice [85], and zoxazolamine paralysis in rats [86]. A direct demonstration of cross-product inhibition in rats has been given by Soda and Levy [87]. Oxyphenylbutazone inhibited the elimination of diphenylhydantoin, and the biotransformation of antipyrine was subject to product inhibition by 4-hydroxyantipyrine. However, neither oxyphenylbutazone nor 4-hydroxyantipyrine affected the elimination kinetics or metabolism of sulfanilamide, a drug undergoing acetylation and glucuronidation, but not subjected to oxidative processes [88].

The observation of product inhibition in the elimination of antipyrine is especially interesting since this drug differs from others in that it is hydrophilic and negligibly bound to plasma proteins. Thus, lipophilicity does not seem to be essential for interaction at the binding site of cytochrome P-450. This conclusion points to the difficulties of predicting metabolic inhibition resulting from drug-drug or drug-metabolite interactions at enzymatic active sites.

In in vitro systems, inhibitory potency is usually reported as the amount of inhibitor necessary to antagonize a reaction by 50% (I_{50}). Although this value is useful for the rapid comparison of large numbers of compounds it is dependent on the substrate concentration and the amount of protein present in the incubate [89]. The inhibitory constant K_i may be more meaningful for purposes of comparison. This value is obtained from Lineweaver-Burk plots; a serious problem, however, is the possibility of obtaining plots that are biased by the decision to use high or low concentrations of substrate. Other procedures to determine the inhibitory constant have been discussed by Mannering [89].

Determination of the dissociation constant K_s of the cytochrome P-450-substrate complex may also serve to estimate the binding capacity of drugs. Great importance was once given to the apparent relationship between the kinetics of drug binding to the cytochrome and the kinetics of drug metabolism [77]. In a number of cases the K_s and K_m values of a given compound were found to be similar indicating that drug binding is an obligatory step in the oxidative metabolism of the drug.

The dissociation constants of the enzyme-substrate complexes of amphetamine, phenobarbital, diphenylhydantoin, and several other compounds

TABLE 2
Spectral Dissociation Constants (K_s) of Drugs which Inhibit Each Others' Metabolism during Coadministrative Drug Treatment in Humans

	K_s
Amphetamine	5×10^{-3}
Aminopyrine	3×10^{-4}
Ethylmorphine	3×10^{-5}
Phenobarbital	1×10^{-5}
Desmethylimipramine	3×10^{-6}
Imipramine	3×10^{-6}
Diphenylhydantoin	1×10^{-6}

Source: Ref. 90.

are given in Table 2 [90]. It can be seen that the K_s values range from 10^{-3} to 10^{-6} M. This wide range seems to be responsible for the different inhibitory capabilities of drugs, compounds with smaller K_s value inhibiting the metabolism of those with higher values. Thus, the metabolism of amphetamine is inhibited by desmethylimipramine [91], chlorpromazine [92], nortriptyline, chlordiazepoxide, and diazepam [93]. These compounds which have relatively low K_s values do inhibit the N-demethylation of aminopyrine and ethylmorphine [89]. Similarly, the clearance of phenobarbital is reduced when diphenylhydantoin is administered concomitantly, while the clearance of the latter drug hardly changes or is even increased when phenobarbital is administered. This can be explained by differences in K_s values since that of phenobarbital is about 10^{-5} M [94] and that of diphenylhydantoin is 10^{-6} M. In summary, diphenylhydantoin inhibits phenobarbital binding to cytochrome P-450 and metabolism. The inhibition may be further aggravated by the formation of hydroxyphenylhydantoin which also occupies a certain percentage of enzymatic sites [80,82]. Although in vitro determination of the K_s values can only provide a very rough estimate of in vivo conditions because it neglects many pharmacokinetic parameters such as differences in intestinal absorption, saturation of the enzyme, steady-state levels, or renal excretion, K_s values may give an indication of whether coadministration of several drugs may lead to inhibitory effects.

If the concepts of alternate substrate inhibition and inhibition by reaction products are correct, then the following preconditions for an inhibitory drug-drug interaction should be met: The drug and the inhibitor must serve as substrates of cytochrome P-450; the K_m or the K_s of the inhibitor, when acting as a substrate, must equal the K_i when acting as an inhibitor [66]; and the inhibitor should not have a V_{max} which greatly exceeds that of the substrate if its presence at the metabolic site is to be maintained [95].

III. GENERAL FEATURES OF ENZYME INDUCTION AND INHIBITION

A. Conditions which Elevate Enzyme Activity

There are more than 200 drugs, carcinogens, and other chemicals which have been shown to stimulate hepatic drug-metabolizing enzymes in laboratory animals and humans [3,96-98]. There are three general types of inducing agents. One group, as typified by phenobarbital, increases the rates of many reactions including oxidation, glucuronidation, and reduction of many other compounds. The second group, primarily certain aromatic polycyclic hydrocarbons with 3-methylcholanthrene or benzo[a]pyrene as prototypes, stimulates a more limited group of reactions. Whereas phenobarbital causes a three- to fourfold increase in microsomal cytochrome P-450 content and NADPH-cytochrome P-450 reductase, 3-methylcholanthrene stimulates formation of a new hemoprotein called cytochrome P_1-450 or P-448, which is distinct from cytochrome P-450 both spectrally and in substrate selectivity, ethyl isocyanide difference spectra, and drug complexing properties [99-102]. In vivo, maximal increases in microsomal enzyme activity following phenobarbital administration are not reached until 3 days, whereas 3-methylcholanthrene doubles enzyme activity within several hours and the maximal increase is reached in 24 hr [43,99]. A third group of inducers may be seen in steroids. In animals pregnenolone-16α-carbonitrile is a more potent inducer than phenobarbital [103,104]. Compounds of the phenobarbital type induce hepatic microsomal enzyme activity in man, and change the rate of drug metabolism necessitating modification of drug therapy. Data currently available are presented in Table 3.

Generally, hypnotics and sedatives in clinical use are known to cause induction of microsomal enzymes in animals. It is very important that these compounds be identified and their effect on the rate of metabolism in man be investigated because sleeping tablets are often given to patients receiving potent specific drug therapy. Thus, phenobarbital reduces the plasma half-life and anticoagulant activity of warfarin [105,106] and other coumarin anticoagulants [107-109]. Nearly all of the commonly used barbiturates exert this action upon warfarin and other anticoagulants. Phenobarbital also decreases the half-life of antipyrine [111]. Shortening of the half-life of aminopyrine due to phenobarbital has been demonstrated on a number of occasions.

Ingestion of phenobarbital shortened the half-life of diphenylhydantoin [109,115,116]. This effect, however, is not observed in all patients

TABLE 3

Drug-metabolizing Enzyme Induction in Humans

	Daily dose (mg)	Day of treatment when altered drug metabolism is determined	Drug affected	Reference(s)
Phenobarbital	120	21	Warfarin	105
Therapeutic daily dose: 50–200 mg	210	2	Warfarin	106
	90	14	Bis-hydroxycoumarin	107
			Bis-hydroxycoumarin	108
	65	21	Bis-hydroxycoumarin	109
	120	14	Prednisolone	110
	2 mg/kg	14	Antipyrine	111
	10–20 μg/ml blood	28	Quinidine	
	300	14	Aminopyrine	112
	300	13	Digitoxin	113
	150	14	Chlorpromazine	114
	1.5–2.5 mg/kg	10	Diphenylhydantoin	115
	65	29	Diphenylhydantoin	109
	1–2 mg/kg		Diphenylhydantoin	116

	100	10	Doxycycline	117
Secobarbital	100	33	Warfarin	118
Therapeutic daily dose: 100 mg	100	8	Warfarin	119
	100	21	Warfarin	120
Pentobarbital Therapeutic daily dose: 50–120 mg	100	10–14	Alprenolol	121
Butabarbital Therapeutic daily dose: 30–60 mg	30–60	21	Phenprocoumon	122
Amobarbital Therapeutic daily dose: 60–150 mg	200	21	Warfarin	120
Combination of Aprobarbital and Vinbarbital Therapeutic daily dose: 50–100 mg	100	18	Bis-hydroxycoumarin	123

(continued)

TABLE 3 (continued)

	Daily dose (mg)	Day of treatment when altered drug metabolism is determined	Drug affected	Reference(s)
Heptabarbital	400	4	Acenocoumarin	124
Therapeutic daily dose: 200 mg	400	3	Bis-hydroxycoumarin	124
	400	3-5	Bis-coumacetate	124
	500	3	Coumarin	124
	400	3	Bis-hydroxycoumarin	125
Glutethimide	1000	21	Warfarin	106
Therapeutic daily dose: 375-750 mg			Warfarin	105
			Ethyl bis-coumacetate	126
			Carbamazepine	127
			Carbamazepine	128
			Carbamazepine	129
Carbamazepine	300-1200	60	Carbamazepine	130
Therapeutic daily dose: 800-1200 mg	400-600	80-190	Antipyrine	131
	200	4	Clonazepam	132

	600	4–14	Diphenylhydantoin	133
	600	14	Warfarin	133
<u>Chlorpromazine</u>	300	14	Chlorpromazine	134
Therapeutic daily dose: 100–1000 mg	300	7–14	Chlorpromazine	114
	300	7–14	Antipyrine	114
	100–450	Long-term	Antipyrine	135
<u>Diphenylhydantoin</u>	600	14	Cortisol	136
Therapeutic daily dose: 600 mg	600	5	Digitoxin	137
	300	3	Dicoumarol	133
	300	22	Antipyrine	131, 138
<u>Spironolactone</u>			Antipyrine	139
Therapeutic daily dose: 100 mg				
<u>Phenylbutazone</u>	300	3–5	Digitoxin	137
Therapeutic daily dose: 200 mg				

(continued)

TABLE 3 (continued)

	Daily dose (mg)	Day of treatment when altered drug metabolism is determined	Drug affected	Reference(s)
Rifampicin	600	Long-term	Rifampicin	140
Therapeutic daily dose: 600 mg	600	7-14	Rifampicin	141
	600	Long-term	Warfarin	142
	900	4-5	Acenocoumarol	143
	600	7	Antipyrine	144
	600	6	Antipyrine	145
	600	28	Tolbutamide	146
	150-600	9	Tolbutamide	147

	150–600	9	Hexobarbital	147
	1200	8	Hexobarbital	145
	1200	8	Digitoxin	148
	600	Long-term	Digitoxin	149
	600	36	Cortisol	150
Testosterone	400	21	Antipyrine	151
Therapeutic daily dose:	400	21	Antipyrine	152
5–15 mg	400	21	Antipyrine	152
Pregnenolone-16α-carbonitrile			Thiopental	153
			Propanidid	153
	750	3	Indomethacin	110

investigated, since the level of diphenylhydantoin has been left unchanged or even raised in some cases [116]. In general, the clinical significance of the interaction between diphenylhydantoin and phenobarbital is uncertain [154-156].

Of other barbiturates, secobarbital [119,120], pentobarbital [121], butobarbital [122], amobarbital [120], a combination of aprobarbital and vinbarbital [123], and heptabarbital [125] have been demonstrated to induce drug metabolism in man. Increased metabolism of the barbiturates themselves results in some degree of tolerance, but increased metabolism of other compounds given simultaneously has also been described. Glutethimide has been shown to shorten the plasma half-life of warfarin [105,106] and of ethyl bis-coumacetate [127].

Tricyclic drugs may also induce liver microsomal oxidizing enzymes as evidenced in Table 3. Thus, carbamazepine enhances its own metabolism [127-129], and at doses between 400 and 600 mg daily reduces antipyrine half-life from 11 to approximately 8 hr [131]. Carbamazepine also shortened half-lives of clonazepam [132], diphenylhydantoin, and warfarin [133].

Rifampicin has a wide spectrum of antibacterial activity, but is principally used in the management of tuberculosis. Studies with patients with biliary T-tubes have shown that repeated administration of rifampicin over a period of 7 days is accompanied by increased biliary excretion [141] and a reduction of its own half-life [140,157]. This has been explained by an enhanced conversion to desacetylrifampicin in the liver during continuous administration.

As observed with anticonvulsant drugs, rifampicin significantly lessens the hypothrombenemia caused by the administration of anticoagulants, requiring an increase in daily dosage [142,143,158,159]. The administration of rifampicin at usual doses decreased the plasma levels and the half-life of warfarin and reduced prothrombin values [142]. Rifampicin has also been shown to reduce the plasma concentration of antidiabetic agents such as tolbutamide and almost to double its rate of disappearance from the plasma [146,147]. Enhanced metabolism of hexobarbital was also observed [145,148], the increased hexobarbital clearance returning to normal 14 days after withdrawal of the drug [145].

The same dose of rifampicin given for 8 days to 6 healthy volunteers significantly reduced the half-life of digitoxin [148]. At the same time, an increased urinary excretion of polar metabolites occurred which lasted for 4 days after termination of rifampicin treatment. A fall in serum digitoxin levels by almost 50% during tuberculostatic treatment with rifampicin (with or without the coadministration of isoniazid and ethambutal) was observed [149]. Correspondingly, the serum half-life of digitoxin was 8.2 ± 1.4 days in untreated subjects, and 4.5 ± 1.5 days in the patients with increased 12β-hydroxylation of digitoxin to digoxin.

Effects of rifampicin on corticosteroid metabolism have also been observed [150]. In the case of Addison's disease which has been treated with corticosteroids, rifampicin treatment resulted in an Addisonian crisis. The most disturbing enzyme-inducing effect of rifampicin, however, is the accelerated metabolism of gonadal steroids. A fourfold increase in the hydroxylation of estradiol and ethinylestradiol in liver microsomes from patients during treatment with rifampicin in therapeutic doses has been demonstrated [19,160]. This was accompanied by a comparable increase in microsomal cytochrome P-450 [160]. Increased ethinylestradiol metabolism could similarly be demonstrated in volunteers taking 0.6 g of rifampicin daily [161].

Since oral contraceptives are frequently prescribed to prevent pregnancy during the management of active tuberculosis, a number of reports have appeared describing symptoms of enhanced metabolism of the oral contraceptive steroids [162-166].

Although diphenylhydantoin is a known enzyme inducer in laboratory animals [167], remarkably few reports exist on its inducing effect in humans. In 1964, Werk and associates [136] observed an abnormal pattern of excretion of cortisol metabolites in the urine of patients receiving diphenylhydantoin therapy for convulsive seizures. This abnormal pattern was characterized by an increased urinary output of the polar unconjugated metabolite 6β-hydroxycortisol and of other polar derivatives. Diphenylhydantoin also increases the metabolism of other drugs (Table 3).

Very little information is available on the persistence of enhanced drug metabolism after withdrawal of the inducing drug. Information presently available is given in Table 4. The figures only indicate the time after withdrawal of the inducer when drug-metabolizing activity has been determined. In no case has the time course of normalization been investigated. The data indicate that enhanced metabolism normalizes approximately one week after withdrawal of the inducer. This is further supported by the observations of Hunter and colleagues [170] who showed normalization of urinary D-glucaric acid excretion within 1 week after removing barbiturates from therapy. Moreover, normal microsomal hexobarbital oxidase activity and cytochrome P-450 content have been found in surgical liver biopsies 6 days after withdrawal of phenobarbital (90 mg daily for a nondefined time, possibly 7-10 days) [171]. However, persistence of induction seems to be dose-dependent. After barbiturate overdosage, evidence of enzyme induction persisted for more than 6 weeks [172].

Besides drugs, environmental contaminants are also known to induce microsomal drug metabolism. Workers in a DDT factory had plasma half-lives of phenylbutazone shorter than those of the control group [173]. Similarly, a decrease in the plasma elimination half-life of phenylbutazone was observed in workers exposed to Lindane [174]. Accelerated elimination of some drugs due to enzyme induction by chlorinated pesticides is long-lasting [175]. However, based on data from fishermen who have been exposed to DDT by eating DDT-contaminated fish, Kolmodin-Hedman [176] suggested that significant acceleration of antipyrine elimination does not occur in

TABLE 4
Persistence of Enhanced Drug Metabolism after Withdrawal of the Inducing Drug

Inducing drug	Drug affected	Days after withdrawal	Reference
Phenylbutazone	Digitoxin	5-7	137
Combination of vinbarbital and aprobarbital	Bis-hydroxycoumarin	7	123
Phenobarbital	Warfarin	7	168
Phenobarbital	Doxycycline	14	117
Carbamazepine	Diphenylhydantoin	10-21	133
Antipyrine	Warfarin	18-24	169
Phenobarbital	Warfarin	28	105
Glutethimide	Warfarin	28	105

humans until the sum of the plasma level of pp-DDA and pp-DDT exceeds 200 ng/ml.

Human food contains numerous nonnutrient lipid-soluble foreign chemicals [177,178], some of which may influence the metabolism of drugs. Pantuck and coworkers [179] demonstrated a stimulatory effect of feeding charcoal-broiled beef to rats on the metabolism of phenacetin in intestine. Feeding a charcoal-broiled diet to volunteers for 4 days also increased the plasma disappearance of phenacetin without influencing the plasma half-life or concentration of the O-deethylated metabolite N-acetyl-para-aminophenol. This effect results in a marked increase in the ratio of the concentration of N-acetyl-para-aminophenol to the concentration of the parent compound phenacetin in plasma. It suggests that charcoal-broiled beef stimulates the metabolism of phenacetin in the gastrointestinal tract and/or during its first pass through the liver. A charcoal-broiled beef diet similarly stimulated the metabolism of antipyrine and theophylline [180].

Additional studies showed that a diet containing large amounts of protein enhances the metabolism of antipyrine and theophylline in humans, whereas a high-carbohydrate diet depresses the rate of metabolism of these drugs [181,182]. Although low-protein diets in animals are known to reduce the concentration of cytochrome P-450 and drug-metabolizing enzymes, dietary protein content does not seem to be a limiting factor on microsomal enzyme activity in humans.

Most human populations ingest about 11% of their daily calorie intake as protein [183]. There is, however, an enormous variation in dietary fat intake, and also in the kinds of fats used [183]. In rats, fats alone without phenobarbital do not have major inducing effects, whereas unsaturated fats and linoleic acid allow phenobarbital to induce high levels of cytochrome P-450. This effect, however, does not parallel the essential fatty acid content of the diet [48,49,184-186]. Since the antioxidant butylated hydroxyanisole partly blocks the facilitating effect of linoleic acid [50], it seems that the effect of fats is more closely linked to their ability to undergo peroxidation than to their content of essential fatty acids. This has led to the assumption that lipid peroxidation of a specific membrane site by singlet oxygen released from cytochrome P-450 may be a common pathway by which a wide variety of molecules will induce the P-450 system (see Sec. II.A.1). Whether or not dietary fatty acid content affects the status of the microsomal enzymes in man is still unknown.

Summarizing the reports of enzyme induction presented so far, several common features concerning drug induction in man become apparent:

1. Only about 10 drugs have been reported to increase their own metabolism or that of other drugs when given at therapeutic doses. Since many hundreds of chemicals are used in drug therapy, this is a remarkably low number (Table 3).
2. Drugs (but not all exogenous inducers) that induce cytochrome P-450 and hence increase the metabolism of other drugs are also metabolized by this poorly selective enzyme.
3. As can be seen in Table 5, the plasma half-life of the inducing agents exceeds 4 hr and is mostly in the range of 1 day or more. This implies a rapid accumulation of the drug providing a constant high concentration in the cellular compartment.

TABLE 5
Plasma Half-lives of Several Inducing Drugs

	Half-life (hr)	Reference
Phenobarbital	70 ± 120	20
Glutethimide	52 ± 7	105
Carbamazepine	37	130
Diphenylhydantoin	24	98
Rifampicin	4	157

4. The time after which enhanced metabolism can be observed after repeated administration of known inducers is approximately 7 days (Table 3). It can be shorter especially when doses above the therapeutic range are administered. This has been pointed out by Breckenridge and colleagues [119]. It indicates that increased synthesis of cytochrome P-450 is the rate-limiting factor since the half-life of this cytochrome is about 1 day [63]. There is no investigation in humans on the exact time course of induction after administering different classes of inducing agents.
5. Similarly, there are no specific investigations on the time required for normalization of drug metabolism after withdrawal of the inducer from therapy. The little data available indicates that enhanced metabolism normalizes within approximately 1 week (Table 4).
6. The metabolism of a wide range of drugs can be enhanced by inducing agents (Table 6). It is remarkable, however, that most of the drugs are subject to aromatic hydroxylation. Of the other possible functionalization reactions, increased desacetylation has been reported in the case of rifampicin and indomethacin, and increased demethylation in the case of propanidid, glycodiazine, and aminopyrine. Unfortunately, this important phenomenon has not been studied further. Among conjugation reactions only glucuronidation seems to be induced. This fact finds an application in the treatment of hyperbilirubinemia.

Whether alcohol has clinically relevant inducing capacity in humans has not been finally evaluated. Although several studies in laboratory animals which have been supplied with high-alcohol-containing diets showed increases in cytochrome P-450 content and drug-metabolizing enzyme activity [201-203], increased enzyme activity in humans has only been demonstrated in heavy drinkers [204].

The inducing effect of steroids is also worth mentioning. Relatively high doses of testosterone induce the metabolism of testosterone itself and antipyrine [151,152]. Pregnenolone-16α-carbonitrile shortened the duration of anesthesia induced by thiopental and propanidid [153], and increased the metabolic rate of indomethacin [110].

B. Conditions which Reduce Enzyme Activity

Many drugs which are metabolized in the liver will, in principle, follow the same biotransformation pathways and will use the same microsomal enzyme systems. In multiple-drug therapy, competition for this system occurs among such drugs. As a consequence, the biotransformation of one drug may be inhibited by another drug given at the same time (Table 7). Particularly representative are the inhibitory effects of oral contraceptives on hepatic drug metabolism [215,232]. For example, Homeida and associates

TABLE 6
Human Functionalization Reactions Which Can Be Accelerated During Treatment with Inducing Agents

Enhanced metabolism	Main reaction	Reference
Alprenolol	Ring-hydroxylation	187
Aminopyrine	4-Hydroxylation (N-demethylation)	188
Antipyrine	4-Hydroxylation	188
Carbamazepine	10,11-Epoxidation	130
Chlorpromazine	3- or 7-Hydroxylation	189
Clonazepam	3-Hydroxylation	190
Cortisol	6-Hydroxylation	136
Coumarin	3- and 7-Hydroxylation	191
Digitoxin	12-Hydroxylation	192
Diphenylhydantoin	Para-hydroxylation	193
Doxycycline	Hydroxylation	117
Estradiol	2- and 4-Hydroxylation	160
17-Ethinylestradiol	2- and 4-Hydroxylation	160
Glycodiazine	O-demethylation	194
Hexobarbital	3-Hydroxylation	195
Indomethacin	N-Desacetylation	196
Methadone	Para-hydroxylation	197
Propanidid	O-demethylation	153
Rifampicin	25-O-desacetylation	198
Testosterone	6β-, 7-, or 16-Hydroxylation	199
Thiopental	Desulfuration	88
Tolbutamide	Hydroxylation	200
Warfarin	7-Hydroxylation	142

TABLE 7
Drugs that Prolong Half-life or Increase Serum Concentration of Other Drugs When Administered Simultaneously

Inhibitory drug	Drug inhibited	Increase in	Complications reported	Reference(s)
Alcohol	Antipyrine	Half-life		152,205
Allopurinol	Antipyrine	Half-life		206
	Bis-hydroxycoumarin	Half-life		206
Aminopyrine	Antipyrine	Half-life		207
Bis-hydroxycoumarin	Chlorpropamide	Half-life	Hypoglycemia	208
	Tolbutamide	Half-life	Hypoglycemia	208,209
	Diphenylhydantoin	Half-life	Ataxia, nystagmus, vertigo, anorexia	133
Chloramphenicol	Chlorpropamide	Half-life		210
	Cyclophosphamide	Half-life		211
	Bis-hydroxycoumarin	Half-life		212
	Diphenylhydantoin	Half-life		212
	Tolbutamide	Half-life	Hypoglycemia	212
Clofibrate	Bis-hydroxycoumarin	Half-life		213
	Diphenylhydantoin	Half-life		213
	Tolbutamide	Half-life		213

Contraceptives (oral) (ethinylestradiol/ dl-norgestrel)	Antipyrine	Half-life		214
	Phenylbutazone	Half-life		215
Dipropylacetate	Phenobarbital	Serum concentration	Phenobarbital intoxication	216
Disulfiram	Antipyrine	Half-life		217
	Diphenylhydantoin	Half-life	Ataxia, nystagmus	218
	Diphenylhydantoin		Cerebellar symptoms	219
Isoniazid	Hexobarbital	Half-life		220
	Diphenylhydantoin	Half-life	Ataxia, nystagmus, cerebellar symptoms	26
Nortriptyline	Antipyrine	Half-life		206
	Bis-hydroxycoumarin	Half-life		206
Oxyphenbutazone	Diphenylhydantoin	Half-life		213
	Tolbutamide	Half-life		221
	Hexobarbital	Half-life		220
Phenprocoumon	Diphenylhydantoin	Half-life		222
Phenylbutazone	Diphenylhydantoin	Half-life		223
	Diphenylhydantoin		Vertigo, anorexia, vomiting, cerebellar damage	224

(continued)

TABLE 7 (continued)

Inhibitory drug	Drug inhibited	Increase in	Complications reported	Reference(s)
	Tolbutamide	Half-life		224
	Tolbutamide		Hypoglycemia	213
	Chlorpropamide		Hypoglycemia	
Phenyramidol	Bis-hydroxycoumarin	Half-life	Hemorrhage	225
	Diphenylhydantoin	Half-life		209
	Tolbutamide	Half-life	Hypoglycemia	209
Sulfadiazine	Diphenylhydantoin	Half-life		213
	Tolbutamide	Half-life		221
Sulfamethizole	Diphenylhydantoin	Half-life		226

	Diphenylhydantoin		Vertigo, cerebellar symptoms	227
	Tolbutamide	Half-life		226
	Warfarin	Half-life		228
Sulfamethoxazole	Tolbutamide	Half-life		228
Sulfamethoxazole and trimethoprim	Diphenylhydantoin	Half-life		213
Sulfaphenazole	Chlorpropamide	Half-life		221
	Tolbutamide	Half-life	Hypoglycemia	221, 229
	Diphenylhydantoin	Half-life		213
Sulthiame	Diphenylhydantoin	Half-life		230
	Diphenylhydantoin		Vertigo, anorexia, vomiting	231

[214] described a 21% decrease in antipyrine clearance in healthy, premenopausal women who received 30 μg ethinylestradiol and 500 μg norgestrel as an oral contraceptive for 6 months. Discontinuation of the contraceptive resulted in a 30% increase in antipyrine clearance. Generalizing these observations, the elimination of any drug which is metabolized by monooxygenases is expected to be impaired during oral contraceptive therapy. Whether the commonly applied schedule of 3 weeks oral contraceptive therapy followed by 1 week without is accompanied by changes in the therapeutic effects of other drugs has not been investigated. However, a reduced efficacy of oral anticoagulants or hypoglycemic agent should be expected during this period.

Plasma half-life and metabolic clearance of antipyrine was impaired when aminopyrine was administered to normal human volunteers [207]. However, the same degree of inhibition of antipyrine metabolism was achieved whether aminopyrine was administered simultaneously at the same time as or 5 hr before antipyrine. Since the half-life of aminopyrine in humans is less than 3 hr while that of its major metabolite 4-aminoantipyrine is approximately 13 hr, inhibition seems to be mediated by this metabolite or possibly by antipyrine to which 4-aminoantipyrine is further metabolized [188]. Several other examples of drug-drug inhibition are given in Table 7 which is obtained from the reviews of Perrin and Fabre [25], Kutt [155], Kristensen [224], Egli [233], and from more recent reports.

However, not all observations of increased serum concentrations or prolonged half-lives are due to drug-drug interaction at the microsomal enzyme level. Especially when drugs with high serum protein binding (such as sulfonamides) are involved, competition at the serum protein binding site may result in displacement of one drug with a consequential increase in blood levels. At the same time the increased concentration of unbound drug may result in enhanced excretion. A similar effect has been observed by Held and Oldershausen [60] in chronic liver disease with reduced serum protein levels when drug protein binding became impaired.

In principle many of the inhibitory drugs should not be given to persons receiving other drugs listed in Table 7. However, if multitherapy is necessary, the dose of the primary drug should be reduced. It is also necessary to carefully monitor the pharmacodynamic effects of the primary drug. If possible, it is ideal to monitor also its blood concentration. However, since alternative drugs are frequently available such combinations should be avoidable.

C. Various Methods Used to Detect Induction or Inhibition

A number of tests have been proposed for the detection of altered drug-metabolizing enzyme activity in humans. Urinary D-glucaric acid excretion may be utilized, but since the sugar is formed by enzymes different from those involved in drug metabolism it is mainly used as a screening test for large groups of patients. The plasma concentration of γ-glutamyltranspeptidase and urine concentration of 6β-hydroxycortisol have also been monitored. Estimation of the changes in the half-life of the drugs antipyrine or aminopyrine are presently widely used indices of altered drug metabolism. However, none of these tests is entirely satisfactory due to the extreme complexity of the monooxygenase system, implying that the activity of some enzymes may be increased while that of others is not.

D-glucaric acid is an end product of glucuronic acid metabolism in humans and guinea pigs, neither of whom are able to synthesize ascorbic acid from glucuronate. In 1965, Aarts observed an increased urinary excretion of D-glucaric acid in patients treated with phenobarbital or aminopyrine [234]. This has subsequently been shown to be a parameter correlating well with hepatic cytochrome P-450 levels in guinea pigs [235]. Increased D-glucaric acid excretion has been observed in workers exposed to dieldrin [170] and in epileptics treated with phenobarbital [236]. However, D-glucaric acid excretion and cytochrome P-450 in liver biopsies do not correlate well [171].

Similarly, D-glucaric acid excretion and antipyrine half-lives in either induced or noninduced subjects did not correlate consistently, indicating that these indices of drug-metabolizing enzyme activity respond differently to the inducing agent. Breimer and coworkers [145] also reported different responses in the excretion of D-glucaric acid and the elimination of hexobarbital and antipyrine. Nevertheless, D-glucaric acid excretion seems to be a useful indicator of induction and has been used extensively for this purpose.

Changes in serum γ-glutamyltranspeptidase have also been associated with alterations in drug metabolism—for example, after the administration of barbiturates [237]. This enzyme occurs in different organs including the liver where it is present in association with the endoplasmic reticulum [238] and is concerned with the intracellular transfer of γ-glutamyl residues. Thus, there is no direct relationship to the cytochrome P-450-dependent enzyme systems, and this enzyme is used mainly as an indicator for function of the liver, the pancreas, and the kidneys. However, increased γ-glutamyltranspeptidase levels in the plasma have been observed in patients receiving anticoagulant therapy [239] and during rifampicin treatment [145]. Increased enzyme levels also correlated with decreased plasma warfarin levels in most of the patients given enzyme inducers [237]. In contrast, patients given benzodiazepines (which have no known inducing effect) showed an increase in plasma levels of the enzyme but not of warfarin. This enzyme consequently does not seem to be a reliable indicator for altered drug-metabolizing activity in humans.

Various inducers such as phenobarbital [240], diphenylhydantoin [136], and DDT [173] increase the excretion of 6β-hydroxycortisol in humans. In workers exposed to DDT, a simultaneous decrease in the plasma half-life of antipyrine occurs; there is, however, no quantitative correlation between these parameters. Furthermore, 6β-hydroxycortisol excretion has also been increased in patients given chlordiazepoxide [241] which is known not to induce drug-metabolizing enzymes at therapeutic doses. Among the endogenous compounds examined, the excretion of 6β-hydroxycortisol nevertheless seems to be best correlated to altered microsomal enzyme activity since 6β-hydroxylation of cortisol is at least a microsomal cytochrome P-450-dependent reaction.

Determination of the plasma half-life of antipyrine has been widely used to estimate drug-metabolizing activity in humans [138,145,242]. It has also been applied to investigate genetic differences in microsomal enzyme activity [111]. However, the half-life of antipyrine does not always correlate with the plasma half-life of other drugs known to be metabolized by the microsomal enzyme system [243], especially when these parameters have been determined in one individual. Thus, antipyrine elimination may not be applicable as a prediction of how an individual will respond to any other drug.

Aminopyrine has been used extensively to study drug metabolism in humans [188,244-246]. In most investigations plasma half-lives of aminopyrine have been determined. Recently, Lauterburg and Bircher [247], Bircher and colleagues [248], and Hepner and Vessell [249,250] proposed a breath test based on a measurement of the methyl group detached from aminopyrine. The released methyl group is further oxidized to formic acid and then to carbon dioxide which is exhaled. If the N-methyl group of aminopyrine is labeled by ^{14}C or ^{13}C, the exhaled carbon dioxide can be easily detected. However, like most of the other indices used to detect drug-metabolizing enzyme activity in humans, the variable responsiveness of aminopyrine metabolism to inducers emphasizes the need of applying several parameters to demonstrate qualitative and quantitative aspects of induction. The use of 6β-hydroxycortisol and D-glucaric acid excretion to afford this additional information has been proposed [246].

D. Clinical Consequences of Induction and Inhibition

1. Complications Arising from Enzyme Induction

Two major aspects must be considered when discussing complications of enzyme induction: (1) altered drug metabolism resulting in either reduced or enhanced drug action; (2) changes in the metabolism of endogenous compounds with consequential production of organic lesions.

Probably the most serious consequences result from the interaction between hypnotics and oral anticoagulants [168]. Plasma concentrations of anticoagulants such as warfarin are reduced by simultaneous application of barbiturates. The obvious danger lies in increased plasma warfarin levels if administration of the hypnotic is interrupted. The maximum inducing effect in humans is usually seen after 2 to 3 weeks of barbiturate administration [169]. The inducing effect of phenobarbital, however, seems to differ in different individuals. In one study, 210 mg/day phenobarbital was given to 21 patients [106]; in only 13 of the subjects was the plasma half-life of warfarin shortened. After withdrawal of the inducing agent anticoagulant concentrations usually return to normal within 18 to 24 days [169]. Although the magnitude of the effect varies between individuals, relatively less variation is observed in the time course.

Because of the serious side effects which result from the simultaneous administration of barbiturates and coumarins, this practice should be discouraged as far as possible. Although careful monitoring may be possible with hospitalized patients it is difficult to control anticoagulant concentration optimally in outpatients. Similar complications will be seen in epileptics being treated with diphenylhydantoin, one of the most potent enzyme-inducing drugs. Benzodiazepines apparently do not have inducing capability in humans. Neither chlordiazepoxide, diazepam, nor nitrazepam had any effects on the anticoagulant response or kinetics of warfarin [241], and may be safely given as tranquilizers and hypnotics to patients taking warfarin. Shortened plasma half-lives of anticoagulant drugs due to enzyme induction must be distinguished from similar effects resulting from a decreased plasma protein binding.

Further complications of enzyme induction due to phenobarbital and diphenylhydantoin have been observed during the long-term treatment of epileptics. Both compounds are known to induce bilirubin conjugation, and consequently low serum bilirubin levels are frequently observed in epileptics treated with these compounds [251]. Diphenylhydantoin and phenobarbital also enhance metabolism of cortisol resulting in the excretion of the more polar 6β-hydroxycortisone [252]. The same mechanism enhances the metabolism of therapeutically applied steroids such as dexamethasone.

Some epileptics (5% among adolescents, 3% of adults) [252a] suffer from osteopathy which develops after months or years of therapy with inducing agents [253-255]. Enzyme induction due to the antiepileptics with the consequence of increased inactivation of cholecalciferol may be the culprit [256], especially when these drugs are given in combination. When serum alkaline phosphatase levels are increased in these patients, vitamin D will cure the osteopathy. Since the antiepileptic therapy cannot be discontinued, high doses of 10 to 100,000 IU vitamin D daily have to be given for weeks [252a]. The subject has been reviewed recently by Kodicek [257]. Recent data on the transformation of vitamin D to the active circulating hormone 1,25-dihydroxycholecalciferol indicate that increased activity of an enzyme can reduce the production of active metabolites by an alternative system. It is suggested that hepatic enzymes responsible for the hydroxylation of vitamin D_3 to 25-hydroxycholecalciferol may be induced so that collateral pathways lead to the formation of inactive metabolites [255,257-259]. These metabolites cannot be used as substrates for the renal microsomal enzyme which normally produces 1,25-dihydroxycholecalciferol from 25-hydroxycholecalciferol [256]. Replacement therapy requires high doses of vitamin D; the therapeutic use of 1,25-dihydroxycholecalciferol appears as an interesting alternative.

Newborn babies of mothers who have been treated with antiepileptic drugs occasionally develop hemorrhage [233,260]. This occurs mostly within the first 24 hr after birth, and hemorrhages are localized atypically in the peritoneum or the pleura. They are explained by vitamin K deficiency with reduced coagulation factors II, VII, IX, and X due to an increased metabolism of vitamin K [33]. Phenobarbital seems to be more frequently involved than diphenylhydantoin. It is recommended that 10 mg vitamin K be administered shortly before partus to mothers receiving antiepileptic therapy, and that 1 mg be administered to the newborn.

In less than 1% of epileptics who have been treated with phenobarbital, diphenylhydantoin, and primidone, a megaloblastic anemia due to folic acid deficiency has been observed [261,262]. The pathogenesis of this deficiency is not clear, but enzyme induction may be involved. Similar to the antiepileptic-induced osteopathy, substitution of the deficient vitamin folic acid in doses between 25 to 500 mg/day remove this side effect. The possible relationship between folate deficiency and mental deterioration in the epileptic is discussed by Richens [263].

Animal studies indicate that chronic inhalation of anesthetics such as methoxyfluorene [264,265] induce microsomal enzyme activity. This was further investigated by Brown [266] who found that anesthetics increase microsomal cytochrome P-450 and NADPH-cytochrome c reductase followed by a slower increase in cytochrome b_5. The clinical implications of this finding are not clear, but anesthetists have a faster rate of halothane biotransformation than do personnel not working in the operating room [22]. Animal experiments also reveal that chronic exposure to one anesthetic can induce the metabolism of other anesthetics [267]. Although trace amounts of anesthetic gases can be found in the atmosphere throughout operating theatres [268,269], and in measurable amounts in exhaled air and blood of anesthesia personnel [270-272], the significance of inhalation of subanesthetic concentrations has not been established. There seems to be no doubt that female operating room personnel have an increased rate of spontaneous abortion [273]. Although this indicates significant inhalation and distribution of the anesthetics in the organism, it is unlikely that the amounts inhaled are sufficient to induce hepatic enzymes. Concentrations of 300 ppm of methoxyfluorene for 10 days cause enzyme induction [266], whereas diethyl ether is only effective at much higher doses, and 3000 ppm of methoxyfluorene result in a decreased activity of microsomal enzymes in the rat. Sensitization of anesthetists to hepatic damage by halothane has been reported [274,275].

Another undesirable effect of treatment with inducing agents is the effect of rifampicin on steroids used for oral contraception [276,277]. In a number of cases, the failure of oral contraceptives was preceded by disturbances of the menstrual cycle (spotting, breakthrough bleeding) which had preceded the pregnancy. In a series of 82 patients, 71% showed menstrual disturbances [163,164]. Out of 88 women taking contraceptive pills during tuberculostatic treatment including rifampicin, 5 became pregnant. Other investigations have also reported pregnancies in women using oral contraceptives taking rifampicin [144,165,278]. It has been suggested, therefore, that the daily dose of the usual oral contraceptives be doubled [279] to correct the abnormalities in the majority of cases. However, since oral contraceptives vary considerably in estrogen and progesterone dosage, it is not possible to make recommendations to cover them all.

2. Complications Arising from Enzyme Inhibition

The competition of drugs for enzyme sites at which they are degraded can result in a variety of adverse effects in humans. Competition can occur at the same site of the microsomal enzyme system or at nonmicrosomal sites such as monoamine oxidase.

In animal studies it has been clearly demonstrated that many analgetics, as well as certain narcotics, antidepressants, and tranquilizers, inhibit the microsomal enzyme system [220]. Isoniazid and oxyphenbutazone prolong the half-life of hexobarbital in humans. Phenyramidol inhibits the metabolism of bis-hydroxycoumarin, of diphenylhydantoin, and of tolbutamide [209,225]. Several patients hemorrhaged when phenyramidol was administered in addition to coumarin therapy which had been previously well tolerated. Phenyramidol also increased the half-life of tolbutamide from approximately 7 to 18 hr with the consequence of hypoglycemia [209]. Furthermore, allopurinol increased the half-life of bis-hydroxycoumarin from 51 to 152 hr [206]. Bis-hydroxycoumarin, disulfiram, methylphenidate, and isoniazid diminished the metabolism of diphenylhydantoin [25,218]. Symptoms of intoxication such as ataxia and nystagmus were observed in these patients. In addition, chloramphenicol inhibited the transformation of tolbutamide, diphenylhydantoin, and dicoumarol [212] explaining the occurrence of hypoglycemia when chloramphenicol was added to tolbutamide therapy. A number of presently known side effects due to drug-drug metabolic inhibition are given in Table 7.

A number of interactions involving enzyme inhibition do not relate to hepatic microsomal enzymes but rather to enzymatic mechanisms located in other subcellular fractions. Monoamine oxidase (MAO) is present in mitochondria and metabolizes biogenic amines such as noradrenaline, dopamine, and 5-hydroxytryptamine [280,281]. MAO can be inhibited by a number of drugs causing accumulation of sympathomimetic amines within the adrenergic neurone. If a patient being treated with a MAO inhibitor takes an indirectly acting sympathomimetic such as ephedrine, amphetamine, phenylpropanolamine, or tyramine, large amounts of stored noradrenaline may be released from the nerve endings leading to a hypertensive crisis. The risk of simultaneous treatment with tricyclic antidepressants like imipramine and MAO inhibitors has long been recognized in psychiatric wards. Tricyclic antidepressants inhibit the neuronal reuptake and hence biological inactivation of noradrenaline, whereas MAO inhibitors decrease the rate of enzymatic degradation of the neurotransmitter. An accumulation of noradrenaline will result in the well-known symptoms corresponding to a rise in plasma catecholamines. The famous so-called cheese reaction is due to the ingestion of cheese with a high content of tyramine. The dietary tyramine is normally metabolized by MAO present in the gut wall and liver before reaching the circulation, but a MAO inhibitor blocks the metabolism of ingested tyramine resulting in release of noradrenaline from adrenergic neurons.

IV. CONCLUSION

A critical factor in assessing adverse drug reactions is the establishment of a causal relationship between the suspected drug and the untoward clinical event. A number of drugs influence the absorption, distribution, metabolism, or excretion of other drugs. Of these various potential causes, interaction at the metabolic site plays a major role resulting in increased or reduced conversion and elimination with possible clinical consequences. Although genetically determined interindividual variations and iatrogenic diseases affect drug metabolism, the observed adverse effects may result from drug-drug interactions at metabolic sites.

Relatively few drugs increase the rate of metabolism in humans. Among them are barbiturates, diphenylhydantoin, phenothiazines, and rifampicin, when chronically administered. The most important interactions are with anticoagulants and hypoglycemic agents. Especially after withdrawal of the inducing drugs when drug metabolism returns to normal levels, hemorrhage and hypoglycemia have to be expected.

More drugs compete for the xenobiotic-metabolizing enzymes and consequently inhibit the biotransformation of others. From pharmacokinetic considerations such effects are expected to occur within hours after application of the inhibitor and will last according to the drug's persistence at the enzyme. Clinically the most important consequences of these interactions again involve the hypoglycemic sulfonylureas, the anticoagulants, and the antiepileptic drug diphenylhydantoin. Of the inhibiting agents, prime attention should be given to intermittently administered oral contraceptives.

Because of the variety of different enzyme reactions involved, none of the tests presently proposed to detect altered drug metabolism is entirely satisfactory, and recourse to several parameters is recommended. These include elimination rate of endogenous compounds and of drugs, but should also involve monitoring of drug-blood concentrations and exact clinical surveillance of the therapy.

Together with the theoretical considerations presented here to predict inducing or inhibitory effects of a drug therapy, a systematic evaluation of all the clinical consequences will provide a framework to recognize adverse drug-drug interactions at the metabolic site and will reduce the ambiguity that in many cases characterizes the assessment of such interactions.

ACKNOWLEDGMENTS

I gratefully acknowledge the excellent and patient secretarial help of Mrs. Elisabeth Pilarski and Ms. Judy Byers.

REFERENCES

1. H. Remmer and M. Siegert, Naunyn-Schmiedebergs Arch. Pharmakol. Exp. Pathol. 247:522 (1964).
2. A. H. Conney, Pharmacol. Rev. 19:317 (1967).
3. A. H. Conney, R. M. Welch, R. Kuntzman, and J. J. Burns, Clin. Pharmacol. Ther. 8:2 (1967).
4. T. K. Basu and J. W. T. Dickerson, Chem.-Biol. Interact. 8:193 (1974).
5. D. L. Azarnoff, Clin. Pharmacol. Ther. 22:817 (1977).
6. A. H. Conney, A. J. Pantuck, K. C. Hsiao, R. Kuntzman, A. P. Alvares, and R. Kappas, Fed. Proc. 36:1647 (1977).
7. B. Testa and P. Jenner, Drug Metabolism: Chemical and Biochemical Aspects. Marcel Dekker, New York, 1976.
8. E. Richter, H. Gallenkamp, B. Keller, D. Brachtel, W. Zilly, and D. D. Breimer, Z. Gastroenterol. 6:381 (1977).
9. L. F. Prescott, in Concepts in Biochemical Pharmacology (J. R. Gillette and J. R. Mitchell, Eds.). Springer-Verlag, New York, 1975, pp. 234-257.
10. D. D. Breimer, Clin. Pharmacokinetics 2:93 (1977).
11. R. Kato, Xenobiotica 7:25 (1977).
12. H. Greim, in The Bile Acids, Vol. 3 (P. P. Nair and D. Kritchevsky, Eds.). Plenum, New York, 1976, p. 53-80.
13. E. S. Vesell, Clin. Pharmacol. Ther. 22:659 (1977).
14. E. S. Vesell and G. T. Passananti, Environ. Health Perspect. 20:159 (1977).
15. W. Kalow, B. K. Tang, D. Kadar, and T. Inaba, Clin. Pharmacol. Ther. 24:576 (1978).
16. E. B. Nelson, P. P. Raj, and K. J. Belfi, J. Pharmacol. Exp. Ther. 178:580 (1971).
17. P. Czygan, H. Greim, A. J. Garro, F. Hutterer, J. Rudick, F. Schaffner, and H. Popper, J. Nat. Cancer Inst. 51:1761 (1973).
18. B. Schoene, R. A. Fleischmann, H. Remmer, and H. F. von Oldershausen, Eur. J. Clin. Pharmacol. 4:65 (1972).

19. H. Remmer, B. Schoene, and R. A. Fleischmann, Drug Metab. Dispos. 1:224 (1973).
20. H. Remmer, R. Fleischmann, and W. Kunz, in The Induction of Drug Metabolism (R. W. Estabrook and E. Lindenlaub, Eds.). Schattauer, Stuttgart and New York, 1979, pp. 555-581.
21. R. Fleischmann, H. Mattenheimer, A. W. Holmes, and H. Remmer, Biochem. Biophys. Res. Commun. 62:289 (1975).
22. H. F. Cascorbi, D. A. Blake, and M. Helrich, Anesthesiology 32:119 (1970).
23. H. Remmer, J. Hirschmann, and I. Greiner, Dtsch. Med. Wschr. 94: 1265 (1969).
24. C. Hoppel, M. Garle, A. Rane, and F. Sjöqvist, Clin. Pharmacol. Ther. 21:294 (1977).
25. L. Perrin and J. Fabre, Schweiz. Rundschau Med. (PRAXIS) 62:846 (1973).
26. H. Kutt, R. Brennan, H. Dehejia, and K. Verebelly, Amer. Rev. Resp. Dis. 101:377 (1970).
27. E. S. Vesell, Advan. Pharmacol. Chemother. 7:1 (1969).
28. B. N. La Du, Hosp. Pract. 6:97 (1971).
29. B. N. La Du, H. G. Mandel, and E. L. Way (Eds.), Fundamentals of Drug Metabolism and Drug Disposition. Williams & Wilkins, Baltimore, 1971.
30. D. W. Nebert and J. E. Gielen, Fed. Proc. 31:1315 (1979).
31. H. V. Gelboin, N. Kinoshita, and F. J. Wiebel, Fed. Proc. 31:1298 (1972).
32. E. T. Cantrell, G. A. Warr, and D. L. Busbee, J. Clin. Invest. 52: 1881 (1973).
33. A. H. Conney and J. J. Burns, Science 178:576 (1972).
34. D. L. Busbee, C. R. Shaw, and E. T. Cantrell, Science 178:315 (1979).
35. G. Kellermann, M. Luyten-Kellermann, and C. R. Shaw, Amer. J. Human Genet. 25:327 (1973).
36. G. Kellermann, C. R. Shaw, and M. Luyten-Kellermann, N. Engl. J. Med. 289:934 (1973).
37. G. K. Tokuhata, Amer. J. Public Health 54:24 (1964).
38. H. Remmer and H. J. Merker, Ann. N.Y. Acad. Sci. 123:79 (1965).
39. J. R. Fouts and L. R. Rogers, J. Pharmacol. Exp. Ther. 147:112 (1965).
40. H. Remmer, J. Mond. Pharm. 3:12 (1969).
41. A. Rubin, T. R. Tephly, and G. J. Mannering, Biochem. Pharmacol. 13:1007 (1964).
42. D. A. Haugen, M. J. Coon, and D. W. Nebert, J. Biol. Chem. 251: 1817 (1976).
43. A. H. Conney, C. Davison, R. Gastel, and J. J. Burns, J. Pharmacol. Exp. Ther. 130:1 (1960).

44. M. B. Yarmolinsky and G. L. de la Haba, Proc. Nat. Acad. Sci. U.S. 45:1721 (1959).
45. A. Reich, R. M. Franklin, A. J. Shaktin, and E. L. Tatum, Science 134:556 (1961).
46. R. Kato, L. Loeb, and H. V. Gelboin, Nature 205:668 (1965).
47. R. Kato, W. R. Jondorf, L. A. Loeb, T. Benn, and H. V. Gelboin, Mol. Pharmacol. 2:171 (1966).
48. W. J. Marshall and A. E. M. McLean, Proc. Nutr. Soc. 30:66A (1971).
49. W. J. Marshall and A. E. M. McLean, Biochem. J. 122:569 (1971).
50. W. J. Marshall and C. Naughton, Biochem. Soc. Trans. 2:992 (1974).
51. A. E. M. McLean and W. J. Marshall, Chem.-Biol. Interact. 3:294 (1971).
52. A. J. Paine and A. E. M. McLean, Biochem. Biophys. Res. Commun. 58:482 (1974).
53. H. K. J. Hahn, D. J. Tuma, A. J. Barak, and M. F. Sorrell, Biochem. Pharmacol. 25:769 (1976).
54. A. P. Poland, E. Glover, and A. S. Kende, J. Biol. Chem. 251:4936 (1976).
55. T. M. Guenther and D. W. Nebert, J. Biol. Chem. 252:8981 (1977).
56. D. W. Nebert, in The Induction of Drug Metabolism (R. W. Estabrook and E. Linden, Eds.). Schattauer, Stuttgart and New York, 1979, pp. 419-452.
57. P. Leder, N. Engl. J. Med. 298:1079 (1978).
58. S. A. Atlas, A. R. Boobis, J. S. Felton, S. S. Thorgeirsson, and D. W. Nebert, J. Biol. Chem. 252:4712 (1977).
59. A. J. Levi, S. Sherlock, and D. Walker, Lancet i:1275 (1968).
60. H. Held and H. F. Oldershausen, Digestion 4:151 (1971).
61. P. B. Andreasen, L. Ranek, B. E. Statland, and N. Tygstrup, Eur. J. Clin. Invest. 4:129 (1974).
62. K. W. Bock, Arch. Toxicol. 39:77 (1977).
63. H. Greim, Naunyn-Schmiedebergs Arch. Pharmakol. Exp. Pathol. 266:261 (1970).
64. R. E. McMahon, J. Pharmacol. Exp. Ther. 138:382 (1962).
65. B. C. Fine and J. D. Molloy, Nature 204:789 (1964).
66. M. W. Anders, An. Rev. Pharmacol. 11:37 (1971).
67. K. Fujii, H. Jaffe, and S. S. Epstein, Toxicol. Appl. Pharmacol. 13:431 (1968).
68. K. Fujii, H. Jaffe, Y. Bishop, E. Arnold, D. Mackintosh, and S. S. Epstein, Toxicol. Appl. Pharmacol. 16:482 (1970).
69. P. S. Graham, R. O. Hellyer, and A. J. Ryan, Biochem. Pharmacol. 19:759 (1970).
70. H. Jaffe and J. L. Neumeyer, J. Med. Chem. 13:901 (1970).
71. S. S. Epstein, J. Andrea, J. A. P. Clapp, and D. Mackintosh, Toxicol. Appl. Pharmacol. 11:442 (1967).

72. S. S. Epstein, S. Joshi, J. Andrea, P. Clapp, H. Falk, and N. Mantel, Nature 214:526 (1967).
73. M. R. Franklin, Biochem. Pharmacol. 21:3287 (1972).
74. M. R. Franklin, Environ. Health Perspec. 14:29 (1976).
75. H. Remmer, J. Schenkman, R. W. Estabrook, H. Sasame, J. Gillette, S. Narasimhulu, D. Y. Cooper, and O. Rosenthal, Mol. Pharmacol. 2:187 (1966).
76. Y. Imai, R. Sato, Biochem. Biophys. Res. Commun. 22:620 (1966).
77. J. B. Schenkman, H. Remmer, and R. W. Estabrook, Mol. Pharmacol. 3:113 (1967).
78. H. B. Matthews, M. Skrinjarić-Spoljar, J. E. Casida, Life Sci. 9(I):1039 (1970).
79. M. R. Franklin, Xenobiotica 1:581 (1971).
80. P. Borondy, T. Chang, and A. J. Glazko, Fed. Proc. 31:582 (1972).
81. C. von Bahr, J. B. Schenkman, and S. Orrenius, Xenobiotica 2:89 (1979).
82. J. J. Ashley and G. Levy, Res. Commun. Chem. Pathol. Pharmacol. 4:297 (1972).
83. P. Jähnchen and G. Levy, Proc. Soc. Exp. Biol. Med. 141:963 (1972).
84. A. J. Glazko, Drug Metab. Dispos. 1:711 (1973).
85. S. A. Stavchansky, W. C. Lubawy, and H. B. Kostenbauder, Life Sci. 14:1535 (1974).
86. W. C. Lubawy, H. B. Kostenbauder, and S. A. Stavchansky, Res. Comm. Chem. Pathol. Pharmacol. 8:75 (1974).
87. D. M. Soda and G. Levy, J. Pharm. Sci. 64:1528 (1975).
88. D. V. Parke, The Biochemistry of Foreign Compounds. Pergamon, Oxford, 1968.
89. G. F. Mannering, in Concepts in Biochemical Pharmacology, Part 2 (B. B. Brodie and J. R. Gillette, Eds.). Springer-Verlag, Berlin, 1971, pp. 452-476.
90. T. B. Vree, P. T. Henderson, E. van der Kleijn, and P. J. M. Guelen, in Clinical Pharmacology of Antiepileptic Drugs (H. Schneider, D. Janz, C. Gardner-Thorpe, H. Meinardi, and A. L. Sherwin, Eds.). Springer-Verlag, New York, 1975, pp. 34-54.
91. J. V. Dingell and A. D. Bass, Biochem. Pharmacol. 18:1535 (1969).
92. L. Lemberger, B. D. Witt, J. M. Davis, and I. Kopin, J. Pharmacol. Exp. Ther. 174:428 (1970).
93. T. Lewander, Eur. J. Pharmacol. 6:38 (1969).
94. I. Jansson, S. Orrenius, L. A. Ernster, and J. B. Schenkman, Arch. Biochem. 151:391 (1972).
95. M. W. Anders and G. J. Mannering, Mol. Pharmacol. 2:341 (1966).
96. S. P. Sher, Toxicol. Appl. Pharmacol. 18:780 (1971).
97. W. A. Ritschel, in Metabolismus (W. A. Rischel, Ed.). Angewandte Biopharmazie, Wissenschaftliche Verlagsgesellschaft, Stuttgart, 1973, pp. 147-161.

98. E. Ebadi, Advan. Neurol. 13:333 (1975).
99. A. G. Hildebrandt, H. Remmer, and R. W. Estabrook, Biochem. Biophys. Res. Commun. 30:607 (1968).
100. R. Kuntzman, W. Levin, M. Jacobsen, and A. H. Conney, Life Sci. 7:215 (1968).
101. D. W. Shoeman, M. D. Chaplin, and G. J. Mannering, Mol. Pharmacol. 5:412 (1969).
102. C. J. Parli and G. J. Mannering, Mol. Pharmacol. 6:178 (1970).
103. H. Selye, Rev. Can. Biol. 29:49 (1970).
104. H. Selye, Experientia 27:1445 (1971).
105. M. G. MacDonald, D. S. Robinson, D. Sylwester, and J. J. Jaffe, Clin. Pharmacol. Ther. 10:80 (1969).
106. M. Corn, Thromb. Diath. Haemorrh. 16:606 (1966).
107. J. E. Goss and D. W. Dickhaus, N. Engl. J. Med. 273:1094 (1965).
108. M. Corn and J. F. Rockett, Med. Ann. D.C. 34:578 (1965).
109. S. A. Cucinell, A. H. Conney, M. Sansor, and J. J. Burns, Clin. Pharmacol. Ther. 6:420 (1965).
110. P. R. Bieck, K. H. Antonin, and U. Klotz, Arzneim.-Forsch. 26:1264 (1976).
111. E. S. Vesell and J. G. Page, J. Clin. Invest. 48:2202 (1969).
112. A. G. Hildebrandt, I. Roots, M. Speck, K. Saalfrank, and H. Kewitz, Eur. J. Clin. Pharmacol. 8:327 (1975).
113. R. W. Jelliffe and D. H. Blankenhorn, Clin. Res. 14:160 (1966).
114. S. Loga, S. Curry, and M. Lader, Brit. J. Clin. Pharmacol. 2:197 (1975).
115. M. Kristensen, J. M. Hansen, and L. Skovsted, Acta Med. Scand. 185:347 (1969).
116. H. Kutt, J. Haynes, and F. H. McDowell, Neurology 15:274 (1965).
117. P. J. Neuvonen and O. Penttilä, Brit. Med. J. 1:535 (1974).
118. A. M. Breckenridge and J. B. Roberts, Pharmacol. Res. Comm. 8:229 (1976).
119. A. Breckenridge, M. L. E. Orme, S. S. Thorgeirsson, and D. S. Davies, Clin. Pharmacol. Ther. 14:514 (1973).
120. D. S. Robinson and D. Sylvester, Ann. Int. Med. 72:853 (1970).
121. G. Alvan, K. Piafsky, M. Lind, and Ch. von Bahr, Clin. Pharmacol. Ther. 22:316 (1977).
122. A. M. Antlitz, M. Tolentino, and M. F. Kosai, Curr. Ther. Res. 10:70 (1968).
123. S. A. Johannson, Acta Med. Scand. 184:297 (1968).
124. P. G. Dayton, Y. Tarcan, T. Chenkin, and M. Weiner, J. Clin. Invest. 40:1797 (1961).
125. P. M. Aggeler and R. A. O'Reilly, J. Lab. Clin. Med. 74:229 (1969).
126. R. E. Van Dam and M. J. H. Bribnau-Overkamp, Folia Med. Neerl. 10:141 (1967).
127. M. Eichelbaum, K. Ikbom, L. Bertilsson, V. A. Ringberger, and A. Rane, Eur. J. Clin. Pharmacol. 8:337 (1975).

128. A. P. Gerardin, F. V. Anadie, J. A. Campestrini, and W. Theobald, J. Pharmacokinet. Biopharm. 4:521 (1976).
129. W. J. Pitlick and R. H. Levy, J. Pharm. Sci. 65:462 (1976).
130. H. G. M. Westenberg, E. van der Kleijn, T. T. Oei, and R. A. de Zeeuw, Clin. Pharmacol. Ther. 23:320 (1978).
131. F. Petruch and R. V. A. Schüppel, Bibl. Psychiat. 151:76 (1975).
132. A. A. Lai, R. H. Levy, and R. E. Cutler, Clin. Pharmacol. Ther. 24:316 (1978).
133. J. M. Hansen, K. Siersback-Nielsen, M. Kristensen, L. Skovsted, and L. K. Christensen, Acta Med. Scand. 189:15 (1971).
134. G. Sakalis, S. H. Curry, G. P. Mould, and M. H. Lader, Clin. Pharmacol. Ther. 13:931 (1972).
135. T. Kolakowska, M. Franklin, and B. Alapin, Brit. J. Clin. Pharmacol. 2:25 (1975).
136. E. E. Werk, J. MacGee, and L. J. Sholiton, J. Clin. Invest. 43:1824 (1964).
137. H. M. Solomon, S. Reich, H. Spirt, and W. B. Abrams, Ann. N.Y. Acad. Sci. 179:362 (1971).
138. F. Petruch, R. V. A. Schüppel, and G. Steinhilber, Eur. J. Clin. Pharmacol. 7:281 (1974).
139. D. H. Huffman, D. W. Shoeman, P. Pentikäinen, and D. L. Azarnoff, Pharmacology 10:338 (1973).
140. V. Nitti, F. D. Vereri, A. Ninni, and G. Meola, Chemotherapy 17:121 (1972).
141. G. Acocella, A. Lamarina, F. B. Nicolis, V. Pagani, and G. Segre, Eur. J. Clin. Pharmacol. 5:111 (1972).
142. R. A. O'Reilly, Fed. Proc. 33:217 (1974).
143. F. Michot, M. Bürgi, and J. Buttner, Schweiz. Med. Wschr. 100:583 (1970).
144. A. Hirsch, J. P. Tillement, and J. Chretien, Rev. Fran. Maladies Resp. 3:174 (1975).
145. D. D. Breimer, W. Zilly, and E. Richter, Clin. Pharmacol. Ther. 21:470 (1977).
146. E. K. G. Syvälahti, K. K. Pihlajamäke, and E. J. Iisalo, Lancet ii:232 (1974).
147. W. Zilly, D. D. Breimer, and E. Richter, Eur. J. Clin. Pharmacol. 9:219 (1975).
148. W. Zilly, D. D. Breimer, E. Richter, Clin. Pharmacokinetics 2:61 (1977).
149. U. Peters, T. U. Hausamen, and F. Grosse-Brockhoff, Dtsch. Med. Wschr. 99:2381 (1974).
150. O. M. Edwards, R. J. Courtenoy-Evans, J. M. Galley, J. Hunter, and A. D. Tait, Lancet ii:549 (1974).
151. S. G. Johnsen, J. P. Kampmann, E. P. Bennett, and F. S. Jørgensen, Clin. Pharmacol. Ther. 20:233 (1976).

152. A. W. Harman, D. B. Frewin, B. G. Priestly, and C. B. J. Alexander, Brit. J. Clin. Pharmacol. 7:45 (1979).
153. S. Szabo, S. Komolos, and Z. Ignjatovic, Z, J. Pharm. Pharmacol. 27:113 (1975).
154. W. D. Diamond and R. A. Buchanan, J. Clin. Pharmacol. 10:306 (1970).
155. H. Kutt, Epilepsia 16:393 (1975).
156. H. Kutt and S. Louis, Drugs 4:256 (1972).
157. V. Nitti, A. Ninni, G. Meola, A. Julians, and G. Curci, Chemotherapy 19:206 (1973).
158. G. Beran, Prax. Pneumol. 26:350 (1972).
159. R. A. O'Reilly, Ann. Intern. Med. 83:506 (1975).
160. H. M. Bolt, H. Kappus, and M. Bolt, Eur. J. Clin. Pharmacol. 8: 301 (1975).
161. H. M. Bolt, M. Bolt, and H. Kappus, Acta Endocrinol. 85:189 (1977).
162. D. Reimers and A. Jezek, Prax. Pneumol. 25:255 (1971).
163. L. Nocke-Finck, H. Breuer, and D. Reimers, Acta Endocrinol. Suppl. 177:136 (1973).
164. L. Nocke-Finck, H. Breuer, and D. Reimers, Dtsch. Med. Wschr. 98:1521 (1973).
165. R. Kropp, Prax. Pneumol. 28:270 (1974).
166. S. L. Altschuler and J. W. Valenteen, Obstetr. Gyn. 44:771 (1974).
167. R. E. Eling, R. D. Harbison, B. A. Becker, and J. R. Fouts, Pharmacologist 11:248 (1969).
168. M. G. MacDonald and D. S. Robinson, J. Amer. Med. Ass. 204:95 (1968).
169. A. Breckenridge and M. L'E. Orme, Ann. N.Y. Acad. Sci. 179:421 (1970).
170. J. Hunter, J. D. Maxwell, M. Carrella, D. A. Stewart, and R. Williams, Lancet i:572 (1971).
171. D. S. Lecamwasam, C. Franklin, and P. Turner, Brit. J. Clin. Pharmacol. 2:257 (1975).
172. A. H. Forrest, P. Roscoe, I. H. Stevenson, and L. F. Prescott, Scot. Med. J. 19:157 (1974).
173. A. Poland, D. Smith, R. Kuntzman, M. Jacobson, and A. H. Conney, Clin. Pharmacol. Ther. 11:724 (1970).
174. B. Kolmodin-Hedman, Eur. J. Pharmacol. 5:195 (1973).
175. A. P. Alvares, A. Tischbein, K. E. Anderson, and A. Kappas, Clin. Pharmacol. Ther. 22:140 (1977).
176. B. Kolmodin-Hedman, Exposure to lindane and DDT and its effects on drug metabolism and serum lipoproteins. Ph.D. Thesis, University of Stockholm, Sweden, 1974.
177. D. G. Crosby, J. Agric. Food Chem. 17:532 (1969).
178. Committee on Food Protection, Food and Nutrition Board, National Research Council, Toxicants Occurring Naturally in Foods. National Academy of Sciences, Washington, D.C., 1973.

179. E. J. Pantuck, K.-C. Hsiao, R. Kuntzman, and A. H. Conney, Science 187:744 (1975).
180. A. Kappas, A. P. Alvares, K. E. Anderson, E. J. Pantuck, C. B. Pantuck, R. Chang, and A. H. Conney, Clin. Pharmacol. Ther. 23: 445 (1978).
181. A. P. Alvares, K. E. Anderson, A. H. Conney, and A. Kappas, Proc. Nat. Acad. Sci. U.S. 73:2501 (1976).
182. A. Kappas, K. E. Anderson, A. H. Conney, and A. P. Alvares, Clin. Pharmacol. Ther. 20:643 (1976).
183. A. E. M. McLean, Fed. Proc. 36:1688 (1977).
184. W. P. Norred and A. E. Wade, Biochem. Pharmacol. 21:2887 (1972).
185. B. Century, J. Pharmacol. Exp. Ther. 185:185 (1973).
186. T. C. Campbell and J. R. Hayes, Pharmacol. Rev. 26:171 (1974).
187. R. Grundin, P. Moldéus, S. Orrenius, K. O. Borg, J. Skänberg, and C. von Bahr, Acta Pharmacol. Toxicol. 35:242 (1974).
188. B. B. Brodie and J. Axelrod, J. Pharmacol. Exp. Ther. 99:171 (1950).
189. A. H. Beckett and G. E. Navas, Xenobiotica 8:721 (1978).
190. S. Garattini, F. Marucci, and E. Mussini, Drug Metab. Rev. 1:291 (1972).
191. M. Kaighen and R. T. Williams, J. Med. Pharm. Chem. 3:25 (1961).
191a. A. Kaldor, G. Somogyi, L. A. Debreczeni, and B. Gachalyi, Int. J. Clin. Pharmacol. 12:403 (1975).
192. L. Storstein, Clin. Pharmacol. Ther. 21:125 (1977).
193. E. Perucca, K. Makki, and A. Richens, Clin. Pharmacol. Ther. 24: 46 (1978).
194. E. Gerhards, Arzneim.-Forsch. 18:704 (1968).
195. M. T. Bush and W. L. Weller, Drug Metab. Rev. 1:249 (1972).
196. R. E. Duggan, A. F. Hogans, K. C. Kwan, and F. G. McMahon, J. Pharmacol. Exp. Ther. 181:563 (1972).
197. H. R. Sullivan and S. L. Due, J. Med. Chem. 16:909 (1973).
198. N. Maggi, S. Furesz, R. Pallanza, and G. Pelizza, Arzneim.-Forsch. 19:651 (1969).
199. A. H. Conney and A. Klutch, J. Biol. Chem. 238:1611 (1963).
200. R. C. Thomas and G. J. Ikeda, J. Med. Chem. 9:507 (1966).
201. C. S. Lieber and L. M. DeCarli, Science 162:917 (1968).
202. P. S. Misra, A. Lefevre, H. Ishii, E. Rubin, and C. S. Lieber, Amer. J. Med. 51:346 (1971).
203. E. Rubin and C. S. Lieber, Science 172:1097 (1971).
204. F. L. Iber, Clin. Pharmacol. Ther. 22:735 (1976).
205. R. Schüppel, Excerpta Med. Int. Congress Ser. 254:52 (1971).
206. E. S. Vesell, G. T. Passananti, and F. E. Greene, New Engl. J. Med. 283:1484 (1970).
207. E. S. Vesell, G. T. Passananti, and G. W. Hepner, Clin. Pharmacol. Ther. 20:661 (1976).

208. M. Kristensen and J. M. Hansen, Acta Med. Scand. 183:83 (1968).
209. H. M. Solomon and J. J. Schrogie, Metabolism 16:1029 (1967).
210. B. Petitpierre and J. Fabre, Lancet i:789 (1970).
210a. F. Petruch and R. V. A. Schüppel, Arzneim.-Forsch. 24:1023 (1974).
211. O. K. Faber, H. T. Mouridsen, and L. Skovsted, Brit. J. Clin. Pharmacol. 2:281 (1975).
212. L. K. Christensen and L. Skovsted, Lancet ii:1397 (1969).
213. L. Skovsted, J. M. Hansen, M. Kristensen, and L. K. Christensen, in Drug Interactions (Morselli, Garattini, and Cohen, Eds.). Raven, New York, 1974, pp. 81-90.
214. M. Homeida, M. Halliwell, and R. A. Branch, Clin. Pharmacol. Ther. 24:228 (1978).
215. K. O'Malley, I. H. Stevenson, and J. Crooks, Clin. Pharmacol. Ther. 13:552 (1972).
216. F. Schobben, E. von der Kleijn, and F. J. M. Gabreels, Eur. J. Pharmacol. 8:97 (1975).
217. E. S. Vesell, G. T. Passananti, and C. H. Lee, Clin. Pharmacol. Ther. 12:785 (1971).
218. T. S. Svendsen, M. B. Kristensen, J. M. Hansen, and L. Skovsted, Eur. J. Clin. Pharmacol. 9:439 (1976).
219. E. Kiørboe, Epilepsia 7:246 (1966).
220. J. J. Burns and A. H. Conney, Proc. Royal Soc. Med. 58:995 (1965).
221. M. Kristensen, Medikament-medikament interaktion. Ph.D. Thesis. Foreningen af Danske Laegestuderendes Forlag, Copenhagen, 1973.
222. L. Skovsted, J. M. Hansen, M. Kristensen, and K. Siersbaek-Nielsen, Acta Med. Scand. 199:513 (1976).
223. P. B. Andreasen, A. Frøland, L. Skovsted, S. A. Anderson, and M. Hauge, Acta Med. Scand. 193:561 (1973).
224. M. B. Kristensen, Clin. Pharmacol. 1:351 (1976).
225. H. M. Solomon and J. J. Schrogie, J. Pharmacol. Exp. Ther. 154:660 (1964).
226. B. Lumholz, K. Siersbaek-Nielsen, L. Skovsted, J. Kampmann, and J. M. Hansen, Clin. Pharmacol. Ther. 17:731 (1975).
227. K. Siersbaek-Nielsen, J. M. Hansen, L. Skovsted, Clin. Pharmacol. Ther. 14:148 (1973).
228. U. C. Dubach, A. Bückert, and F. Raaflaub, Schweiz. Med. Wschr. 96:1483 (1966).
229. L. K. Christensen, J. M. Hansen, and M. Kristensen, Lancet ii:1298 (1963).
230. J. M. Hansen, M. Kristensen, and L. Skovsted, Epilepsia 9:17 (1968).
231. G. W. Houghton and A. Richens, Brit. J. Clin. Pharmacol. 1:59 (1974).
232. D. E. Carter, R. Bressler, M. R. Hughes, M. R. Haussler, C. S. Christian, and M. W. Heine, Clin. Pharmacol. Ther. 18:700 (1974).
233. M. Egli, Schweiz. Med. Wschr. 107:1513 (1977).

234. E. M. Aarts, Biochem. Pharmacol. 14:359 (1965).
235. J. Hunter, J. D. Maxwell, D. A. Stewart, M. Carella, and R. Williams, Biochem. Pharmacol. 22:743 (1973).
236. M. Davies and D. Lebadarios, in Urinary D-glucaric Acid Excretion and Screening for Enzyme Induction (A. Richens and F. P. Woodford, Eds.). Elsevier, Amsterdam, 1976, p. 13.
237. B. Whitfield, D. W. Moss, G. Neale, M. Orme, and A. Breckenridge, Brit. Med. J. 1:316 (1973).
238. A. Szewczuk, Clin. Chim. Acta 14:608 (1966).
239. S. B. Rosalki, D. Parlow, and D. Rau, Lancet ii:376 (1971).
240. S. Burstein and E. L. Klaiber, J. Clin. Endocrinol. 25:293 (1965).
241. M. L. E. Orme, A. Breckenride, and R. V. Brooks, Brit. Med. J. 3:611 (1972).
242. R. Schüppel, F. Petruch, and K. Fleischer, in Alcohol and Aldehyde Metabolizing Systems, Vol. 3 (R. G. Thurman, J. R. Williamson, H. R. Drott, and B. Chance, Eds.). Academic, New York, 1977, pp. 385-390.
243. D. Kadar, T. Inaba, L. Endrenyi, G. E. Johnson, and W. Kalow, Clin. Pharmacol. Ther. 14:552 (1973).
244. J. R. Gillette, B. B. Brodie, and B. N. La Du, J. Pharmacol. Exp. Ther. 119:532 (1957).
245. H. Remmer, Naunyn-Schmiedebergs Arch. Pharmakol. Exp. Pathol. 235:279 (1959).
246. A. G. Hildebrandt, J. Roots, G. Heinemeyer, S. Nigam, and H. Helge, in The Induction of Drug Metabolism (R. W. Estabrook and E. Lindenlaub, Eds.). Schattauer, Stuttgart and New York, 1979, pp. 615-626.
247. B. H. Lauterburg and J. Bircher, J. Pharmacol. Exp. Ther. 196: 501 (1976).
248. J. Bircher, A. Küpfer, I. Gikalov, and R. Preisig, Clin. Pharmacol. Ther. 20:484 (1976).
249. G. W. Hepner and E. S. Vesell, N. Engl. J. Med. 291:1384 (1974).
250. G. W. Hepner and E. S. Vesell, Clin. Pharmacol. Ther. 21:620 (1977).
251. R. P. H. Thompson, A. L. W. F. Eddleston, and R. Williams, Lancet i:21 (1969).
252. Y. Choi, K. Trasher, E. E. Werk, L. J. Sholiton, and C. Olinger, J. Pharmacol. Exp. Ther. 141:157 (1971).
252a. R. Kruse, in Antiepileptische Langzeitmedikation (H. Helenchen, Ed.). Karger, Basel, 1975, pp. 114-143.
253. F. Schmid, Fortschr. Med. 85:381 (1967).
254. A. Richens and D. J. F. Rowel, Brit. Med. J. 4:73 (1970).
255. C. E. Dent, A. Richens, D. J. F. Rowe, and T. C. B. Stamp, Brit. Med. J. 4:69 (1970).

256. T. C. B. Stamp, J. M. Round, D. J. F. Round, and J. G. Haddad, Brit. Med. J. 4:9 (1972).
257. E. Kodicek, Lancet i:325 (1974).
258. T. J. Hahn, S. J. Birge, C. R. Scharp, and L. V. Avioli, J. Clin. Invest. 51:741 (1972).
259. J. Silver, G. Neal, D. Davies, A. Breckenridge, and G. R. Thompson, Clin. Sci. 42:12 (1972).
260. H. G. Kohler, Lancet i:267 (1966).
261. J. Chanarin, in The Megaloblastic Anaemias. Blackwell, Oxford, 1969, p. 830.
262. E. H. Reynolds, Lancet i:1376 (1973).
263. A. Richens, Brit. J. Clin. Pharmacol. 1:185 (1974).
264. M. L. Berman and J. E. Bochantin, Anesthesiology 32:500 (1970).
265. H. W. Linde and M. L. Berman, Anesth. Analg. (Cleveland) 50:656 (1971).
266. B. R. Brown, Jr., Anesthesiology 39:178 (1973).
267. R. A. Van Dyke, J. Pharmacol. Exp. Ther. 154:364 (1966).
268. H. W. Linde and D. L. Bruce, Anesthesiology 30:363 (1969).
269. D. L. Bruce and H. W. Linde, Anesthesiology 36:517 (1972).
270. T. Corbett and G. T. Ball, Anesthesiology 34:532 (1971).
271. B. Hallen, H. Ehrner-Samuel, and M. Thomason, Acta Anaesthesiol. Scand. 14:17 (1970).
272. C. E. Whitcher, E. N. Cohen, and J. R. Trudell, Anesthesiology 35:348 (1971).
273. E. N. Cohen, J. W. Bellville, and B. W. Brown, Jr., Anesthesiology 35:343 (1971).
274. S. Belfrage, I. Ahlgren, and S. Axelson, Lancet ii:1466 (1966).
275. G. Klatskin and D. V. Kimberg, N. Engl. J. Med. 280:515 (1968).
276. D. M. Burley, in Drug Interactions (Grahame-Smith, Ed.). Macmillan, London, 1977, pp. 293-299.
277. M. Davies, R. Williams, and D. M. Burley, Med. Chir. Dig. 5:341 (1976).
278. J. L. Skolnick, B. S. Stoler, D. B. Katz, and W. H. Anderson, J. Amer. Med. Ass. 236:1382 (1976).
279. E. Hempel and W. Klinger, Drugs 12:442 (1976).
280. A. F. Lant, in Transactions of the Medical Society of London. London, 1974, pp. 142-155.
281. P. A. van Zwieten, Int. J. Clin. Pharmacol. 15:217 (1977).

Chapter 5

GENETIC ASPECTS OF DRUG METABOLISM RELATING TO DRUG ACTION

Armanda Jori

"Mario Negri" Institute for Pharmacological Research
Milan, Italy

Variability in drug response is controlled by environmental and hereditary factors and forms the object of study of the relatively new field known as pharmacogenetics. Genetic control may act through the different kinetic processes responsible for variability in drug response, namely, absorption, distribution, biotransformation, and excretion, as well as the actual mechanisms of action. But because drug metabolism is a major variable in influencing the biological response, it is on this aspect that pharmacogeneticists have focused most of their attention.

This chapter reviews genetically controlled metabolic reactions which lead to variability in drug response. General aspects of hereditary control in drug metabolism are analyzed, and situations are distinguished in which (1) genetic polymorphism is responsible for the polymodal variability in drug responses expressed by discontinuous curves; and (2) hereditary control is maintained by genes at multiple loci, yielding unimodal variability curves.

The review of pharmacogenetics in animals discusses data where the differences in drug response between species and strains and within strains are explained by genetic factors controlling drug biotransformation or endogenous substrates on which drugs act. The importance of genetic control is underlined not only in drug metabolism, but also in drug interactions.

Pharmacogenetics in humans concern contributions obtained from analysis of drug responses recorded in twins, entire families, and populations. The advantages and disadvantages of these approaches are discussed, together with the utility of experimental animal studies as a model for evaluating the hereditary factors responsible for human variability.

I. INTRODUCTION

The effect of a drug is determined not only by specific drug-receptor interactions, but also by a number of events which indirectly modulate the amount of drug available at receptor sites. The rate of absorption, the amount of protein binding, metabolic reactions, tissue uptake, and excretion rates all play important roles. It is perhaps not surprising, therefore, that individual variability in drug responses is a widely accepted concept in pharmacological studies.

Both environmental and genetic factors can modify these processes, causing changes in drug response. For a long time the effect of the environment superimposed upon genetic factors made it difficult to assess the real importance of hereditary control over variability in response to drugs. Thus, only over the past 20 years has attention been focused on how drug effects and genetic characteristics are interrelated. "Pharmacogenetics," a term coined by Vogel in 1959 [1], is the relatively new field dealing with the variability in drug response under hereditary control. This variability, according to Vesell [2], may depend on genetic conditions altering the manner in which the body acts on drugs, or drugs act upon the body. The first aspect might be labeled "genetics of drug kinetics," because it concerns the genetic features which govern the processes affecting drug disposition in the body, such as absorption, protein binding, excretion, and metabolism. In these processes drugs interact with proteins by means including ionic or covalent binding, passage through membranes, and receptor site interactions.

Genetic mutations which alter the quality and/or quantity of the specific proteins concerned can affect the rate and extent of these mechanisms. For example, genetically determined low levels of [3], or structural differences in [4], serum proteins mean that the binding affinity for certain drugs is reduced, thus explaining large individual variations in unbound drug concentrations in the blood of some patients [5]. This variability can be a source of difference in pharmacological activity [6, 7].

Unfortunately, our knowledge of genetic control in these various kinetic processes is limited, as only a few studies of this type have been undertaken. Pharmacogeneticists have focused their attention mainly on drug metabolism since it is a major variable in determining drug response. This is perhaps useful as far as genetic control is concerned since other processes governing the pharmacokinetic profile of a drug such as renal excretion do not differ so markedly from one individual to another or from one animal species to another. The foundations of pharmacogenetics were laid in studies on laboratory animals, where large differences in drug response were seen between animal species and between different strains of a single species. These differences have been investigated in detail since they are closely connected with the difficulty of extrapolating to humans pharmacological data obtained in animals. However, as the modern system of drug development is still based on demonstrating pharmacological and toxicological activities in animals before projecting the results to humans, these differences between animal species constitute a currently topical question which must be considered when new drugs are submitted to pharmacological screening. Initial reports on genetic aspects of drug response in humans described the hypersensitivity of some individuals to therapeutic agents. Pharmacogeneticists provided the explanation of adverse reactions and abnormal toxicity in humans by demonstrating hereditary alterations of enzymatic proteins involved in the metabolic degradation of drugs. Examples of the early pharmacogenetic discoveries include identification of the phenotypes for isoniazid acetylation [8], inherited atypical human serum cholinesterases responsible for abnormal responses to succinylcholine [9], and glucose 6-phosphate dehydrogenase deficiency in hemolysis induced by a variety of agents [10,11].

More recently not only drug hypersensitivity but also drug resistance has been investigated from this angle. A lack of, or reduced activity of, an enzymatic system makes a person less able than others to metabolize drugs, and increases drug toxicity, but the opposite defect can also have untoward consequences. People with faster-than-normal drug metabolism may not obtain the desired therapeutic effect to the same degree, and may suffer a kind of genetically induced resistance to drug action. These aspects have been reviewed by a number of authors [4,12-14].

II. CONCEPTS OF HEREDITARY CONTROL IN DRUG METABOLISM

Variability of response to drugs is common to mammals and can reflect variability in the reactions involved in drug metabolism. Measurements of the pharmacological effects of a drug, its toxic reactions, its blood disappearance curves, as well as the activity of drug-metabolizing enzymes in different individuals are parameters offering differing degrees of specificity to evaluate this phenomenon. The frequency distribution curves that can be constructed from measurements of these parameters appear to be of two types. The first is a discontinuous polymodal curve (bi- or trimodal) and the second type is a unimodal Gaussian curve of continuous variability.

The study of how genetic factors contribute to this variability, the analysis of the variability by genetic techniques, and the application of these findings to therapeutics is the basis of pharmacogenetics.

A. Unimodal Distribution

When a drug is given to individuals to obtain a given effect (excluding the situations described in Sec. II.B), the frequency distribution in terms of quantitative response, or of plasma drug concentrations, or of biological half-life, or of any other quantitative parameters related to drug availability is broadly expressed as a unimodal curve. This means that the trait considered is controlled by genes at multiple loci. In other words, a character which is repeatable and which gives rise to a continuous Gaussian distribution curve is under polygenic control.

As regards drug metabolism, it is difficult to determine the exact contribution of this continuous variability because of environmental factors which also exert an effect. According to Falconer [15], in a given population the observed phenotypic variance (Vp) is the sum of genetic and environmental contributions to variance (Vg + Ve). By partitioning the genetic contribution to variance (Vg), such as the portion of the total phenotypic variation attributable to any genetic cause, a factor called "heritability" can be identified which more specifically designates that portion of the total phenotypic variance attributable to additive genetic effects alone. To estimate how much of the variability of the character in the population can be ascribed to genetic factors, more specifically to its heritability, the character must be measured in whole families or in twins. For example, Whittaker and Price-Evans [16] have applied the formulas suggested by Falconer [15] to data collected in a family study of genetic contributions to variability in phenylbutazone metabolism. They concluded that 65% of phenotypic variance was caused by heritability.

Much information on genetic determination can be obtained more easily in experiments with animals. Several approaches have been used to estimate the degree of genetic determination. One of the most widely used approaches involves comparison of two inbred strains, and their F1, F2, and backcross generations. As within the two parental strains and the F1 hybrids, no genetic but only environmental variance can be detected, the genetic determination can be assessed from the ratio of variance of the segregating F2 generation (VF2) minus F1 variance (index of environmental variance) to the F2 variance (VF2) [(VF2 - VF1)/VF2]. From these findings the minimum number of loci affecting the character can also be approximated.

Other approaches used in experimental pharmacogenetics are:

1. Comparisons of many highly inbred strains [17]. This method is based on measurement of the character and on the estimate of the

between- and within-strain variance components ($\sigma_g^2 + \sigma_e^2$) by means of an analysis-of-variation design. The reliability of the estimate of the relative importance of genetic and environmental factors by this method depends on the number of unrelated inbred strains.

2. The diallele cross technique [18], a method useful for studying the additive and nonadditive components of genetic variance, consists of making all possible crosses between a number of inbred strains and investigating the general combining ability of each line and specific combining ability of each pair of strains. The average response of a strain represents the general combining ability, while the deviation in response from the average combining ability of the two strains is the specific combining ability of the cross. The specific combining ability component is attributable to non-additive genetic variance. Differences in general combining ability are attributable to additive genetic variance.

B. Polymodal Distribution

Polymodal variability in a quantitative trait may be due to genetic polymorphism, meaning the occurrence of a character having two or more discontinuous forms within a given population of individuals. These genetic conditions are due to the action of a single gene acting at a single locus and are transmitted in Mendelian fashion.

The discontinuous curves produced by genes at a single locus on the chromosome can be analyzed by considering that discrete portions of the curve represent different phenotypes. As regards the polymorphism of drug metabolism, there are two types of distribution, one in which all phenotypes are common and another in which one phenotype is rare [19]. Vesell [2] has summarized "all the pharmacogenetic conditions known to behave as a single factor resulting from a single point mutation affecting a single protein" (Table 1). Among these, adverse reactions to phenacetin, sensitivity to dicoumarol, and resistance to warfarin are examples of pharmacogenetic polymorphism of drug metabolism in which one phenotype is rare. Such cases are usually discovered by chance although occasionally as the result of very extensive population studies.

In contrast, glucose 6-phosphate deficiency, slow inactivation of isoniazid, and atypical pseudocholinesterase are conditions which occur widely in the population, to the extent that in some ethnic groups the normal allele occurs less frequently than the "aberrant" allele [20]. However, the 13 examples of polymorphism in human drug metabolism reported by Vesell [2] are the only situations known in which a gene acting at a single locus is responsible for an abnormal response. Therefore, it can be stated that genetic polymorphism is only one particular aspect of the more general variability in drug response.

TABLE 1
Pharmacogenetic Conditions with Putative Aberrant Enzyme, Mode of Inheritance, Frequency, and Drugs that can Elicit the Signs and Symptoms of the Disorder

Name of condition	Aberrant enzyme and location	Mode of inheritance	Frequency	Drugs that produce the abnormal response
Genetic conditions probably transmitted as single factors altering the way the body acts on drugs (altered drug metabolism)				
Acatalasia	Catalase in erythrocytes	Autosomal recessive	Mainly in Japan and Switzerland, reaching 1% in certain small areas of Japan	Hydrogen peroxide
Slow inactivation of isoniazid	Isoniazid acetylase in liver	Autosomal recessive	Approximately 50% of U.S. population	Isoniazid, sulfamethazine, sulfamaprine, phenelzine, dapsone, hydrazine, procainamide
Suxamethonium sensitivity or atypical pseudocholinesterase	Pseudocholinesterase in plasma	Autosomal recessive	Several aberrant alleles; most common disorder occurs 1 in 2500	Suxamethonium or succinylcholine
Diphenylhydantoin toxicity due to deficient parahydroxylation	?Monooxygenase in liver microsomes that parahydroxylates diphenylhydantoin	Autosomal or X-linked dominant	Only one small pedigree	Diphenylhydantoin
Bis-hydroxycoumarin	?Monooxygenase in liver microsomes that hydroxylates bis-hydroxycoumarin	Unknown	Only one small pedigree	Bis-hydroxycoumarin

Acetophenetidine-induced methemoglobinemia	?Monooxygenase in liver microsomes that deethylates acetophenetidine	Autosomal recessive	Only one small pedigree	Acetophenetidin
Genetic conditions probably transmitted as single factors altering the way drugs act on the body				
Warfarin resistance	?Altered receptor or enzyme in liver with increased affinity for vitamin K	Autosomal dominant	Two large pedigrees	Warfarin
Glucose 6-phosphate dehydrogenase deficiency, favism, or drug-induced hemolytic anemia	Glucose 6-phosphate dehydrogenase	X-linked incomplete codominant	Approximately 100,000,000 affected in world; occurs in high frequency where malaria is endemic; 80 biochemically distinct mutations	A variety of analgesics [acetanilide, acetylsalicylic acid, acetophenetidine (phenacetin), antipyrine, aminopyrine (Pyramidon)], sulfonamides and sulfones [sulfanilamide, sulfapyridine, N_2-acetylsulfanilamide, sulfacetamide sulfisoxazole (Gantrisin), thiazolsulfone, salicylazosulfapyridine (Azulfidine), sulfoxone, sulfamethoxypyridazine (Kynex)], antimalarials [primaquine, pamaquine, pentaquine, quinacrine (Atabrine)], nonsulfonamide antibacterial agents [furazolidone, nitrofurantoin (Furadantin), chloramphenicol, para-aminosalicylic acid], and miscellaneous drugs [naphthalene, vitamin K, probenecid, trinitrotoluene, methylene blue, dimercaprol (BAL), phenylhydrazine, quinine, quinidine]

(continued)

TABLE 1 (continued)

Name of condition	Aberrant enzyme and location	Mode of inheritance	Frequency	Drugs that produce the abnormal response
Drug-sensitive hemoglobins Hemoglobin Zurich	Arginine substitution for histidine at the 63rd position of the β-chain of hemoglobin	Autosomal dominant	Two small pedigrees	Sulfonamides
Hemoglobin H	Hemoglobin composed of four β-chains	Autosomal recessive	Approximately 1 in 300 births in Bangkok	Same drugs as listed above for G 6-PD deficiency
Inability to taste phenylthiourea or phenylthiocarbamide	Unknown	Autosomal recessive	Approximately 30% of Caucasians	Drugs containing the N—C=S group such as phenylthiourea, methyl, and propylthiouracil
Glaucoma due to abnormal response of intraocular pressure to steroids	Unknown	Autosomal recessive	Approximately 5% of U.S. population	Corticosteroids
Malignant hyperthermia with muscular rigidity	Unknown	Autosomal dominant	Approximately 1 in 20,000 anesthesized patients	Various anesthetics, especially halothane
Methemoglobin reductase deficiency	Methemoglobin reductase	Autosomal recessive heterozygous carriers affected	Approximately 1 in 100 are heterozygous carriers	Same drugs as listed above for G 6-PD deficiency

Source: From Ref. 2. Reproduced with permission.

III. PHARMACOGENETICS IN LABORATORY ANIMALS

Observation of species differences in response to drugs led to the idea that hereditary factors might influence the control of the enzyme systems responsible for drug metabolism. Originally, variations in pharmacological response had been attributed entirely to differences in sensitivity of receptor sites. However, the development of basic pharmacological tests and the increasingly appropriate methodology for drug assay has made it possible to determine meaningful relationships between drug dosage, plasma drug concentrations, and intensity of response. As a result, the widely observed species differences in drug response could be explained on the basis of varying bioavailability. Further, variation in drug availability was found to depend mainly on the different behavior of xenobiotic-metabolizing enzymes in various animal species [21].

The hypothesis that the different sensitivity to drugs of various species including humans depended mainly on the kinetics of the drug, rather than its interaction with the receptors, was further supported by plasma level data. Thus, despite several-hundredfold differences among species in the duration or intensity of the effects of drugs such as barbiturates [22], tranquilizers [23], and antirheumatic agents [24], reaction to and recovery from the effects of these drugs occur at similar plasma levels. These findings showed that the application of animal data to humans or the prediction of drug response in humans from laboratory animal data can only be made on the basis of an appropriate correlation between the pharmacological activity and the kinetic profile of the drug in the animal species studied.

Different reactions to drugs have also been observed between strains within one species [25-27]. These correlate with differences in activity of the enzymatic systems responsible for drug metabolism [27,28]. Therefore, animal studies using selected strains are considered useful not only for preliminary investigations before preclinical trials, but also as suitable models for research on hereditary factors implicated in drug metabolism.

Experiments in animals have numerous advantages over human investigations: environmental factors affecting the drug response, such as temperature, pathology, drug interactions, and circadian rhythms, can be controlled; sex, age, and body weight can be selected, mating can be planned, and litters can be obtained according to needs. Moreover, the use of inbred strains offers parental lines of subjects which are really homozygous.

In the following sections examples of differences in drug metabolism between species, between strains, and within strains will be reviewed, and animal data will be presented to illustrate the genetic factors controling biotransformation and the resulting altered response to drugs.

A. Species Differences

Drug metabolism reactions may be divided into conjugation and functionalization reactions. The former, which include conjugation with glucuronic acid, acetic acid, sulfate, and amino acids, exhibit species patterns which can be distinguished on a qualitative basis and can be correlated with phylogenetic development. In laboratory animals, the discovery of species differences such as a lack of glucuronyltransferase activity in the cat [29] or a poor ability to conjugate aromatic hydrocarbons with mercapturic acid in the guinea pig, were pioneer steps in this field. Comparative aspects of drug metabolism including conjugation have been reviewed in great detail by Mellet [31] and will not be discussed further in this chapter.

More attention will be focused on functionalization reactions, which include oxidation, reduction, and hydrolysis. These reactions occur, with few substantial qualitative differences, in either laboratory animals or humans. Of greater interest are the quantitative differences in these reactions, which depend directly on the different rates of enzymatic activity. A higher rate of metabolism in one species can result in reduced pharmacological or toxicological properties of an active substrate, or in potentiation of activity when an inactive precursor is transformed into an active agent. Differences in duration of drug action were described many years ago. Quinn and collaborators [26] reported that the half-lives of antipyrine, hexobarbital, and aniline were very long in humans, and shorter in the mouse than in other animal species examined (Table 2). In the species listed in Table 3 a clear relationship was found between the half-lives in vivo and enzyme activity for these substrates in vitro. Therefore, although the half-life of a drug is the result of many kinetic factors, the large interspecies differences in duration of drug action can be attributed to a broad variability in the rate of biotransformation between species. From Table 2, it can be seen that species-related differences in enzyme activity arise not only for classes of drugs having similar pharmacological activity or chemical structure, but are common to many otherwise unrelated drugs. Furthermore, the data in Table 2 indicate that drugs are eliminated faster in small animals such as mice than in larger species such as the dog or monkey. Therefore, with some exceptions, a negative correlation has been proposed between the rate of drug metabolism, or more generally the rate of drug disappearance, and body size [31].

The situation is more involved for a drug having a complex metabolic pattern. In such cases, differences in metabolic rate for the various reactions may lead to completely different ratios between the parent drug and each of its metabolic products. This may produce different pharmacological pictures, particularly when the metabolites have activities of their own. In this situation differences in metabolic routes as well as differences in drug metabolism rates must be considered for different animal species. For example, amphetamine can be C-hydroxylated, oxidatively deaminated, and N-oxidized [32]. The rat, in which para-hydroxylation is the prevalent pathway [33], can accumulate the two hydroxylated metabolites para-hydroxyamphetamine and para-hydroxynorephedrine [34] in specific areas of the brain. These metabolites have been suggested as mediators of some of the

TABLE 2
Biological Half-life ($t_{1/2}$) of Various Drugs in Different Animal Species

Drug	Humans	Rat	Guinea pig	Rabbit	Dog	Mouse	Horse	Monkey	Reference
Hexobarbital (min)	360 ± 7	140 ± 54	—	60 ± 11	260 ± 20	19 ± 7	—	—	26
Antipyrine (min)	600	141	110	63	107	11	—	109	26
Aniline (min)	—	71	45	35	167	35	—	—	26
Phenylbutazone (hr)	72	6	5	3	6	—	6	8	189
Cytoxan (min)	216	43	—	—	32	17	—	47	190
Amethopterin (min)	134	—	—	—	90	25	—	75	31
Digoxin (hr)	44	9	16	—	27	—	—	—	191
Isoniazid (hr)	4	0.4	—	—	2.5	—	—	1.2	192
Caffeine (min)	297	130	—	95	—	—	—	—	Latini (unpublished)

TABLE 3
Relationship between Biological Half-life ($t_{1/2}$) and Metabolism by Liver Microsomes of Antipyrine and Hexobarbital in Different Animal Species

	Antipyrine		Hexobarbital	
Species	$t_{1/2}$ (min)	Relative enzyme activity (μg/g/hr)	$t_{1/2}$ (min)	Relative enzyme activity (μg/g/hr)
Mouse	11	170	19	598
Rabbit	63	39	60	196
Rat (female)	141	58	140	134
Dog	107	29	260	36

Source: Data obtained from Ref. 26

drug's dopaminergic and noradrenergic effects [35]. In view of their prolonged presence in the dopamine and noradrenaline nerve endings, these metabolites may act as false catecholaminergic mediators responsible for the tolerance to central effects which repeated administration produces in rats [36,37]. Interestingly, animal species such as the mouse which do not accumulate hydroxylated metabolites of amphetamine do not show tolerance [38]. However, in the urine of human amphetamine addicts, hydroxylated basic metabolites such as para-hydroxyamphetamine, para-hydroxynorephedrine, and norephedrine have been detected, suggesting that these metabolites may also have some role in the paranoid psychoses of chronic abusers [39].

Imipramine also has a complex, species-dependent metabolic pattern [40]. In the rat and humans demethylation is the preferential pathway converting imipramine to desipramine (DMI), an active metabolite responsible for many of the parent compound's central effects; DMI is then slowly metabolized to other products. In contrast, rabbits and mice rapidly metabolize imipramine by reactions other than demethylation, forming hydroxylated compounds with no central activity. The antisedative effect of imipramine is therefore not apparent in the rabbit [41] which, conversely, is very sensitive to the peripheral cardiotoxic effects of this and several other tricyclic drugs [42].

Diazepam [43], and benzodiazepines in general [44], follow different metabolic patterns in different animal species. For diazepam, demethylation predominates in the guinea pig whereas hydroxylation prevails in the rat. The metabolites formed are further transformed by species-dependent pathways, so that although in vivo diazepam disappears from the bloodstream at the same rate, metabolites are present in the brain in different ratios and for different lengths of time. As these metabolites participate in some of diazepam's pharmacological properties the differences reported are of importance when interpreting pharmacological results obtained in various animal species.

These examples raise the question of whether pharmacological research on new drugs conducted with laboratory animals can in fact provide data extrapolable to humans. Had imipramine been investigated only in rabbits and mice it would not have been disclosed as a potential antidepressant since these species do not transform it into the active metabolite. Likewise desipramine, which is too rapidly inactivated in these animals, would not have been discovered as an antidepressant agent [40]. Similarly, phenylbutazone was initially considered to have negligible antiinflammatory action, as in animals its half-life was 3-6 hr as opposed to 3 days in humans [45].

The mythical search for an animal species which is similar to the human in its drug-metabolizing activity and which as a consequence is more suitable than other species for drug screening is, in my opinion, utopian. However, thorough drug screening in various animal species can provide the integrated background information required as a basis for preclinical pharmacological trials only if the results of metabolic and kinetic research have shown a correlation with observed pharmacological activity.

Much attention has been paid recently to the genotoxic action of some labile metabolites formed by aryl-oxidation of drugs or polycyclic hydrocarbons mediated by monooxygenases. The carcinogenic, hepatotoxic, and mutagenic effects of the intermediate epoxides formed are due to their covalent binding to nucleic acid and other cellular macromolecules [46-47]. Alternatively, the epoxides may be metabolized by conjugation with glutathione or hydration to diols [48-49]. Therefore, the genotoxic properties of polycyclic hydrocarbons depend on the ratio of epoxide formation (through epoxide synthetase) to epoxide inactivation (through hydrase and glutathione transferase).

Epoxide synthetase and hydrase are both present in the endoplasmic reticulum in liver and other organs such as the lung, heart, spleen, and kidney [50-51]. Recently epoxide synthetase activity has also been found in nuclear membranes [52].

Different animal species, however, have different ratios of activating to inactivating enzymatic activity in their various tissues [53]. This can lead to varying toxicity in different species as illustrated by the metabolism of the carcinogen styrene (Table 4) [51]. The rat, an animal widely used in metabolic and toxicological studies, should, on the basis of this data, be the species most resistant to styrene-mediated toxicity, while the rabbit and mouse should have the least ability to inactivate styrene epoxide and consequently should be the most sensitive to its toxic effects. Analysis of the data reported in Table 4 indicates that the lungs of the mouse and rabbit

TABLE 4
Ratios of Styrene Oxide Hydrase to Styrene Monooxygenase Activity in Male and Female Animals[a]

		Hydrase/monooxygenase activity				
Species	Sex	Liver	Heart	Lungs	Spleen	Kidneys
Rat	M	4.44	8.64	4.79	4.79	9.14
	F	6.49	7.65	3.23	0.58	2.12
Mouse	M	1.55	2.73	0.27	1.62	2.11
	F	1.53	1.32	0.80	2.97	1.76
Guinea pig	M	1.61	17.91	1.44	9.16	5.19
	F	3.04	1.32	1.88	8.60	5.75
Rabbit	M	2.41	0.58	0.24	1.31	1.67
	F	2.35	5.12	0.72	3.10	1.75

[a] Ratios calculated on the results of the enzymatic activity evaluated from three determinations conducted on separate tissue pools.
Source: From Ref. 51. Reproduced with permission.

have the lowest ratios of inactivation to formation of styrene epoxide and consequently show the highest sensitivity to styrene toxicity. As inhalation is the main route of entry of styrene into the body, mouse and rabbit lungs can be regarded as the most sensitive target organs for its toxic action.

These findings provide a general explanation of how differences in the rates of formation and inactivation of labile metabolites can render different animal species more or less sensitive to the toxicity of environmental contaminants. They are also important when it comes to selecting a particular species as a model for toxicity or carcinogenicity studies.

Finally, marked species differences in drug metabolism can be related to drug interactions which are metabolic in origin. Thus, inducers or inhibitors of drug metabolism have different activities in various species. Conney [54], reviewing the problems of enzyme induction more than a decade ago, reported that polycyclic hydrocarbons increase drug metabolism in the rat, mouse, guinea pig, hamster, and cat, while phenobarbital stimulates drug metabolism in the rat, mouse, guinea pig, rabbit, dog, and humans. Nikethamide induces metabolism in rats, rabbits, and mice, but has no such effect in guinea pigs [55]. DDT stimulates metabolism in virtually all animal species, but is without effect in mice [56]. Contraceptive steroids increase metabolism in the rat and mouse, but not in the guinea pig [57,58], or in humans [59].

The effect of a classical inhibitor of drug metabolism, SKF-525A, seems to be greatest in rats and least in rabbits, but the magnitude of the species difference depends on the substrate used [60]. These effects may be due to species variability in the metabolism of the inducing or inhibiting agents. However, evidence for qualitative and quantitative differences in drug metabolism and in drug interaction between animal species arising from differences in some steps of the electron-transfer chain is demonstrated by the following in vitro biochemical and enzymatic studies. Inhibition of substrate metabolism by agents such as DPEA (2,4-dichlorophenyl-phenoxyethylamine), SKF-525A (diethylaminoethyl-2,2-diphenylvalerate), and chlorcyclizine was found to be competitive or noncompetitive depending on the species examined [60]. Similarly, the effects of phenobarbital and 3-methylcholanthrene (representing the two main classes of inducing agents) on the spectral properties of cytochrome P-450 from rats, mice, guinea pigs, and rabbits suggested that species differences in the inducibility of microsomal drug metabolism might be due to qualitative differences in the rate-limiting component of the hydroxylase system [61]. Further, the kinetic properties of cytochrome P-450 differ widely from one species to another, while the species differences in the metabolism of ethylmorphine parallel those in the content and functional activity of the components of the electron-transport system [62].

The equilibrium between the low and the high spin state of cytochrome P-450 ferric iron also seems to differ among mammalian species [63]. This point is of interest as interaction of a type I substrate is associated with conversion of hemoprotein iron from the low to the high spin state, whereas in the interaction with a type II substrate low-spin cytochrome P-450 is favored. In order of decreasing amounts of high-spin cytochrome P-450 the species can be ranked as follows: rabbit $>$ guinea pig $\simeq$ hamster $\simeq$ mouse $>$ rat (64].

Other species differences concern the distribution of enzyme activity in microsomal subfractions [65]. It has been observed that the components of the monooxygenase system are concentrated in smooth microsomal membranes in the liver fractions, but the magnitude of this concentration varies with the animal species investigated [65]. The smooth-to-rough ratios for the specific enzyme activities were as high as 4-5 in rabbit liver microsomes, from 1.5 to 3 in rat, and $\sim$2 in monkey and guinea pigs. In mouse liver, specific enzyme activities and electron-transfer components of drug metabolism were evenly distributed between smooth and rough membranes. Other biochemical components of liver microsomal subfractions also vary widely between different animal species. For instance the cholesterol/phospholipid ratio in smooth and rough microsomal membrane fractions is $\sim$4 in mice and $\sim$1 in monkeys and guinea pigs [65].

B. Strain Differences

Strain-dependent variations in drug response and in drug metabolism occur in rabbits, rats, and mice, but apparently not in hamsters [66]. Variations in the drug response of guinea pigs, cats, and dogs have not been examined in detail since pure strains of these animals bred under rigid genetic control are not commonly available.

1. Rabbit

Up to 20-fold variation exists in the basal activity of hepatic microsomal enzymes from a number of rabbit strains [27]. Examination of different substrates, each representing a different metabolic pathway, revealed broad differences in metabolic rates for some reactions, but very little for others. Moreover, when microsomal enzymatic activity was stimulated by an inducer such as phenobarbital, qualitative and quantitative differences appeared between strains, so the ratio of stimulated to basal metabolism differed widely for each substrate between strains and between substrates within the strain. Most of the more significant results are reported in Table 5, suggesting that strain-dependent variability in drug response results not only from basal differences in drug metabolism but also from differences in the manner in which each strain interacts with drugs or environmental factors. Differences have also been reported in the rates of metabolism of morphine, atropine, and cocaine by enzymatic systems other than monooxygenases, such as esterases [67,68].

2. Rat

Interstrain variability in drug-metabolizing enzymes in rats showed a two- to threefold difference between metabolic rates for a single drug studied in the most common strains [26,69-71]. This is considerably less than the variability reported in different strains of rabbits [27] or mice [25, 72]. These differences, although occurring to a lesser extent, nevertheless account for many of the observed interstrain differences in pharmacological response. The following examples support this assertion. The significant differences in sleeping time following hexobarbital administration to commonly used strains do not depend on differences in central nervous system sensitivity to barbiturates, since the awakening brain concentrations are similar [73] (see Table 6). The variability appears to be mainly correlated with differences in basal hexobarbital hydroxylase activity. Similarly, the poor antireserpine activity of imipramine in female Long-Evans rats can be explained by the fact that imipramine demethylase is lower in this strain than in others [74,75]; the brain concentration of the active metabolite desipramine (DMI) is thus low and correlates with the poor activity of imipramine in reversing reserpine-induced hypothermia (see Fig. 1). Differences between Sprague-Dawley and Long-Evans rats were sex- and

TABLE 5
Interstrain Differences in the Metabolism of Various Substrates by Rabbit Liver[a]

Enzymatic reaction	Dutch		English		Jacks		California		New Zealand		Cottontails	
	B	S	B	S	B	S	B	S	B	S	B	S
Hexobarbital oxidation	141	329	173	339	220	540	248	490	254	520	19	490
Amphetamine para-hydroxylation	154	154	87	104	102	104	55	48	82	90	8	14
Nitrobenzoic acid reduction	89	249	67	148	92	689	22	15	122	314	50	170
Zoxazolamine ring oxidation	155	253	153	219	71	274	200	321	162	308	139	312
Chlorpromazine sulfur oxidation	152	141	139	140	100	137	159	161	143	158	147	170
Aminopyrine dealkylation	73	160	221	235	—	—	122	308	78	190	15	66

[a]Results expressed as substrate metabolized by the 9000g supernatant fraction of rabbit liver (nmol/g liver/hr). B = basal metabolism levels; S = level of induced metabolism (animals were treated with phenobarbital 15 mg/kg daily × 3 days).

Source: Data from Ref. 27.

TABLE 6
Hexobarbital Effect in Various Rat Strains[a]

Strain	Hexobarbital-induced sleeping time (min)	Hexobarbital blood concentration at awakening (μg/ml)	Hexobarbital metabolism in vitro (μmol/g liver per 15 min)
Long-Evans	56 ± 4	36 ± 3	1.2 ± 0.1
Wistar	24 ± 5	36 ± 3	1.9 ± 0.3
Holtzman	58 ± 7	39 ± 2	0.9 ± 0.1
Sprague-Dawley	28 ± 7	31 ± 3	1.4 ± 0.1

[a]Hexobarbital injected at the dose of 100 mg/kg i.p.

Source: Data from Ref. 73.

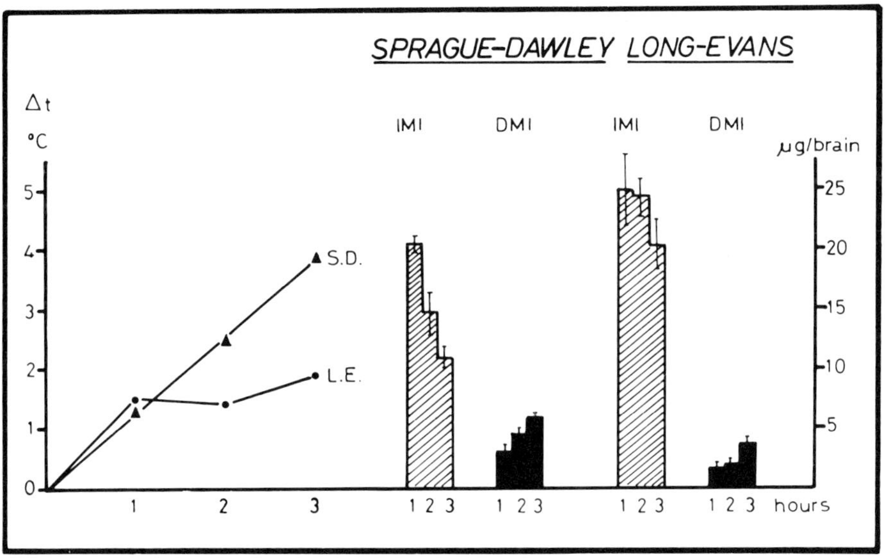

FIGURE 1 Effect of imipramine (20 mg/kg i.p.) on the body temperature of Sprague-Dawley (S.D.) and Long-Evans (L.E.) rats receiving reserpine (5 mg/kg i.v.) (on the left). Brain concentrations of imipramine (IMI) and of its metabolite desipramine (DMI) have been determined 1, 2, and 3 hr after the IMI administration. (Reproduced from Ref. 75 with permission.)

substrate-dependent [76]. In these experiments female Long-Evans rats metabolized several substrates such as para-nitroanisole, aminopyrine, imipramine, and hexobarbital to a lesser extent than Sprague-Dawley rats, but this difference was not apparent for aniline. Male Long-Evans rats conversely had higher enzyme activity for the same substrates as male Sprague-Dawley rats. Long-Evans rats of both sexes were insensitive to the inducing properties of phenobarbital, but normally sensitive to 3-methylcholanthrene (3MC) induction [77]. Kinetic studies showed that 3MC increased the V_{max} for aniline hydroxylase and stimulated the formation of cytochrome P-448 (or P_1-450) to a similar extent in the two strains of rats, whereas phenobarbital enhanced enzymatic activity and increased cytochrome P-450 concentrations only in Sprague-Dawley rats [78].

Illustrating the difficulties involved in this type of genetic study, other workers found contrasting results showing that while phenobarbital stimulated metabolism in all the strains studied (including Long-Evans rats), the effect of 3MC varied with strain [73]. Despite the qualitative differences between these results they are consistent with the notion that induction by phenobarbital and 3MC involves processes which differ in some events and are controlled by genetic factors. This is in agreement with similar data obtained in mice, as discussed more extensively later [79].

We have found that in Sprague-Dawley but not in Long-Evans rats phenobarbital induced the activity of a soluble hepatic enzyme, aldehyde dehydrogenase [75]. The inducibility of this enzyme is inherited as a dominant characteristic, but it is not under the same genetic control as the induction of aniline hydroxylase activity [80]. At variance with our results, Deitrich [80] showed that Long-Evans rats were the most reactive of the strains studied to the induction of aldehyde dehydrogenase by phenobarbital.

These contradictory results can be explained by the use of Long-Evans rats from different sources. Long-Evans rats (B) from Italian stock differ from the Long-Evans rats (A) provided by French laboratories and used in the above experiments. In terms of basal metabolic activity and induced enzyme function, Long-Evans (B) behave similarly to Sprague-Dawley rats (see Table 7). Thus, these differences which show variation even within strains may explain the contradictory results obtained by different authors, and should be taken into account when results from different laboratories are compared. It has however been adequately demonstrated [77] that the insensitivity of Long-Evans (A) rats to induction is not due to a reduced bioavailability of phenobarbital, which is in fact higher than in Sprague-Dawley rats. Induction by phenobarbital does not occur in Long-Evans rats even when the drug concentrations in peripheral and central tissues [77] are comparable with the levels causing induction in the other strains. Other inducers with unrelated structure but belonging to the phenobarbital inducer-type category are also only weakly active in Long-Evans (A) rats [77].

TABLE 7
Basal and Phenobarbital-induced Aminopyrine Metabolism in Long-Evans Rats from Two Different Sources Compared to Sprague-Dawley Rats[a]

Strain	Aminopyrine Metabolism	
	Saline	Phenobarbital
Sprague-Dawley	260 ± 19	908 ± 78
Long-Evans (A)	138 ± 25*	224 ± 49*
Long-Evans (B)	246 ± 7	801 ± 117

[a] Results express the metabolite formed (4×NH_2-antipyrine) (nmol/g/hr) after incubation of aminopyrine with the 9000<u>g</u> fraction of liver homogenates obtained from female rats treated with saline or phenobarbital (50 mg/kg I.P. daily for 3 days).
*$p < 0.01$ versus Sprague-Dawley and Long-Evans (B) groups.
Source: Data from Ref. 77.

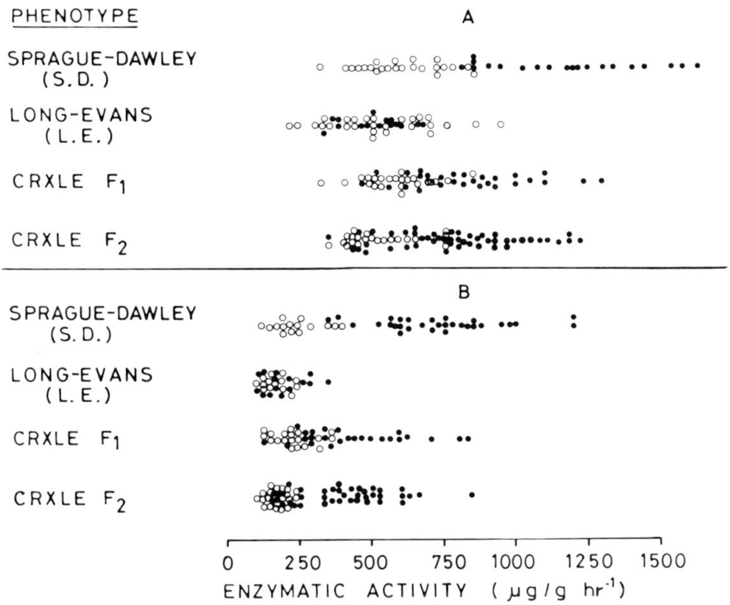

FIGURE 2 Genetic variability between liver microsomal enzyme activity in female rats: (A) aniline hydroxylase; (B) aminopyrine demethylase. ● Determination of enzymatic activity on the 9000g liver homogenate fraction from individual rats given phenobarbital (50 mg/kg); ○ Control value from an untreated rat. (From Jori, unpublished.)

Preliminary data obtained by crossing Sprague-Dawley (S.D.) and Long-Evans (L.E.) rats suggest that sensitivity to phenobarbital induction is probably genetically determined as a dominant trait. As shown in Fig. 2, the specific enzymatic activity of aniline hydroxylase and aminopyrine demethylase is significantly increased by phenobarbital in S.D. rats, but is unaffected in L.E. rats. The F1 hybrids behave similarly to the S.D. strain, whereas in the F2 hybrids the enzymatic activity after phenobarbital treatment appears to be distributed in a bimodal pattern. Approximately a quarter of the animals appear to have noninducible drug-metabolizing enzyme systems.

The importance of strain as far as differences in enzyme reduction are concerned is not limited to interactions with various inducing agents, but also affects responses to forced environmental changes. Thus the degree of microsomal enzyme induction for the side chain oxidation of hexobarbital and the aromatic hydroxylation of aniline, produced by various stresses such as cold, forced swimming, or movement restriction, is strain-dependent [81]. Table 8 illustrates the interactions between specific stress situations and metabolic pathways in two different rat strains.

TABLE 8
Effect of Stress on the Metabolism of Aniline (A) and Hexobarbital (H) in Two Rat Strains[a]

	Strain			
	Long-Evans		Holtzman	
Stress	H	A	H	A
Swim	$\nearrow$	—	$\searrow$	—
Restriction	$\underline{\nearrow}$	—	$\searrow$	—
Cold	$\nearrow$	$\nearrow$	$\underline{\nearrow}$	—

[a]Key: $\nearrow$ increase of activity; $\searrow$ decrease of activity; $\underline{\nearrow}$ little but significant increase of activity; — no effect.
Source: Data from Ref. 81.

3. Mouse

Most pharmacogenetic investigations in animal species have utilized the mouse. The widespread use of this species in pharmacological and biochemical laboratories has permitted the accumulation of much information on the responsiveness of various mouse strains to drugs. Data illustrating the strain-dependent susceptibility to the pharmacological and toxicological effects of chloroform [82, 83], amphetamine [84], hexobarbital [25], chlorpromazine [85], and morphine [86] form a historical background to the development of interest in this field. The mouse has thus become the most useful species for studying hereditary factors controlling drug response. This is mainly because of its low cost, since large numbers are used in cross-mating experiments, and because numerous inbred strains are available. Inbred strains obtained by more than 20 generations of brother-sister matings have more than a 99% probability of being homozygous [87].

Early research in this field showed that the response to hexobarbital varied widely between several inbred strains of mice which, however, gave uniform within-strain individual responses [25]. Later, measurements of hexobarbital oxidase activity in hepatic microsomes showed that the pharmacological response was related to the degree of enzymatic activity rather than to different sensitivity of the receptor sites [72]. When reactive and low-reactive strains were mated the level of hexobarbital oxidase activity responsible for sleeping time was seen to be polygenically inherited.

More recently, interest has centered on the genetic factors which regulate the responsiveness of aryl hydrocarbon hydroxylase activity to inducing agents. Interest in these enzymatic systems is based on their importance in the metabolism of foreign compounds and the fact that they are stimulated by chemical and environmental pollutants. Basic contributions to these findings have been made by a restricted number of authors, in particular Nebert and his colleagues. These findings will be extensively reviewed in view of the originality of the research and the importance of the results, the latter supporting the hypothesis that in mice, individual susceptibility to drug toxicity and carcinogenesis is regulated by the genetic system controling monooxygenase activity. Nebert and Gielen in 1972 [88] found that in some mouse strains 3-methylcholanthrene (3MC) induced hepatic aryl hydrocarbon hydroxylase (AHH) activity and cytochrome P_1-450 content, but in others the inductive effect was absent [88]. The responsiveness of AHH activity and cytochrome P_1-450 content to aromatic hydrocarbons, which was found to be inherited as a simple autosomal dominant trait, was designated the Ah locus, the allele Ah^b was used to denote the locus in the responsive C57B1/6 strain (abbreviation B6), and the allele Ah^d in the unresponsive DBA/2 strain (abbreviation D2) mice. Similar conclusions were reached independently by other authors [89], and the genetic expression for AHH activity induction was also found to affect extrahepatic tissues [90-92].

Nebert and colleagues obtained evidence that unlike 3MC-inducible AHH activity, basal activity is inherited additively [93]. It therefore appears that basal and 3MC-inducible AHH activity are controled by different genetic regulatory systems. This agrees with the hypothesis formulated following other approaches such as spectral [94] and paramagnetic [95] studies, indicating that the enzyme active site differs in the basal and the aromatic hydrocarbon-inducible hydroxylase system.

Induction of AHH activity by phenobarbital treatment results in a similar increase of enzymatic activity in both responsive and unresponsive inbred strains [88]. These results show that the induction of AHH activity by the two types of inducers is also under different genetic control, in line with the common knowledge [96,97] that induction of monooxygenase activity by phenobarbital differs from that by aromatic hydrocarbons as was noted earlier for rats [78].

Further research by Nebert on the degree of 3MC-inducible hydroxylase activity in seven inbred strains of mouse, and in the progeny resulting from their possible backcrosses and intercrosses, showed that at least two genetic loci are involved in aromatic hydrocarbon responsiveness [93]. A more complicated hypothetical model for AHH induction was consequently proposed with three alleles at each of two nonlinked genetic loci. However, as pointed out in several recent reviews [98-101], when a responsive strain is appropriately crossed with a nonresponsive one, a simplified scheme depicting an autosomal dominant expression is valid for all investigations related to aromatic hydrocarbon responsiveness.

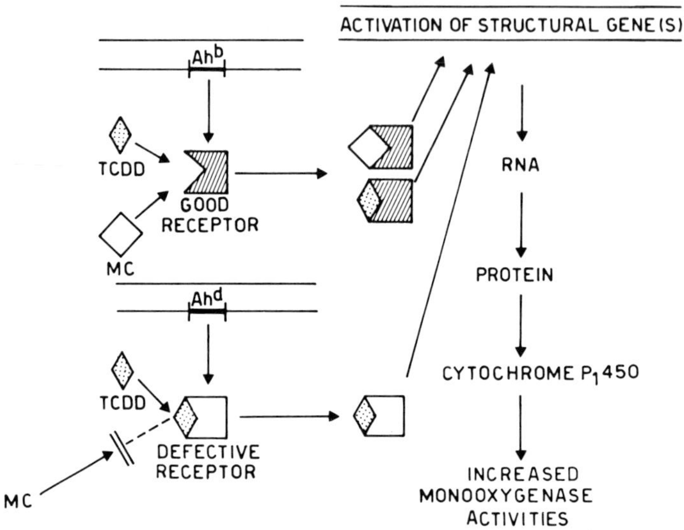

FIGURE 3 Hypothetical scheme indicating the involvement of a receptor as a gene product associated with a locus responsible for aromatic hydrocarbon "responsiveness." Although the Ah locus was suggested [94,193], two or more nonlinked loci in the mouse are most likely involved [93]. In this figure, Ah^b represents C57B1/6 (B6) as the prototype strain for aromatic hydrocarbon "responsiveness" and Ah^d represents DBA/2 (D2) as the prototype strain for aromatic hydrocarbon "nonresponsiveness" [94,193]. (Reproduced from Ref. 102 with permission.)

To explain the presence or the absence of AHH inducibility by 3MC, Nebert [102] proposed a model (Fig. 3) in which a gene product associated with the Ah locus is suggested as a cytosolic receptor able to bind aromatic hydrocarbon inducers. The inducer-receptor complex activates structural genes which induce protein synthesis necessary for cytochrome P_1-450 formation. According to this hypothesis, the unresponsiveness of the D2 strain to 3MC-mediated AHH activity induction could arise from a mutation involving a defective cytosolic receptor with diminished binding affinity for polycyclic aromatic inducers. Poland and coworkers [103] have shown that TCDD (tetrachlorodibenzo-para-dioxin), a compound 30,000 times more potent than 3MC as a hydroxylase inducer, induces AHH and cytochrome P_1-450 formation in hepatic and extrahepatic tissues of both responsive and nonresponsive mice. According to the Nebert model, this very potent halogenated polycyclic compound may act at the same defective receptor, but binding is sufficient to cause the induction responsive process even in nonresponsive strains. Efforts have been made to clarify some of the factors controlling the processes which lead to the induction response, including synthesis of new heme in the mitochondrion and its transport into the endoplasmic reticulum. Recent studies have attempted to determine whether a relationship exists between an Ah locus and some of these factors. For example, plasma concentrations of hemopexin, a possible carrier in intracellular heme transport [104], were seen to increase to a similar extent following treatment with phenobarbital in all mouse strains examined. Conversely, after 3MC pretreatment the increase of hemopexin was lower in strains nonresponsive to AHH induction. These data could be indicative of an association between the Ah locus and hemopexin induction [105] although, because of large individual variations, no such correlation has as yet been statistically demonstrated. From a pharmacological point of view, the importance of these numerous studies lies in the relationship found between the Ah locus, which regulates the inducibility of cytochrome P_1-450 and the subsequent increase of monooxygenase activity, and susceptibility of mice to drug toxicity. In other words, they demonstrate that in mice at least, the sensitivity to environmental pollutants, carcinogens, and teratogens, as well as immunological reactions, can be genetically inherited and regulated by a single or a very small number of genes.

These statements will be clarified by the following remarks. Different forms of cytochrome P-450 exist and generate different ratios of metabolites from the same substrate [101]. Many reactive intermediates from polycyclic hydrocarbons and other xenobiotics have been associated with the induction of cytochrome P_1-450 [99,106]. Mice (Ah^b locus) responsive to the polycyclic hydrocarbons are likely to have higher levels of reactive intermediates resulting from increased cytochrome P_1-450 content and greater P_1-450/P-450 ratio. Consequently, as the enzymatic pathways responsible for inactivation of these reactive metabolites (e.g., epoxide hydrase and glutathione transferase) are only slightly affected by polycyclic hydrocarbon induction, responsive mice are maximally exposed to the carcinogenic and toxicological reactions mediated by these labile metabolites. It is interesting that in stimulated responsive mice the ratio of cytochrome P_1-450 to P-450 is larger in extrahepatic than in hepatic tissues, where it never reaches unity. This could explain the high incidence of polycyclic hydrocarbon-mediated tumors in extrahepatic tissues such as lung, skin, and lymphatic tissues as opposed to the rare cases in the liver.

It appears that the route of administration can also play a role in increasing or decreasing the susceptibility of responsive mice to chemicals. For instance, when benzo[a]pyrene is administered orally, it can be detoxified in the liver where the cytochrome P_1-450 content does not exceed the P-450; consequently accumulation of the compound is prevented in the target organ where metabolic production of reactive metabolites by P_1-450 could occur to a larger extent. This phenomenon, called first-pass elimination [107], explains for instance the greater resistance of responsive mice to aplastic anemia produced by oral benzo[a]pyrene. In contrast, these animals are markedly affected by the teratogenic effects of polycyclic hydrocarbons administered systemically. All these aspects have been extensively reviewed recently by Nebert and colleagues [100-102].

Differences in drug response result not only from genetically determined differences in drug metabolism but also from genetically determined differences in the metabolism of endogenous substrates with which they interact. The latter situation applies to interstrain differences in specific neurochemical parameters, particularly the turnover of putative neurotransmitters, and the binding to receptor sites [2]. Two examples of this type of genetically mediated difference in drug response will be discussed.

The first example concerns the genetically determined sensitivity to amphetamine. From various strains reported to show poor reactivity to the drug [108,109], we selected C3H mice because they react normally to amphetamine as regards some peripheral and central effects, but do not specifically respond to its stimulant properties causing hypermotility, stereotypy, and hyperthermia [110]. C3H mice were mated with BALB/C, a normally reactive inbred strain, and the offspring of the various crosses (F1, F2, and backcrosses) were examined. We found that for the hyperthermic effect at least, sensitivity to amphetamine was inherited as a partially additive dominant trait, partially modified by a maternal effect from the C3H females [111] (Fig. 4). This genetic factor, however, does not control amphetamine bioavailability, as disappearance from the blood and metabolite formation and accumulation are similar in both sensitive and unresponsive strains [112]. These findings agree with amphetamine's ability to evoke some normal responses even in C3H mice [110].

Further investigations were therefore undertaken to explore the origin of this unresponsiveness in C3H mice. As amphetamine hyperthermia is thought to be of central origin and mediated by dopaminergic structures [113], the lack of amphetamine hyperthermic effect could hypothetically originate from differences in the dopaminergic system with which amphetamine interacts. Indeed, C3H mice do not respond to the dopamine-releasing action of amphetamine with the expected increase in concentration of striatal homovanillic acid (HVA), the main dopamine metabolite [114].

There were also significant differences between the basal metabolism of dopamine in sensitive and insensitive mice. In a typical dopamine-containing area such as the striatum, dopamine levels were in the normal range, but dopamine turnover was lower in C3H mice than in responsive mice and turnover time was approximately 40% more than that in a sensitive strain [114]. In support of our findings, it should be recalled that interstrain differences in brain dopamine levels [115] or in tyrosine hydroxylase activity [116-118] have also been described. It was thus concluded that in the C3H strain basic differences in dopamine metabolism could be responsible for the insensitivity to the effects of amphetamine which, like hyperthermia, are mediated by interactions with central dopamine mechanisms.

Strain-dependent sensitivity to morphine is a second example of genetically controlled drug response due to differences not in the metabolic pattern

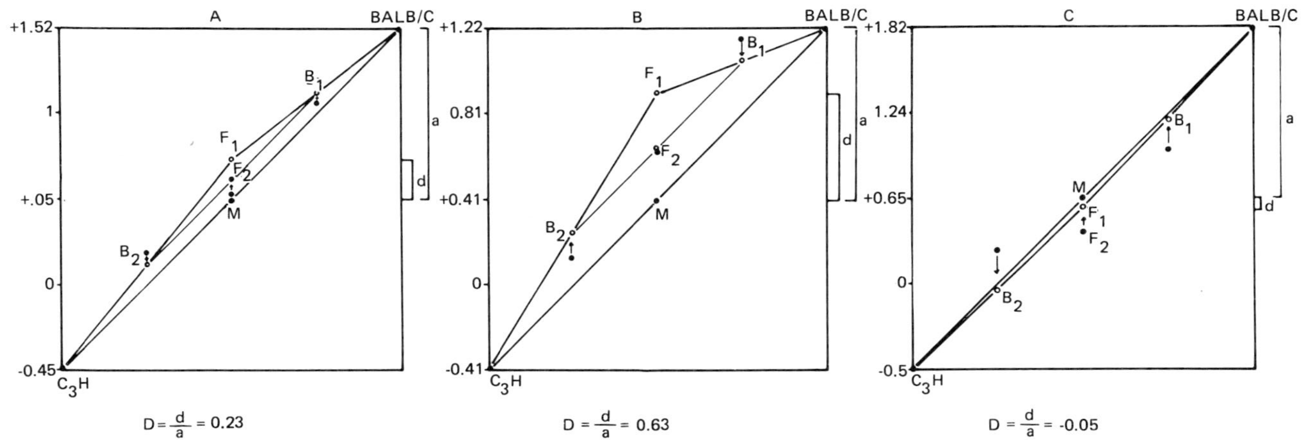

FIGURE 4 Genetic triangles representing the observed and expected population means for the hyperthermic effect of amphetamine. The mean values for the nonsegregating populations (Balb/c; C3H and F_1) are the corner points of the triangle, which is inscribed in a square. The F_1 mean is entered on the vertical line, which bisects the square at a distance d above the midparent (M) value. The expected means for the backcrosses B_1 and B_2 lie on the midpoint of Balb/C F_1 and F_1 C3H, respectively. F_2 is at a distance d/2 above the midparent. The observed B_1, B_2, and F_2 values are shown in filled-in circles and an arrow points from the observed to the expected means. D = degree of dominance [194]. (A) The values are the means of ♀ and ♂. (B) The values are the means of ♀. (C) The values are the means of ♂. (From Ref. 111.)

of the drug itself, but in the specific neurochemical structures on which it acts. Quantitative differences between the response of different mouse strains to morphine, and opiates in general, vary with the individual effects of opiates [86,119-122]. For instance, the strain presenting the highest motility response (running behavior) is the least sensitive to the analgesic effect. A negative statistical correlation between the degree of running and the analgesic effect caused by morphine was demonstrated [122] in nonsegregating strains and in backcrossed mice obtained by mating strains showing different sensitivity to these two parameters. This negative correlation, which excludes the possibility of any difference in reactivity depending on different absorption, metabolism, or blood barrier permeability to morphine, was large enough to suggest that both effects are influenced by many of the same genes. However, other attempts to define the genetic basis for variability in response to morphine effects by examining the response of several recombinant-inbred strains showed that the genetic determinants for running activity were different from those for analgesia [123], although the link between these strong genetic determinants was not satisfactorily clarified. The mode of inheritance of morphine sensitivity is characterized by partial or full dominance [124]. The development of tolerance to locomotor stimulation and analgesia, which appeared to be strain-dependent, is also under genetic control [121,122]. Genetic analysis seems complex, as probably more than three loci are responsible for this trait [125]. Attempts to obtain biochemical bases to explain these genetically controlled responses to morphine highlighted the importance in analgesia of opiate binding ability and of the size of some limbic structures which have both been found to vary in different strains of mice [126,127]. A positive correlation exists between the amount of narcotic receptor proteins and the analgesic responses [128]. These receptor sites are closely associated with the limbic system which is an important area for the analgesic effects [129,130].

Thus it has been suggested that genetic differences in brain structures resulting in differences in morphine receptor sites or in morphine receptor affinity could account for differences in sensitivity or tolerance to morphine effects.

IV. PHARMACOGENETICS IN HUMANS

The importance of genetic factors affecting drug response in humans, the methods employed to study inherited drug sensitivity, and the knowledge available on human genetics have already been extensively reviewed [2,4, 14,131,132].

In humans the genetic component of the wide interindividual variability in drug response has been investigated mainly by comparison of drug disappearance from the blood of twins, family units, or populations. Each of these approaches offers advantages and drawbacks which must be considered before reaching a conclusion. By comparing the drug half-life in identical (homozygous) and fraternal (dizygous) twins, the variability in drug response due to environmental factors can be distinguished from that arising from genetic factors. This approach was first introduced by Francis Galton in 1875 [133], and was successfully used by Vesell to study the disappearance curves for a number of drugs. Greater differences were found between fraternal than identical twins and these results have been offered as evidence that the main mechanisms for elimination of drugs such as phenylbutazone [28], antipyrine [134], and dicoumarol [135] are genetically rather than environmentally controlled. A formula suggested by Neel and Schull [136] and Osborne and De George [137] has been applied to show that the contribution of heredity influence on the rate of metabolism of these drugs was almost 100%.

The identical twin model presents the advantage of automatically eliminating differences in age and sex that, in animals at least [138,139], have been found to influence the rate of drug metabolism. A drawback, however, is that in general identical twins are more likely than fraternal twins to be exposed to a similar environment, as a consequence of similar habits and tastes. In addition, while it enables researchers to establish the hereditary basis for differences in drug response, it is of little use in clarifying genetic aspects such as the mode of inheritance of the genetically controlled trait [14].

Vesell [131] suggests that this last deficiency can be overcome if a distribution curve of drug response is constructed based on the twin studies. The type of curve obtained can help to distinguish the mode of inheritance. However, it seems difficult to collect enough data from twin models in order to plot a clear distribution curve, particularly when a trait appears extremely rare in a type of polymodal distribution. Family studies must therefore be undertaken to clarify the mode of inheritance. The study of a trait in the individuals of a family can reveal whether it is dominant or recessive, sex-linked, or associated with an autosomal chromosome. Disadvantages in family studies, however, lie in the difficulty of testing all family members, ethical problems, differences in drug metabolism due to different ages of children, parents, and grandparents, and the influence of the environment in which the members live as a consequence of their age and work.

The information obtained through twin and family approaches can help define the genetic origin of an abnormal or unusual drug response, and can serve as the basis for larger studies involving entire populations. The prevalence of a pharmacogenetic trait and the frequency of the genes responsible for them in populations of unrelated persons can be of great importance from the epidemiological point of view. One of the more complete examples of the utility of these integrated studies is the pharmacogenetic investigation of isoniazid acetylation. An abnormal toxic effect in some subjects undergoing isoniazid therapy was first observed by Hughes and coworkers [140] who suggested that such individuals were unable to rapidly acetylate the drug.

Comparison of the elimination of acetylated isoniazid in urine from fraternal and identical twins showed that this trait was under genetic control [141]. Family studies by Knight and coworkers [142], and subsequently on a larger number of families by Evans and coworkers [8], led to the conclusion that rapid acetylation is a dominant trait and slow acetylation a recessive trait inherited in classical Mendelian fashion. Population studies by many authors [143-146] showed that the porportion of slow acetylators greatly varied throughout the world, ranging from about 5% among Canadian Eskimos to about 83% among Egyptians. Approximately one-half the population of the United States and of groups of European origin are slow acetylators. These data mean that the recessive gene for slow acetylation has an unusually high frequency, calculated as close to 72% [8].

Acetylation of isoniazid is catalyzed by N-acetyltransferase, a hepatic enzyme present in smaller amounts in the livers of slow as opposed to rapid acetylators [147]. All drugs metabolized by this enzyme should present the same polymorphism as isoniazid. Sulfamethazine [148], hydralazine [147], and phenelzine [149] are in fact acetylated by the same N-acetyltransferase and both the therapeutic effectiveness [150] and side effects [151,152] of these drugs have been reported mainly in slow inactivators of isoniazid.

Another classical example of a genetic factor affecting drug response is glucose 6-phosphate dehydrogenase deficiency, chromosome X-linked genetic defect responsible for drug-induced hemolytic anemia (see Table 1) [10]. The hereditary trait is not directly associated with drug metabolism, but affects the biological substrate on which the drug acts. The first family study, by Childs and collaborators [153], showed that the pattern of response among family members appeared compatible with sex-linked transmission without dominance. Population investigations showed that this genetic defect, with many variants for certain ethnic groups [154,155], affects millions of people all over the world [156,157].

Conversely, other genetic traits which affect drug-metabolizing enzymes or the environment through which drugs act on the body are extremely rare. Some inborn errors of metabolism responsible for abnormal resistance to anticoagulants [158-160], for hypersensitivity to diphenylhydantoin [161], or for malignant hyperthermia following general anesthesia [162, 163] present an autosomal recessive or dominant character but are found in only a few families. Many of these pharmacogenetic conditions transmitted as Mendelian recessives or dominants have been recorded by Vesell [2] (Table 1); each of the conditions listed yields a discontinuous polymodal distribution curve.

However, a more general consideration of how individuals produce the expected response to a given drug yields a continuous unimodal distribution curve.

Several environmental factors contribute to the wide differences in the rates of drug metabolism between individuals which govern drug response when large populations are examined. Therefore, twin studies, in which the weight of environmental factors can be assessed better, have proved particularly useful in determining the influence of genetic factors on interindividual variability.

Among monooxygenase-metabolized xenobiotics such as ethanol [164], halothane [165], and nortriptyline [166], differences in the rate of blood disappearance are much greater between fraternal than between identical twins. It has thus been concluded that most of the variability in drug metablism mediated by hepatic microsomal enzymes is genetically determined in humans. Family studies with phenylbutazone [16], dicoumarol [20], and nortriptyline [167] showed that the distribution curves of drug half-lives after single doses, or of the steady-state levels in chronic treatments, were continuous and unimodal. These results are compatible with the hypothesis, suggested by animal experiments, that interindividual variability in the biooxidation of these drugs is polygenically inherited.

If, then, the rate of hepatic microsomal drug metabolism is mainly under genetic control, a hypothesis of particular clinical value that it should be possible in a given individual to find correlations between metabolic rates of many different drugs. Data available at present neither support not refute this hypothesis. In fact, when as a measure of metabolic rate the half-lives of various drugs were compared in the same subjects, no uniform correlation was obtained. Positive correlations were found for the half-lives of desipramine, amitriptyline, and oxyphenbutazone [168], for dicoumarol and phenylbutazone [135], for glutethimide and sulfinpyrazone [169], and for glutethimide and amobarbital [169]. However, no correlation was obtained between the half-lives of antipyrine and aminopyrine [170], antipyrine and dicoumarol [135], antipyrine and glutethimide or sulfinpyrazone [169]. These discrepancies may find a biochemical explanation in the known existence of multiple forms of cytochrome P-450, each displaying distinct substrate selectivities [171]. In contrast, these discrepancies undermine the validity of a proposal to classify individuals into various "types" according to their rates of drug metabolism in order to reduce toxicity or underdosage [172].

Interactions between drugs also appear to be under genetic control. An interesting example is the appearance of signs of diphenylhydantoin overdosage in patients also receiving isoniazid [173]. As isoniazid is an inhibitor of diphenylhydantoin metabolism [174], slow isoniazid acetylators have a greater likelihood of accumulating diphenylhydantoin to an extent producing toxicity [175,176]. Similarly, phenobarbital was found to increase hemolysis induced by acetophenetidine in two patients genetically hypersensitive to the drug [177]. This occurs probably through induction of the microsomal hydroxylase, thereby increasing formation of the toxic metabolite responsible for the adverse reaction [177].

Of more general interest, however, is the possible genetic control of the response of monooxygenase systems to inhibitors or inducers. Little data is available for inhibitors. Thus, broad interindividual differences in the ability to reduce the metabolism of antipyrine and dicoumarol have been reported for nortriptyline, allopurinol [178], and disulfiram [179]. The differences do not seem to depend on differences in plasma concentrations of the inhibitors, but data concerning the genetic component of this variability are lacking.

More documented investigations concern sensitivity to inducing agents where the response of individuals also shows a high degree of variability. As found in different animal strains [77], in humans also these interindividual variations are not dependent on the absolute blood concentration of the inducers. Twin studies showed that at least concerning the inducing effect of phenobarbital, this variability is under very rigid genetic control [180].

The inducibility of AHH by 3MC was investigated in vitro in human cultured lymphocytes. In agreement with findings in mice (where regulation of AHH inducibility is under genetic control at a single locus Ah) [91], wide interindividual variability in the extent of AHH induction in humans was found to be under monogenic control, the distribution curve of this effect having a trimodal pattern (low-, intermediate-, and high-inducible groups) [181]. Kellerman et al. [181] therefore postulated a genetic model for AHH inducibility in humans in which two alleles (for low and high inducibility) operate codominantly at the Ah locus. Although very stimulating, these data have not yet been confirmed because of the great variability in the results of lymphocyte assays [182,183]. Consequently the monogenic variation was never corroborated by other authors.

Twin studies by Atlas and collaborators [184] confirmed that interindividual variability in AHH inducibility by 3MC in human lymphocytes was controled by genetic rather than environmental factors, but suggested the control might be more compatible with the hypothesis of a polygenic pattern of inheritance. Thus, according to these authors, a continuous rather than a trimodal frequency distribution of inducibility can be expected from a human population study. Kellerman et al. in 1973 [185] and Trell et al. in 1976 [186] reported that bronchogenic carcinoma and laryngeal carcinoma frequency was associated with high inducibility. In particular, the frequency of the high-inducible allele in patients with bronchogenic carcinoma was twice that found in a control population. More recently, other studies failed to confirm that AHH inducibility in pulmonary macrophages or in cultured lymphocytes differed in patients with primary lung tumor and in healthy controls [187]. These data, however, are fairly recent; larger population studies and more rigorous experimental procedures are required before the concept can be rejected or accepted.

The inheritable component of AHH inducibility in humans, as shown with cultured lymphocytes—and more recently cultured monocytes—[188] is already well documented [101]. Whatever control—monogenic or polygenic—is eventually confirmed, these experimental approaches to AHH inducibility will be of some predictive value in assessing whether certain types of cancer are likely to develop.

V. CONCLUSIONS

A large number of pharmacogenetic investigations have ascertained that wide variations in drug response arise from the genetic factors affecting drug metabolism. Earlier observations of different reactivity to drugs in various experimental animal species and in selected strains are now understood within this context. Such a knowledge has enabled us to carry out better oriented drug screening.

The discovery that some animal species have a greater capacity to accumulate reactive intermediates than others suggests the use of these animals in studies of potential carcinogenic agents. The availability of mouse strains found to be genetically tolerant to opiates and to amphetamine could represent an interesting experimental tool for studying the mechanisms of addiction to these drugs and for investigating possible genetical predisposition to addiction in man.

Using selected inbred strains of mice and their crosses, it has been possible to demonstrate that the allelic differences in a single gene, the Ah locus, or in a very small number of genes can influence the susceptibility of mice to drug toxicity. Thus the predisposition of some mouse strains or of individuals in segregating populations to cancer mutation, hepatotoxicity, or even birth defects produced by environmental chemicals can be predicted by measuring phenotypic aryl hydrocarbon hydroxylase (AHH) activity. The large interindividual variations in drug response in man, arising from differences in drug disposition and more specifically in drug metabolism, have also been seen to be under genetic control. Drug metabolism in basal conditions is affected by multiple genetic factors (polygenic control) much more than by environmental factors.

These findings have given rise to the interesting hypothesis that individuals could be classified according to their metabolic capacity. Although this concept has been shown to be true for some biotransformation reactions not involving cytochrome P-450 (e.g., acetylation of drugs by N-acetyltransferase), it does not hold for drugs metabolized by monooxygenases. Correlations between the pharmacokinetic data of several drugs in the same subject were in fact unsatisfactory and their use to predict the behavior of other drugs in clinical practice does not seem warranted.

A more interesting prospect is that pharmacogenetics could be of value in predicting cancer predisposition. The extent of cytochrome P_1-450 induction by chemicals has been found to be genetically regulated in humans. Whether this control is exerted by a single genetic locus or is polygenically mediated is at present debated. Improved biological assays are required if we are to extend our knowledge.

But whether the distribution frequency of AHH inducibility in a given population is expressed by a polymodal or by a Gaussian curve, individuals in the higher portion of the inducibility spectrum will probably be more likely to develop cancer from exposure to chemicals and other environmental pollutants.

REFERENCES

1. F. Vogel, Ergeb. Inn. Med. Kinderheilkd. 12:52 (1959).
2. E. S. Vesell, Biochem. Pharmacol. 24:445 (1975).
3. G. P. Lewis, H. Jick, D. Slone, and S. Shapiro, Ann. N.Y. Acad. Sci. 179:729 (1971).
4. B. N. La Du, An. Rev. Med. 23:453 (1972).
5. H. M. Triedman, R. A. Fishman, and M. D. Yahr, Trans. Amer. Neurol. As. 85:166 (1960).
6. A. H. Anton, Clin. Pharmacol. Ther. 9:561 (1968).
7. C. H. Kunin, N. Engl. J. Med. 281:1188 (1969).
8. D. A. P. Evans, K. A. Manley, and V. A. McKusick, Brit. Med. J. 2:485 (1960).
9. W. Kalow and N. Staron, Can. J. Biochem. Physiol. 35:305 (1957).
10. E. Beutler, in The Metabolic Basis of Inherited Disease, 2nd ed. (J. B. Stanbury, J. B. Wyngaarden, and D. S. Fredrickson, Eds.). McGraw-Hill, New York, 1966, pp. 1060-1089.
11. A. G. Motulsky, J. Am. Med. Ass. 165:835 (1957).
12. B. N. La Du and W. Kalow (Eds.), Ann. N.Y. Acad. Sci. 151:691 (1968).
13. E. S. Vesell (Ed.), Ann. N.Y. Acad. Sci. 179 (1971).
14. S. N. Cohen and W. W. Weber, Pediatr. Clin. North Amer. 19:21 (1972).
15. D. S. Falconer, Introduction to Quantitative Genetics. Ronald, New York, 1960.
16. J. A. Whittaker and D. A. Evans, Brit. Med. J. 4:323 (1970).
17. T. H. Roderick, Radiat. Res. 20:631 (1963).
18. T. H. Roderick and G. Schlager, in Biology of the Laboratory Mouse, 2nd ed. (E. L. Green, Ed.). McGraw-Hill, New York, 1966, pp. 151-164.
19. D. A. P. Evans, in The Scientific Basis of Medicine, Annual Reviews. Athlone, London, 1969, pp. 166-182.
20. A. G. Motulsky, Ann. N.Y. Acad. Sci. 123:167 (1965).
21. B. B. Brodie, in Absorption and Distribution of Drugs (T. B. Binns, Ed.). Livingstone, Edinburgh, 1964, pp. 199-251.
22. B. B. Brodie and W. D. Reid, Fed. Proc. 26:1062 (1967).
23. J. R. Gillette, Ann. N.Y. Acad. Sci. 123:42 (1965).
24. M. Yourish, B. Paton, B. B. Brodie, and J. J. Burns, Arch. Ophthalmol. 53:264 (1955).
25. G. E. Jay, Jr., Proc. Soc. Exp. Biol. Med. 90:378 (1955).
26. G. P. Quinn, J. Axelrod, and B. B. Brodie, Biochem. Pharmacol. 1:152 (1958).
27. R. L. Cram, M. R. Juchau, and J. R. Fouts, Proc. Soc. Exp. Biol. Med. 118:872 (1956).
28. E. S. Vesell and J. G. Page, Science 159:1479 (1968).

29. D. Robinson and R. T. Williams, Biochem. J. 68:23P (1958).
30. E. K. Marshall, Jr., K. Emerson, Jr., W. G. Cutting, and D. Babbitt, J. Am. Med. Ass. 108:953 (1937).
31. L. B. Mellett, Progr. Drug Res. 13:136 (1969).
32. R. L. Smith and L. G. Dring, in Amphetamines and Related Compounds (E. Costa and S. Garattini, Eds.). Raven, New York, 1970, pp. 121-139.
33. M. Goldstein and B. Anagnoste, Biochim. Biophys. Acta 107:166 (1965).
34. A. Jori and S. Caccia, J. Pharm. Pharmacol. 26:746 (1974).
35. E. Costa and A. Groppetti, in Amphetamines and Related Compounds (E. Costa and S. Garattini, Eds.). Raven, New York, 1970, pp. 231-255.
36. B. B. Brodie, A. K. Cho, and G. L. Gessa, in Amphetamines and Related Compounds (E. Costa and S. Garattini, Eds.). Raven, New York, 1970, pp. 217-230.
37. A. Jori, S. Caccia, and E. Dolfini, in Central Mechanisms of Anorectic Drugs (S. Garattini and R. Samanin, Eds.). Raven, New York, 1978, pp. 179-189.
38. A. Jori and D. Bernardi, Eur. J. Pharmacol. 19:276 (1972).
39. E. Anggård, L. E. Jonsson, A. L. Hogmark, and L. M. Gunne, Clin. Pharmacol. Ther. 14:870 (1973).
40. J. V. Dingell, F. Sulser, and J. R. Gillette, J. Pharmacol. Exp. Ther. 143:14 (1964).
41. S. Garattini, A. Bonaccorsi, A. Jori, and R. Samanin, Rev. Neurol. (Paris) 127:265 (1972).
42. E. Elonen, M. Linnoila, I. Lukkari, and M. J. Mattila, Acta Pharmacol. Toxicol. 37:274 (1975).
43. S. Garattini, E. Mussini, F. Marcucci, and A. Guaitani, in The Benzodiazepines (S. Garattini, E. Mussini, and L. O. Randall, Eds.). Raven, New York, 1973, pp. 75-97.
44. M. A. Schwartz, in The Benzodiazepines (S. Garattini, E. Mussini, and L. O. Randall, Eds.). Raven, New York, 1973, pp. 53-74.
45. J. J. Burns, in Metabolic Factors Controlling Duration of Drug Action, Vol. 6 (B. B. Brodie and E. G. Erdös, Eds.). Pergamon, Oxford, 1962, pp. 277-288.
46. P. L. Grover, A. Hewer, K. Pal, and P. Sims, Int. J. Cancer 18:1 (1976).
47. E. S. Reynolds, M. T. Moslen, S. Szabo, R. J. Jaeger, and S. D. Murphy, Amer. J. Pathol. 81:219 (1975).
48. F. Oesch, Xenobiotica 3:305 (1973).
49. H. Mukhtar and E. Bresnick, Chem.-Biol. Interact. 15:59 (1976).
50. F. Oesch, H. Glatt, and H. Schmassmann, Biochem. Pharmacol. 26:603 (1977).
51. L. Cantoni, M. Salmona, T. Facchinetti, C. Pantarotto, and G. Belvedere, Toxicol. Lett. 2:179 (1978).

52. W. A. Bornstein, H. Chuang, E. Bresnick, H. Mukhtar, and J. R. Bend, Chem.-Biol. Interact. 21:343 (1978).
53. C. L. Litterst, E. G. Mimnaugh, R. L. Reagan, and T. E. Gram, Drug Metab. Dispos. 5:259 (1975).
54. A. H. Conney, Pharmacol. Rev. 19:317 (1967).
55. F. G. Brazda, S. Heidingsfelder, and M. Martin, Comp. Biochem. Physiol. 14:239 (1965).
56. L. G. Hart and J. R. Fouts, Naunyn-Schmiedebergs Arch. Pharmakol. Exp. Pathol. 249:486 (1965).
57. A. Jori, G. Guiso, and C. Ravazzani, J. Pharm. Pharmacol. 28:714 (1976).
58. G. Briatico, G. Guiso, A. Jori, and C. Ravazzani, Brit. J. Pharmacol. 58:173 (1976).
59. A. Breckenridge, in Pharmacology of Steroid Contraceptive Drugs (S. Garattini and H. W. Berendes, Eds.). Raven, New York, 1977, pp. 307-311.
60. R. Kato, K. Onoda, and G. M. Takayana, Jap. J. Pharmacol. 19:438 (1969).
61. A. P. Alvares, G. Schilling, and W. Lewin, J. Pharmacol. Exp. Ther. 175:4 (1970).
62. D. S. Davies, P. L. Gigon, and J. R. Gillette, Life Sci. 8(2):85 (1969).
63. K. Kumaki and D. W. Nebert, Pharmacology 17:262 (1978).
64. K. Kumaki, M. Sato, H. Kon, and D. W. Nebert, J. Biol. Chem. 253:1048 (1978).
65. T. E. Gram, D. H. Schroeder, D. C. Davis, R. L. Reagan, and A. M. Guarino, Biochem. Pharmacol. 20:1371 (1971).
66. H. Meier, Experimental Pharmacogenetics: Physiopathology of Hereditary and Pharmacologic Responses. Academic, New York, 1963.
67. S. Ellis, J. Pharmacol. Exp. Ther. 94:130 (1948).
68. G. Werner, Naunyn-Schmiedebergs Arch. Pharmakol. Exp. Pathol. 251:320 (1965).
69. J. L. Page and E. S. Vesell, Pharmacologist 10:179 (1968).
70. J. L. Page and E. S. Vesell, Proc. Soc. Exp. Biol. Med. 131:256 (1969).
71. R. L. Furner, T. E. Gram, and R. E. Stitzel, Pharmacology 2:181 (1969).
72. E. S. Vesell, Pharmacology 1:81 (1968).
73. R. L. Furner, T. E. Gram, and R. E. Stitzel, Biochem. Pharmacol. 18:1635 (1969).
74. A. Jori, D. Bernardi, C. Pugliatti, and S. Garattini, Biochem. Pharmacol. 19:1315 (1970).
75. A. Jori, D. Bernardi, and C. Pugliatti, paper presented at the 2nd Riunione Nazionale della Società Italiana di Neuropsicofarmacologia, Tieernia, Italy, June 14-16, 1969.

76. A. Jori, R. Pescador, and C. Pugliatti, Biochem. Pharmacol. 20: 2695 (1971).
77. A. Jori, C. Pugliatti, and V. Santini, Pharmacology 7:296 (1972).
78. A. Jori and R. Pescador, Chem.-Biol. Interact. 8:297 (1974).
79. J. E. Gielen and D. W. Nebert, Science 172:167 (1971).
80. R. A. Deitrich, Science 173:334 (1971).
81. R. E. Stitzel and J. S. McCarthy, Biochem. Pharmacol. 21:755 (1972).
82. P. Shubik and A. C. Ritchie, Science 117:285 (1953).
83. M. K. Deringer, T. B. Dunn, and W. E. Heston, Proc. Soc. Exp. Biol. Med. 83:474 (1953).
84. L. C. Weaver and T. L. Kerley, J. Pharmacol. Exp. Ther. 135:240 (1962).
85. S. D. Huff, Roscoe B. Jackson Memorial Laboratory Annual Report (1961-1962), No. 33, 1962.
86. J. Jacob and C. Barthelemy, Therapie 22:1435 (1960).
87. E. L. Green, in Biology of the Laboratory Mouse, 2nd ed. (E. L. Green, Ed.). McGraw-Hill, New York, 1966, pp. 11-22.
88. D. W. Nebert and J. E. Gielen, Fed. Proc. 31:1315 (1972).
89. P. E. Thomas, R. E. Kouri, and J. J. Hutton, Biochem. Genet. 6: 157 (1972).
90. J. E. Gielen, F. M. Goujon, and D. W. Nebert, J. Biol. Chem. 247:1125 (1972).
91. D. W. Nebert, F. M. Goujon, and J. E. Gielen, Nature N. Biol. 236:107 (1972).
92. A. Niwa, K. Kumaki, D. W. Nebert, and A. P. Poland, Arch. Biochem. Biophys. 166:559 (1975).
93. J. R. Robinson, N. Considine, and D. W. Nebert, J. Biol. Chem. 249:5851 (1974).
94. D. W. Nebert, J. E. Gielen, and F. M. Goujon, Mol. Pharmacol. 8: 651 (1972).
95. D. W. Nebert and H. Kon, J. Biol. Chem. 248:169 (1973).
96. N. E. Sladek and G. J. Mannering, Mol. Pharmacol. 5:174 (1969).
97. J. R. Gillette, Advan. Enzyme Regul. 1:215 (1963).
98. S. A. Atlas and D. W. Nebert, Semin. Oncol. 5:89 (1978).
99. D. W. Nebert, R. C. Levitt, M. M. Orlando, and J. S. Felton, Clin. Pharmacol. Ther. 22:640 (1977).
100. D. W. Nebert, R. C. Levitt, N. M. Jensen, G. H. Lambert, and J. S. Felton, Arch. Toxicol. 39:109 (1977).
101. S. S. Thorgeirsson and D. W. Nebert, Advan. Cancer Res. 25:149 (1977).
102. D. W. Nebert, J. R. Robinson, A. Niwa, K. Kumaki, and A. P. Poland, J. Cell. Physiol. 85:393 (1975).
103. A. Poland and E. Glover, J. Biol. Chem. 249:5599 (1974).

104. U. Muller-Eberhard and H. H. Liem, in Structure and Function of Plasma Proteins, Vol. 1 (A. C. Allison, Ed.). Plenum, London, 1974, pp. 35-53.
105. I. S. Owens, D. W. Nebert, H. H. Liem, and U. Muller-Eberhard, Biochem. Pharmacol. 27:1665 (1978).
106. R. E. Kouri, T. H. Rude, R. Joglekar, P. M. Dansette, D. M. Jerina, S. A. Atlas, I. S. Owens, and D. W. Nebert, Cancer Res. 38:2777 (1978).
107. M. Gibaldi, R. N. Boyers, and S. Feldman, J. Pharm. Sci. 60: 1338 (1971).
108. A. M. Brown, Lab. Anim. Care 15:111 (1965).
109. E. Dolfini, S. Garattini, and L. Valzelli, Eur. J. Pharmacol. 7:220 (1969).
110. A. Jori and S. Garattini, in Frontiers in Catecholamine Research (E. Usdin and S. Snyder, Eds.). Pergamon, New York, 1973, pp. 939-941.
111. A. Jori and M. Rutczynski, Psychopharmacology 59:199 (1978).
112. A. Jori and S. Caccia, J. Pharm. Pharmacol. 27:886 (1975).
113. C. Matsumoto and W. Griffin, J. Pharm. Pharmacol. 23:710 (1971).
114. S. Caccia, G. Cecchetti, S. Garattini, and A. Jori, Brit. J. Pharmacol. 49:400 (1973).
115. G. M. Everett, in Frontiers in Catecholamine Research (E. Usdin and S. H. Snyder, Eds.). Pergamon, New York, 1973, pp. 657-659.
116. R. D. Ciaranello, R. Barchas, S. Kessler, and J. D. Barchas, Life Sci. 11(1):565 (1972).
117. R. D. Ciaranello, H. J. Hoffman, J. G. M. Shire, and J. Axelrod, J. Biol. Chem. 249:4528 (1974).
118. D. S. Segal, R. T. Kuczenski, and A. J. Mandell, Behav. Biol. 7: 75 (1972).
119. K. Eriksson and K. Kiihnmaa, Ann. Med. Exp. Biol. Fenn. 49:73 (1971).
120. G. F. Gebhart and C. L. Mitchell, Arch. Int. Pharmacodyn. Ther. 201:128 (1973).
121. A. Goldstein and P. Sheehan, J. Pharmacol. Exp. Ther. 169:175 (1969).
122. A. Oliverio and C. Castellano, Psychopharmacologia 39:13 (1974).
123. L. Shuster, G. W. Webster, G. Yu, and B. E. Eleftheriou, Psychopharmacologia 42:249 (1975).
124. C. Castellano and A. Oliverio, Psychopharmacologia 41:197 (1975).
125. A. Oliverio, C. Castellano, and B. E. Eleftheriou, Psychopharmacologia 42:219 (1975).
126. A. Baran, L. Shuster, B. E. Eleftheriou, and D. W. Bailey, Life Sci. 17:633 (1976).
127. C. C. Wimer, R. E. Wimer, and T. H. Roderick, J. Comp. Physiol. Psychol. 76:57 (1971).

128. L. Shuster, A. Baran, and B. E. Eleftheriou, Fed. Proc. 34:713 (1975).
129. M. J. Kuhar, C. B. Pert, and S. H. Snyder, Nature 245:447 (1973).
130. A. Herz, K. Albus, J. Metys, P. Schubert, and H. Teschemaker, Neuropharmacology 9:539 (1970).
131. E. S. Vesell, Fed. Proc. 31:1253 (1972).
132. E. S. Vesell, An. Rev. Pharmacol. 14:249 (1974).
133. F. Galton, J. Brit. Anthropol. Inst. 5:391 (1875).
134. E. S. Vesell and J. G. Page, Science 161:72 (1968).
135. E. S. Vesell and J. G. Page, J. Clin. Invest. 47:2657 (1968).
136. J. V. Neel and W. J. Schull, Human Heredity. University of Chicago Press, Chicago, 1954.
137. R. H. Osborne and F. V. De George, Genetic Basis of Morphological Variation on Evaluation and Application of the Twin Study Method. Harvard University Press, Cambridge, 1959.
138. R. Kato, Drug Metab. Rev. 3:1 (1974).
139. W. Klinger, Arch. Int. Pharmacodyn. Ther. 184:5 (1970).
140. H. B. Hughes, L. H. Schmidt, and J. P. Biehl, Trans. Conf. Chemother. Tubercol. 14:217 (1955).
141. R. Bönicke and B. P. Lisboa, Naturwissenschaften 44:314 (1957).
142. R. A. Knight, M. J. Selm, and H. W. Harris, Trans. Conf. Chemother. Tubercol. 18:52 (1959).
143. W. W. Weber, in Metabolic Conjugation and Metabolic Hydrolysis, Vol. 3 (W. H. Fishman, Ed.). Academic, New York, 1973.
144. N. Hashem, S. Khalifa, and A. Nour, Amer. J. Physiol. Anthropol. 31:97 (1969).
145. A. G. Motulsky, in Genetics Today: 11th International Congress, Vol. 3. The Hague, Netherlands, 1963, p. 875.
146. A. R. Armstrong and H. E. Peart, Amer. Rev. Respir. Dis. 81:588 (1960).
147. J. W. Jenne, J. Clin. Invest. 44:1992 (1965).
148. D. A. P. Evans and T. A. White, J. Lab. Clin. Med. 63:394 (1964).
149. G. R. Gordon, J. H. Peters, R. Gelber, and L. Levy, Proc. West. Pharmacol. Soc. 13:17 (1970).
150. E. C. Johnstone, Mod. Probl. Pharmacopsychiatry 10:30 (1975).
151. D. A. P. Evans, K. Davison, and R. T. C. Pratt, Clin. Pharmacol. Ther. 6:430 (1965).
152. H. M. Perry, Jr., A. Sakamoto, and E. M. Tan, J. Lab. Clin. Med. 70:1020 (1967).
153. B. Childs, W. Zinkham, E. A. Browne, E. L. Kimbro, J. V. Torbert, J. Hinnant, and M. Sachs, Bull. Johns Hopkins Hosp. 102:21 (1958).
154. H. N. Kirkman, S. A. Doxiadis, T. Valaes, N. Tassopoulos, and A. G. Brinson, J. Lab. Clin. Med. 65:212 (1965).
155. A. G. Motulsky, Fed. Proc. 31:1286 (1972).

156. A. R. Tarlov, G. J. Brewer, P. E. Carson, and A. S. Alving, Arch. Intern. Med. 109:209 (1962).
157. H. N. Kirkman, Ann. N.Y. Acad. Sci. 151:753 (1968).
158. R. A. O'Reilly, P. M. Ageller, M. S. Hoag, L. S. Leong, and M. L. Kropatkin, N. Engl. J. Med. 271:809 (1964).
159. R. A. O'Reilly and P. M. Aggeler, Fed. Proc. 24:1266 (1965).
160. R. A. O'Reilly, N. Engl. J. Med. 282:1448 (1970).
161. H. Kutt, M. Wolk, R. Scherman, and F. McDowell, Neurology 14: 542 (1964).
162. W. Kalow, B. A. Britt, M. E. Terreau, and C. Haist, Lancet ii:895 (1970).
163. B. A. Britt and W. Kalow, Ann. N.Y. Acad. Sci. 151:947 (1968).
164. E. S. Vesell, J. G. Page, and G. T. Passananti, Clin. Pharmacol. Ther. 12:192 (1971).
165. H. F. Cascorbi, E. S. Vesell, D. A. Blake, and M. Helrich, Clin. Pharmacol. Ther. 12:50 (1971).
166. B. Alexanderson, D. A. Evans, and F. Sjöqvist, Brit. Med. J. 4:764 (1969).
167. M. Åsberg, D. A. P. Evans, and F. Sjöqvist, J. Med. Genet. 8:129 (1971).
168. W. Hammer, S. Martens, and F. Sjöqvist, Clin. Pharmacol. Ther. 10:44 (1969).
169. D. Kadar, T. Inaba, L. Endrenyi, G. E. Johnson, and W. Kalow, Clin. Pharmacol. Ther. 14:552 (1973).
170. G. W. Hepner and E. S. Vesell, N. Engl. J. Med. 291:1384 (1974).
171. D. A. Haugen, T. A. Van der Hoeven, and M. J. Coon, J. Biol. Chem. 250:3567 (1975).
172. E. S. Vesell, Clin. Pharmacol. Ther. 22(2):659 (1977).
173. H. Kutt, W. Winters, and F. H. McDowell, Neurology 16:594 (1966).
174. H. Kutt, K. Verebely, and F. H. McDowell, Neurology 18:706 (1968).
175. H. Kutt, R. Brennan, H. Dehejia, and K. Verebely, Am. Rev. Respir. Dis. 101:377 (1970).
176. R. W. Brennan, H. Dehejia, H. Kutt, K. Verebely, and F. McDowell, Neurology 20:687 (1970).
177. N. T. Shahidi, Ann. N.Y. Acad. Sci. 151:822 (1968).
178. E. S. Vesell, G. T. Passananti, and F. E. Greene, N. Engl. J. Med. 283:1484 (1970).
179. E. S. Vesell, G. T. Passananti, and C. H. Lee, Clin. Pharmacol. Ther. 12:785 (1971).
180. E. S. Vesell and J. G. Page, J. Clin. Invest. 48:2202 (1969).
181. G. Kellermann, M. Luyten-Kellermann, and C. R. Shaw, Amer. J. Hum. Genet. 25:327 (1973).
182. R. E. Kouri, H. Ratrie III, S. A. Atlas, A. Niwa, and D. W. Nebert, Life Sci. 15:1585 (1974).

183. H. L. Gurtoo, N. Bejba, and J. Minowada, Cancer Res. 35:1235 (1975).
184. S. A. Atlas, E. S. Vesell, and D. W. Nebert, Cancer Res. 36:4619 (1976).
185. G. Kellermann, C. R. Shaw, and M. Luyten-Kellermann, N. Engl. J. Med. 289:934 (1974).
186. E. Trell, R. Korsgaard, B. Hood, P. Kitzing, G. Norden and B. G. Simonsson, Lancet ii:140 (1976).
187. T. L. McLemore, R. R. Martin, D. L. Busbee, R. C. Richie, R. R. Springer, K. L. Toppell, and E. T. Cantrell, Cancer Res. 37: 1175 (1977).
188. T. Okuda, E. S. Vesell, E. Plotkin, R. Tarone, R. C. Bast, and H. V. Gelboin, Cancer Res. 37:3904 (1977).
189. J. J. Burns, in Conference on Non-human Primate Toxicology, Vol. 86 (C. O. Miller, Ed.). Department of Health, Education, and Welfare, Washington, D.C., 1966.
190. L. B. Mellett, Fed. Proc. 22:305 (1963).
191. G. T. Okita, Fed. Proc. 26:1125 (1967).
192. J. H. Peters, Amer. Rev. Respir. Dis. 81:485 (1960).
193. Committee on Standardized Genetic Nomenclature for Mice, Biochem. Genet. 9:369 (1973).
194. J. H. Bruell, in Roots and Behaviour (E. L. Bliss, Ed.). Hoeber-Harper, New York, 1962, pp. 48-67.

Chapter 6

DRUG METABOLISM AND DRUG TOXICITY: SOME EVOLUTIONARY CONSIDERATIONS

W. Robert Jondorf

Institute of Pharmacology
University of Berne
Berne, Switzerland

After considering evolutionary concepts which focus attention on linear and cyclical events in the emergence of biological systems and homologies, this chapter deals with the versatility of the drug-metabolizing enzymes in the context of the aquatic and terrestrial habitat.

In discussing the range of drug-metabolizing activities which tend to convert lipophilic compounds into more polar excretable entities, it is inferred that some of these activities might be considered as "primordial" compared with others, and it would seem that reducing enzymes and sulfate conjugation mechanisms would have to be included among the primordial pathways.

Rationalization of what might contribute to the "terrestrial drive" in freshwater vertebrate species or the "aquatic drive" in terrestrial species, and the migrations between fresh water and seawater, leads to the recognition of the importance of steroids, thyroid hormones, and prolactin in integrating vertebrate physiological responses to the environment. These in turn are regulated by the drug-metabolizing enzyme system for which steroids and thyroid hormones can serve as endogenous substrates.

In terrestrial invertebrates such as insects, the regulation of life cycles is dependent on juvenile hormone and ecdysone, and the action of these appears to be regulated in great measure by the insect drug-metabolizing enzymes for which these hormones can serve as substrates.

Although relatively few chemical pathways can achieve the metabolism of key endogenous substrates and a multitude of exogenous lipid-soluble compounds taken in from the environment, certain polychlorinated (or polybrominated) aromatic compounds, though lipid-soluble, are themselves resistant to biotransformation despite the fact that they induce the drug-metabolizing enzymes. In vertebrates they accumulate in adipose tissues and skin, producing various characteristic biochemical, physical, and behavioral lesions which affect reproduction.

The body burdens of cumulated compounds are handed from one generation to the next via the egg yolk (in birds) or the milk (in mammals). In terms of evolution, these cumulating chemicals (including specific isomeric polychlorinated biphenyls, cyclodiene insecticide epoxides, dibenzofurans, and dibenzodioxins) neutralize the heritage of the drug-metabolizing enzymes which enabled aquatic forms of life to colonize terrestrial habitats.

I. INTRODUCTION TO EVOLUTIONARY CONCEPTS

The historical developments of ideas on evolution [1,2] were concerned with procedures for recognizing morphological homologies, and constructing classifications from them. Other features of thinking in the nineteenth century were concerned with the way in which additions to unaltered ancestral ontogenies might occur, and how inherited variations and natural selection could produce differential advantages for the survivors of given species.

Size, structure, and dynamics of species populations and interactions with the substrate environment [3,4] are more recent preoccupations that have come into prominence, particularly with respect to the allocation of innate resources by organisms to produce progeny or to restrict progeny in order to increase survival rate in a saturated environment.

However, present techniques and discoveries have changed the emphasis in evolutionary thinking toward molecular biology and a concern with the biochemical unity of life [5-7] in terms of composition of cellular material, methods of replication, and the biochemical pathways for energy metabolism.

What appears to emerge as a recognizable outline which is relevant for the general themes of this chapter is that life depends on the cell as a unit. Viruses, although they are not cellular, parasitize cells and switch the host cell metabolism to propagate viral needs.

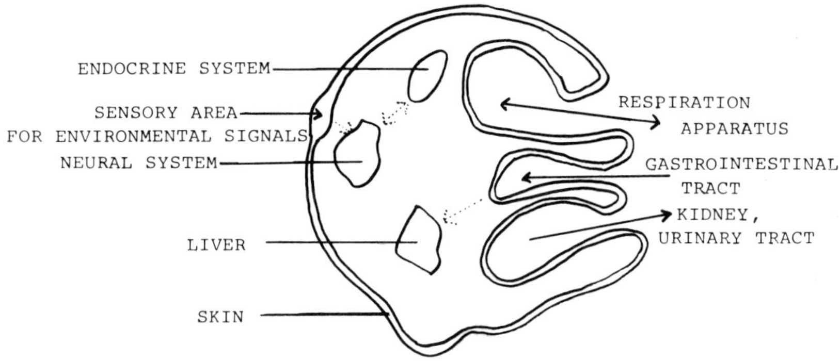

FIGURE 1 A generalized multicellular vertebrate organism simplified and represented as a unicellular form of life. Various tissues replace subcellular components. Neuroendocrinological coordination is seen to respond to environmental signals. The liver assumes the role of the intracellular metabolic enzymes. The skin which delineates the cell has specialized properties in a sensory area and in the invaginations that serve as channels for anabolic and catabolic exchange with the substrate or habitat.

In some respects multicellular vertebrate organisms whose origins from lower forms are still obscure, since nature only leaves traces and provides no witnesses of events unhurried by time, could be represented in the guise of a single cell as shown in Fig. 1. This would not distract from the recognition of the metabolic characteristics that all cells have in common:

They contain reactions which utilize polyphosphates, particularly ATP, for exchanging increments of energy between the integrated metabolic pathways balancing anabolism and catabolism.

They synthesize and store similar building blocks for macromolecular structures in reactions catalyzed mainly by proteins which themselves are linear polymers of definite structure. A number of catalytically functional and structural proteins have recognizable molecular homologies in cell lines from different organisms.

Biological information for protein synthesis is controlled by a complex coding process enshrined in the genetic material of the cell.

There are some characteristic compounds including porphyrins, pyridoxal, and other heterocyclic molecules, glutathione, and certain trace elements which act as focal catalytic centers for enhancing enzyme activity.

Despite these similarities, profound biochemical differences must also exist, for species function differently and are obviously as different from one another as they are from the basic aggregate morphology of Fig. 1.

Moreover, the several tissues of any one species differ in their biochemical adaptations.

What began in the previous century as a quest for establishing morphological homologies and classifications has been replaced by a scientific quest for establishing the molecular basis for transitions that must have taken place between prebiological and biological events on the one hand [8-12] and for understanding the events that led to evolutionary homologous molecular differentiations in living systems on the other hand [6,13].

Whereas Prigogine [8] and Stucki [9] postulate that prebiochemical and biochemical systems would become optimized and yet stabilized by essentially linear sequences of bifurcations and fluctuations, Eigen and Schuster [10-12] postulate a quality or self-correction factor leading to selective optimization of a hypercycle system of functionally cooperating units.

With regard to the emergence of recognizable molecular homologies consistent with the growth of a phylogenetic tree of life, the amino acid sequence analysis of proteins such as cytochrome c [6,13] represents a remarkable advance compared with the mere biochemical demonstration of similarities in amino acid composition between paleolithic and corresponding modern specimens [14].

By concentrating on the metabolic fate of drugs and other exogenous compounds in various organisms we can gain an understanding of what constitutes a response to a functional need, in evolutionary terms. In a study of this kind, it becomes apparent that there is a threshold appearance of drug-metabolizing enzyme activity on the evolutionary scale. What is perhaps less clear is the nature of the primordial drug-metabolizing enzymes, since it is unlikely that all the drug-metabolizing capabilities were simultaneously acquired as a cluster of versatile nonspecific enzymes.

This chapter will also try to define the implications attendant on the spread of unmetabolizable lipid-soluble environmental chemicals as contaminants of the biosphere. These chemicals scatter and undo what the magic hand of chance had brought together.

We have come this far through the gates of time, with genetically perfected devices to explore all the terrestrial possibilities. The heritage of the drug-metabolizing enzyme systems characteristic of the higher forms of terrestrial life is now irreversibly threatened [15-18], for the effects of these unmetabolizable chemicals mimic the pitiful condition that land-living species ingesting ordinary lipophilic foreign compounds would experience in the absence of the protective detoxifying xenobiotic-metabolizing enzymes which made the transition from aquatic to terrestrial life triumphantly possible.

II. THRESHOLDS

Basing his ideas on experiments where drugs were administered to intact animals or incubated with appropriately fortified liver homogenates, Brodie

[19] established various important generalizations characterizing the special nonspecific enzymes responsible for the biotransformation of foreign compounds in vertebrates.

At that time already, it was appreciated that these enzymes were localized in the liver, that they had unusual cofactor requirements for NADPH and O_2, and that they did not wastefully metabolize normally occurring endogenous substrates required by the body for maintaining homeostasis.

It was recognized that the various pathways of metabolic transformation could be inhibited by the same inhibitors and that these inhibitors tended to prolong the duration of action of the drugs tested. Furthermore, there were quite astounding species differences in drug-metabolizing enzyme activity. Thus, dealkylation and hydroxylation reactions, easily monitored when mammalian liver homogenates were incubated with drugs, were not observed in parallel experiments with turtle, frog, or fish liver homogenates. Although other explanations were at first considered, it was apparent that the drug-metabolizing enzymes might be missing in the lower vertebrates which excreted drugs and foreign compounds unchanged.

Lipid solubility of drugs and foreign compounds was recognized as a rate-limiting factor in urinary excretion [20] and it then became clear that the nonspecific drug-metabolizing enzymes in general converted relatively lipophilic foreign compounds into more polar more readily excretable entities [21].

The absence of drug-metabolizing enzyme activity noted in experiments with fish and certain amphibia [19,22,23] could be explained on that basis, for lipid solubility of drugs or exogenous environmental compounds is not a barrier to their excretion in those aquatic species capable of eliminating them unchanged by continuous dialysis through the lipoidal membranes of gills or skin. Conversely, lipid solubility is not a barrier for the entry of exogenous compounds into these species [22] and since various halogenated environmental contaminants now persist in most ecosystems [15,18,24-27], aquatic vertebrates lacking drug-metabolizing enzyme systems can at best do no more than equilibrate with such contaminants.

The drug-metabolizing enzymes can be considered in terms of biochemical evolution accompanying the transition from aquatic to terrestrial life [22,23]. They provide the means for disposing of lipid-soluble foreign compounds in organisms where water retention priorities have led to anatomical modifications of the skin and to the physicochemical adaptation of kidney filtration and concentration systems facilitating excretion of polar substances [20].

To illustrate this, drug metabolism was studied in toads [22,23] which in their adult form are primarily terrestrial while the free-swimming larval forms are obviously aquatic. When test drugs were administered to adult toads, metabolism took place. Judging from the low recoveries of unchanged compounds from whole animal experiments and from incubation of liver homogenates with appropriate test compounds, it was clear that exogenous phenols could be conjugated with glucuronide or sulfate. The toad tadpoles did not have the capacity for metabolism under these circumstances. In corresponding experiments with reptiles [22,23] in vivo and in vitro, evidence was obtained that snakes, alligators, and tortoises could metabolize appropriate test drugs by NADPH- and O_2-dependent enzymes associated with the liver microsomal subcellular fraction.

III. ENZYME SYSTEMS FOR DRUG METABOLISM

Although some drugs and environmental chemicals may be excreted unchanged by terrestrial species of animals, they are more usually converted to more polar metabolites by nonspecific NADPH- and O_2-dependent enzymes before excretion, unless they resemble endogenous intermediate substrates sufficiently to become enmeshed in the network of enzymes regulating intermediary homeostatic metabolism, and thereby become incorporated into cellular macromolecular material as indicated in general diagrammatic form (Fig. 2) to emphasize the detoxifying principles of the drug-metabolizing system.

The fate of most drugs and foreign compounds undergoing metabolic biotransformation in higher vertebrates was conveniently classified by

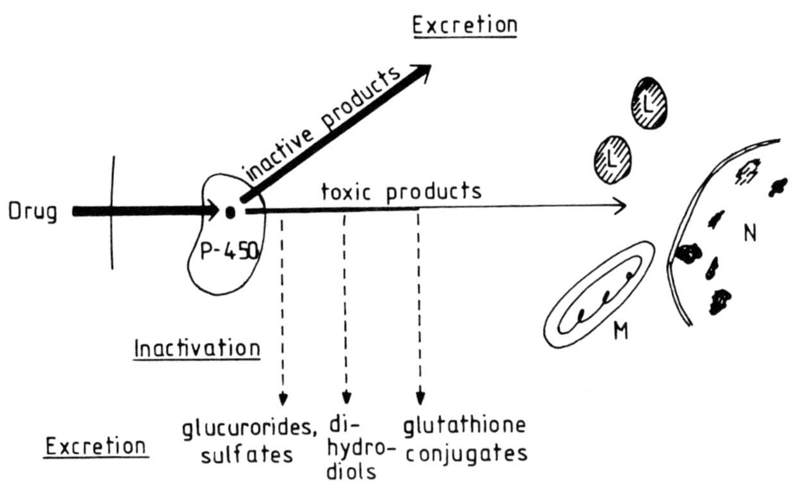

FIGURE 2 Schematic representation of the formation of predominantly inactive excretable metabolites when lipid-soluble drug entering liver cell(s) interacts with the cytochrome P-450 system. Some active intermediate may become incorporated into macromolecular material in subcellular components such as lysosomes (L), mitochondria (M), or nucleus (N). (Slightly modified from Ref. 28.)

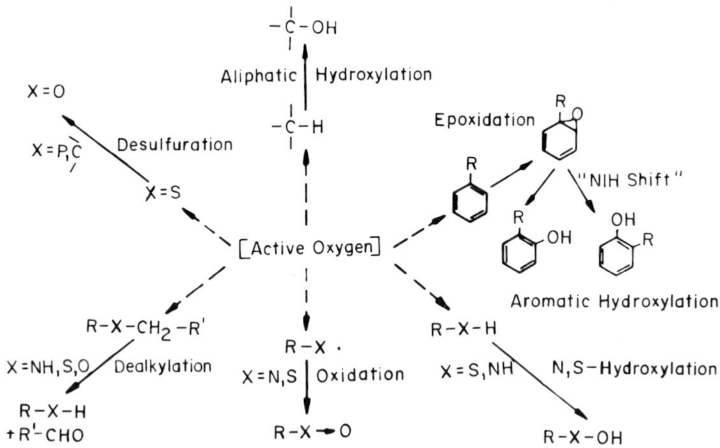

FIGURE 3 Characteristic reactions catalyzed by the drug-metabolizing enzyme system through the mediation of "active oxygen." The versatility of the system as here depicted does not in general extend to dehalogenations of aromatic chloro compounds. (From Ref. 35.)

Williams [29,30] into phase I and phase II reactions. The phase I reactions were those that converted one functional group into another or introduced some polar groups(s) into nonpolar substrates. The phase II reactions were the synthetic mechanisms that conjugated existing or newly introduced polar groups with endogenous entities to form glucuronides, sulfates, mercapturic acids, and so on. The range of oxidative phase I reactions [23,29, 31-34] includes aromatic and aliphatic hydroxylations, N- and O-dealkylation, deamination, sulfoxidation, and desulfuration reactions which can be represented in their most general form as different kinds of hydroxylation reactions [35] as shown in Fig. 3.

Obviously, a great deal depends on the nature of the "active oxygen." As formulated by Gillette [32], the microsomal drug-metabolizing system is considered as a monooxygenase mechanism where NADPH reduces a microsomal component (A) which then reacts with molecular oxygen to form the active oxygen intermediate. This intermediate is capable of transferring active oxygen to the lipophilic drug substrate according to reactions that can be summarized as follows:

$$\text{NADPH} + \text{A} + \text{H}^+ \longrightarrow \text{AH}_2 + \text{NADP}^+$$

$$\text{AH}_2 + \text{O}_2 \longrightarrow \text{active oxygen}$$

$$\text{Active oxygen} + \text{drug} \longrightarrow \text{oxidized drug} + \text{A} + \text{H}_2\text{O}$$

$$\text{NADPH} + \text{O}_2 + \text{drug} + \text{H}^+ \longrightarrow \text{NADP}^+ + \text{H}_2\text{O} + \text{oxidized drug}$$

In this representation, A and AH_2 are considered to be the oxidized and reduced forms of cytochrome P-450. It can be seen that for each molecule of O_2 consumed, one molecule of substrate is oxidized by introduction of one of the atoms of oxygen, while the other oxygen atom undergoes two-equivalent reduction to water.

A greater understanding of the complexities of cytochrome P-450 interactions with lipophilic, relatively nonpolar substrates [36-38] had led to elaborations in current concepts of oxidative drug-metabolizing events in the liver which are illustrated by the schemes of Nebert et al. [39] or of Orrenius [28] as shown in Fig. 4. It should be emphasized that cytochrome P-450 is not exclusively localized in liver cells, for some oxidative metabolic transformations mediated by the cytochrome P-450 complex also occur, for example, in the adrenal cortex, intestinal mucosa, kidney tissue, lung, and placenta.

Even the scheme illustrated in Fig. 4 may have to be revised in view of the exciting implications of the discovery of superoxide radical and dismutase enzyme involvement in the biological handling of molecular oxygen [40], their possible role in cytochrome P-450-linked oxidations [41,42], and in the induction of drug-metabolizing enzyme activities [42].

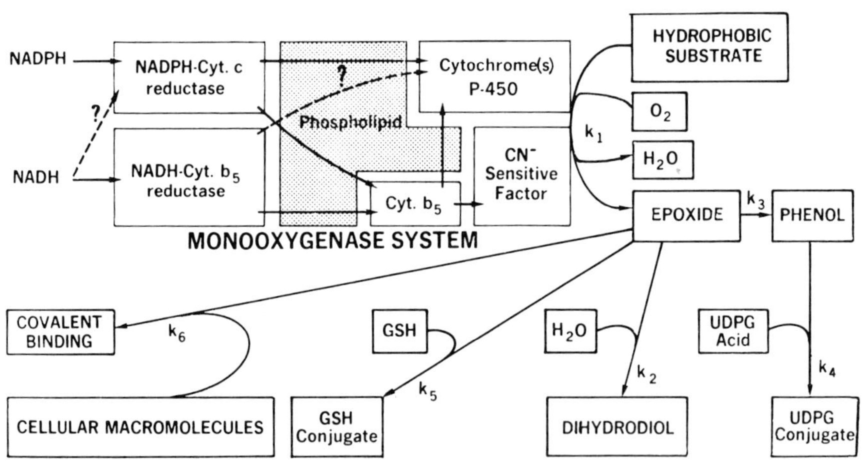

FIGURE 4 Scheme for membrane-bound multicomponent cytochrome P-450-mediated monooxygenase system, and possible metabolic pathways followed by hydrophobic exogenous drug substrate(s). For any particular drug substrate the relative reaction rates k_1-k_6 are not easily determined, and would be expected to be dependent on factors related to strain, species age, diurnal and seasonal variables, as well as hormonal and nutritional status. (From Ref. 39.)

IV. REDUCTION REACTIONS

It is worth remembering that in addition to the oxidative pathways of drug metabolism, there are capabilities for reductive and hydrolytic metabolism which have to be considered. Studies on the metabolism of azo and nitro compounds in the organism have had an enormous influence on the development of new drugs and toxicological problems. The key was the recognition by Tréfouël and colleagues [43] that the lipid-soluble azo dye Prontosil was reductively cleaved to sulfanilamide in the body. A compound that had relatively little biological activity in vitro was transformed in vivo into an antibacterial metabolite. However, as we shall see, the reduction of nitro compounds by the higher vertebrates in vivo can give rise to toxic intermediates.

Let us assume for the moment, as we have done with the oxidative pathways, that Fig. 1 is an approximation of reality, and that what holds for drug-metabolizing events in the subcellular fractions of a particular organ reflects the capability in drug metabolism of the whole "unicellular" organism.

Then, with regard to enzymatic azo-reduction and nitro-reduction of exogenous compounds, it is known that mammalian liver microsomal preparations also contain NADPH-dependent enzymes which under anaerobic conditions catalyze the reduction of azo compounds [44-49] and nitro compounds [49-51].

Nitro compounds such as nitrobenzene, para-nitrobenzoic acid, chloramphenicol [50], niridazole [52], and nitrazepam [53] are reduced enzymatically by nitro-reductase of mammalian liver (or kidney) homogenates. The NADPH-dependent reaction is inhibited by oxygen and promoted by flavins. There is evidence that nitroso compounds and hydroxylamines are reduced by the same enzyme system [49] so that the overall reduction of a nitro compound ($R{-}NO_2$) can be assumed to proceed stepwise:

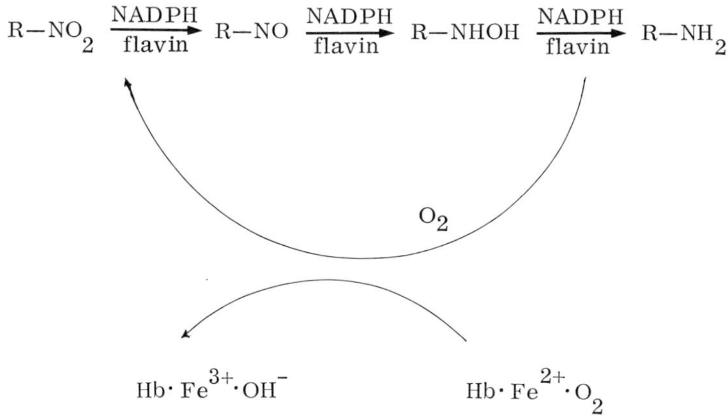

The formation of the intermediates shown explains the relationship between drug-metabolizing enzyme activity and the toxic manifestations of methemoglobinemia observed after nitrobenzene administration [27,54,55] or exposure.

A great deal of research has been done on the similarities between nitro-reductase and azo-reductase, on the one hand, and between azo-reductase and NADPH-cytochrome c reductase, on the other, in the mammalian liver systems that have been most extensively studied [47-49]. It is accepted that there are differences. Part of the confusion arises from the realization [46-48] that the reductive scission of the —N=N— double bond in azo compounds is also a stepwise phenomenon and is subject to autooxidation as indicated:

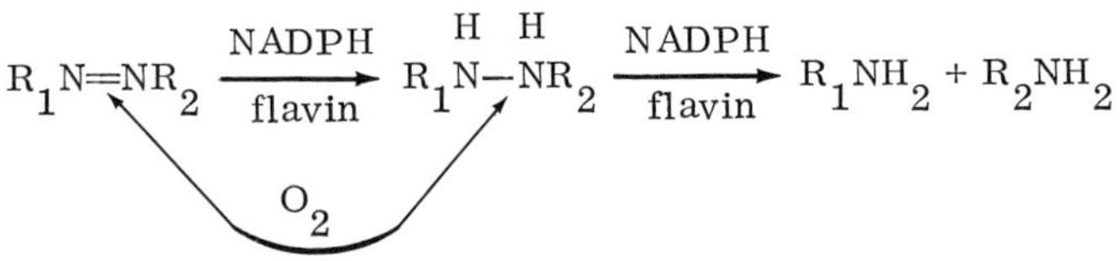

The early experiments on comparative evolutionary and developmental aspects of drug-metabolizing enzyme activity already referred to [22,23, 56] concentrated on the oxidative phase I pathways of metabolism, and guidelines were established for the threshold appearance on the evolutionary scale of these oxidative enzyme activities. In more recent studies of the reduction of nitro and azo compounds in various types of fish [57-59] both nitro-reductase and azo-reductase activities could be measured in most of the liver homogenates incubated anaerobically in the presence of substrates and NADPH under the appropriate conditions. Although nitro-reductase activity appears to be absent in amphibia, it was shown that higher vertebrates could reduce nitro compounds [57].

The metabolism of drugs and exogenous compounds by fish and amphibia will be discussed more fully in a later section in terms of what is known about hormonal regulation in these vertebrates [60-64].

Terrestrial insect microsomal preparations such as those of the housefly [65] have both nitro- and azo-reductase activities, and insect NADPH-cytochrome c reductase activities are well documented [66]. Drug-metabolizing activities of insects will also be dealt with more fully in a later section.

The supposition that liver (or kidney) microsomal reactions reflect what might be taking place in the whole vertebrate organism now has to be challenged.

It has been known for some time that aromatic nitro compounds are also reduced by bacterial flora in the intestine [67], but the bacterial enzymes differ in some respects from the mammalian system [68-70] and require NADPH, Mn^{2+} and reduced glutathione for activity.

The role of intestinal bacteria in the reduction of nitro compounds, which has practical and evolutionary significance, was investigated by comparing the methemoglobinemia in response to nitrobenzene in animals some of which had been treated with an antibiotic [55]. The methemoglobinemia was absent in antibiotic-treated and germfree animals, indicating that the bacterial nitro-reduction predominates in mammals. Further, very thorough studies by Zachariah and Juchau [71] and Wheeler et al. [72] in connection with para-nitrobenzoic acid administered to rats showed quite clearly that the reductive formation of para-aminobenzoic acid was drastically reduced in germfree or antibiotic-pretreated animals.

The selective reassociation of bacterial types with germfree animals indicated that in vivo and in vitro reducing activity was primarily associated with S. faecalis and Clostridium spp. [72]. Different species of animals have different complex ecosystems of intestinal bacterial symbionts [73] which in turn have various proportions of anaerobic types reducing different kinds of terminal electron acceptors [74]. Therefore, it is not at all surprising that there are profound species differences in the overall capabilities for reducing nitro compounds.

It is ironic that the original awareness of azo-reductase activity in vivo occasioned by the realization that an azo compound, Prontosil, was metabolized to sulfanilamide [43] has since been superseded by experimental evidence that azo-reductase activity of the bacterial intestinal flora [75-78] probably accounts for the greatest proportion of cleavage reduction of both lipid-soluble and water-soluble azo compounds.

The bacterial intestinal flora are also involved in other reductive pathways of drug metabolism [73,79,80] including dehydroxylation of catechols and phenolic acids [81-84] which display characteristic features of anaerobic respiration [74].

Unlike the photosynthetic bacteria or algae which would obtain their energy from light in reducing reactions [85,86], the intestinal bacteria are dependent on chemical compounds as the source of energy for bioconversions under anaerobic conditions [74].

It would seem likely that the reduction of organic nitro and azo compounds by intestinal microorganisms is related to the primordial mechanisms of nitrogen fixation [87] and assimilatory nitrate-reductase activities [88].

V. HYDROLYTIC REACTIONS

The hydrolysis of exogenous esters and amides is an important pathway in drug biotransformation. There are diverse esterases in body fluids and in various tissues, and these appear to have overlapping selectivities and variable activities depending on species [89,90].

Whereas procaine is hydrolyzed fairly readily by plasma esterases [91,92], the amide analog undergoes hydrolysis much more slowly and this is reflected in the duration of observed therapeutic effects of these drugs.

Some amides are not hydrolyzed by amidases until they have undergone some initial microsomal biotransformation [93-96], and this also appears to hold for certain carbamate insecticides [97-100] which are less readily hydrolyzed than their dealkylated metabolites. This is illustrated by the general scheme:

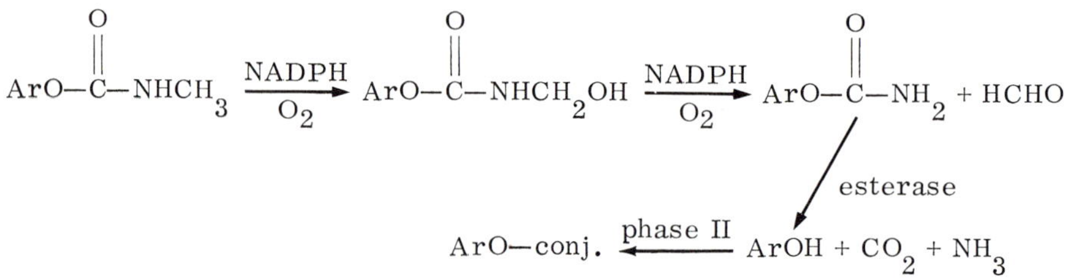

Substrates for the hydrolytic enzymes are compounds with important toxicological effects such as the organophosphorus and carbamate insecticides [101-106]. With such a vast literature, there is no chance to do more than indicate how resistance or susceptibility to toxic effects may be related to esterase activity.

Some of the variables involved in the metabolism of malathion are illustrated in Fig. 5. Malathion which appears to be more toxic to insects than to mammals, can be degraded by carboxyesterase or phosphatase activities. In mammals [101,105] the lower toxicity is ascribable to the greater rate of carboxyesterase degradation. Microsomal oxidation of malathion to malaoxon occurs in both susceptible and resistant insects, but the phosphatase degradation of malaoxon is faster in resistant insects [107,108]. In other species of insects, however, resistance is associated with increased carboxyesterase activity [109-111]. This carboxyesterase activity conferring resistance is sufficiently selective to distinguish between ethyl esters and methyl or other alkyl analogs [112]. The toxicity of malathion for resistant strains of insects and for mammals can be enhanced dramatically by inhibitors of carboxyesterase activity [109,110,113].

Not all esters that might be expected to be hydrolyzed in vivo in fact are. Notable exceptions are the pyrethroid-type compounds, as shown in Fig. 6. The metabolism of these derivatives in insects [114,115] and in mammals [116] showed no evidence of ester hydrolysis but instead pointed to the involvement of microsomal enzymes in the stepwise oxidative metabolism of the terminal cis or trans methyl group to the corresponding carboxylic acid [117]. Microsomal oxidation also takes place on the side chain adjacent to the cyclopentenone ring [118].

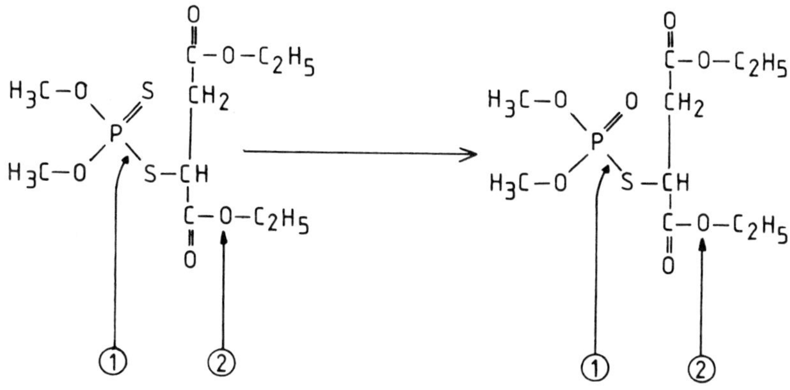

FIGURE 5 Some factors involved in the metabolism of malathion (>P=S compound), showing microsomal conversion to malaoxon (>P=O compound) and sites of degradation by phosphatase (1), and carboxyesterase (2).

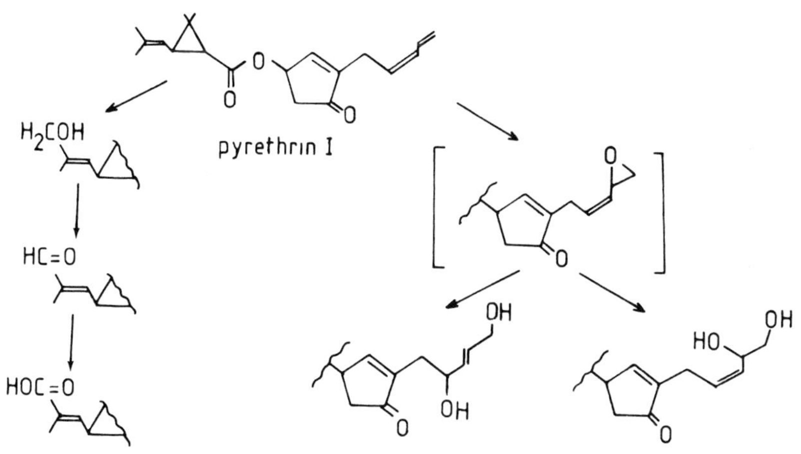

FIGURE 6 Oxidative metabolic transformations undergone by pyrethrin I in rats and houseflies showing how the isobutenyl side chain of the acid moiety is hydroxylated. The hydroxymethyl metabolite of pyrethrin may be (conjugated or) further oxidized. Microsomal oxidation also occurs on the cyclopentenone ring in the alcohol entity. The ester link remains intact. The wavy lines in the illustration according to Nakatsugawa and Morelli [117] merely emphasize the portions of the molecule subject to oxidation.

VI. CONJUGATION REACTIONS

A. Glucuronide Formation

The synthetic conjugation reactions which drugs and exogenous compounds or their phase I products of biotransformation undergo have been exhaustively and encyclopedically reviewed. These reviews also emphasize that there are normal endogenous substrates for conjugation whose biological activity is terminated by the conjugation reactions and subsequent excretion [119,120].

Conjugation reactions involve the formation of an active intermediate and a transferring enzyme. In the case of glucuronide formation [121-124] in mammals, the liver contains enzymes that catalyze the synthesis of uridine diphosphate-glucuronic acid (UDPGA) which serves as a donor of the glucuronic acid entity to the various phenolic, alcoholic, or carboxylic acceptors in the transfer reaction. This transfer reaction is mediated by microsomal transferase enzymes localized predominantly in the liver, but also in other tissues. Aromatic amides [125] and sulfhydryl compounds [126] can also be acceptor molecules in the transfer reaction.

The general sequence of the reactions with a substrate R<u>A</u>H can be simply represented as:

$$\alpha\text{-glucose-1-phosphate} + \text{UTP} \longrightarrow \text{UDP-glucose} + \text{PP}_i$$

$$\text{UDP-glucose} + 2\text{NAD}^+ + \text{H}_2\text{O} \xrightarrow[\text{dehydrogenase}]{\text{UDP-glucose}} \text{UDPGA} + 2\text{NADH} + 2\text{H}^+$$

$$\text{UDPGA} + \text{R}\underline{\text{A}}\text{H} \xrightarrow[\text{transferase}]{\text{glucuronyl-}} \text{R}\underline{\text{A}}\text{-glucuronic acid} + \text{UDP}$$

(<u>A</u> is part of the acceptor group and in the context here can be O, COO, NH, or S.)

Glucuronide conjugation occurs in a great variety of birds and mammals [121], in reptiles such as the alligators and snake [22], and in adult terrestrial amphibia [22,23,127,128].

The widespread distribution of this conjugation mechanism may well be related to the relatively ready availability of carbohydrate entities, the solubility of the glucuronic acids, as well as their polarity and lack of toxicity [129].

Among mammals, cats and other felines are deficient in their capacity for forming glucuronide conjugation products with exogenous compounds [130] and in many instances alternative conjugation mechanisms predominate in these species [131], although endogenous entities such as bilirubin and certain steroids can be excreted in the bile as glucuronides even in these "deficient" species [132,133].

The deficiency of glucuronidation in felines is ascribed to a lack of UDP-glucuronyltransferase activity for certain specific acceptors. It is not clear whether one transferase or a group of related transferases with varying and possibly overlapping acceptor specificities is involved in glucuronidation [129].

In terrestrial amphibia a similar situation has been recorded where hepatic UDP-glucuronyltransferase activity leads to conjugation of exogenous phenols [22,128] but not of endogenous acceptors like bilirubin [119,128].

With regard to glucuronidation in fish, certain endogenous substrates appear to be excreted as glucuronides [134-136] in some species investigated. Exogenous lipid-soluble substrates have been shown to be conjugated as glucuronides by trout liver [137,138].

Recent work with other species of fish in vivo has established that some exogenous substrates can indeed be conjugated and excreted as glucuronides [139-141].

However, there is no question that phenols appear to be unexpectedly toxic to other species of fish [22] which are unable to conjugate exogenous phenolic substrates [23,127]. Failure to form glucuronides in vivo was thought to be due to the absence of UDP-glucose dehydrogenase leading to formation of UDPGA [22] since fish liver had some microsomal glucuronyltransferase activity. There is confirmatory evidence that some of the enzyme components in the glucuronic acid pathway of glucose metabolism may be missing in fish [142].

What is not clear at this stage is whether these at times conflicting results reflect species differences in drug-metabolizing enzyme activities in the various types of fish investigated, or whether some of the results showing that conjugation may be taking place could be explained by induction of enzyme activities brought about by unknown environmental contaminants [143]. An alternative explanation may be sought in seasonal, migratory hormone-dependent salt- or freshwater adaptations [61,144,145] which could have quite profound effects on the status of drug-metabolizing activity of particular species that may be under investigation in different laboratories.

In insects, UDP-glucosyltransferase must be assumed to be involved in the detoxifying conjugations since glucosides are formed with various exogenous substrates that are conjugated as glucuronides in other species [121,146,147]. Glucoside conjugation also occurs in marine arthropods [148,149] which cannot dispose of exogenous lipid-soluble foreign compounds through their gills [23].

B. Sulfate Conjugation

The biosynthesis of sulfate ester derivatives of exogenous compounds or their phase I metabolites and of normal endogenous substrates such as steroids has been the subject of authoritative reviews [33,150-153].

The formation of an active intermediate sulfate donor molecule (3'-phosphoadenosine-5'-phosphosulfate, PAPS) and subsequent transfer of sulfate to the acceptor molecule involves the following sequence of reactions:

$$\text{ATP} + \text{SO}_4^{2-} \xrightarrow{\text{ATP sulfurylase}} \text{adenosine-5'-phosphosulfate (APS)} + \text{PP}_i$$

$$\text{ATP} + \text{APS} \xrightarrow[\text{phokinase}]{\text{APS phos-}} \text{3'-phosphoadenosine-5'-phosphosulfate (PAPS)} + \text{ADP}$$

$$\text{PAPS} + \text{R}\underline{\text{A}}\text{H} \xrightarrow[\text{transferase}]{\text{Sulfo-}} \text{R}\underline{\text{A}}\text{—SO}_3\text{H} + \text{3'-phosphoadenosine-5'-phosphate (PAP)}$$

A is part of the acceptor group and in the context here can be O or NH. Phenols, aliphatic alcohols, and certain aromatic amines may form excretable sulfate derivatives; PAP is further degraded to AMP.

It is surprising that the formation of the active intermediate, PAPS (structure II in Fig. 7), requires the transformation of a primary active intermediate, APS (structure I in Fig. 7), into a secondary active compound with further expenditure of energy as represented by the second ATP-requiring step.

It is possible that the primary active intermediate APS is a "primordial" intermediate in microorganisms engaged in the dissimulatory reduction of inorganic sulfate to sulfide [74,153]. The further phosphorylation of APS to PAPS may be related to the specific sulfate donor function of such a molecule, and the emergence of enzymes capable of catalyzing the hydrolysis of PAPS.

Enzymes hydrolyzing PAPS to PAP and transferable sulfate occur in mammalian tissues [154-157], in hen oviduct [158], and in marine mollusks [159].

The transfer of sulfate to steroidal and phenolic acceptors has received a great deal of attention particularly with regard to the presence of sulfate esters in the excreta of many types of organisms, although the specificities of the various sulfotransferases may not have been studied in detail, largely because of difficulties involved in isolation and purification of these enzymes [150,153].

Enzymes capable of transferring sulfate to phenolic acceptors are widely distributed in the animal kingdom and occur in mammalian tissues [146,160,161]. Sulfate conjugation of phenolic substrates also occurs in birds [146,162], reptiles [22,146], amphibia [22], insects [146,163], arachnids [146], and even mollusks [146,164,165].

Sulfotransferase activity with PAPS as sulfate donor and steroid as acceptor is also widespread in mammalian tissues [153], although it is recognized that enzymes of different selectivities are implicated [160,166].

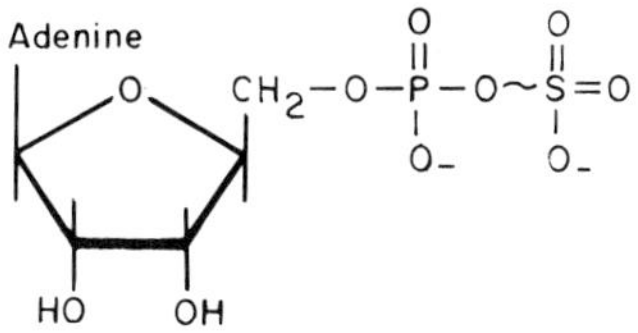

(I)

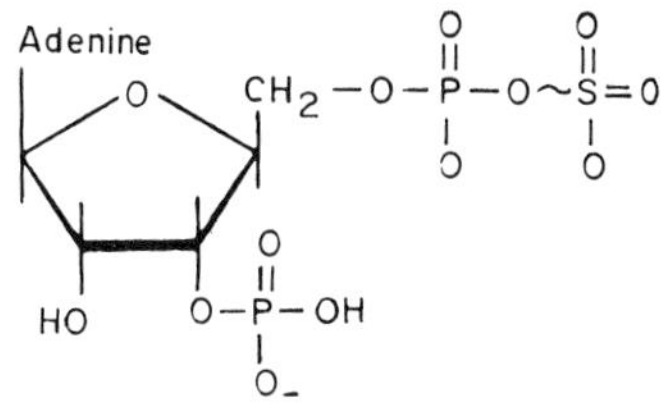

(II)

FIGURE 7 Structures of the two principal activated forms of sulfate: APS (I) and PAPS (II). (From Refs. 153a, 153b.)

While fish do not conjugate exogenous phenols as sulfates [23,127], steroid alkyl sulfates—particularly of those steroids with a primary or secondary alcohol function in the C-17 side chain—occur in the bile of various species of fish [167,169,171,172], even those as primitive and primordial as the coelacanth [168].

Sulfate salts of bile alcohols also occur in frog bile [170] and in the bile of humans [173].

Steroidal insect hormones (which will be discussed in Sec. X) yield sulfates and this type of conjugation serves as a regulatory mechanism in insect development [174-177].

From the widespread occurrence of active sulfate in nature and the transfer of sulfate to exogenous and endogenous acceptors, it can be inferred that the functional and structural integrity of various organisms ranging from anaerobic bacteria such as Desulfovibrio desulfuricans [74] to the higher mammals [152,153] depend on the integration of their sulfate status with their general metabolism.

The drug-metabolizing activity leading to the formation of sulfate conjugates is but one aspect of a phenomenon of the greatest evolutionary significance. The great hypercycles of sulfate activation and transfer [153] began to gather momentum long before they were required for maintaining cartilaginous structures [178] in vertebrates or cerebrosidal awareness [179,180] in the higher forms of life.

C. Conjugations Involving Amide Synthesis

The biosynthesis of phase II metabolites involving condensation of an amine drug ($R'—NH_2$) with a carboxylic acid, or conversely a drug containing a carboxyl group (R—COOH) with an amino acid [30,33,146], require the formation of an active intermediate involving coenzyme A. The activation system was discovered in a study of the acetylation of sulfanilamide [181].

The reactions may be represented in their most general form:

$$R{-}COOH + ATP \xrightarrow[\text{synthetase}]{\text{acyl}} R{-}CO{-}AMP + PPi$$

$$R{-}CO{-}AMP + CoA{-}SH \xrightarrow[\text{thiokinase}]{\text{acyl}} R{-}CO{-}S{-}CoA + AMP$$

$$R{-}CO{-}S{-}CoA + R'{-}NH_2 \xrightarrow{\text{transacylase}} R{-}CO{-}NHR' + CoA{-}SH$$

Amino compounds that can be acetylated tend to be aromatic amines, exogenous α-amino acids and S-arylcysteines, hydrazines, and sulfonamides.

The acetyl conjugation of sulfonamides has been shown to occur in different tissues of various species of mammals [30,146] and in birds [30]. Species differences in acetylation among the higher vertebrates are in part explained by deacetylating enzymes occurring in liver and kidney [182-184], although there appears to be considerable substrate selectivity in amines for the types of compounds that can be acetylated [33,146].

Toads and tree frogs can acetylate exogenous aromatic amino compounds [185]. Fish also have this capacity [139,186].

Among invertebrates, insects can acetylate exogenous amine substrates [187-189].

In the converse reaction involving aromatic or heterocyclic exogenous carboxylic drugs, amide formation takes place by conjugation with endogenous glycine in most mammalian species. The active intermediate in these reactions is the activated exogenous acid which is then transacylated according to the overall reaction sequence shown above.

Conjugations with glycine also occur in pigeons, in reptiles, and in certain amphibia [146], but the conjugation with other endogenous amino acids is well documented.

Conjugation with glutamine has been shown to occur in humans and nonhuman primates, particularly with exogenous carboxylic acids related to phenylacetic acid [190-194]. In these primate species, a characteristic acylating enzyme in liver and kidney tissue facilitates the particular glutamine conjugation [195].

In reptiles [146,196] and birds such as hens, ducks, turkeys, and geese, administered carboxylic acids were conjugated with ornithine [197].

In studies with the isomeric aminobenzoic acids in chickens [198], administration of these compounds in vivo gave rise to urinary ornithine conjugates, some glucuronide conjugates, and N-acetyl derivatives. Incubations of these substrates with liver tissue gave rise to ornithine conjugates and some N-acetylated products. When the aminobenzoates were injected into egg yolk before incubation of fertilized eggs, N-acetylation conjugates were detected before ornithine conjugates developmentally.

This type of study helps to establish some kind of primordial sequence in conjugation reactions. In view of the critical importance of coenzyme A as a two-carbon group carrier in intermediary metabolism and in initiation of the tricarboxylic acid cycle [199] in the oxidative breakdown of fatty acids and other biosynthetic processes, it is not altogether surprising that exogenous compounds can interact with such important intermediates in the early metabolic pool during development.

However, the true significance of ornithine conjugation in some types of reptiles and birds has not yet been satisfactorily explained. What is clear is that amphibia only conjugate exogenous carboxylic acid with glycine. Since uric acid is an end product of nitrogen metabolism in birds and in reptiles, and biosynthesis of uric acid involves glycine as a precursor, it is conceivable that alternative phase II conjugation/detoxication mechanisms were thrown into prominence in nature's selection experiments [146,196]. Having considered this, it is nonetheless equally true that not all species of birds can form ornithine conjugates with appropriate test compounds [200]. Taurine conjugation appears to be a replacement pathway in birds which do not metabolize exogenous carboxylic acids with ornithine [201,202].

D. Mercapturic Acid Formation

Mercapturic acids are N-acetylcysteine conjugates found as metabolites of exogenous organic compounds. The biosynthetic pathway leading to these derivatives and the types of compounds which are second substrates for glutathione S-transferase have been comprehensively reviewed quite recently [203-205].

The overall scheme in mercapturic acid formation in rodents can be represented as shown in Fig. 8. It is recognized that those compounds undergoing metabolic conversion to mercapturic acids are first conjugated with glutathione by glutathione S-transferases which are known to have distinctive but broadly overlapping substrate selectivities [206]. The terminal amino acids of the S-conjugated glutathione are removed sequentially by enzymes which have been found to be abundant in kidney microsomal preparations [207,208]. The cysteine derivatives are then acetylated as described in the previous section through the intervention of an "active intermediate," acetyl-CoA [209,210].

The types of exogenous organic compounds that serve as substrates for the glutathione S-transferase [204,205] include halogenated nitrobenzenes and polycyclic hydrocarbon epoxides.

With regard to polycyclic hydrocarbons which are metabolized via epoxides in the so-called K region [211], the bile of rats given naphthalene [212], phenanthrene [213,214], or benzanthracene [215] contained the hydroxymercapturic acids as well as the cysteine, cysteinylglycine, and glutathione

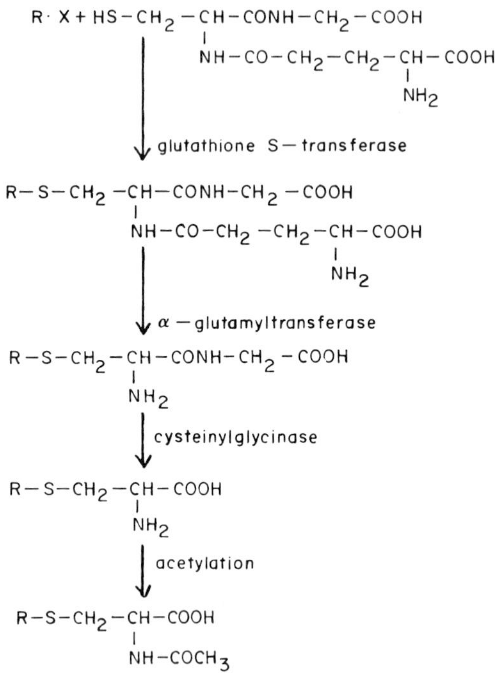

FIGURE 8 Stages in the formation of mercapturic acid conjugates upon interaction of substrate R·X and glutathione (see Ref. 205).

conjugates of the respective polycyclic hydrocarbon epoxides, which provided convincing evidence for the reaction sequence in mercapturic acid synthesis.

Figure 9 shows the pathways of phenanthrene metabolism in the rat [214], which has since been expanded and confirmed by studies of the metabolism of the key intermediate, 9,10-epoxy-9,10-dihydrophenanthrene [216], which proved beyond all doubt that epoxides were intermediates in the metabolism of polycyclic hydrocarbons leading to mercapturic acid formation.

Since epoxides serve as substrates for the glutathione S-transferase system, it was of interest that the insecticide dieldrin, a stable epoxide, could not be metabolized further by mammalian enzyme preparations [217] or by insects [218].

Other exogenous substrates for the glutathione S-transferase system are various halogenated nitrobenzenes [204] which depending on the number of halogen atoms in the molecule may display an otherwise rare type of aromatic dehalogenation:

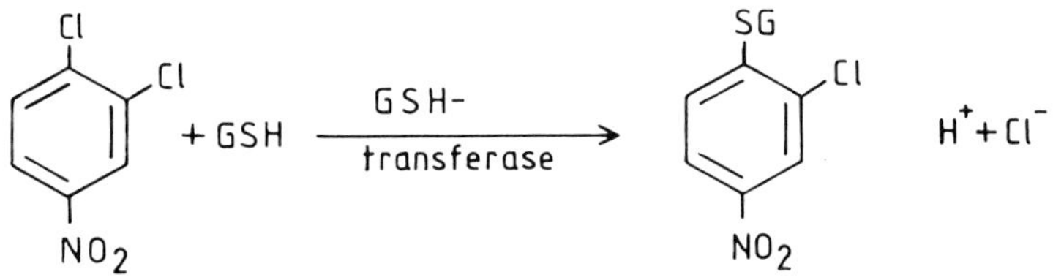

This reaction takes place in the soluble fraction of mammalian, avian, reptilian, and amphibian liver under appropriate conditions [219-222].

Moreover, insects such as locusts and houseflies [223,224] can conjugate this type of substrate.

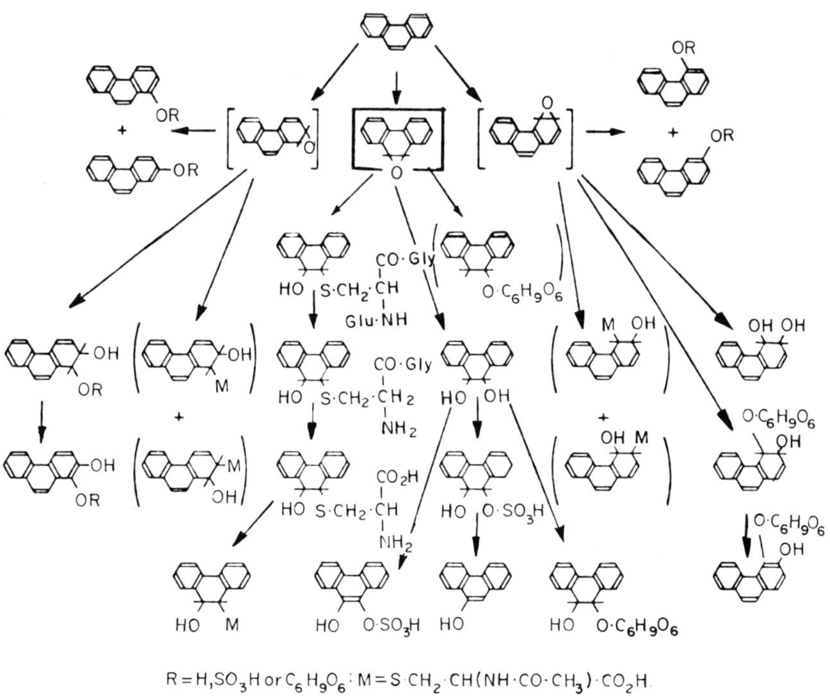

FIGURE 9 Pathways of phenanthrene metabolism in the rat showing hypothetical epoxide intermediates (in square brackets). One of these epoxides (heavy outline) subsequently became available for a study of its metabolism [216]; the general scheme of mercapturic acid and hydroxymercapturic acid formation, as well as the formation of other metabolites via respective intermediates, were thus elegantly confirmed. (From Ref. 214.)

It is all the more surprising, therefore, that insects are unable to metabolize heptachlor epoxide [225] or dieldrin [218] further. It is more surprising still when it is realized that the glutathione S-transferase activity (measured with chlorocyclohexene breakdown products of gammexane as second substrates) is induced in dieldrin-resistant strains of houseflies [226]. These matters will be discussed further in sections dealing more specifically with drug-metabolizing enzyme activities in insects (Sec. X) and with the cumulation in the environment of unmetabolizable compounds, many of which are inducers of the drug-metabolizing enzymes (Sec. XI).

It has recently become clear that the glutathione S-transferases have unexpectedly wide distribution in different mammalian tissues, and in addition they are widely distributed in the animal kingdom [205]. The biological importance of the mercapturic acid conjugation system looks as if it may be primarily related to a strategy for preventing potentially harmful exogenous compounds and their active phase I intermediate metabolites from binding to cellular macromolecules (see Fig. 2).

VII. FISH, DRUG METABOLISM, AND HORMONE REGULATION

Many of the pathways of drug metabolism have now been considered, and some patterns have begun to emerge of how the various drug-metabolizing enzyme capabilities are distributed in species of varying complexity on the evolutionary scale. In order to clarify some evolutionary concepts in terms of drug metabolism, certain well-defined groups in the animal kingdom will be discussed separately, with particular reference to hormonal factors.

Attention has already been drawn to some of the conflicting data obtained in drug metabolism studies with different species of fish. In a sense this is hardly surprising since there are over 30,000 species of fish [62], only a few of which have been studied at all methodically.

In drug metabolism studies with mammals, factors that are likely to influence the overall metabolic transformation of exogenous lipid-soluble compounds are known, and in consequence are taken into consideration. These factors would include age, strain, sex, general hormonal and nutritional status of a species that is being studied, and such environmental factors as real or simulated seasonal variation.

In corresponding studies with fish, relatively little attention has been paid to such important biochemical parameters.

Quite apart from the general needs for food, maintaining contact with their own species, and escaping from predators, fish have to be able to adapt to changes in the degree of salinity and of temperature in their habitat, and they must be able to respond to such environmental cues as change of light intensity and pressure.

Most fish species are restricted to spending their lives in waters within a quite limited range of salinity. They may be adapted for a freshwater or a marine existence. Other species are capable of seasonal migrations connected with their reproductive cycles. Examples readily come to mind. Salmon migrate from salt water to fresh water, and eels migrate from fresh water to a marine environment for spawning.

The hormonal influences that regulate osmotic balance in fish are now reasonably well understood. The dominant factor in fresh water adaptation appears to be prolactin [60,144,227,228], while cortisol affects all the osmoregulatory organs of fish for adaptation to seawater [145,229,230]. These respective influences are compared in Table 1.

The balance of prolactin- and corticosteroid-mediated effects may be liable to seasonal adjustments and these lead to migratory movement and anatomical as well as biochemical adaptations.

There are changes in thyroid activity which are associated with migratory movements of fish [231-235]. These thyroid changes are not primarily related to, or interacting with, prolactin-mediated effects in osmoregulation. Fish thus differ in important respects from the higher vertebrates such as the amphibia [63] (see discussion in Sec. VIII) and mammals [60,61].

It may well be that thyroid hormone activity in fish primarily determines the stimulation of certain cellular functions concerned with the basal metabolic rate [236,237] which facilitate adjustments to changes in environmental temperature or to generalized activity in major migrations. There is, however, another feature of thyroid hormone activity in fish which is concerned with biochemical metamorphosis, particularly with reference to visual pigments [238,239] and changes in hemoglobin [240].

The interrelationship of rhodopsin and porphyropsin visual pigments based respectively on $retinal_1$ and $retinal_2$ [241,242], the oxidized forms of retinols found respectively in livers of marine and freshwater fishes (Fig. 10), have important implications for evolutionary development [241]. What has to be assumed is that even in fish and especially in migratory fish or deep-sea species, oxidative and reductive NADH- and possibly NADPH-dependent [243] metabolic pathways exist which permit the subtle adaptations of retinol (vitamin A) metabolism [242] to the needs of the organism at any particular season, and to the primordial requirements at the spawning sites whether these be freshwater or marine.

Wald [241] recognized the unities of metamorphosis in vertebrates and realized that what land was to the frog, the sea was to the salmon. Since thyroid hormones probably play a significant role in the seaward migration of freshwater fish, and since freshwater adaptation is predominantly under the influence of prolactin, it might be expected that marine species have a higher drug-metabolizing capability than freshwater species of fish [63].

TABLE 1
Influences of Prolactin and Cortisol in Fish[a]

Target organ	Cortisol	Prolactin
Gills	Increased Na permeability; increased Na influx in FW and efflux in SW (increased Na pump, Na,K-ATPase); increased water permeability (Pos)	Decreased Na permeability; decreased Na pump (Na,K-ATPase); Na retention (increased Na pump), when given with cortisol; decreased water permeability (Pos)
Intestine	Increased NaCl and water absorption (increased Cl pump, PNa, PCl, Pos, Na,K-ATPase, HCO_3-ATPase)	Decreased NaCl and water absorption (decreased Cl pump, PNa or Pos?)
Kidney	Antinatriuresis (increased Na pump, Na,K-ATPase)	Diuresis (decreased Pos?); increased Na pump (Na,K-ATPase)
Urinary bladder	Increased water absorption (increased Na pump, Pos)	Decreased water absorption (decreased Pos); increased Na pump (Na,K-ATPase, synergism with cortisol?)

[a] Prolactin is a "broad-spectrum" anterior pituitary hormone with wide-ranging effects in vertebrates [60]. Among the actions of prolactin are those that regulate osmolarity in freshwater-adapted fish. Cortisol appears to act as an antagonist to prolactin, and fish are prepared for seawater adaptation under the influence of this corticosteroid. These influences and counterinfluences affect all the organs involved in hydromineral balance [145].
Key: FW = fresh water; SW = seawater; PNa = permeability for Na^+; PCl = permeability for Cl^-; Pos = osmotic permeability.
Source: Adapted from Ref. 145.

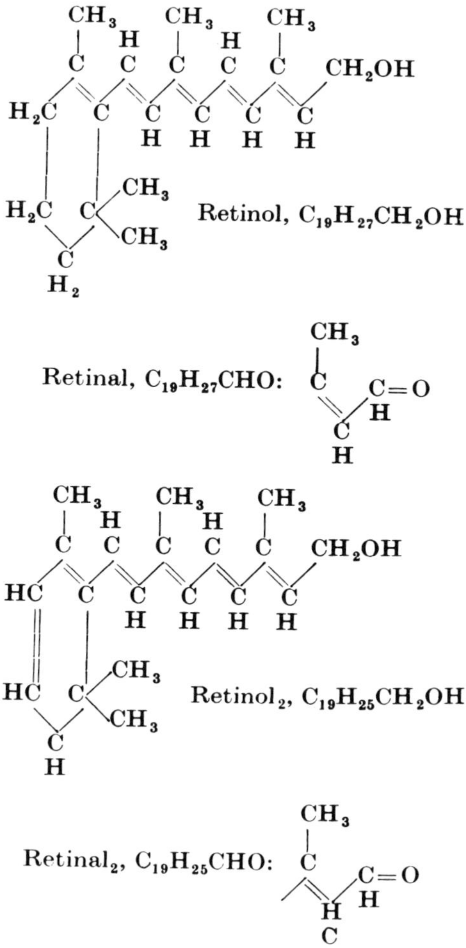

FIGURE 10 Formulas of retinol and the corresponding aldehyde retinal$_1$ showing how these are related to retinol$_2$ and retinal$_2$. The implications for eye pigment formation (and drug metabolism) in marine- and freshwater-adapted fish are discussed in the text. (From Ref. 242.)

Studies on intact freshwater fish exposed to various lipid-soluble exogenous drugs and chemicals under defined conditions [22],244] showed that in many instances drugs which are not appreciably bound by tissue proteins distribute evenly between fish and surrounding water.

Furthermore, regardless of what may or may not be found in terms of drug-metabolizing enzyme activity in vitro with subcellular fractions from liver or other organs appropriately fortified, various methoxytriazines and phenyl ureas were highly toxic to five different species of freshwater fish [244]. In extension of the same series of tests, Bathe et al. [244] found as shown in Table 2 that different species of freshwater fish differed in their sensitivity to a selection of phosphorus and carbamate insecticides, but were almost equally sensitive to pp'-DDT which accumulated in the tissues.

Compounds which do not accumulate and which are not specifically neurotoxic will tend to diffuse from the fish unchanged [22]. This supports the original idea [22,23] that the oxidative xenobiotic-metabolizing enzyme systems disposing of lipid-soluble foreign compounds were developed in species or with species that could not dialyze such compounds through the lipid membranes of gill or skin. Furthermore, since this type of experiment is conducted on species of fish adapted for a freshwater existence under the predominant influence of prolactin, as we have just seen, little if any drug-metabolizing enzyme activity is to be expected [63]. However, it is well documented that hepatic subcellular fractions obtained from various marine species, when incubated under appropriate fortified conditions, have azo-reductase [57] and nitro-reductase [58] activities. This reducing capability may be an extension of the preexisting capability for reducing the series of retinol$_2$-retinal$_2$ compounds to the corresponding dihydro compounds that contribute to the characteristic visual pigments in marine species of fish.

In view of the corticosteroid mediation to saltwater physiological adaptation in fish, it is not surprising that various in vitro preparations have been shown to oxidatively metabolize steroid substrates [135,245].

Pohl et al. [245a] have looked into the in vitro oxidative drug-metabolizing enzyme activity of a number of marine species of fish, and detected limited hydroxylation and dealkylation of various substrates, which did not respond appreciably to the usual inducing substances known to affect mammalian liver microsomal drug-metabolizing activity. Even dogfish shark which upon removal from their marine environment were shown to have accumulated polychlorobiphenyls in their tissues [246] had relatively little oxidative drug-metabolizing activity demonstrable in metabolic studies in vitro, and could not metabolize administered ^{14}C-pentachlorobiphenyl.

Results with a freshwater fish, the brook trout, were even more decisive [25]. When the metabolism of certain isomeric chlorobiphenyls was compared in trout, pigeon, and rat in vivo and the excreta examined (Fig. 11) for metabolites, it was found that the rodent and avian species could hydroxylate 4-chloro-, 4,4'-dichloro-, and 2,2',5,5'-tetrachlorobiphenyl as shown, but the trout could not. No 2,4,5,2',4',5'-hexachlorobiphenyl metabolites were detected in the rat, pigeon, or trout. The whole question of unmetabolizable lipid-soluble exogenous compounds will be discussed in Sec. XI, for these cumulative isomers have grave implications for the survival of terrestrial species [17,64].

TABLE 2

Results of Acute Fish Toxicity Studies in Different Freshwater Species Exposed to Various Insecticides and to Acetone

Substance	Solubility in water	Exposure (hr)	LC_{50} (ppm) Trout	Crucian carp	Catfish	Perch	Guppy
Phosphamidon (Dimicron 100): O-(2-chloro-2-diethylcarbamoyl-1-methyl-vinyl)O, O-dimethylphosphate	Miscible	48	20	650	360	200	100
		96	20	600	360	150	54
Diazinon (Basudin 60 EC): O, O-diethyl O-(2-isopropyl-6-methyl-4-pyrimidinyl) phosphorothioate	Active ingr.	48	8	5	8	—	6
	40 ppm	96	8	5	8	—	3
GS 13005 (Supracide 40 EC): O, O-dimethyl s-[5-methoxy-2-oxo-1, 3, 4-thiadiazol-3(2H)-ylmethyl]-phosphorodithioate	Active ingr.	48	0.08	30	30	—	0.5
	240 ppm	96	0.08	30	30	—	0.06
CGA 13608: 2-(methylpropargyl-amino)-phenylmethylcarbamate	850 ppm	48	0.16	10	7	0.8	—
		96	0.16	9	5	0.6	—
p, p'-DDT WHO-standard	Approx.	48	0.030	0.030	> 0.080	0.030	0.040
	0.02 ppm	96	0.028	0.025	0.038	0.015	0.037
Acetone	∞	48	8,000	12,000	16,000	11,000	10,000
	Soluble	96	8,000	12,000	16,000	11,000	5,600

Source: Adapted from Ref. 244.

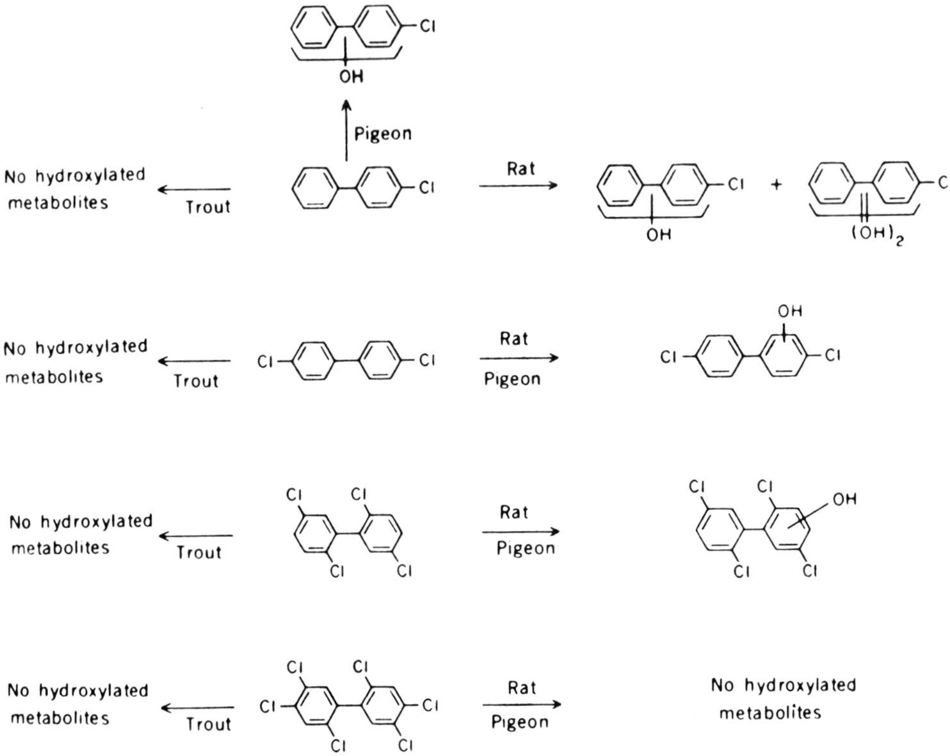

FIGURE 11 Scheme for the metabolic biotransformation of pure isomers of the various chlorinated biphenyls shown in rat, pigeon, and brook trout in vivo. Rat and pigeon can oxidatively metabolize the mono-, di-, and tetra-substituted isomers, but fail to metabolize 2,4,5,2',4',5'-hexachlorobiphenyl. Brook trout does not metabolize any of the chlorinated biphenyls. (From Ref. 25, © 1972 by the American Association for the Advancement of Science.)

What seems to have escaped general attention in applying criteria of mammalian drug metabolism to fish, even in reviews which set out to catalog whatever was ever attempted in terms of drug metabolism in vitro in various species of fish [59], is an application of the careful standards that operate in studies with mammals where hormonal and environmental factors are controlled.

It should be possible to select a migratory species of fish and compare the freshwater-adapted with the marine-adapted phase, and to manipulate the hormone status either by surgical intervention or by treatments with prolactin, corticosteroids, and possibly thyroid hormones or one of the retinols to optimize conditions, especially for studying reductive pathways of drug metabolism. It should then be possible to rationalize drug metabolism studies in fish. It would be predictable that the marine form of the species would show higher drug-reducing activity than its freshwater-adapted seasonal variant. This prediction is based on effects that prolactin might exert not only on the general physiology of fish and various biochemical parameters attendant on membrane permeability [60,61,144], but on possible prolactin-directed inhibitory effects on drug metabolism [63] which need further investigation.

In general evolutionary terms, prolactin would facilitate the excretion of lipid-soluble compounds through lipoidal membranes.

It is remarkable that the hormones so vital in initiating and supporting milk secretion in mammals—prolactin and corticosteroids [60]—should be the same that regulate osmoregulation in fish tissues. Since lipid-soluble drugs can be excreted via the milk [247], it is no surprise that lipid-soluble exogenous compounds can be excreted unchanged in freshwater fish [22,23].

VIII. AMPHIBIA, THYROXINE, AND PROLACTIN

It is important at this stage to reconsider the question of drug-metabolizing activity in amphibia in the general context of hormonal regulation of metamorphosis [63,64].

Although tadpoles of toads and of frogs did not metabolize exogenous drug substrates by functionalization or conjugation reactions [23,127], the adult forms of toads could metabolize some exogenous test substrates [23] but not apparently by the same mechanisms as mammals [22]. Adult toads and some frogs that were terrestrially adapted could conjugate exogenous phenolic compounds [22,23,128].

Clearly something has happened in terms of a biochemical metamorphosis accompanying the physical metamorphosis, which led to the development or acquisition of a drug-metabolizing capability. How is this brought about?

It has to be admitted that the biochemistry of amphibian metamorphosis has been studied more methodically with respect to other parameters such as visual pigments and hemoglobin characteristics [241,248], nitrogen excretion patterns [249-252], protein synthesis [253] and morphogenic determinants [254]. It has been established in studies with those biochemical, enzymatic parameters and with observations on the overt physical signs of amphibian metamorphosis that the so-called terrestrial drive of amphibia could be induced or accelerated by thyroid hormones [63,253,254] and impeded by chemical inhibitors of thyroid hormone action [254-256].

It was also recognized that prolactin exerted a juvenilizing effect on tadpoles [60,257,258] which overcame the terrestrial drive induced by thyroxine, and in effect led to the prolongation of the larval aquatic phase of growth. Furthermore, prolactin induced a secondary metamorphosis in some adult, terrestrially adapted amphibia, enabling them to pursue an "aquatic drive" leading to a return to a watery environment for breeding and spawning [60,259-261]. What is remarkable is that the primary thyroid-hormone-induced physical [259] and biochemical metamorphosis [262] of amphibia can be inhibited by prolactin, a hormone which could be considered as a special kind of larval growth factor [263,264]. Not only that, the secondary prolactin-induced metamorphosis in the red-spotted newt or "red eft" is correspondingly inhibited by thyroxine [259,265].

From the evolutionary point of view, the realization that hormones obtained from mammalian sources have such profound morphological and biochemical effects on lower vertebrates undergoing metamorphosis is astonishing.

Thyroxine and its closely related natural congeners, the "terrestrial drive" thyroid hormones [237,253,266-29] and prolactin [60,61,258,270], are "broad-spectrum" hormones which have tissue-specific but nonetheless very varied biochemical activities in different target organs of vertebrates.

For example, in major reviews on the known biochemical and physiological actions of prolactin [60,61] there are well-documented effects on growth, on reproduction, on osmoregulation and membrane permeabilities, on amphibian metamorphosis, on ectodermal structures, on synergism with steroids and antagonistic but nonetheless coordinated interaction with thyroid hormones. Moreover, there are parental behavioral effects which appear to be well synchronized with mammary development and antigonadal stimuli in mammals. These latter properties are well illustrated by the work of Renfree [271] with marsupials.

The point that has to be made, since it is not stressed sufficiently in previous reviews, is that prolactin has effects in mammals on the estrous cycle, lactation, mammary development, and other manifestations of the "eternally feminine" principle, and yet the hormone has primarily osmoregulatory effects on fish [62,145] and characteristic effects on primary and secondary metamorphosis in amphibia [258].

This means that the hormone had a relatively primordial existence in the "generalized unicellular vertebrate" long before the specific mammalian target tissues for its biological expression had evolved. In terms of homology, human prolactin polypeptide [272] has considerable regional homology of amino acid sequences with human growth hormone and with sheep prolactin [273,274].

Conservation of homologies has to be invoked to account for the response to mammalian hormones in amphibia, and the presumed response of mammals to amphibian prolactin.

The arguments with respect to thyroid hormones are less complex since the molecules are identical and simpler thanks to "the accidental chemical affinity of tyrosine for iodine" [258] in a marine environment, and the incorporation of these derivatives into the life processes at the cellular level when primordial vertebrates shifted to fresh water and to terrestrial habitats.

Steroids were already committed in fish, as we have discussed in a previous section, and the balance of prolactin and steroid hormones merely helped to guide the seasonal migrations of these aquatic vertebrates to habitats with different salinities [62].

The tyrosine-sequestered iodine, in the event, acquired the function of a definitive cue for the emergence of terrestrial vertebrates. It is possible that circumstances were governed by the light sensitivity of flavin-catalyzed reactions involving iodotyrosines [275,276] which would be instrumental in reflecting environmental circumstances.

The thyroid hormones are known to stimulate drug-metabolizing enzymes under certain circumstances [124,277-279] and themselves are known to undergo metabolic transformations as substrates for these enzymes in terrestrial vertebrates [280,281]. Therefore, the development of drug-metabolizing enzyme activity in metamorphozing amphibia ought to be correlated with thyroid-hormone dependent effects. A detailed study with drug-metabolizing enzyme activity ought to be conducted in metamorphozing amphibia, by analogy with other work [255,256,259], on thyroid-mediated effects on levels of urea cycle enzymes in tadpoles.

An incidental finding of such a study is likely to be the recognition that prolactin, the juvenilizing hormone which promotes growth without differentiation in tadpoles, actually inhibits drug-metabolizing enzyme activity. Indeed, it is already known that tadpoles do not oxidatively metabolize or subsequently conjugate exogenous test compounds [22,23].

What has to be remembered when predictions like this are made is that although prolactin and thyroid hormones act respectively to inhibit and promote metamorphosis, the antagonism between these hormones does not operate at all levels during tadpole development [264,282]. This is probably because secretion and control of prolactin release [267,283] and the regulation of thyroid hormone metabolism [268] in higher vertebrates, complex though they may be, are nonetheless mediated by the same small centrally acting peptide, thyrotropin-releasing hormone (TRH), which is surprisingly nonspecific in that respect [284].

IX. AVIAN SPECIES

There are more than 8000 species of birds [285], which differ greatly among themselves developmentally, behaviorally, and in their seasonal adjustments to diet and habitat. Less than 100 species have been studied at all systematically with respect to metabolism of drugs, environmental chemicals, and pesticides [162,222]. However, a great deal has been learned from research with chickens, pigeons, and quails in particular [22,123,162,286] which taken in conjunction with more sporadic and incidental studies on other species [222] allow for certain tentative generalizations to be made.

Birds appear to be capable in varying degrees of all the major functionalization and conjugation biotransformations. Species differences appear to be quantitative rather than qualitative [162] except for certain distinctive conjugation reactions [200, 201]. Birds have been shown to metabolize a very wide range of experimentally administered lipid-soluble xenobiotics [162]. Furthermore, liver microsomal preparations from avian species can metabolize a variety of drug substrates under NADPH- and O_2-dependent conditions [22, 286-289].

As with mammals [280, 290], steroid hormones are natural endogenous substrates for the drug-metabolizing enzymes also in birds [291-293]. Their metabolism in birds is stimulated by pretreatment with, or exposure to, polychlorinated hydrocarbon inducers [24] that have become part of the global ecosystem [294-296]. What may be involved for a particular species of bird is illustrated in Table 3, which shows that the inducing effects on the metabolism of endogenous steroids in pigeons brought about by two different chlorinated hydrocarbon insecticides may be additive or synergistic [294]. Pretreatment of chickens or ducks with dieldrin or pp'-DDT also selectively induced liver microsomal drug-metabolizing activity with respect to various exogenous test substrates [297, 298].

When fed to laying birds over a period covering seasonal egg production, these inducers reduced eggshell thickness [299]. Reduction of eggshell thickness and correspondingly diminished hatching success is also a feature

TABLE 3
Respective Increases in ^{14}C-Testosterone or ^{14}C-Progesterone Metabolism in Male and Female Pigeon Liver Microsomal Preparations[a]

	Amount of polar metabolites formed (nmol)	
	Testosterone	Progesterone
Control	28.7 ± 4.7 (8)	30.1 ± 8.4 (8)
DDT	75.4 ± 18.0 (6)	78.3 ± 8.4 (6)
Dieldrin	111.4 ± 12.7 (6)	90.3 ± 6.1 (6)
DDT + dieldrin	168.2 ± 9.9 (4)	155.4 ± 17.8 (4)

[a] Microsomal preparations were from control birds and from others that had ingested predetermined amounts of pp'-DDT and/or dieldrin added to their feed. The mean and the standard deviation are given with the number of birds shown in parentheses. In all cases 500 nmol of labeled substrate was present, incubation time was 30 min, and weight of microsomal fraction used was 300 mg.
Source: Data from Ref. 294.

of wild bird reproduction affected by exposure to persistent chlorinated hydrocarbons in the environment [300]. These facts draw attention to important differences between avian and mammalian drug-metabolizing capability.

They also serve as warnings, for such unexpected lesions and as yet incompletely understood biochemical aberrations in the reproductive cycle of wild birds [300,301] have brought about a sudden and timely awareness of the deterioration of the environment through chemicals. These, despite their inducing effects on the drug-metabolizing enzymes [24,294], accumulate in vertebrate tissues and interfere with vital functions. Pigeon liver preparations fortified with an NADPH-generating system can metabolize aldrin to dieldrin [302-304], and the oxidative metabolism in vivo of specific mono-, di-, and tetrachlorobiphenyls in pigeons is well documented [25] (Fig. 11). Here again, though, there is an awareness that the higher terrestrial (or aerial) vertebrates cannot metabolize certain lipophilic substrates. Reference to Fig. 11 will show that neither the pigeon nor the rat could oxidatively metabolize 2,4,5,2',4',5'-hexachlorobiphenyl.

The metabolic biotransformation of pp'-DDT has also been studied in detail in nonlaying chicks [305] and a whole range of metabolites has been identified (Fig. 12). Yet despite the fact that polychlorinated biphenyls, dieldrin, and pp'-DDT induce drug-metabolizing enzyme activities in birds, polychlorinated biphenyls accumulated in the tissues of pigeons [306,307] and dieldrin and pp'-DDT tended to accumulate in adipose tissues of hens fed diets containing these insecticides [308], while Ludke [309] found that one of the metabolites of pp'-DDT, namely, pp'-DDE, accumulated in the tissues of quail treated with both dieldrin and pp'-DDT.

What is particularly well documented and what must be regarded as a major sex difference in drug-metabolizing capability of all species of birds is that female laying birds have the opportunity for excreting lipid-soluble exogenous compounds into their eggs [24,300,310-315]. Since fertilized eggs develop as closed systems independently of the circulation of the mother birds, it is of obvious interest to determine how development proceeds with a burden of lipid-soluble exogenous contaminants.

When the developmental aspects of avian phase I drug-metabolizing enzyme activity [22,286,316] and glucuronide formation [123,317,318] are compared with those of more usually investigated mammalian species [22, 58,63,319,320], they are seen to differ in important respects.

Liver microsomal preparations from chick embryos have prehatching competence to perform oxidative drug metabolism [22,286,321]. Conjugations with sulfate [322] and glucuronic acid of acceptors such as ortho-aminophenol [318] have also been demonstrated before hatching. After hatching, there is a surge of oxidative drug-metabolizing activity [286] and newly hatched chicks have the highest capacity for oxidatively metabolizing lipid-soluble drug substrates, as shown in Fig. 13. This elevated capacity gradually declines toward the 7-day posthatching levels, which more closely resemble the adult capacity.

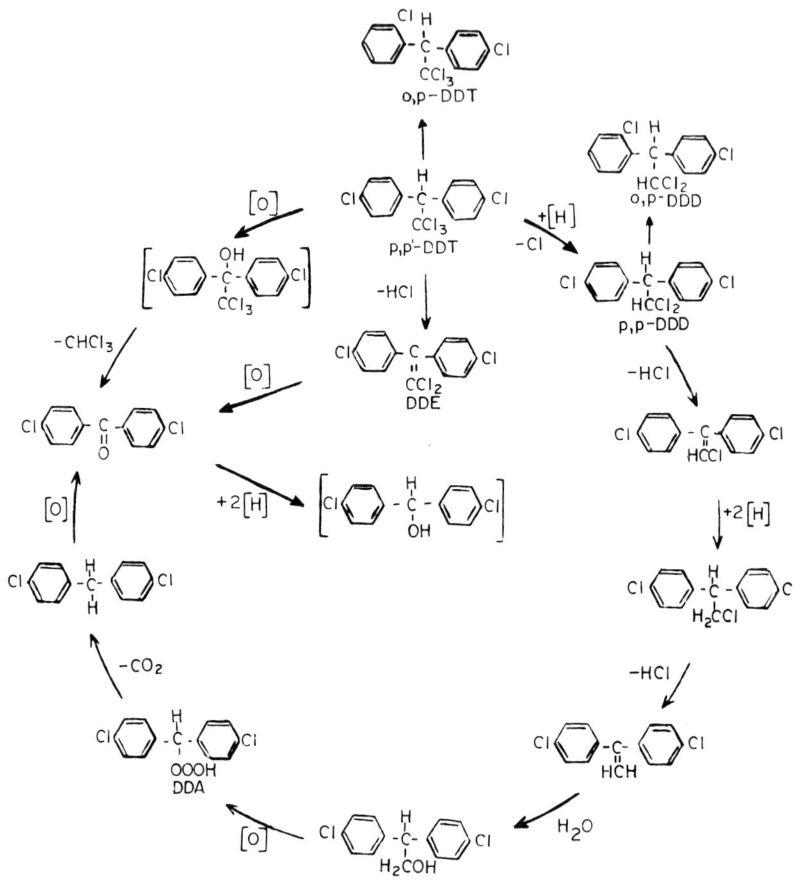

FIGURE 12 Metabolic pathways of pp'-DDT in chicks. (From Ref. 305.)

The absorption of the residual yolk possibly containing endogenous inducers as well as food reserves, as the chicks hatch, may contribute to the surge of drug-metabolizing activity in the newly hatched bird [286].

In birds incubated from fertile eggs injected with pp'-DDT or pp'-DDE [288], the oxidative liver microsomal drug-metabolizing activity was greater than that of corresponding preparations from chicks hatched from control eggs. Whereas pp'-DDT can be metabolized by the chick [305] to various polar metabolites as shown in Fig. 12, dieldrin is a greater burden since this is a stable epoxide which merely induces the metabolism of other drugs and exogenous chemicals.

Dieldrin injected into fertilized eggs [323] does not prevent the development of chicks, but on hatching and resorbing the yolk, the chick acquires a burden of lipid-soluble exogenous inducing substance which will affect its steroid metabolism [294] and neurological condition particularly when temporarily deprived of feeding opportunities [323]. Under those conditions the blood levels of the unmetabolizable inducer, dieldrin, continue to rise, as the chick uses up its nutritional reserves in the resorbed residual egg yolk (Fig. 14). The passage of chlorinated lipophilic environmental chemicals from mother bird to egg [297,314,324] obviously puts the survival of the next generation at risk.

However, by sharing the exogenous compound burden with several of the progeny which upon hatching have the highest xenobiotic-metabolizing activity, the arrangements of nature could be interpreted as benign attempts at trying to ensure the survival of the survivors under existential circumstances.

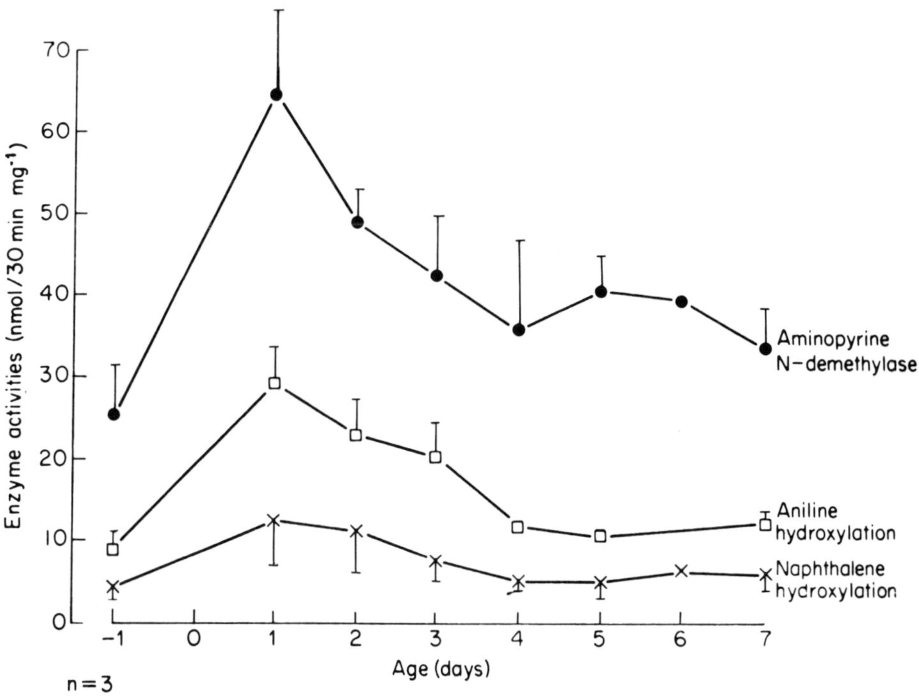

FIGURE 13 Oxidative drug-metabolizing enzyme activity of liver microsomal preparations obtained from female chicks ranging in age from 1 to 7 days, and from embryos on the day before hatching. The elevation of the drug-metabolizing activity in incubations with the three substrates shown corresponds to a peaking in the neonatal NADPH-cytochrome P-450 reductase activity but is not associated with any fluctuations in microsomal cytochrome b_5 or cytochrome P-450 content. (From Ref. 286.)

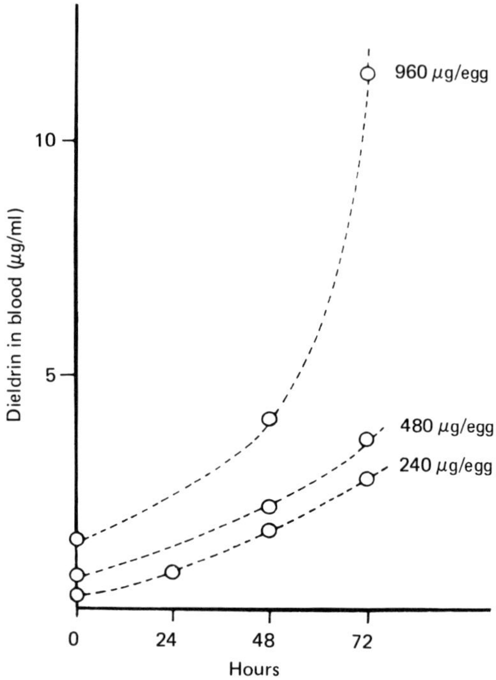

FIGURE 14 Concentrations of dieldrin in the blood in starved chicks newly hatched from eggs dosed with various amounts of dieldrin before incubation. As the chicks live off the food resource of the resorbed egg yolk, the blood levels of unmetabolizable dieldrin rise. (Data from Ref. 323.)

X. INSECTS

A. Insects and the Higher Vertebrates

In the previous discussion on birds, an attempt was made to assess the effects of various environmental chemicals including chlorinated hydrocarbon insecticides on the drug-metabolizing capabilities of nontarget species. It is now necessary to discuss drug metabolism in insects in some detail, with particular reference to the characteristic hormonal regulation of insect development.

It may be unwise to generalize about more than 700,000 species of insects [285] which have successfully colonized the biosphere. The diversity implicit in these numbers leads to caution when scientific data from one species are extrapolated to others. The variety of habitats and life cycles often complicated by metamorphosing changes during development nonetheless point to some characteristic biochemical features of insect organization and homeostatic control.

The recognition of some of these features [325,326] has enabled scientists to diminish the impact of insect disease vectors and undesirable agricultural competitors by devising selective toxicants for their control [102,327-330]. These selective toxicants in effect create desperate biochemical conditions, from which, more often than not, resistant strains of insects emerge [331,332].

The taxonomic gulf between insects and the higher vertebrates is reflected in the composition of hemolymph [326,333] where proline plays a role as an extra energy source, and together with other small organic molecules contributes to osmoregulation [326].

The integument of insects is of great interest developmentally. Its formation is dependent on distinctive characteristics of tyrosine metabolism [334-336]. Some of the features of this distinctive tyrosine metabolism leading to chitinous exocuticle formation is under the activator control of ecdysone [326,337], as is the development of the fat body [338], the hub of insect metabolism which determines the physiological activity of the other tissues. Other, inhibitory features of developmental control of insects are exercized by juvenile hormones [337].

Another characteristic feature of insect biochemistry is the inability to synthesize the steroid skeleton from precursors such as mevalonate [330, 337,339,340]. Insects require exogenous sources of preformed steroids from plant sources or from symbiotic organisms. Precursors such as sitosterol, camposterol, stigmasterol, or cholesterol, however, can be metabolized by insects to ecdysone [339-341].

Important in their own right, but of more interest in the past from the point of view of selective insecticide development, are the characteristics of the insect nervous system [102,342] and of the volatile chemical communication system that orientates different species of insects with respect to aggregation [343-347], food plants [348-352], and predator threats [353].

B. Insects and the Range of Drug Metabolism

The detoxication mechanisms which tend to convert relatively nonpolar lipid-soluble drugs, environmental chemicals, or endogenous hormonal substrates into more polar excretable forms are present in insects. Insects also have organs appropriate for the filtration and subsequent concentration of the metabolites [147] which are compatible with the water conservation priorities of terrestrial as opposed to aquatic life.

The characteristics of insect monooxygenase reactions in vitro have been worked out and reviewed in considerable detail [66,117,354, 355] for some of the more readily accessible species. The insect enzymes localized in the microsomal subcellular fractions obtained from whole insect or insect organ homogenates require NADPH and oxygen for activity and are inhibited by carbon monoxide. This type of similarity

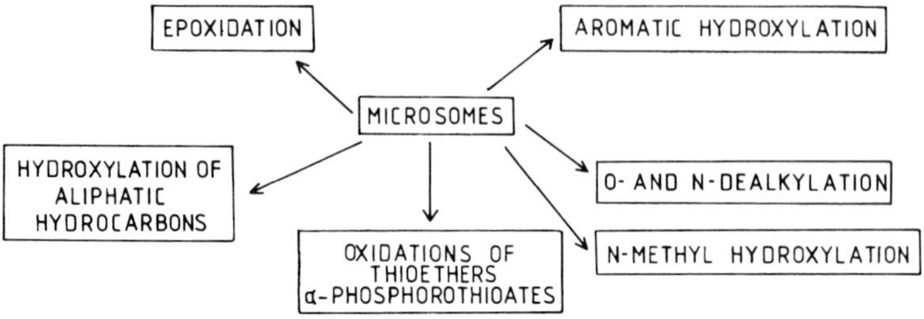

FIGURE 15 Range of oxidative reactions carried out by monooxygenases in insects. (From Ref. 354.)

supports the overall conclusion that the range of insect enzyme activities shown in Fig. 15 can be summarized by the general equation:

$$\text{Substrate} + O_2 + H_2X \longrightarrow \text{substrate-O} + X + H_2O$$

where H_2X represents an electron donor such as NADPH (or NADH) and the oxygen molecule is divided between metabolite and water [354].

It should be emphasized that suitably fortified drug-metabolizing experiments with given substrates in vitro, using whole insect homogenates, homogenates obtained from abdomens, fat body, or gut tissue, may give widely varying results even for the same species of insect [66]. In part this may be due to the presence of endogenous inhibitors like the xanthommatin eye pigment of housefiles, as shown in Fig. 16 [356], or digestive proteinases in the gut of the armyworm [357]. In part also, the tissue distribution of enzyme activity is not as clearly established for insects as it is for mammals, although it is recognized that fat body preparations tend to have considerable metabolic versatility for processing various substrates [66,354], including DDT [358].

In insects also, there is a whole range of extramicrosomal drug-metabolizing activities which includes various esterases, in particular carbamate esterases, epoxide hydrases, and nitro-reductases [106].

With regard to the enzymatic conjugation reactions in insects [146, 147,355], these are also well documented. A wide range of insects conjugate phenols with glucose. The formation of glucoside metabolites is dependent on UDPG as the glucose donor [359]. Sulfate conjugation of phenolic metabolites in insects appears to require ATP and inorganic sulfate [147]. Glutathione is involved in conjugation mechanisms for some organophosphate dearylations [355]. Furthermore, glutathione is required for stabilizing the quaternary form of the enzyme that dehydrochlorinates DDT, and for the biotransformation of hexachlorocyclohexane to pentachlorocyclohexene [105].

C. Insects and Their Hormonal Control

In vertebrates it is thought that steroid hormones might be the normal substrates for the nonspecific hepatic drug-metabolizing enzymes [280,290]. It is not altogether surprising, therefore, that the hormones regulating insect function and development should also serve as substrates for drug-metabolizing enzymes located in the insect fat body, gut tissue, hemolymph, or in the cytosol of other tissues.

Thus juvenile hormone of the silkmoth (Hyalophora cecropia) which is relatively nonspecific in the sense that it inhibits metamorphosis in a variety of insects [360] is thought to undergo the sequence of metabolic biotransformations in the southern armyworm (Prodenia eridania) shown in Fig. 17 [361].

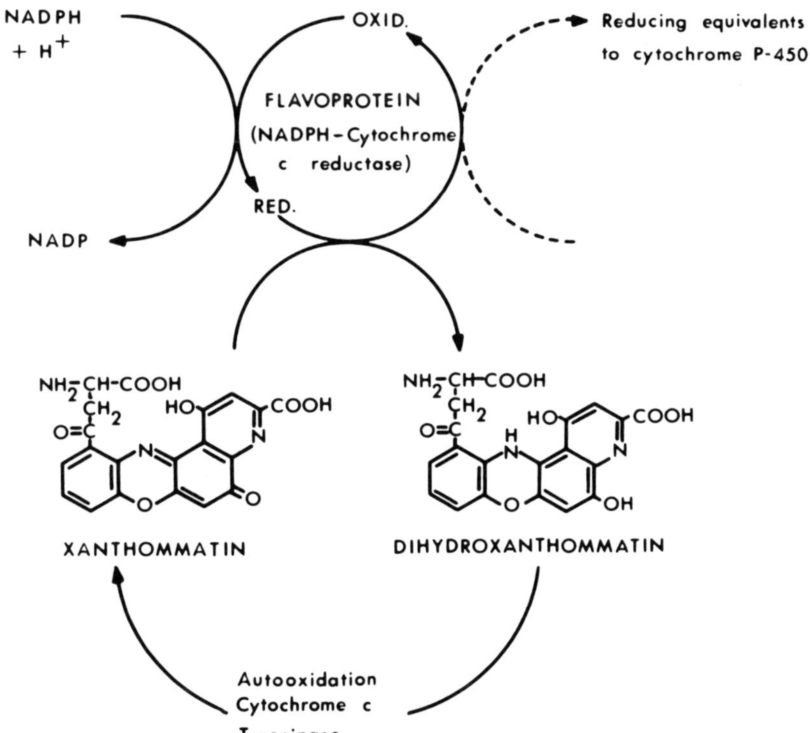

FIGURE 16 Inhibition of monooxygenase activity by an endogenous eye pigment factor, xanthommatin, in insects. (From Ref. 66.)

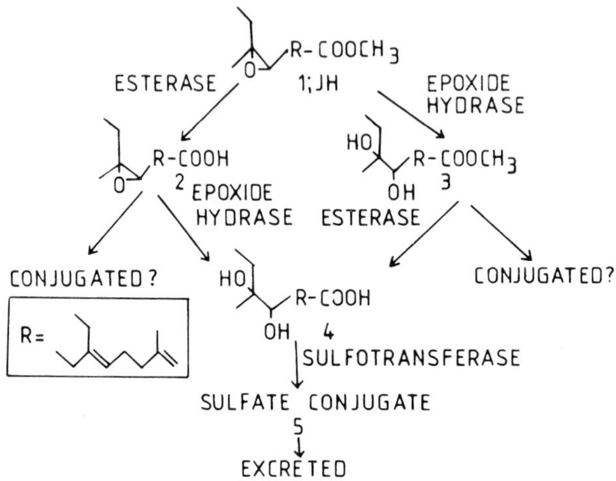

FIGURE 17 The major metabolic pathways of silkmoth juvenile hormone (JH) in the southern armyworm (Prodenia eridania) showing how deactivation by esterase and epoxide hydrase lead to precursors that can be conjugated. (From Ref. 361.)

What is very striking is that esterase, epoxide hydrase, and sulfotransferase activities occur in a number of tissues in the armyworm and in other insects. However, the esterase activity in the hemolymph appears to fluctuate according to the stage of insect development [362].

The original isolation of compounds with juvenile hormone activity from excreta of insects [363] suggests that metabolism of juvenile hormone may go further, at least in Tenebrio molitor, to yield farnesol and farnesal as end products.

Other closely related natural juvenile hormones [364] might be expected to undergo similar biotransformations in vivo, thereby contributing to the orderly and gradated regulatory activity of development in the various tissues. A very large number of synthetic juvenile hormone analogs has become available [337]. Many of these compounds would have insect-directed "antimetabolite" potential for what must turn out to be their critically important interlocking gene-action system [326,365,366] programming the subtleties of differentiation, morphogenesis, and mating maturity.

As for steroid hormone metabolism [337,339,340], insects have the capacity to esterify free sterols, hydrolyze sterol esters, hydroxylate, dealkylate, cleave side chains, reduce and oxidize, and conjugate with glucose or sulfate in ways which also ensure that ecdysone control of molting is achieved without aberration (Fig. 18).

The first requirement is that steroids from exogenous sources are metabolized to the key intermediate, cholesterol. Clearly, different insect species will have different capabilities in biotransformation of such precursors, which differ from one food plant to another [367]. Injected ^{3}H-cholesterol, depending on species of insect, is metabolized in vivo to α-ecdysone [341], 20-hydroxyecdysone [368], or both of these ecdysones [369].

Rapid changes in ecdysone levels during metamorphosis imply that biosynthesis, utilization, and inactivation processes are rigorously controlled. The evidence [339] suggests that inactivation occurs via conjugation reactions, as indicated in Fig. 19.

Conjugation reactions have also been demonstrated in vitro with ecdysones in appropriate incubations with insect fat body [370] or larval gut tissue preparations [176].

D. Insecticide Metabolism

The greatest interest in drug metabolism in insects is still centered on the toxicology of the various major categories of insecticides such as the

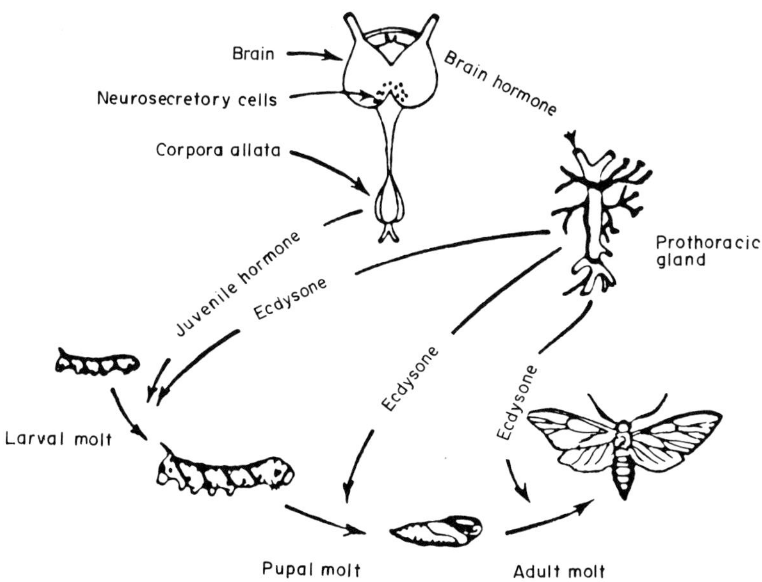

FIGURE 18 Scheme showing hormonal regulation of molting and metamorphosis in an insect. While a great deal is now known about juvenile hormone and the ecdysones, the nature of the brain hormone has not yet been determined. (From Ref. 339.)

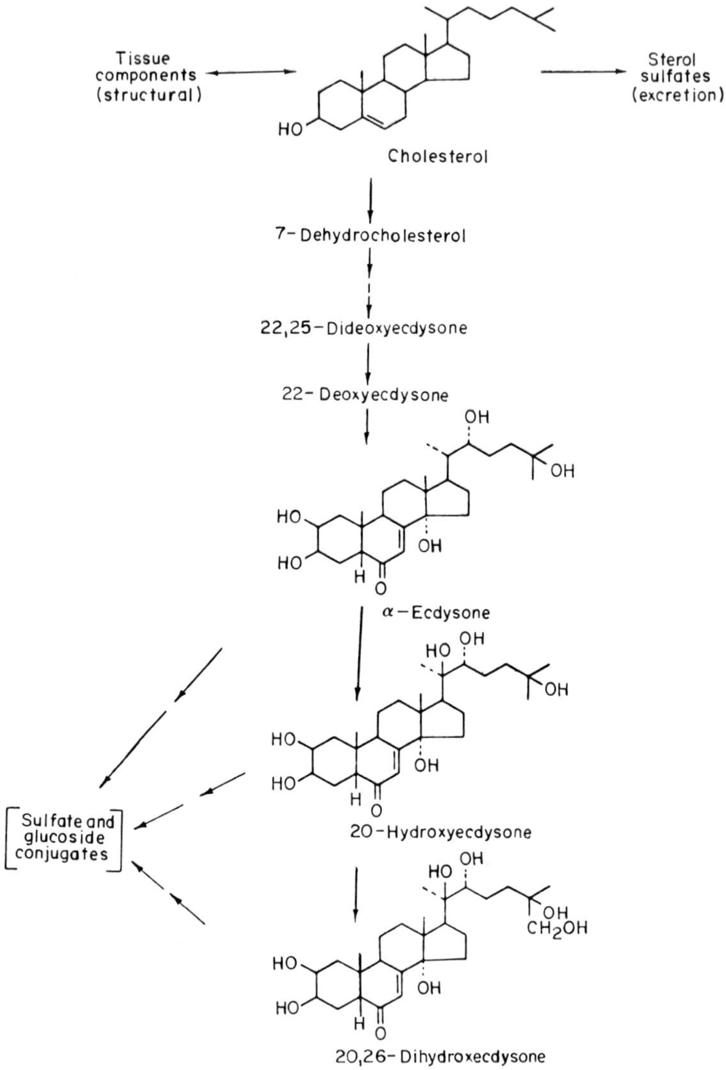

FIGURE 19 Steroid metabolism in the tobacco hornworm (Manduca sexta) showing how cholesterol is a precursor of α-ecdysone and related compounds. (Modified from Ref. 339.)

chlorinated hydrocarbons, organophosphorus compounds, carbamates, pyrethroids, and insect hormone analogues [66,102,105,354,371,372].

The problems of insecticide metabolism are naturally related to the variation in susceptibility of target and nontarget species and to the development of resistance in target species [105,330-332]. Inevitably, somewhat controversial evolutionary considerations are invoked when the progress of insecticide challenge and response is observed as a triumph or a disaster, depending on the vantage point.

The range of oxidative drug-metabolizing activities carried out by various insect species has already been indicated (Fig. 15). It is now necessary to draw attention to the formulas of some of the different types of insecticide to show that many of these compounds possess multiple sites where metabolic transformations can occur and where a combination of several biotransformations could make predictions about preferred pathways in any given species quite unreliable. The net toxicological effects in any given situation would depend on the relative biological potency of metabolites and parent insecticide. In the context of this chapter it is not possible to give more than one or two detailed illustrations of what may be involved in terms of differential toxicities when these are related to net differences in drug metabolism.

Diazinon (Fig. 20) is one of the organophosphorus insecticides. According to O'Brien [101], all organophosphates are hydrolyzed, with rates of hydrolysis that are more rapid in mammals than in insects. The hydrolysis products of the organophosphates are detoxification products which do not inhibit cholinesterase, but not all organophosphates are direct inhibitors of cholinesterase. The largest group of latent inhibitors, phosphorothionates with the general formula R—P=S, need to be metabolically activated to the corresponding R—P=O analogues for cholinesterase inhibition.

By using judiciously labeled ^{32}P- and ^{14}C-diazinon and -diazoxon in incubation experiments with rat and cockroach tissue preparations, Shishido and colleagues [373-375] were able to plot the respective metabolic pathways, demonstrating as shown in Fig. 21 how the NADPH- and O_2-dependent microsomal enzymes, as well as the esterases and glutathione transferase reactions, were relatively apportioned in the vertebrate and the invertebrate species.

Although microsomal activation of diazinon to diazoxon appears to be relatively greater in rat liver than in cockroach fat body, the vertebrate esterase activity more than compensates for the initial toxicological disadvantage [373]. Moreover, the glutathione-conjugative degradation reaction of diazoxon has a much higher activity in rat liver and blood than the analogous enzyme activities in cockroach tissues. Consequently the differentially greater toxicity of diazinon for the cockroach is connected with the greatly enhanced detoxication of the initially activated insecticide in the rat.

From what has been said already (Sec. X.C.) about insect hormones serving as substrates for the drug-metabolizing enzymes, we would expect

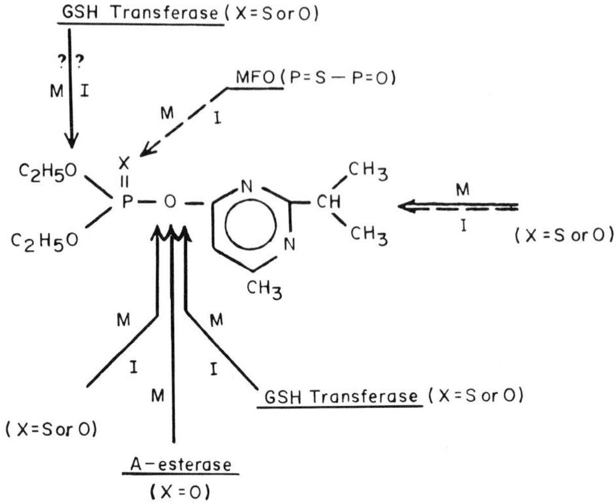

FIGURE 20 The possible target sites of drug-metabolizing enzyme attack on diazinon (X≡S) and diazoxon (X≡O) demonstrable by incubating mammalian (M) liver and insect (I) fat body preparations with substrate under appropriately fortified conditions in vitro. Dashed lines indicate activation, solid lines detoxication. (From Ref. 330.)

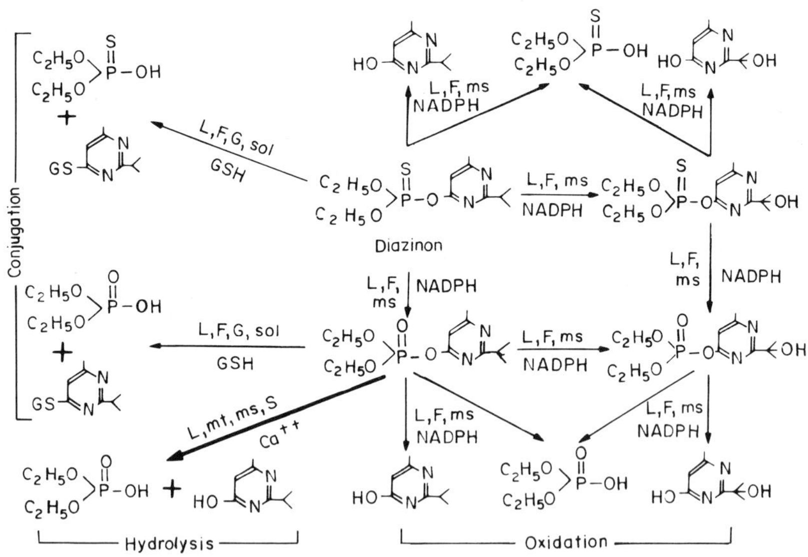

FIGURE 21 Metabolic pathways of diazinon in the rat and the American cockroach as determined by studies in vitro: L = rat liver; S = rat serum; F = American cockroach gut, using mitochondrial (mit), microsomal (ms), or cytosol (sol) preparations. (From Ref. 373.)

epoxidation reactions to be at least as important as any other pathway of metabolism for insects, if indeed one of the functions of the drug-metabolizing enzyme system in terrestrial species is to protect their overall physiological integrity.

Epoxidation reactions with exogenous substrates do in fact occur in insects. Chlorinated Diels-Alder reaction products, the cyclodiene insecticides heptachlor, and the stereoisomers aldrin and isodrin are metabolized to epoxides, as shown in Fig. 22. Thus Giannotti et al. [376] showed that aldrin was metabolized to dieldrin in the American cockroach (Periplaneta americana). Cohen and Smith [218] followed the biotransformation of aldrin in locusts (Schistocerca gregaria) and showed that the compound was slowly and almost exclusively metabolized to dieldrin. Dieldrin when administered to locusts was slowly excreted unchanged. Work with other insect species [377-380] again showed that aldrin was converted mainly to dieldrin. Perry et al. [225] found that both resistant and susceptible houseflies converted heptachlor to heptachlor epoxide.

The NADPH- and O_2-requiring microsomal system of insects is involved in aldrin conversion to dieldrin, as was shown by Ray [381] on incubating whole housefly microsomal preparations with the substrate under suitably fortified conditions. Carbon monoxide inhibited the metabolism, but this inhibition could be reversed in part by ultraviolet light. An explanation for this can be found in the photoalteration of cyclodiene compounds when irradiated [382,383].

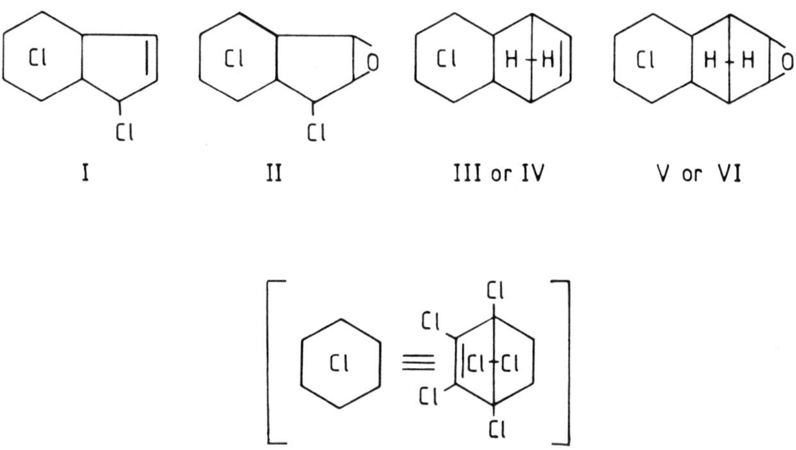

FIGURE 22 The cyclodiene insecticides heptachlor (I) and the stereoisomeric aldrin and isodrin (III, IV) are metabolized to heptachlor epoxide (II) and dieldrin and endrin (V and VI, respectively) as shown in a simplified two-dimensional representation. (From Ref. 375a.)

Williamson and Schechter [384] confirmed the microsomal nature of aldrin epoxidation in several species of lepidopterous larvae and made the important discovery that the darkening reaction catalyzed by the phenolase complex [326] inhibited the epoxidation of aldrin to dieldrin. When an inhibitor of the phenolase reaction was included in the incubation systems there was an increase in epoxidation. Furthermore, in agreement with earlier findings in intact insects [218], microsomal incubation with dieldrin as substrate yielded no further metabolite. We have therefore in dieldrin a very striking and unusually stable epoxide.

What is more usual is that epoxides are transient intermediates which are further metabolized by epoxide hydrases [211,385]. This is illustrated by the findings of Schonbrod et al. [386], Boose and Terriere [387], Khan and Terriere [388], and Khan [389] who showed quite clearly that various strains of houseflies which had the microsomal capability for metabolizing aldrin to its epoxide also hydroxylated naphthalene to 1-naphthol. It is well known that this metabolic biotransformation of naphthalene proceeds via an obligatory epoxide and 1,2-dihydrodiol intermediate pathway [211,390]. Curiously enough, the housefly naphthalene hydroxylating capability is related to its degree of resistance to DDT [386,387], but there is no clear-cut link with resistance to cyclodiene insecticides, the mechanisms of which does not appear to be known [105,332].

However, bearing in mind that biotransformations involving epoxide and dihydrodiol formation are of critical importance in juvenile hormone metabolism [361], it is worth considering the effect of age and stage of development on microsomal epoxidation activity [66]. Something emerges particularly clearly from the studies of Benke et al. [391] on age-activity profiles with gut preparations from the Madagascar cockroach (Gromphadorania portentosa) where epoxidation and hydroxylation activities were followed over several instars. The activities follow a characteristic rhythm cycle, being low during the molt and passing through maxima about halfway through each development phase. What these findings and somewhat simpler results with gut preparations of Prodenia eridania [357] imply is that microsomal epoxidation and hydroxylation appear to be synchronized with the processes of metamorphosis, as shown in Fig. 23. It remains to be determined with precision to what extent the cyclodiene epoxides interfere with the parameters of metamorphosis.

It would be possible to go into further exhaustive details of insects and their drug-metabolizing enzyme activities, particularly with reference to insecticide metabolism [105,354,371]. However, from what has been said and from what has been suggested, it has already been possible to recognize that the drug-metabolizing enzymes are important regulatory factors in maintaining the hormone-dependent physiological integrity of the higher terrestrial invertebrates in the various stages of their life cycles.

As such, they act in concert with ecdysones and juvenile hormones, the harmonized opposing principles which appear to be the invertebrate equivalents of thyroid hormones and prolactin in the higher vertebrates.

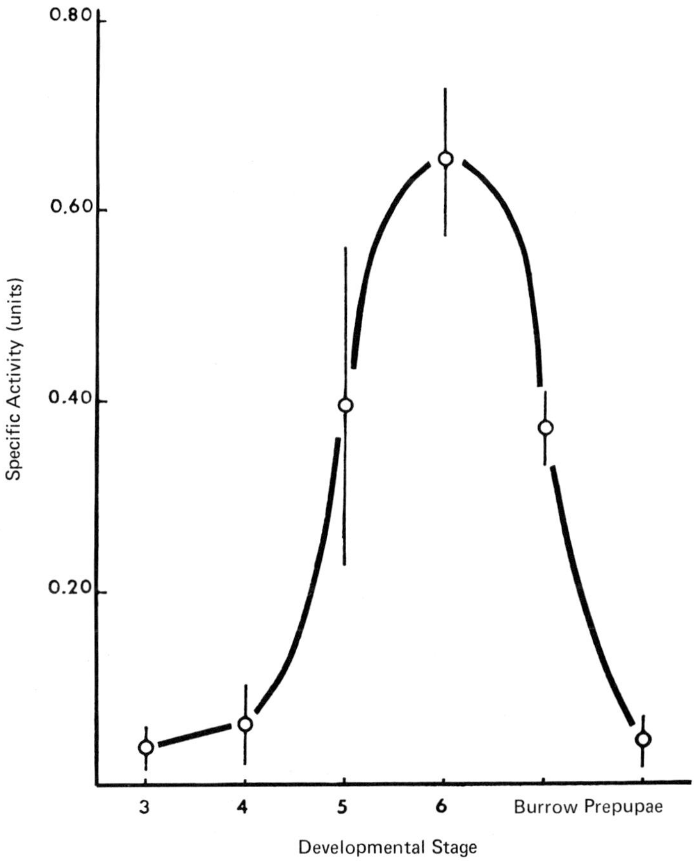

FIGURE 23 Developmental profile through several instars, of NADPH- and O_2-dependent metabolism of aldrin to dieldrin by gut homogenates of southern armyworm (P. eridania) incubated with substrate under appropriately fortified conditions. Epoxidation activity is low initially, rises dramatically to reach a maximum at the sixth instar, and then declines as the larvae prepare to pupate. (From Ref. 357.)

XI. UNMETABOLIZABLE LIPID-SOLUBLE COMPOUNDS; EVOLUTION, WHAT NOW?

In the previous sections, we have seen that a great variety of exogenous compounds which are relatively lipid-soluble tend to be substrates for the drug-metabolizing enzymes in terrestrial species of animals.

The exogenous compounds are rendered more polar by these enzymes and are thereby converted into excretable entities. Some water-soluble or volatile lipophilic exogenous compounds can be excreted unchanged by terrestrial species without any prior interaction with the drug-metabolizing enzymes [17,392].

These evolutionary arrangements of nature have been interpreted [22, 23] as protective devices for the higher terrestrial organisms against the persistence and accumulation of naturally occurring lipid-soluble compounds which, although they may not be nutrients, are taken up from the environment. Such lipophilic compounds in the absence of the drug-metabolizing enzymes "would be trapped in the body, and would be doomed, like the Flying Dutchman, to wander throughout the protoplasmic seas for evermore" [22].

The range of metabolic pathways characterizing the versatility of the drug-metabolizing enzymes which thus protect the higher terrestrial species (Fig. 3) [35] anticipates that relatively few pathways suffice to metabolize an enormous number of possible substrates. However, as already mentioned, the aromatic C—Cl (or C—Br) bond appears to be almost completely resistant to biotransformation, possibly in order to safeguard the evolutionary priorities of aromatic C—I bond metabolism in the delicately balanced formation and interconversions of the iodotyrosines and iodothyronines in the higher vertebrates [393-395].

A full appreciation of the consequences of the metabolic stability of the aromatic C—Cl bond has only recently emerged, when it became apparent on analysis of tissues and in the detection of biological and behavioral lesions in various species that the global ecosystem had become contaminated with unmetabolizable aromatic chloro compounds. These were related to insecticides [312,313,396], polychlorinated biphenyls [15,17,24,311,397], and impurities in herbicides [398-401].

The activities of humans had brought about something which might be described as "chemical fallout" or a "Flying Dutchman" situation (Fig. 24) from which humans themselves have no protection. What was very striking about the observations 10 years ago was that the organochlorine insecticide residues in seabirds were comparable with those in land birds [313] despite the fact that insecticides were applied to a terrestrial environment, and the sea might have been expected to dilute agricultural runoff. Furthermore, there are no insect pests in Antarctica, and yet fish, birds, and seals had insecticide residues in their tissues [312] even in these the remotest parts of the world. The identification of polychlorinated biphenyl residues in birds' livers and birds' eggs [311,396] prompted the question of why it was that these materials accumulated in greater quantities than chlorinated insecticides and why they accumulated in seabirds and seals and not in domestic animals which shared a habitat with man.

It was clear at the outset that the persistent environmental chemicals could not be confined to the areas where they were applied, and that uncontrolled ocean dumping had contributed to extraction and concentration of organochlorine compounds by marine organisms. What Koeman et al. [397] realized was that the polychlorinated biphenyls found as residues in fish

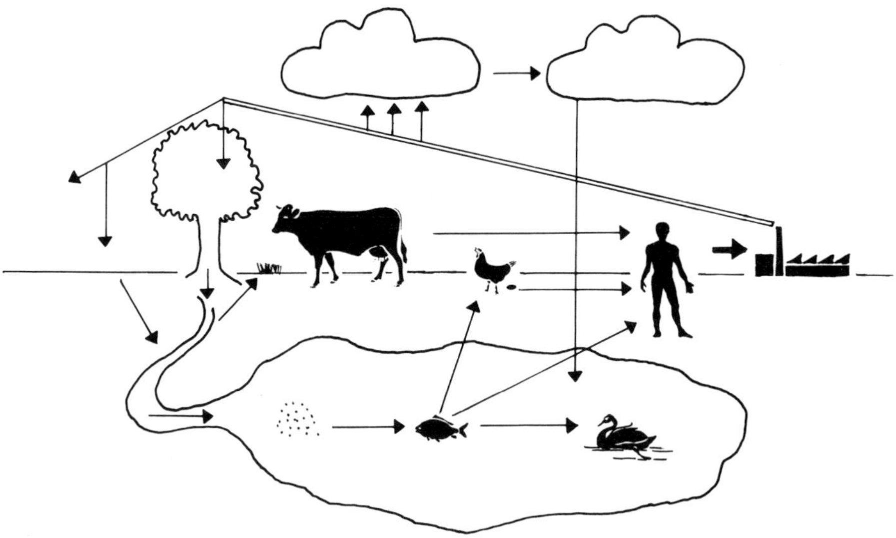

FIGURE 24 Scheme showing generation of environmental "chemical fall-out" affecting the global ecosystem. Man and seabirds are shown at the somewhat foreshortened ends of their respective food chains, bioconcentrating unmetabolizable chlorinated insecticides, herbicide contaminants, and polychlorinated biphenyl inducers of drug metabolism. Man contributes to the generation of these environmental chemicals; the seabird does not. (Adapted from Ref. 27.)

were not the same as those found in seabird tissues. The lower polychlorinated biphenyls were not metabolized by fish tissues together with the more highly chlorinated biphenyls. Seabirds metabolized the lower polychlorinated biphenyl isomers, as might have been expected [25,402,403], so that only the more chlorinated unmetabolizable isomers appeared as detectable tissue residues.

What is it that contributes toward the tissue accumulation of certain lipophilic isomeric aromatic chloro compounds in the "Flying Dutchman" situation, even in species with drug-metabolizing enzymes which are inducible moreover by the very compounds that are not themselves metabolized [24,294,404,405]? An early answer to this was provided by systematically comparing the metabolic fate of monochlorobenzene, the various isomeric di-, tri-, and tetrachlorobenzenes and penta- and hexachlorobenzene in rabbits [406-411]. As the number of chloro substituents increased, the excretion of polar metabolites declined, and there was a tendency for 1,2,4,5-tetrachlorobenzene [411] and penta- and hexachlorobenzene [409] to accumulate in body fat and skin.

Another feature of these studies was the recognition that for appreciable oxidative metabolism to take place, there had to be two adjacent unsubstituted positions on the aromatic ring to allow for postulated intermediate formation of epoxide [410,411] in accordance with more general later concepts [412,413].

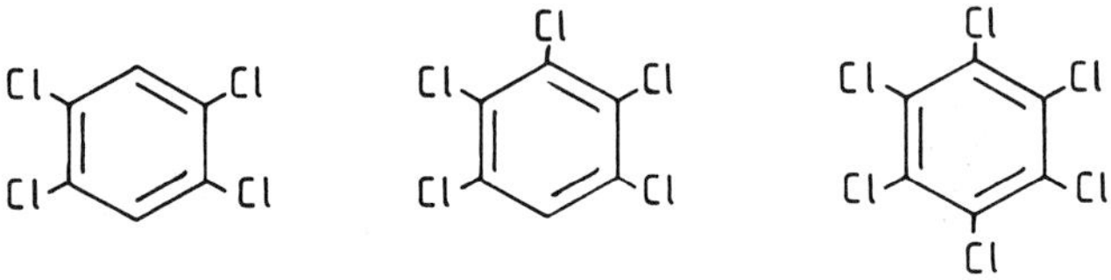

Accumulating chlorobenzenes

The consequences of this kind of tissue accumulation of unmetabolizable lipid-soluble compounds, which may be overtly symptomless and which may show up in a population only on routine analysis of body fat [26,414,415], depend on the degree of exposure, the toxicity of the cumulating material, and the relative stability of the proportion of fat to other tissues in the body. The seriousness of the situation arising, and a foretaste of the future, can be gauged from the symptoms seen in humans inadvertently exposed to acute or chronic poisoning by one or more of these accumulating organochlorine compounds.

Thus, in a population eating bread made from wheat dressed with the fungicide hexachlorobenzene [416,417], there was an epidemic outbreak of porphyria cutanea tarda, the symptoms of which [418,419] include neurological disorders, disturbances in porphyrin metabolism, and hemorrhagic dermal lesions. It was shown subsequently in animal experiments that although hexachlorobenzene is not metabolized, drug-metabolizing enzyme activity is induced in the liver, as is the microsomal content of cytochrome P-450 [404] and mitochondrial heme precursor synthesis.

In pregnant animals, delivery of normal litters is superseded by the convulsive death of the young on suckling. Normal neonatal rats fostered by mothers predosed with hexachlorobenzene also die of convulsions on ingesting lipid-soluble hexachlorobenzene excreted in the foster mothers' milk [417].

The adaptive responses in mammals to lipid-soluble accumulating substances taken in from the environment include induction of the drug-metabolizing enzymes, skin lesions to permit some losses of the accumulating substance through an otherwise impermeable barrier, induction of precursor heme synthesis [420], and, in the case of nursing females, excretion via the milk. These responses are characteristic symptoms seen on exposure to other unmetabolizable aromatic polyhalogenated environmental chemicals.

Other major inadvertent human exposures to polychlorinated biphenyls [421,422], polybrominated biphenyls [423,424], and 2,3,7,8-tetrachlorodibenzo-para-dioxin (TCDD) [425] have given rise to great anxieties about public health and the future.

These anxieties coupled with the insidious onset and the persistence and the strangeness of the symptoms were compounded by the initial uncertainties connected with the realization that the population most immediately affected by polyhalogenated biphenyls was in effect exposed to complex mixtures of compounds. Only a few of these, according to animal experiments subsequently performed on various species, had the characteristic drug-metabolizing enzyme-inducing, acengenic, skin lesions and porphyria-producing, mortality-accelerating properties [405,426,427].

With regard to the rules established for the cumulating isomers in the chlorinated benzene series, these appear to hold in the polyhalogenated biphenyl series of compounds, and the unmetabolizable cumulating isomers appear to be those which lack adjacent unsubstituted positions in at least one of the rings in the molecule (Fig. 11) [25,428,429]. The cumulation in adipose tissue and the hepatic and other biochemical effects, in part at any rate, may not be subject to rationalization according to rules defining structure-activity relationships, for in the preparation of the various isomeric chlorinated biphenyls, contamination with trace amounts of high-potency polychlorinated dibenzofurans may occur [422,430,431]. Figure 25 showing the structures of biphenyls, dibenzofurans, and dibenzodioxins helps to clarify such findings.

The potency of 2,3,7,8-tetrachlorodibenzofuran in bringing about delayed death from composite unknown causes in experimental animals [432] is comparable with that of the corresponding dibenzodioxin (TCDD) [425]. Although TCDD has been studied in various biological systems for its persistence and enzyme induction [433,434] and has been compared on a structure-activity basis with other chlorinated dioxins [435] (most of which were inactive) for effects on porphyrin precursor synthesis and on drug-metabolizing enzymes, none of this information is as yet available in any kind of systematic form for the chlorinated dibenzofurans.

What is inescapable, as explanations are still sought and sometimes persuasively offered [42] for the phenomenon of persistent induction by lipid-soluble compounds which themselves are poor cytochrome P-450 substrates and thus have a correspondingly prolonged "Flying Dutchman" biological half-life, is that the endogenous steroid substrate metabolism becomes abnormal not only in birds as already discussed (Table 3) [24,294] but in mammals [436,437] including primates [438]. These abnormalities in steroid metabolism are threats to the present generation.

Yet the next generation is also at risk with the passage of unmetabolizable lipid-soluble polychlorinated environmental inducers into eggs [24, 300,314,439] or milk [247,417,424] by the higher vertebrates burdened

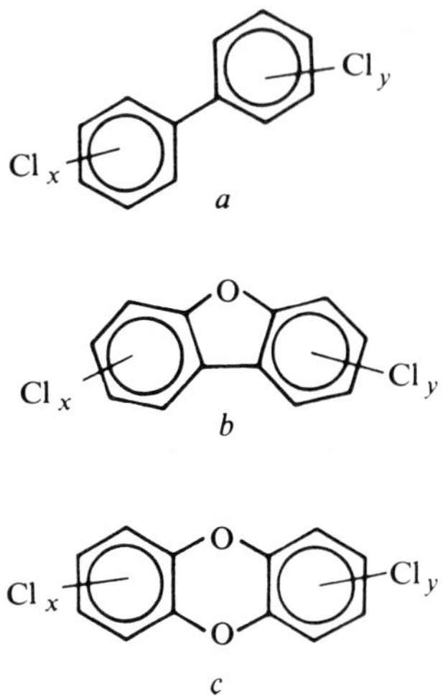

FIGURE 25 Comparison of the structures of (a) chlorinated biphenyls, $x + y = 1\text{–}10$; (b) chlorinated dibenzofurans, $x + y = 1\text{–}8$; (c) chlorinated dibenzodioxins, $x + y = 1\text{–}8$. (From Ref. 430.)

with these chemicals. Severe problems also arise during parturition [440].

The lipid-soluble cumulating chloro and bromo compounds are neutralizing the evolutionary endowment of the drug-metabolizing enzymes in the higher terrestrial vertebrates.

Induction of the drug-metabolizing enzyme system by these exogenous compounds does not bring about resistance, as would sometimes happen in a corresponding situation with a terrestrial insect population confronted with a new insecticide [331]. On the contrary, induction merely creates additional burdens of aberrant endogenous steroid and possibly thyroid hormone [441] and vitamin A metabolism for the terrestrial and aerial vertebrates.

No species has come to the rescue. No aerobic bacteria have appeared to add biphenyls, dibenzofurans, and dibenzodioxins to their repertoire of ring fission [442]. Nothing in the food chain has taken the initiative to break up these compounds which are doomed to wander throughout the protoplasmic seas for evermore.

The NIH shift has not come to the rescue [413].

None of the possibilities for restoring the appropriate balance of prolactin- and thyroid hormone-dependent control systems in the higher vertebrates can be readily invoked in situations which dramatically but selectively affect membranes in skin, stomach, and liver.

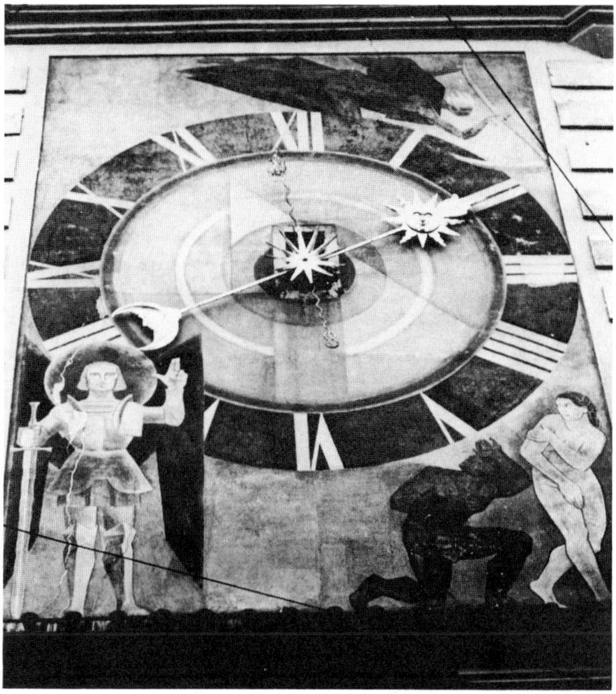

FIGURE 26 "And the Lord God said, Behold the man is become as one of us, to know good and evil: and now, lest he put forth his hand and take also of the tree of life, and eat, and live forever: Therefore the Lord God sent him forth from the Garden of Eden to till the ground from whence he was taken. So he drove out the man; and he placed at the east of the garden of Eden Cherubims, and a flaming sword which turned every way, to keep the way of the tree of life" (Genesis 4:22-24). The clockface in Berne illustrating these verses from Genesis, and combining sun, moon, and stars, and concepts of time which are both linear and cyclical, summarizes the main features of this chapter, which are ultimately concerned with keeping the way of the tree of life.

The long-term prospects for the global ecosystem contaminated by a peculiarly persistent chemical fallout [17,64] are reminiscent of certain biblical passages which show concern for the integrity of the tree of life (Fig. 26).

ACKNOWLEDGMENTS

This chapter is dedicated with great affection to Professor Marcel Bickel and to my other friends in the Institute of Pharmacology at the University of Berne. I am also mindful of the indirect influence of the late Professor Walther Wilbrandt in whose garden, after a sudden thunderstorm at one of his hospitable gatherings, a golden salamander unexpectedly told me some of the things I had wanted to know about prolactin.

REFERENCES

1. P. G. Fothergill, Historical Aspects of Organic Evolution. Hollis and Carter, London, 1952.
2. S. J. Gould, Ontogeny and Phylogeny. Belknap Press, Harvard University Press, Cambridge, 1977.
3. L. C. Cole, Quart. Rev. Biol. 29:103 (1954).
4. S. J. McNaughton, Amer. Naturalist 109:251 (1975).
5. D. A. Karnofsky and C. W. Young, Fed. Proc. 26:1139 (1967).
6. M. O. Dayhoff and R. V. Eck, in Atlas of Protein Sequence and Structure, Vol. 5 (M. O. Dayhoff, Ed.). National Biomedical Research Foundation, Silver Spring, Md., 1972, p. 1.
7. A. Albert, Intra-Science Chem. Rept. 8:55 (1974).
8. I. Prigogine, Science 201:777 (1978).
9. J. W. Stucki, Progr. Biophys. Mol. Biol. 33:99 (1978).
10. M. Eigen and P. Schuster, Naturwissenschaften 64:541 (1977).
11. M. Eigen and P. Schuster, Naturwissenschaften 65:7 (1978).
12. M. Eigen and P. Schuster, Naturwissenschaften 65:341 (1978).
13. M. O. Dayhoff, C. M. Park, and P. J. McLaughlin, in Atlas of Protein Sequence and Structure, Vol. 5 (M. O. Dayhoff, Ed.). National Biomedical Research Foundation, Silver Spring, Md., 1972, p. 7.
14. P. H. Abelson, Ann. N.Y. Acad. Sci. 69:276 (1957).
15. Environmental Protection Agency, Proceedings of the National Conference on Polychlorinated Biphenyls, November 1975, Chicago, EPA-560/6-75-004. Washington, D.C., 1976.
16. Department of Health, Education, and Welfare, Final Report of the Subcommittee on the Health Effects of Polychlorinated Biphenyls and Polybrominated Biphenyls, July 1976. Washington, D.C., 1976.
17. M. H. Bickel, in Industrial and Environmental Xenobiotics (J. R. Fouts and I. Gut, Eds.). Excerpta Medica, Amsterdam, 1978, p. 156.
18. B. N. Ames, Science 204:587 (1979).
19. B. B. Brodie, J. Pharm. Pharmacol. 8:1 (1956).
20. B. B. Brodie and C. A. M. Hogben, J. Pharm. Pharmacol. 9:345 (1957).

21. L. E. Gaudette and B. B. Brodie, Biochem. Pharmacol. 2:89 (1959).
22. B. B. Brodie and R. P. Maickel, in Proceedings of the First International Pharmacology Meeting, Vol. 6 (B. B. Brodie and E. G. Erdös, Eds.). Pergamon, London, 1962, p. 299.
23. B. B. Brodie, R. P. Maickel, and W. R. Jondorf, Fed. Proc. 17: 1163 (1958).
24. R. W. Risebrough, P. Rieche, D. B. Peakall, S. G. Herman, and M. N. Kirven, Nature 220:1098 (1968).
25. O. Hutzinger, D. M. Nash, S. Safe, A. S. W. DeFreitas, R. J. Norstrom, D. J. Wildish, and V. Zitko, Science 178:312 (1972).
26. W. B. Deichmann, Arch. Toxikol. 29:1 (1972).
27. D. Henschler, in Allgemeine und Spezielle Pharmakologie und Toxikologie, 2nd ed. (W. Forth, D. Henschler, and W. Rummel, Eds.). Bibliographisches Institut, Mannheim, 1977, p. 572.
28. S. Orrenius, in Proceedings of the Sixth International Congress of Pharmacology, Vol. 6 (N. T. Kärki, Ed.). Pergamon, Oxford, 1976, p. 39.
29. R. T. Williams, Detoxication Mechanisms, 2nd ed. Chapman and Hall, London, 1959.
30. R. T. Williams, Fed. Proc. 26:1029 (1967).
31. B. B. Brodie, J. R. Gillette, and B. N. La Du, Ann. Rev. Biochem. 27:427 (1958).
32. J. R. Gillette, Progr. Drug Res. 6:11 (1963).
33. H. G. Mandel, in Fundamentals of Drug Metabolism and Drug Disposition (B. N. La Du, H. G. Mandel, and E. L. Way, Eds.). Williams & Wilkins, Baltimore, 1971, p. 149.
34. G. J. Mannering, in Fundamentals of Drug Metabolism and Drug Disposition (B. N. La Du, H. G. Mandel, and E. L. Way, Eds.). Williams & Wilkins, Baltimore, 1971, p. 206.
35. V. Ullrich, in Industrial and Environmental Xenobiotics (J. R. Fouts and I. Gut, Eds.). Excerpta Medica, Amsterdam, 1978, p. 3.
36. T. Omura, E. Sanders, R. W. Estabrook, D. Y. Cooper, and O. Rosenthal, Arch. Biochem. Biophys. 117:660 (1966).
37. T. Omura, R. Sato, D. Y. Cooper, O. Rosenthal, and R. W. Estabrook, Fed. Proc. 24:1181 (1965).
38. A. Hildebrandt and R. W. Estabrook, Arch. Biochem. Biophys. 143: 66 (1971).
39. D. W. Nebert, J. S. Felton, and J. R. Robinson, Proc. Eur. Soc. Toxicol. 16:82 (1975).
40. I. Fridovich, Science 201:875 (1978).
41. M. J. Coon, H. W. Strobel, and R. F. Boyer, Drug Metab. Dispos. 1:92 (1973).
42. A. J. Paine, Biochem. Pharmacol. 27:1805 (1978).

43. J. Tréfouël, J. Tréfouël, F. Nitti, and D. Bovet, Compt. Rend. Séanc. Soc. Biol. 120:756 (1935).
44. G. C. Mueller and J. A. Miller, J. Biol. Chem. 180:1125 (1949).
45. G. C. Mueller and J. A. Miller, J. Biol. Chem. 185:145 (1950).
46. J. R. Fouts, J. J. Kamm, and B. B. Brodie, J. Pharmacol. Exp. Ther. 120:291 (1957).
47. P. H. Hernandez, J. R. Gillette, and P. Mazel, Biochem. Pharmacol. 16:1859 (1967).
48. P. H. Hernandez, P. Mazel, and J. R. Gillette, Biochem. Pharmacol. 16:1877 (1967).
49. J. R. Gillette, in Handbook of Experimental Pharmacology, Vol. 28, Part 2 (B. B. Brodie and J. R. Gillette, Eds.). Springer-Verlag, New York, 1971, p. 349.
50. J. R. Fouts and B. B. Brodie, J. Pharmacol. Exp. Ther. 119:197 (1957).
51. J. R. Gillette, J. J. Kamm, and H. A. Sasame, Mol. Pharmacol. 4: 541 (1968).
52. J. N. Faigle and H. Keberle, Ann. N.Y. Acad. Sci. 160:544 (1969).
53. M. Mitchard, Xenobiotica 1:469 (1971).
54. M. Kiese, Ann. N.Y. Acad. Sci. 123:141 (1965).
55. B. G. Reddy, L. R. Pohl, and G. Krishna, Biochem. Pharmacol. 25: 1119 (1976).
56. W. R. Jondorf, R. P. Maickel, and B. B. Brodie, Biochem. Pharmacol. 1:352 (1958).
57. R. H. Adamson, R. L. Dixon, F. L. Francis, and D. P. Rall, Proc. Nat. Acad. Sci. U.S. 54:1386 (1965).
58. D. R. Buhler and M. E. Rasmusson, Arch. Biochem. Biophys. 124: 582 (1968).
59. S. M. Sieber and R. H. Adamson, in Drug Metabolism: From Microbe to Man (D. V. Parke and R. L. Smith, Eds.). Taylor and Francis, London, 1977, p. 233.
60. C. S. Nicoll, in Handbook of Physiology, Sec. 7, Vol. 4, Part 2 (E. Knobil and W. H. Sawyer, Eds.). American Physiological Society, Washington, D.C., 1974, p. 253.
61. C. S. Nicoll and H. A. Bern, in Lactogenic Hormones (G. E. W. Wolstenholme and J. Knight, Eds.). Churchill Livingstone, Edinburgh, 1972, p. 299.
62. J. Maetz and B. Lahlou, in Handbook of Physiology, Sec. 7, Vol. 4, Part 1 (E. Knobil and W. H. Sawyer, Eds.). American Physiological Society, Washington, D.C., 1974, p. 521.
63. W. R. Jondorf, in Drug Toxicity (J. W. Gorrod, Ed.). Taylor and Francis, London, 1979, p. 25.
64. W. R. Jondorf, Trends Biochem. Sci. 4:141 (1979).
65. L. Shargel, S. Akov, and P. Mazel, J. Toxicol. Appl. Pharmacol. 14:645 (1969).

66. C. F. Wilkinson and L. B. Brattsten, Drug Metab. Rev. 1:153 (1972).
67. H. G. Bray, Z. Hybs, S. P. James, and W. V. Thorpe, Biochem. J. 53:266 (1953).
68. A. K. Saz and L. M. Martinez, J. Biochem. 223:285 (1956).
69. A. K. Saz and R. B. Slie, J. Biol. Chem. 210:407 (1954).
70. A. K. Saz and R. B. Slie, Arch. Biochem. Biophys. 51:5 (1954).
71. P. K. Zachariah and M. R. Juchau, Drug Metab. Dispos. 2:74 (1974).
72. L. A. Wheeler, F. B. Soderberg, and P. Goldman, J. Pharmacol. Exp. Ther. 194:135 (1975).
73. P. Goldman, Ann. Rev. Pharmacol. Toxicol. 18:523 (1978).
74. H. W. Doelle, Bacterial Metabolism, 2nd ed. Academic, New York, 1975, p. 157.
75. J. J. Roxon, A. J. Ryan, and S. E. Wright, Food Cosmet. Toxicol. 4:419 (1966).
76. J. J. Roxon, A. J. Ryan, and S. E. Wright, Food Cosmet. Toxicol. 5:367 (1967).
77. J. J. Roxon, A. J. Ryan, and S. E. Wright, Food Cosmet. Toxicol. 5:645 (1967).
78. R. Gingell, J. W. Bridges, and R. T. Williams, Xenobiotica 1:131 (1971).
79. R. R. Scheline, J. Pharm. Sci. 57:2021 (1968).
80. R. T. Williams, Toxicol. Appl. Pharmacol. 23:769 (1972).
81. J. C. Dacre, R. R. Scheline, and R. T. Williams, J. Pharm. Pharmacol. 20:619 (1968).
82. B. R. Goldin, M. A. Peppercorn, and P. Goldman, J. Pharmacol. Exp. Ther. 186:160 (1973).
83. M. Sandler, B. L. Goodwin, C. R. J. Ruthven, and D. B. Calne, Nature 229:414 (1971).
84. M. Sandler, F. Karoum, C. R. J. Ruthven, and D. B. Calne, Science 166:1417 (1969).
85. H. W. Doelle, Bacterial Metabolism, 2nd ed. Academic, New York, 1975, p. 84.
86. P. Candau, C. Manzano, and M. Losada, Nature 262:715 (1976).
87. E. K. Jackson, G. W. Parshall, and R. W. F. Hardy, J. Biol. Chem. 243:4952 (1968).
88. R. H. Garrett and A. Nason, J. Biol. Chem. 244:2870 (1969).
89. W. Kalow, in Proceedings of the First International Pharmacology Meeting, Vol. 6 (B. B. Brodie and E. G. Erdös, Eds.). Pergamon, London, 1962, p. 137.
90. R. T. Williams, Proc. Eur. Soc. Study Drug Toxicity 4:9 (1964).
91. W. Kalow, J. Pharmacol. Exp. Ther. 104:122 (1952).
92. M. H. Aven, A. Light, and F. F. Foldes, Fed. Proc. 12:299 (1953).
93. G. Hollunger, Acta Pharmacol. Toxicol. 17:356 (1960).
94. G. Hollunger, Acta Pharmacol. Toxicol. 17:365 (1960).
95. G. Hollunger, Acta Pharmacol. Toxicol. 17:374 (1960).

96. G. Hollunger, Acta Pharmacol. Toxicol. 17:384 (1960).
97. E. Hodgson and J. E. Casida, Biochem. Pharmacol. 8:179 (1961).
98. E. Hodgson and J. E. Casida, Biochim. Biophys. Acta 42:184 (1960).
99. L. W. Dittert and T. Higuchi, J. Pharm. Sci. 52:852 (1963).
100. T. R. Fukuto, M. A. H. Fahmy, and R. L. Metcalf, J. Agr. Food Chem. 15:273 (1967).
101. R. D. O'Brien, Ann. N.Y. Acad. Sci. 123:156 (1965).
102. R. D. O'Brien, Insecticides: Action and Metabolism. Academic, New York, 1967.
103. W. N. Aldridge, Brit. Med. Bull. 25:236 (1969).
104. T. R. Fukuto, Drug Metab. Rev. 1:117 (1972).
105. A. S. Perry and M. Agosin, in The Physiology of Insecta, 2nd ed., Vol. 6 (M. Rockstein, Ed.). Academic, New York, 1974, p. 3.
106. W. C. Dauterman, in Insecticide Biochemistry and Physiology (C. F. Wilkinson, Ed.). Plenum, New York, 1976, p. 149.
107. F. J. Oppenoorth, Entomol. Exp. Appl. 2:304 (1959).
108. R. B. March, Entomol. Soc. Amer. Misc. Publ. 1:13 (1959).
109. F. Matsumara and A. W. A. Brown, J. Econ. Entomol. 54:1176 (1961).
110. F. Matsumara and C. J. Hogendijk, Entomol. Exp. Appl. 7:179 (1964).
111. M. G. Townsend and J. R. Busvine, Entomol. Exp. Appl. 12:243 (1969).
112. W. C. Dauterman and F. Matsumara, Science 138:694 (1962).
113. F. W. Seume and R. D. O'Brien, Toxicol. Appl. Pharmacol. 2:495 (1960).
114. I. Yamamoto and J. E. Casida, J. Econ. Entomol. 59:1542 (1966).
115. I. Yamamoto, E. C. Kimmel, and J. E. Casida, J. Agr. Food Chem. 17:1227 (1969).
116. J. E. Casida, E. C. Kimmel, M. Elliott, and N. F. James, Nature 230:326 (1971).
117. T. Nakatsugawa and M. A. Morelli, in Insecticide Biochemistry and Physiology (C. F. Wilkinson, Ed.). Plenum, New York, 1976, p. 61.
118. M. Elliott, N. F. Janes, E. C. Kimmel, and J. E. Casida, J. Agr. Food Chem. 20:300 (1973).
119. R. Schmid and R. Lester, in Glucuronic Acid (G. J. Dutton, Ed.). Academic, New York, 1966, p. 493.
120. M. F. Jayle and J. R. Pasqualini, in Glucuronic Acid (G. J. Dutton, Ed.). Academic, New York, 1966, p. 507.
121. G. J. Dutton, in Glucuronic Acid (G. J. Dutton, Ed.). Academic, New York, 1966, p. 186.
122. G. J. Dutton, in Handbook of Experimental Pharmacology, Vol. 28, Part 2 (B. B. Brodie and J. R. Gillette, Eds.). Springer-Verlag, New York, 1971, p. 378.

123. G. J. Dutton, G. J. Wishart, J. E. A. Leakey, and M. A. Goheer, in Drug Metabolism: From Microbe to Man (D. V. Parke and R. L. Smith, Eds.). Taylor and Francis, London, 1977, p. 71.
124. T. A. Miettinen and E. Leskinen, in Metabolic Conjugation and Metabolic Hydrolysis, Vol. 1 (W. H. Fishman, Ed.). Academic, New York, 1970, p. 157.
125. J. Axelrod, J. K. Inscoe, and G. M. Tomkins, J. Biol. Chem. 232: 835 (1958).
126. J. W. Clapp, J. Biol. Chem. 223:207 (1956).
127. R. P. Maickel, W. R. Jondorf, and B. B. Brodie, Fed. Proc. 17: 390 (1958).
128. R. Lester and R. Schmid, Nature 190:452 (1961).
129. G. J. Dutton, in Drug Metabolism in Man (J. W. Gorrod and A. H. Beckett, Eds.). Taylor and Francis, London, 1978, p. 81.
130. D. Robinson and R. T. Williams, Biochem. J. 68:23P (1958).
131. P. C. Hirom, J. R. Idle, and P. Millburn, in Drug Metabolism: From Microbe to Man (D. V. Parke and R. L. Smith, Eds.). Taylor and Francis, London, 1977, p. 299.
132. G. H. Lathe and M. Walker, Biochem. J. 70:705 (1958).
133. S. E. H. Archer, T. Scatcherd, and W. Taylor, Biochem. J. 94:778 (1965).
134. I. M. Arias, Bull. Mt. Desert Island Biol. Lab. 4:17 (1962).
135. E. H. Charreau and M. Tesone, J. Steroid Biochem. 5:65 (1974).
136. J. G. Eales and D. A. R. Sinclair, Comp. Biochem. Physiol. 49A: 661 (1974).
137. G. J. Dutton and J. P. Montgomery, Biochem. J. 70:17P (1958).
138. J. J. Lech, Toxicol. Appl. Pharmacol. 24:114 (1973).
139. K. C. Huang and S. F. Collins, J. Cell Comp. Physiol. 60:49 (1962).
140. R. H. Adamson and A. M. Guarino, Comp. Biochem. Physiol. 42A: 171 (1972).
141. A. M. Guarino and J. B. Anderson, Xenobiotica 6:1 (1976).
142. M. M. Salseduc, Biochem. Pharmacol. 17:1163 (1968).
143. J. T. Ahokas, O. Pelkonen, and N. T. Kärki, Xenobiotica 7:104 (1977).
144. T. J. Lam, Gen. Comp. Endocrinol., Suppl. 3:328 (1972).
145. T. Hirano and N. Mayer-Gostan, in Comparative Endocrinology (P. J. Gaillard and H. H. Boer, Eds.). Elsevier/North Holland, Amsterdam, 1978, p. 209.
146. J. N. Smith, in Comparative Biochemistry, Vol. 6 (M. Florkin and H. S. Mason, Eds.). Academic, New York, 1964, p. 403.
147. J. N. Smith, in Drug Metabolism: From Microbe to Man (D. V. Parke and R. L. Smith, Eds.). Taylor and Francis, London, 1977, p. 219.
148. T. Gessner and T. H. Elmamlouk, Xenobiotica 7:106 (1977).

149. T. H. Elmamlouk and T. Gessner, Xenobiotica 7:111 (1977).
150. K. S. Dodgson, in Drug Metabolism: From Microbe to Man (D. V. Parke and R. L. Smith, Eds.). Taylor and Francis, London, 1977, p. 91.
151. K. S. Dodgson and F. A. Rose, in Metabolic Conjugation and Metabolic Hydrolysis, Vol. 1 (W. H. Fishman, Ed.). Academic, New York, 1970, p. 239.
152. K. S. Dodgson and F. A. Rose, in Metabolism of Sulfur Compounds, Vol. 7 (D. M. Greenberg, Ed.). Academic, New York, 1975, p. 359.
153. R. H. DeMeio, in Metabolism of Sulfur Compounds, Vol. 7 (D. M. Greenberg, Ed.). Academic, New York, 1975, p. 287.
153a. H. Hilz and F. Lipmann, Proc. Nat. Acad. Sci. U.S. 41:880 (1955).
153b. P. W. Robbins and F. Lipmann, J. Biol. Chem. 229:837 (1957).
154. B. Spencer, Biochem. J. 77:294 (1960).
155. J. B. Adams, Biochim. Biophys. Acta 83:127 (1964).
156. A. S. Balasubramanian and B. K. Bachhwat, Biochim. Biophys. Acta 59:389 (1962).
157. A. S. Balasubramanian, L. S. Polter, L. I. Rice, J. B. Sharon, and W. Marx, Anal. Biochem. 21:22 (1967).
158. S. Suzuki and J. L. Strominger, J. Biol. Chem. 235:257 (1960).
159. H. Yoshida and F. Egami, J. Biochem. 57:215 (1969).
160. J. S. Holcenberg and S. W. Rosen, Arch. Biochem. Biophys. 110: 551 (1965).
161. H. Boström and B. Wengle, Acta Endocrinol. 56:691 (1967).
162. H. P. Pan and J. R. Fouts, Drug Metab. Rev. 7:1 (1978).
163. J. N. Smith, Biochem. J. 60:436 (1955).
164. S. Bouchilloux and J. Roche, Bull. Soc. Chim. Biol. 37:37 (1955).
165. I. H. Goldberg and A. Delbrück, Fed. Proc. 18:235 (1959).
166. Y. Nose and F. Lipmann, J. Biol. Chem. 233:1348 (1958).
167. I. G. Anderson, T. Briggs, and G. A. D. Haslewood, Biochem. J. 90:303 (1964).
168. I. G. Anderson and G. A. D. Haslewood, Biochem. J. 93:34 (1964).
169. I. G. Anderson, G. A. D. Haslewood, A. D. Cross, and L. Tökés, Biochem. J. 104:1061 (1967).
170. G. A. D. Haslewood, Biochem. J. 90:309 (1964).
171. G. A. D. Haslewood, Biochem. J. 100:233 (1966).
172. G. A. D. Haslewood, J. Lipid Res. 8:535 (1967).
173. T. Laatikainen, P. Peltokallio, and R. Vihko, Steroids 12:407 (1968).
174. R. F. N. Hutchins and J. N. Kaplanis, Steroids 13:605 (1969).
175. J. Koolman, J. A. Hoffmann, and P. Karlson, Hoppe-Seyler's Z. Physiol. Chem. 354:1043 (1973).
176. R. S. H. Yang and C. F. Wilkinson, Biochem. J. 130:487 (1972).
177. R. S. H. Yang and C. F. Wilkinson, Comp. Biochem. Physiol. 46B: 717 (1973).

178. F. D'Abramo and F. Lipmann, Biochim. Biophys. Acta 25:211 (1957).
179. F. A. Cumar, H. S. Barra, H. J. Maccioni, and R. Caputto, J. Biol. Chem. 243:3807 (1968).
180. J. L. Nussbaum and P. Mandel, J. Neurochem. 19:1789 (1972).
181. F. Lipmann, J. Biol. Chem. 160:173 (1945).
182. B. B. Brodie and J. Axelrod, J. Pharmacol. Exp. Ther. 94:29 (1948).
183. H. G. Bray, S. P. James, W. V. Thorpe, and M. R. Wasdell, Biochem. J. 47:483 (1950).
184. J. M. Schaffer and R. N. Bieter, J. Pharmacol. Exp. Ther. 100: 192 (1950).
185. R. B. Failey, R. C. Anderson, F. G. Henderson, and K. K. Chen, J. Pharmacol. Exp. Ther. 78:336 (1943).
186. J. T. Litchfield, J. Pharmacol. Exp. Ther. 67:212 (1939).
187. C. M. Myers and J. N. Smith, Biochem. J. 54:276 (1953).
188. M. Bouchy-Urison, Bull. Soc. Chim. Biol. 36:525 (1954).
189. M. Boccacci and S. Bettini, Experientia 12:432 (1956).
190. C. P. Sherwin and M. Helfand, J. Biol. Chem. 40:17 (1919).
191. F. W. Power, Proc. Soc. Exp. Biol. Med. 33:598 (1936).
192. J. B. Jepson, Biochem. J. 69:22P (1958).
193. R. Z. Patel and M. A. Crawford, Biochem. J. 89:81P (1963).
194. R. L. Smith and J. Caldwell, in Drug Metabolism: From Microbe to Man (D. V. Parke and R. L. Smith, Eds.). Taylor and Francis, London, 1977, p. 331.
195. K. Moldave and A. Meister, J. Biol. Chem. 229:463 (1957).
196. J. N. Smith, Biochem. J. 69:509 (1958).
197. B. C. Baldwin, D. Robinson, and R. T. Williams, Biochem. J. 76: 595 (1960).
198. H. J. Wolfe and K. C. Huang, J. Cell Comp. Physiol. 54:243 (1959).
199. H. W. Doelle, Bacterial Metabolism, 2nd ed. Academic, New York, 1975, p. 38.
200. J. W. Bridges, M. R. French, R. L. Smith, and R. T. Williams, Biochem. J. 118:47 (1970).
201. J. W. Bridges, M. E. Evans, J. R. Idle, P. Millburn, F. O. Osiyemi, R. L. Smith, and R. T. Williams, Xenobiotica 4:645 (1974).
202. M. O. James, R. L. Smith, R. T. Williams, and M. Reidenberg, Proc. Roy. Soc., Ser. B 182:25 (1972).
203. E. Boyland, in Handbook of Experimental Pharmacology, Vol. 28, Part 2 (B. B. Brodie and J. R. Gillette, Eds.). Springer-Verlag, New York, 1971, p. 584.
204. L. F. Chasseaud, Drug Metab. Rev. 2:185 (1973).
205. P. L. Grover, in Drug Metabolism: From Microbe to Man (D. V. Parke and R. L. Smith, Eds.). Taylor and Francis, London, 1977, p. 105.

206. M. J. Pabst, W. H. Habig, and W. B. Jakoby, Biochem. Biophys. Res. Commun. 52:1123 (1973).
207. G. Semenza, Biochim. Biophys. Acta 24:401 (1957).
208. T. Suga, H. Kumaoka, and M. Akagi, J. Biochem. 60:133 (1966).
209. J. S. Elce, Biochem. J. 116:913 (1970).
210. R. M. Green and J. S. Elce, Biochem. J. 147:283 (1975).
211. D. M. Jerina and J. W. Daly, in Drug Metabolism: From Microbe to Man (D. V. Parke and R. L. Smith, Eds.). Taylor and Francis, London, 1977, p. 13.
212. E. Boyland, G. S. Ramsay, and P. Sims, Biochem. J. 78:376 (1961).
213. E. Boyland and P. Sims, Biochem. J. 84:564 (1962).
214. E. Boyland and P. Sims, Biochem. J. 84:571 (1962).
215. E. Boyland and P. Sims, Biochem. J. 91:493 (1964).
216. E. Boyland and P. Sims, Biochem. J. 95:788 (1965).
217. E. Boyland and K. Williams, Biochem. J. 94:190 (1965).
218. A. J. Cohen and J. N. Smith, Nature 189:600 (1961).
219. J. Booth, E. Boyland, and P. Sims, Biochem. J. 79:516 (1961).
220. P. L. Grover and P. Sims, Biochem. J. 90:603 (1964).
221. E. Boyland and L. F. Chasseaud, Biochem. J. 115:985 (1969).
222. J. G. Wit, in Drug Metabolism: From Microbe to Man (D. V. Parke and P. L. Smith, Eds.). Taylor and Francis, London, 1977, p. 247.
223. A. J. Cohen and J. N. Smith, Biochem. J. 90:449 (1964).
224. A. J. Cohen, J. N. Smith, and H. Turbert, Biochem. J. 90:457 (1964).
225. A. S. Perry, A. M. Mattson, and A. J. Buckner, J. Econ. Entomol. 51:346 (1958).
226. P. Sims and P. L. Grover, Biochem. J. 95:156 (1965).
227. G. E. Pickford and J. G. Phillips, Science 130:454 (1959).
228. J. H. Ball, Gen. Comp. Endocrinol., Suppl. 2:10 (1969).
229. S. Utida and T. Hirano, in Response of Fish to Environmental Changes (W. Chavin and N. Egami, Eds.). Thomas, Springfield, Ill., 1973, p. 240.
230. T. Hirano, M. Morisawa, M. Ando, and S. Utida, in Intestinal Ion Transport (J. W. L. Robinson, Ed.). Medical and Technical Publ., Lancaster, Pa., 1975, p. 300.
231. A. J. Matty, Symp. Zool. Soc. London 2:1 (1960).
232. D. R. Swift, Symp. Zool. Soc. London 2:17 (1960).
233. M. Fontaine and J. Leloup, Gen. Comp. Endocrinol. 3:317 (1962).
234. J. G. Eales, Can. J. Zool. 41:811 (1963).
235. A. D. Woodhead, J. Zool. 146:238 (1966).
236. J. R. Tata, L. Ernster, and O. Lindberg, Nature 193:1058 (1962).
237. J. R. Tata, L. Ernster, O. Lindberg, E. Arrhenius, S. Pedersen, and R. Hedman, Biochem. J. 86:408 (1963).
238. G. Wald, J. Gen. Physiol. 40:901 (1956-57).
239. D. D. Beatty, Vision Res. 9:855 (1969).

240. H. J. A. Koch, in Perspectives in Endocrinology (E. J. W. Barrington and C. B. Jorgensen, Eds.). Academic, New York, 1968, p. 305.
241. G. Wald, Science 128:1481 (1958).
242. G. Wald, Nature 219:800 (1968).
243. S. Futterman, J. Biol. Chem. 238:1145 (1963).
244. R. Bathe, K. Sachsse, L. Ullmann, W. D. Hormann, F. Zak, and R. Hess, Proc. Eur. Soc. Toxicol. 16:113 (1975).
245. R. Reinboth, J. Steroid Biochem. 6:341 (1975).
245a. R. J. Pohl, J. R. Bend, A. M. Buarino, and J. R. Fouts, Drug Metab. Dispos. 2:545 (1974).
246. J. R. Bend, L. G. Hart, A. M. Guarino, D. P. Rall, and J. R. Fouts, in Environmental Protection Agency, Proceedings of the National Conference on Polychlorinated Biphenyls, November 1975, Chicago, EPA-560/6-75-004. Washington, D.C., 1976, p. 292.
247. T. P. Bennett and E. Frieden, in Comparative Biochemistry, Vol. 4 (M. Florkin and H. S. Mason, Eds.). Academic, New York, 1962, p. 483.
249. A. F. Munro, Biochem. J. 54:29 (1953).
250. G. W. Brown, W. R. Brown, and P. P. Cohen, J. Biol. Chem. 234: 1775 (1959).
251. G. W. Brown and P. P. Cohen, Biochem. J. 75:82 (1960).
252. P. P. Cohen and G. W. Brown, in Comparative Biochemistry, Vol. 2 (M. Florkin and H. S. Mason, Eds.). Academic, New York, 1960, p. 161.
253. J. R. Tata, Curr. Top. Dev. Biol. 6:79 (1971).
254. R. Weber, in The Biochemistry of Animal Development, Vol. 2 (R. Weber, Ed.). Academic, New York, 1967, p. 227.
255. W. K. Paik and P. P. Cohen, J. Biol. Chem. 236:531 (1961).
256. W. K. Paik and P. P. Cohen, J. Gen. Physiol. 43:683 (1960).
257. H. A. Bern and C. S. Nicoll, Rec. Progr. Horm. Res. 24:681 (1968).
258. W. Etkin and A. G. Gona, in Handbook of Physiology, Sec. 7, Vol. 3 (M. A. Greer and D. H. Solomon, Eds.). American Physiological Society, Washington, D.C., 1974, p. 5.
259. W. C. Grant and G. Cooper, Biol. Bull. 129:510 (1965).
260. W. C. Grant and G. E. Pickford, Biol. Bull. 116:429 (1959).
261. C. W. Hoffman and J. N. Dent, J. Morphol. 157:79 (1978).
262. A. K. Medda and E. Frieden, Endocrinol. 87:356 (1970).
263. W. Etkin and R. Lehrer, Endocrinol. 67:457 (1960).
264. W. Etkin and A. G. Gona, J. Exp. Zool. 165:249 (1967).
265. A. G. Gona, T. Pearlman, and W. Etkin, Endocrinol. 48:585 (1970).
266. F. L. Hoch, in Handbook of Physiology, Sec. 7, Vol. 3 (M. A. Greer and D. H. Solomon, Eds.). American Physiological Society, Washington, D. C., 1974, p. 391.

267. A. G. Gilman and F. Murad, in The Pharmacological Basis of Therapeutics 5th ed. (L. S. Goodman and A. Gilman, Eds.). Macmillan, New York, 1975, p. 1372.
268. A. G. Gilman and F. Murad, in The Pharmacological Basis of Therapeutics 5th ed. (L. S. Goodman and A. Gilman, Eds.). Macmillan, New York, 1975, p. 1398.
269. P. W. Nathanielsz, Brit. Med. Bull. 31:51 (1975).
270. K. von Werder and H. K. Rjosk, Klin. Wochenschr. 57:1 (1979).
271. M. B. Renfree, Nature 278:549 (1979).
272. B. Shome and A. F. Parlow, J. Clin. Endocrinol. 45:1112 (1977).
273. H. D. Niall, M. L. Hogan, G. W. Tregear, G. V. Segre, P. Hwang, and H. Friesen, Rec. Progr. Horm. Res. 29:387 (1973).
274. C. H. Li, in Handbook of Physiology, Sec. 7, Vol. 4, Part 2 (E. Knobil and W. H. Sawyer, Eds.). American Physiological Society, Washington, D.C., 1974, p. 103.
275. D. Reinwein and J. E. Rall, J. Biol. Chem. 241:1636 (1966).
276. T. J. Visser, I. van der Does-Tobé, R. Docter, and G. Hennemann, Biochem. J. 150:489 (1975).
277. R. Kato and A. Takahashi, Mol. Pharmacol. 4:109 (1968).
278. E. S. Vesell, Clin. Pharmacol. Ther. 22:659 (1977).
279. J. Fishman and H. L. Bradlow, Clin. Pharmacol. Ther. 22:721 (1977).
280. A. H. Conney and R. Kuntzman, in Handbook of Experimental Pharmacology, Vol. 28, Part 2 (B. B. Brodie and J. R. Gillette, Eds.). Springer-Verlag, Berlin, 1971, p. 401.
281. L. Van Middlesworth, in Handbook of Physiology, Sec. 7, Vol. 3 (M. A. Greer and D. H. Solomon, Eds.). American Physiological Society, Washington, D.C., 1974, p. 215.
282. H. A. Bern, C. S. Nicoll, and R. C. Strohman, Proc. Soc. Exp. Biol. Med. 126:518 (1967).
283. J. D. Neill, in Handbook of Physiology, Sec. 7, Vol. 4, Part 2 (E. Knobil and W. H. Sawyer, Eds.). American Physiological Society, Washington, D.C., 1974, p. 469.
284. W. Vale, R. Blackwell, G. Grant, and R. Guillemin, Endocrinol. 93:26 (1973).
285. R. Freeman, Classification of the Animal Kingdom. Lion Library, London, 1975.
286. G. Powis, A. H. Drummond, D. E. MacIntyre, and W. R. Jondorf, Xenobiotica 6:69 (1976).
287. P.-C. Fink and B. Keréjartó, Hoppe-Seyler's Z. Physiol. Chem. 345:272 (1966).
288. M. B. Abou-Donia and D. B. Menzel, Biochemistry 7:3788 (1968).
289. C. H. Walker, in Environmental Quality and Safety, Vol. 3 (F. Coulston and F. Korte, Eds.). Academic, New York, 1974, p. 113.

290. A. H. Conney, K. Schneidman, M. Jacobson, and R. Kuntzman, Ann. N.Y. Acad. Sci. 123:98 (1965).
291. R. S. Mathur, R. H. Common, D. C. Collins, and D. S. Layne, Biochim. Biophys. Acta 176:394 (1969).
292. G. A. Quamme, D. S. Layne, and D. G. Williamson, Comp. Biochem. Physiol. 39B:25 (1971).
293. A. R. Robinson, G. O. Henneberry, and R. H. Common, Biochim. Biophys. Acta 326:93 (1973).
294. D. B. Peakall, Nature 216:505 (1967).
295. H. G. Nowicki and A. W. Norman, Steroids 19:85 (1972).
296. W. M. Britton, Bull. Environ. Contamin. Toxicol. 13:698 (1975).
297. K. L. Davison and J. L. Sell, J. Agr. Food Chem. 20:1198 (1972).
298. J. L. Sell and K. L. Davison, Fed. Proc. 32:2003 (1973).
299. K. L. Davison and J. L. Sell, Arch. Environ. Contamin. Toxicol. 2:302 (1974).
300. I. Newton and J. Bogan, Nature 249:582 (1974).
301. L. F. Stickel and L. I. Rhodes, in The Biological Impact of Pesticides in the Environment. Oregon State University Press, Corvallis, 1970, p. 31.
302. K. A. Hassal, Pest. Biochem. Physiol. 1:259 (1971).
303. J. M. Runnels and M. A. Q. Khan, Amer. Zool. 13:1308 (1973).
304. J. M. Runnels and M. A. Q. Khan, Gen. Pharmacol. 6:97 (1975).
305. M. B. Abou-Donia and D. B. Menzel, Biochem. Pharmacol. 17:2143 (1968).
306. J. L. Lincer and D. B. Peakall, Environ. Pollut. 4:59 (1973).
307. A. S. DeFreitas and R. J. Norstrom, Can. J. Physiol. Pharmacol. 52:1080 (1974).
308. J. G. Cummings, M. Eidelman, V. Turner, D. Reed, K. T. Zee, and R. E. Cook, J. Ass. Offic. Anal. Chem. 50:418 (1967).
309. J. L. Ludke, Bull. Environ. Contamin. Toxicol. 11:297 (1974).
310. E. M. Thompson, G. J. Mountney, and G. W. Ware, J. Econ. Entomol. 60:235 (1967).
311. D. C. Holmes, J. H. Simmons, and J. O'G. Tatton, Nature 216:227 (1967).
312. J. O'G. Tatton and J. H. A. Ruzicka, Nature 215:346 (1967).
313. J. Robinson, A. Richardson, A. N. Crabtree, J. C. Coulson, and G. R. Potts, Nature 214:1307 (1967).
314. I. H. Wiese, N. C. J. Basson, J. H. Van der Vyver, and J. H. Van der Merwe, Phytophylactica 1:161 (1969).
315. I. Brandt, P.-G. Högman, Y. Larsson, and S. Olsson, Acta Vet. Scand. 19:368 (1978).
316. W. R. Jondorf, D. E. MacIntyre, and G. Powis, Brit. J. Pharmacol. 47:624P (1973).
317. G. J. Dutton, Enzyme 15:304 (1973).

318. G. J. Dutton and V. Ko, Biochem. J. 99:550 (1966).
319. J. R. Fouts and R. H. Adamson, Science 129:897 (1959).
320. K. J. Netter, in Proceedings of the Sixth International Congress of Pharmacology, Vol. 6 (N. T. Karki, Ed.). Pergamon, Oxford, 1976, p. 3.
321. C. F. Strittmatter and F. T. Umberger, Biochim. Biophys. Acta 180:18 (1969).
322. B. Spencer and J. Raftery, Biochem. J. 99:35P (1966).
323. J. H. Koeman, R. C. H. M. Oudejans, and E. A. Huisman, Nature 215:1094 (1967).
324. R. C. Stendell, in Environmental Protection Agency, Proceedings of the National Conference on Polychlorinated Biphenyls, November 1975, Chicago, EPA-560/6-75-004. Washington, D.C., 1976, p. 262.
325. M. Rockstein, Ed., The Physiology of Insects, Vols. 1-6, 2nd ed. Academic, New York, 1974.
326. H. H. Rees, Insect Biochemistry. Chapman and Hall, London, 1977.
327. R. L. Metcalf, Organic Insecticides. Interscience, New York, 1955.
328. E. Y. Spencer, Symposium on metabolism of insecticides, Can. J. Biochem. Physiol. 37:1090 (1959).
329. G. B. Staal, Ann. Rev. Entomol. 20:417 (1975).
330. R. M. Hollingworth, in Insecticide Biochemistry and Physiology (C. F. Wilkinson, Ed.). Plenum, New York, 1976, p. 431.
331. F. J. Oppenoorth and W. Welling, in Insecticide Biochemistry and Physiology (C. F. Wilkinson, Ed.). Plenum, New York, 1976, p. 508.
332. F. W. Plapp, Annu. Rev. Entomol. 21:179 (1976).
333. M. Florkin and C. Jeuniaux, in The Physiology of Insecta, 2nd ed., Vol. 5 (M. Rockstein, Ed.). Academic, New York, 1974, p. 255.
334. P. Karlson and C. E. Sekeris, Acta Endocrinol. 53:505 (1966).
335. M. Locke, in The Physiology of Insecta, 2nd ed., Vol. 6 (M. Rockstein, Ed.). Academic, New York, 1974, p. 123.
336. R. H. Hackman, in The Physiology of Insecta, 2nd ed., Vol. 6 (M. Rockstein, Ed.). Academic, New York, 1974, p. 215.
337. K. Slama, M. Romanuk, and F. Sorm, Insect Hormones and Bioanalogues. Springer-Verlag, Vienna, 1974.
338. L. L. Keeley, Annu. Rev. Entomol. 23:329 (1978).
339. M. J. Thompson, J. N. Kaplanis, W. E. Robbins, and J. A. Svoboda, Advan. Lipid Res. 11:219 (1973).
340. J. A. Svoboda, J. N. Kaplanis, W. E. Robbins, and M. J. Thompson, Annu. Rev. Entomol. 20:205 (1975).
341. P. Karlson and H. Hoffmeister, Z. Physiol. Chem. 331:298 (1963).
342. R. D. O'Brien, in Insecticide Biochemistry and Physiology (C. F. Wilkinson, Ed.). Plenum, New York, 1976, p. 271.
343. D. J. Nolte, S. H. Eggers, and I. R. May, J. Insect. Physiol. 19:1547 (1973).

344. H. H. Shorey, Animal Communication by Pheromones. Academic, New York, 1976.
345. R. M. Silverstein, in Chemical Control of Insect Behavior (H. H. Shorey and J. J. McKelvey, Eds.). Wiley, New York, 1977, p. 231.
346. Y. Tamaki, in Chemical Control of Insect Behavior (H. H. Shorey and J. J. McKelvey, Eds.). Wiley, New York, 1977, p. 253.
347. K. Munakata, in Chemical Control of Insect Behavior (H. H. Shorey and J. J. McKelvey, Eds.). Wiley, New York, 1977, p. 93.
348. J. E. Baker, D. P. Rainey, and D. M. Norris, Forest Sci. 14:91 (1968).
349. B. L. Gilbert and D. M. Norris, J. Insect Physiol. 14:1063 (1968).
350. D. M. Norris, Nature 222:1263 (1969).
351. J. W. Hanover, Ann. Rev. Entomol. 20:75 (1975).
352. M. Berenbaum, Science 201:532 (1978).
353. E. Sondheimer and J. B. Simeone, Chemical Ecology. Academic, New York, 1970.
354. M. Agosin and A. S. Perry, in The Physiology of Insecta, 2nd ed., Vol. 5 (M. Rockstein, Ed.). Academic, New York, 1974, p. 537.
355. R. S. H. Yang, in Insecticide Biochemistry and Physiology (C. F. Wilkinson, Ed.). Plenum, New York, 1976, p. 177.
356. R. D. Schonbrod and L. C. Terriere, J. Econ. Entomol. 64:44 (1971).
357. R. I. Krieger and C. F. Wilkinson, Biochem. Pharmacol. 18:1403 (1969).
358. S. S. Miyake, C. W. Kearns, and H. Lipke, J. Econ. Entomol. 50:359 (1957).
359. G. J. Dutton, Comp. Biochem. Physiol. 7:39 (1962).
360. H. Röller and K. H. Dahm, Progr. Horm. Res. 24:651 (1968).
361. M. Slade and C. F. Wilkinson, Comp. Biochem. Physiol. 49B:99 (1974).
362. L. L. Sanburg, K. J. Kramer, F. J. Kézdy, J. H. Law, and H. Oberlander, Nature 253:266 (1975).
363. P. Schmialek, Z. Naturforsch., Ser. B. 16:461 (1961).
364. K. J. Judy, D. A. Schooley, L. L. Dunham, M. S. Hall, B. J. Bergot, and J. P. Siddall, Proc. Nat. Acad. Sci. U.S. 70:1509 (1973).
365. C. M. Williams, in The Nature of Biological Diversity (J. M. Allen, Ed.). McGraw-Hill, New York, 1963, p. 243.
366. H. V. Gelboin, Advan. Cancer Res. 10:1 (1967).
367. R. I. Krieger, P. P. Feeny, and C. F. Wilkinson, Science 172:579 (1971).
368. M. N. Galbraith, D. H. S. Horn, E. J. Middleton, and J. A. Thomson, Chem. Commun. 1970, p. 179.
369. A. Willig, H. H. Rees, and T. W. Goodwin, J. Insect Physiol. 17:2317 (1971).
370. G. Heinrich and H. Hoffmeister, Z. Naturforsch. 25B:358 (1970).

371. C. F. Wilkinson, Insecticide Biochemistry and Physiology. Plenum, New York, 1976.
372. J. E. Casida, Science 146:1011 (1964).
373. T. Shishido and J.-I. Fukami, Pest. Biochem. Physiol. 2:39 (1972).
374. T. Shishido, K. Usui, and J.-I. Fukami, Pest. Biochem. Physiol. 2:27 (1972).
375. T. Shishido, K. Usui, M. Sato, and J.-I. Fukami, Pest. Biochem. Physiol. 2:51 (1972).
375a. G. T. Brooks, A. Harrison, and J. T. Cox, Nature 197:311 (1963).
376. O. Giannotti, R. L. Metcalf, and R. B. March, Ann. Entomol. Soc. Amer. 49:588 (1956).
377. F. Korte, G. Ludwig, and J. Vogel, Justus Liebig Ann. Chem. 656: 139 (1962).
378. A. S. Perry, G. W. Pearce, and A. J. Buckner, J. Econ. Entomol. 57:867 (1964).
379. M. C. Bowman, F. Acree, C. S. Lofgren, and M. Beroza, Science 146:1480 (1964).
380. P. Gerolt, J. Econ. Entomol. 58:849 (1965).
381. J. W. Ray, Biochem. Pharmacol. 16:99 (1967).
382. L. C. Mitchell, J. Ass. Offic. Anal. Chem. 44:643 (1961).
383. J. Roburn, Chem. Ind., No. 38, 1555 (1963).
384. R. L. Williamson and M. S. Schechter, Biochem. Pharmacol. 19: 1719 (1970).
385. F. Oesch, D. M. Jerina, and J. W. Daly, Biochim. Biophys. Acta 227:685 (1971).
386. R. D. Schonbrod, W. W. Philleo, and L. C. Terriere, J. Econ. Entomol. 58:74 (1965).
387. R. B. Boose and L. C. Terriere, J. Econ. Entomol. 60:580 (1967).
388. M. A. Q. Khan and L. C. Terriere, J. Econ. Entomol. 61:732 (1968).
389. M. A. Q. Khan, J. Econ. Entomol. 62:388 (1969).
390. J. Booth and E. Boyland, Biochem. J. 70:681 (1958).
391. G. M. Benke, C. F. Wilkinson, and J. N. Telford, J. Econ. Entomol. 65:1221 (1972).
392. R. T. Williams, in Handbook of Experimental Pharmacology, Vol. 28, Part 2 (B. B. Brodie and J. R. Gillette, Eds.). Springer-Verlag, New York, 1971, p. 226.
393. A. Taurog, Rec. Progr. Horm. Res. 26:189 (1970).
394. A. Taurog, in Handbook of Physiology, Sec. 7, Vol. 3 (M. A. Greer and D. H. Solomon, Eds.). American Physiological Society, Washington, D.C., 1974, p. 101.
395. K. Sterling and J. H. Lazarus, Ann. Rev. Physiol. 39:349 (1977).
396. A. V. Holden and K. Marsden, Nature 216:1274 (1967).
397. J. H. Koeman, M. C. ten Noever de Brauw, and R. H. De Vos, Nature 221:1126 (1969).

398. B. Nelson, Science 166:977 (1969).
399. Editorial Nature 226:309 (1970).
400. K. D. Courtney, D. W. Gaylor, M. D. Hogan, H. L. Falk, R. R. Bates, and I. Mitchell, Science 168:864 (1970).
401. D. Shapley, Science 180:285 (1973).
402. K. Ueda, in PCB Poisoning and Pollution (K. Higuchi, Ed.). Kodansha, Tokyo, 1976, p. 25.
403. Y. Yoshimura and S. Yoshihara, in PCB Poisoning and Pollution (K. Higuchi, Ed.). Kodansha, Tokyo, 1976, p. 41.
404. O. Wada, Y. Yano, G. Urata, and K. Nakao, Biochem. Pharmacol. 17:595 (1968).
405. D. J. Ecobichon, in Environmental Protection Agency, Proceedings of the National Conference on Polychlorinated Biphenyls, November 1975, Chicago, EPA-560/6-75-004. Washington, D.C., 1976, p. 57.
406. J. N. Smith, B. Spencer, and R. T. Williams, Biochem. J. 47:284 (1950).
407. W. M. Azouz, D. V. Parke, and R. T. Williams, Biochem. J. 50:702 (1952).
408. D. V. Parke and R. T. Williams, Biochem. J. 59:415 (1955).
409. D. V. Parke and R. T. Williams, Biochem. J. 74:5 (1960).
410. W. R. Jondorf, D. V. Parke, and R. T. Williams, Biochem. J. 61:512 (1955).
411. W. R. Jondorf, D. V. Parke, and R. T. Williams, Biochem. J. 69:181 (1958).
412. D. R. Boyd, J. W. Daly, and D. M. Jerina, Biochemistry 11:1961 (1972).
413. J. W. Daly, D. M. Jerina, and B. Witkop, Experientia 28:1129 (1972).
414. W. Durham, Ann. N.Y. Acad. Sci. 160:183 (1969).
415. F. W. Kutz and S. C. Strassman, in Environmental Protection Agency, Proceedings of the National Conference on Polychlorinated Biphenyls, November 1975, Chicago, EPA-560/6-75-004. Washington, D.C., 1976, p. 139.
416. R. K. Ockner and R. Schmid, Nature 189:499 (1961).
417. F. DeMatteis, B. E. Prior, and C. Rimington, Nature 191:363 (1961).
418. H. S. Marver and R. Schmid, in The Metabolic Basis of Inherited Disease, 3rd ed. (J. B. Stanbury, J. B. Wyngaarden, and D. S. Frederickson, Eds.). McGraw-Hill, New York, 1972, p. 1087.
419. G. D. Sweeney and K. G. Jones, in Industrial and Environmental Xenobiotics (J. R. Fouts and I. Gut, Eds.). Excerpta Medica, Amsterdam, 1978, p. 229.
420. J. J. T. W. A. Strik, Environ. Health Persp., 23:167 (1978).
421. M. Kuratsune, in PCB Poisoning and Pollution (K. Higuchi, Ed.). Kodansha, Tokyo, 1976, p. 9.

422. M. Kuratsune, Y. Masuda, and J. Nagayama, in Environmental Protection Agency, Proceedings of the National Conference on Polychlorinated Biphenyls, November 1975, Chicago, EPA-560/6-75-004. Washington, D.C., 1976, p. 14.
423. Editorial Lancet ii:19 (1977).
424. L. B. Brilliant, G. Van Amburg, I. Isbister, H. Humphrey, K. Wilcox, J. Eyster, A. W. Bloomer, and H. Price, Lancet ii:643 (1978).
425. A. Hay, Nature 262:639 (1976).
426. M. Biocca, J. A. Moore, B. N. Gupta, and J. D. McKinney, in Environmental Protection Agency, Proceedings of the National Conference on Polychlorinated Biphenyls, November 1975, Chicago, EPA-560/6-75-004. Washington, D.C., 1976, p. 67.
427. A. Poland and E. Glover, Mol. Pharmacol. 13:924 (1977).
428. H. B. Matthews and M. W. Anderson, Drug Metab. Dispos. 3:371 (1975).
429. S. Mühlebach and M. H. Bickel, Experientia 35:951 (1979).
430. G. W. Bowes, M. J. Mulvihill, B. R. T. Simoneit, A. L. Burlingame, and R. W. Risebrough, Nature 256:305 (1975).
431. J. A. Goldstein, J. R. Hass, P. Linko, and D. J. Harvan, Drug Metab. Dispos. 6:258 (1978).
432. J. A. Moore, B. N. Gupta, and J. G. Vos, in Environmental Protection Agency, Proceedings of the National Conference on Polychlorinated Biphenyls, November 1975, Chicago, EPA-560/6-75-004. Washington, D.C., 1976, p. 77.
433. A. Niwa, K. Kumaki, and D. W. Nebert, Mol. Pharmacol. 11:399 (1975).
434. A. Poland and E. Glover, Mol. Pharmacol. 10:349 (1974).
435. A. Poland and E. Glover, Mol. Pharmacol. 9:736 (1973).
436. D. Wasserman, M. Wasserman, S. Cucos, and M. Djavaherian, Environ. Res. 6:334 (1973).
437. L. Fishbein, Ann. Rev. Pharmacol. 14:139 (1974).
438. J. R. Allen, Fed. Proc. 34:1675 (1975).
439. S. Jensen and G. Sundström, Nature 251:219 (1974).
440. T. F. Jackson and F. L. Halbert, J. Amer. Vet. Med. Assoc. 165:437 (1974).
441. S. D. Sleight, S. Mangkoewidjojo, B. T. Akoso, and V. L. Sanger, Environ. Health Persp. 23:341 (1978).
442. H. W. Doelle, Bacterial Metabolism, 2nd ed. Academic, New York, 1975, p. 490.

Chapter 7

IN VIVO ASSESSMENT OF HEPATIC DRUG DISPOSITION

Johannes Bircher and Rudolf Preisig

Department of Clinical Pharmacology
University of Berne
Berne, Switzerland

When studying drug disposition, the jump from in vitro to in vivo conditions implies a considerable increase in the complexity of underlying biological phenomena. The liver as the main organ of xenobiotic biotransformation occupies a pivotal position in this interplay of biological processes, and an assessment of hepatic drug disposition requires a detailed analysis of influencing factors.

The present chapter discusses hepatic drug disposition in vivo by integrating two distinct viewpoints. In a first approach, many important factors influencing hepatic drug disposition are considered; these include extrahepatic mechanisms affecting the fate of foreign compounds, drug transport to the liver, hepatic uptake, biotransformation, and elimination. In a second approach, major and most recent methodological concepts are discussed in detail, stressing their benefits, limits, and shortcomings. The methods used to assess in vivo hepatic drug disposition are mainly centered on elimination studies. Biliary excretion being a direct elimination route provides a particularly useful means of investigation, while elimination into blood and indirectly into breath, urine, and saliva may all yield valuable information.

Results of studies from our own laboratory included in this review have been supported by the Swiss National Science Foundation.

I. INTRODUCTION

The in vivo study of hepatic drug disposition is fraught with many obstacles. Most of the presently available methods are time-consuming and impose inconvenience on the investigated individuals, and the interpretation of resulting data is subject to narrow limitations. Despite these constraints, investigation of drug disposition in the intact organism—be it normal subjects or patients—is ultimately pertinent, because only such studies can produce the kind of data which are needed for rational drug therapy.

In vivo investigation of drug disposition generally requires due planning. All available information about chemical and biochemical properties of a drug under study has to be included in the formulation of the hypotheses on which the design of a protocol is to be based. Alternatively, results obtained in animals must be evaluated to properly plan studies in humans. Often the usefulness of a particular approach has to be verified in pilot studies. An optimal experimental design, however, will also consider all those factors which are specific for the intact organism: drug dosages, the quality, number, and size of samples, etc. Furthermore, the investigated individuals should be appropriately characterized. On the basis of these considerations it becomes obvious that in vivo investigations have to be optimized in every possible way. Thus, they combine science, art, and service in an almost ideal way.

The present chapter has not been intended as an exhaustive review covering all the pertinent literature. The expressed ideas rather have resulted from experiences made by the authors during the past few years while actively studying hepatic drug disposition in vivo.

II. EXTRAHEPATIC FACTORS DETERMINING DRUG DISPOSITION

When investigating drug disposition in vivo the whole organism may be involved in many ways. In order to understand the specific contribution of the liver it is necessary, therefore, to consider to what extent extrahepatic processes may modify the overall disposition of a drug, and how the part played by the liver can be assessed separately. Obviously, selection of appropriate test substances may simplify the problem: many xenobiotics are eliminated almost exclusively by the liver and have therefore been considered as model compounds. In other instances simple corrections—e.g., for urinary output—may for practical purposes be adequate (Fig. 1) [1]. With other drugs, each component contributing to their overall disposition needs to be evaluated.

The special anatomical arrangement of the liver between the gastrointestinal tract and the systemic circulation adds to the importance of extrahepatic factors which may determine the fate of a drug [2]. Depending on the route of administration, a particular compound may distribute itself within the organism either before being transported to the liver or after a first passage through the intestinal epithelium and the liver. For some drugs, both the intestine and the liver may remove and metabolize a large

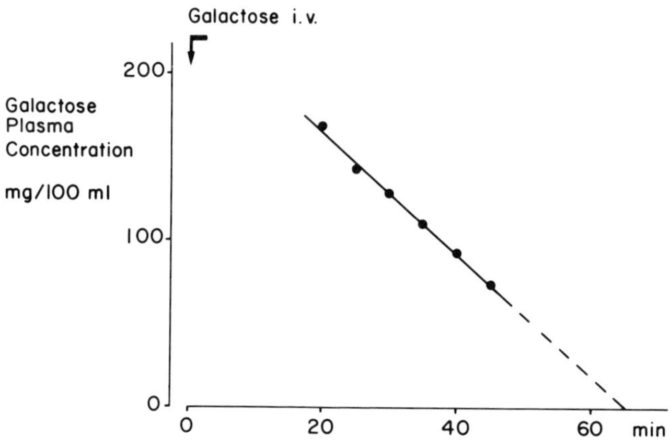

FIGURE 1 Determination of the hepatic galactose elimination capacity (GEC). The calculations assume zero-order elimination, a correction factor of 5 min for sampling of peripheral venous plasma instead of the average body content, and a simple correction for urinary output. The further assumption that the rest of the injected amount of galactose is metabolized in the liver is not fully valid because in the normal adult about 2.0 to 2.5 mg/min may be metabolized extrahepatically. Since this value is relatively constant, it does not interfere with the practical usefulness of the galactose elimination capacity as a quantitative test of hepatic function. Calculations (for a male subject, 25 years old, 55 kg) are as follow: 27,500 mg (amount injected) - 3880 mg (amount eliminated in urine) = 23,620 mg (amount presumably eliminated by metabolism). GEC = 23,620/(65 + 5) = 337 mg/min = 6.1 mg/min/kg.

fraction of the dose before it can reach the systemic circulation. The hepatic contribution to presystemic elimination becomes particularly prominent with drugs having a high hepatic extraction. Other compounds undergo biliary elimination and reabsorption from the intestine, leading to a degree of enterohepatic circulation which may decisively influence their fate within the organism.

Once distribution has occurred, the study of hepatic drug disposition requires consideration of those extrahepatic factors which determine the availability of a drug for hepatocellular uptake and metabolism. Within this context the volume of distribution, the degree of plasma protein binding, penetration into formed elements of the blood, as well as the total amount of blood flowing to the liver may all be pertinent [2-4]. As these factors can change for instance with age, sex, or disease, they may modify the in vivo rate of drug metabolism without necessarily reflecting an altered function of the liver [5].

Comparing data between subjects or between species is often desirable. In this case the question will arise whether rates of drug metabolism should be expressed per kg of body weight or per g of liver weight. The two procedures will give similar results under many circumstances, yet the liver-to-body weight ratio varies with age, and with many diseases such as obesity, emaciation, or acromegaly [6]. In liver disease, liver weight may be increased with or without a change in total amount of cytochrome P-450 [7-9]. The most pertinent way to express the results of a study must therefore be evaluated in each instance.

III. HEPATIC DRUG METABOLISM AND DISPOSITION

In order to undergo hepatic elimination, a drug must first be transported to the liver, then be taken up by the hepatocytes, and eventually combine with the metabolizing enzymes or the canalicular membranes. The relative importance of each of these sequential events differs for various drugs and must therefore be considered separately in more detail (Table 1). Current experience with hepatic handling of foreign compounds shows that some drugs exhibit a high degree of rate limitation of one specific process. Such drugs may therefore be used to study this particular step with little interference by other factors which may determine rates of hepatic drug disposition. It must be pointed out, however, that the specificity of all test compounds is relative. Interferences, therefore, must always be anticipated and properly evaluated in each instance. Furthermore, as the fate of different chemical compounds may vary to a large extent, extrapolations from so-called model compounds to other drugs require great caution.

A. Hepatic Blood Flow

Several kinetic models accounting for the contribution of blood flow to hepatic drug disposition have been proposed. One model considers the hepatic sinusoids as a series of parallel tubes [10], whereas another refers to accessible spaces within the liver as a well-stirred single compartment [11] (Fig. 2). While the former model was useful to describe hepatic disposition of galactose [12], the latter appeared more suitable for lidocaine [13,14].

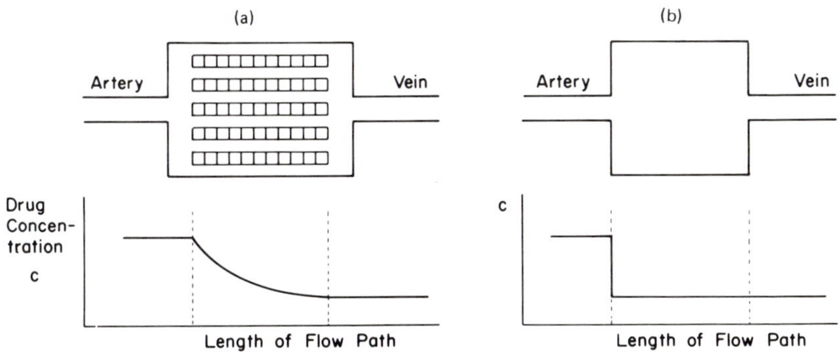

FIGURE 2 Schematic diagram of two models which have been used to explain hepatic clearance of foreign compounds: (a) The "parallel tube model" [10] implies that the concentration of the test compound falls exponentially along the length of hepatic sinusoids. Consequently the hepatocytes lining the sinusoids are exposed to decreasing substrate concentrations. To calculate organ clearance it has been proposed to divide hepatic removal by the logarithmic average ($\bar{c}$) of the inflow (c_i) and the outflow (c_o) concentration: $\bar{c} = (c_i - c_o)/(\ln c_i - \ln c_o)$. (b) In the "well-stirred compartment model" [11] the liver is depicted as a single well-stirred compartment. Sinusoidal concentrations therefore equal hepatic venous concentrations and the hepatic clearance is calculated as the ratio of the removal rate to the hepatic venous concentrations. Assumptions for both models are that portal and hepatic arterial blood mix instantaneously, that only unbound drug traverses hepatocyte membranes, that hepatic perfusion rather than diffusion of compounds from the blood to the intracellular enzymes is rate-limiting, and that the rate of metabolism or biliary elimination depends on the concentration. The parallel tube model has been successfully applied to hepatic galactose removal [12], whereas the well-stirred compartment model appears to be more appropriate to explain lidocaine kinetics [13,14].

TABLE 1
In Vivo Assessment of Hepatic Drug Disposition

Mechanism to be assessed	Special features of test compound	Examples of test compounds	Reference(s)
Hepatic blood flow	High hepatic extraction	Indocyanine green	16, 23
	High protein binding	Sulfobromophthalein	17
		Taurocholate	18
		Lidocaine	23, 173
		Propranolol	20, 66, 174
	Low protein binding	Galactose	21
		Ethanol	22
Hepatic uptake	Membrane-bound transport system	Indocyanine green	16
		Sulfobromophthalein	17
		Bile salts	36
		Ouabain	37
	Intracellular binding	Imipramine	32
		Methadone	34
Metabolism: Functionalization reactions	Low clearance, low protein binding	Antipyrine	50–56
		Aminopyrine	142, 143, 145
	Low clearance, high protein binding	Tolbutamide	63, 171
		Phenylbutazone	175
		Phenytoin	64
	High clearance, high protein binding	Propranolol	20, 66
		Lidocaine	11, 13, 14, 66
	Saturation kinetics	Phenytoin	75–77
		Salicylic acid	78
	Stereoselectivity	Warfarin	87

		Nirvanol	154
		Mephenytoin	46
Conjugation reactions	Polymorphic acetylation	Procainamide	177
		Sulfadimidine	95,178
		Isoniazid	179
		Sulfapyridine	180,181
	Glucuronidation	Menthol	182
Route of elimination:			
Into bile	Conjugation with glutathione	Sulfobromophthalein	108
	Measurement of transport maximum	Sulfobromophthalein	108,183
	No metabolic change	Indocyanine green	184
	Assessment of canalicular bile formation	Erythritol	125
		Mannitol	124
	Osmotic choleresis	Ioglycamide	185
		Ethacrynic acid	
		Bile acids and derivatives	98
Into breath	$^{14}CO_2$ exhalation	Aminopyrine	137,142,143
		Diazepam	152
		Mephenytoin	46
		Glycodiazine	148
Into blood	Pharmacologically active metabolites	Nirvanol	46
		Procainamide	177
Into urine	Conjugated metabolites	Debrisoquine	90–92
		Amobarbital	89
		Sulfadimidine	95,186

The assumptions underlying these two models may be modified to account for uneven distribution of enzymes within hepatic acini or uneven flow through hepatic sinusoids [15]. This may render them more attractive physiologically, but also more difficult to apply in practice. Since these models have been tested in isolated liver preparations, their relevance for the study of drug metabolism in vivo is as yet ill defined.

Even though various models may give numerically different results, they agree in that hepatic extraction of a compound—defined as the ratio of the arteriohepatic venous concentration difference to the arterial concentration—determines the extent to which its elimination by the liver is flow-dependent. A drug with a practically complete extraction in a single passage through the liver and without interference by extrahepatic elimination has the potential to serve as a test compound to measure hepatic blood flow. Unfortunately no such substance has become established so far. The presently used compounds such as indocyanine green [16], sulfobromophthalein [17], or taurocholic acid [18] have extractions between 0.6 and 0.9. Their clearance will therefore underestimate hepatic perfusion. A direct measurement of the hepatic arteriovenous concentration difference is needed, if the hepatic plasma or blood flow is to be calculated. Similar considerations also apply to such drugs and substances as lidocaine [19], propranolol [20], galactose [21], or ethanol [22].

Despite these limitations, a recent study in patients with abnormalities in hepatic blood flow has shown that assessment of the clearance of a high-extraction drug may be used to predict the clearance of another similar drug. Specifically, in patients with heart failure of varying severity, the ICG clearance was numerically similar to the clearance of lidocaine. On the basis of an ICG plasma disappearance curve it has therefore been possible to determine the infusion rate of lidocaine to achieve a desired steady-state plasma concentration [23].

If it is possible to catheterize a hepatic vein, hepatic blood flow can be measured with the Fick principle: An appropriate test compound is injected or infused intravenously and its arterial and hepatic venous plasma concentration is assessed [24]. In addition, the hepatic extraction of a drug under study may be measured simultaneously and its hepatic uptake or clearance may be calculated. This procedure is obviously invasive and subject to a number of limitations [24], especially in liver disease [25,26], but it may yield information which cannot be obtained in any other way. In particular hepatic removal or clearance may be related to total elimination of a drug, thereby directly assessing the contribution of the liver to its overall disposition (Fig. 3).

B. Hepatic Uptake

Even though hepatocellular uptake is an essential prerequisite for biotransformation and/or biliary elimination of any compound, the mechanisms

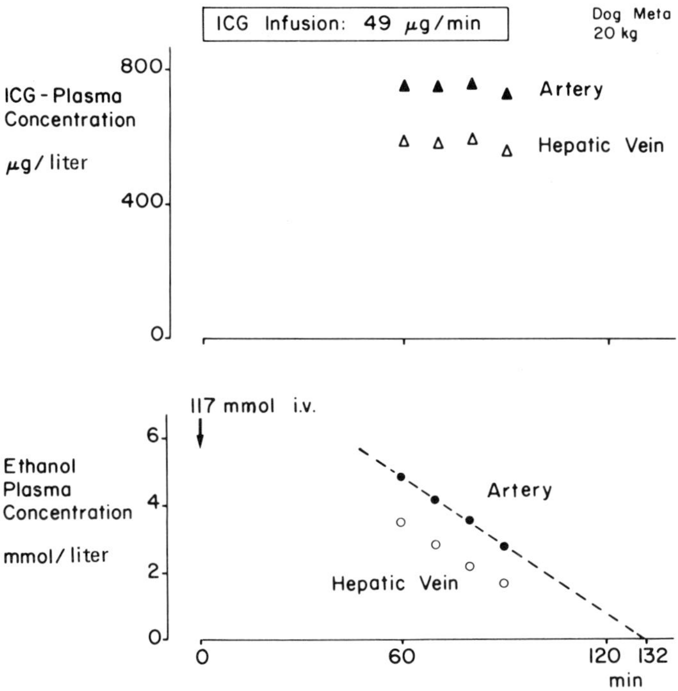

FIGURE 3 Estimation of hepatic blood flow and splanchnic removal of ethanol in a dog by hepatic vein catheterization. During a steady state achieved by a continuous infusion of ICG, hepatic removal of the dye equals its infusion rate. Consequently, hepatic plasma flow may be estimated as the ratio of the infusion rate to the mean arteriohepatic venous concentration difference (49 μg/min ÷ 165 μg/liter = 0.30 liter/min). With a hematocrit of 49% the estimated blood flow amounts to 0.58 liter/min. If this value is multiplied by the mean arteriohepatic venous difference in ethanol concentration, hepatic ethanol uptake may be estimated (0.58 liter/min × 1.28 mmol/liter = 0.75 mmol/min). Dividing the injected amount of ethanol by the extrapolated time to reach zero concentration yields an estimate of its total elimination (117 mmol ÷ 132 min = 0.88 mmol/min). Consequently hepatic removal of ethanol in this experiment amounted to 84% of total ethanol elimination. A critical analysis of assumptions and limitations of such calculations have been given by Bradley [24] and Gillette and Pang [2,4].

involved in the uptake process have received relatively little attention. Only recently has it been shown that uptake may occur completely independently of the further disposition of the investigated compounds. In many instances it has been assumed that the compounds pass the hepatocellular membrane because of their lipophilicity and subsequent binding to subcellular components such as ligandin [27], lysosomes [28-31], or lipid membranes [32]. In such instances, it appears that these subcellular components serve as a reservoir from which the drugs may be released either to undergo biotransformation or biliary excretion, or to return to the general circulation [32-34]. Apart from such passive mechanisms an increasing number of foreign compounds have been found to be taken up by a saturable, sodium- and energy-dependent transport system. Cholephilic dyes such as ICG [35] and bile acids [36], but also ouabain [37], morphine, and nalorphine [38], belong to this category.

The relevance of these highly effective passive or active hepatic uptake processes for in vivo drug disposition is as yet insufficiently defined. They may be important, for instance, in producing a high hepatic extraction of some drugs. If a hepatocellular uptake mechanism effectively competes with plasma protein binding, hepatic extraction is not necessarily restricted to the free (unbound) fraction, but may remove a high percentage of the total amount of drug present in blood even in a single passage through the liver. This type of extraction has been called "nonrestrictive." Thus, some of these hepatic uptake processes could explain that even highly protein-bound compounds may exhibit flow limitations of hepatic elimination and a high degree of presystemic elimination [3,39,40].

By contrast, many other substances diffuse into hepatocytes only to the extent that they are dissolved in plasma water and unbound to plasma proteins. Their hepatic extraction, therefore, is "restricted" to the free or unbound fraction and may correspondingly be quite small. In such instances the degree of plasma protein binding may be an important determinant for the rate of hepatocellular uptake and metabolism [3,41].

C. Functionalization Reactions

1. General Considerations

One of the problems in the evaluation of hepatic biotransformation of xenobiotics is the large variability in the type and kinetics of the chemical reactions involved. Evidence from in vitro studies is accumulating to indicate that multiple forms of cytochrome P-450 exist, and that the different forms may have overlapping substrate selectivities [42,43]. Consequently, it has not been possible so far to predict rates of metabolism of a given drug on the basis of the rates of metabolism of model compounds. This difficulty has been illustrated recently by in vitro studies in human livers, where the correlations among rates of metabolism of different drugs was found to vary widely. As shown in Table 2, benzo[a]pyrene hydroxylation

TABLE 2
Correlation between Rates of Metabolism of Different Drugs in 32 Human Livers in Vitro[a]

	Zoxazolamine hydroxylation	Coumarin hydroxylation	7-Ethoxycoumarin O-dealkylation	Antipyrine hydroxylation	Hexobarbital hydroxylation
Benzo[a]pyrene hydroxylation	0.69	0.57	0.35	0.85	0.72
Zoxazolamine hydroxylation		0.72	0.75	0.82	0.64
Coumarin hydroxylation			0.61	0.72	0.71
7-Ethoxycoumarin O-dealkylation				0.47	0.37
Antipyrine hydroxylation					0.79

[a] Numbers represent correlation coefficients derived from linear regression analysis. Levels of statistical significance are 0.45 for $p < 0.01$ and 0.55 for $p < 0.001$.
Source: Adapted from Ref. 44.

closely paralleled antipyrine hydroxylation (r = 0.85), but not 7-ethoxycoumarin O-dealkylation (r = 0.35) [44]. It has been generally accepted, therefore, that results obtained with one drug are regarded as representative only for that particular drug and that extrapolation to other drugs is hazardous [45].

A further difficulty for in vivo studies is related to the fact that most drugs are simultaneously transformed into several different metabolites, some of which are further transformed into other compounds. The proportions among the different primary and secondary metabolites is likely to vary from subject to subject. Consequently, the investigator has to deal with a multiplicity of, and a variability in, metabolic routes which may occur in parallel and/or in series. The metabolites themselves may either accumulate in blood or be eliminated more or less rapidly in bile or urine.

The consequences of these complexities are multiple:

1. Elimination of a compound by metabolism is generally the sum of several metabolic transformations. Measurement of a drug clearance therefore, may not adequately reflect the rate of formation of individual metabolites. For instance, N-demethylation of mephenytoin to nirvanol in the dog is not dose-dependent as opposed to hydroxylation (Fig. 4). This dose dependence of a minor metabolite is not reflected in the plasma clearance of mephenytoin [46].

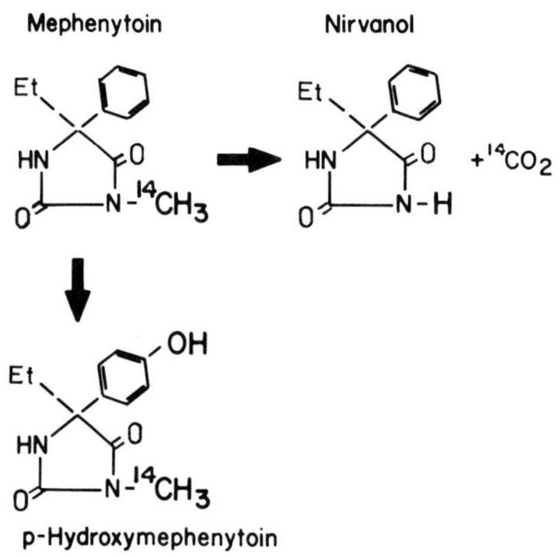

FIGURE 4 The two main pathways of mephenytoin metabolism can be assessed easily with ([^{14}C]methyl)-mephenytoin. Demethylation leads to nirvanol which accumulates in plasma, and to $^{14}CO_2$ which may be collected in exhaled air. Hydroxylation does not remove the label and can therefore be assessed simply by counting urinary radioactivity.

2. Metabolites accumulating in plasma may influence the rate of metabolism of the unchanged compound. This phenomenon has been well documented, for instance, with primidone [47] and also observed with mephenytoin. N-Demethylation of mephenytoin is inhibited in the presence of the demethylated metabolite nirvanol [46].
3. Evaluation of a single major metabolite is likely to neglect the more or less variable importance of minor metabolites (Fig. 5).
4. If an experimental design requires that metabolic end products are sampled, it should be realized that the kinetics of formation of secondary metabolites—resulting from further metabolism of primary metabolites—may be related to the disposition of the administered compound only in an indirect manner. Therefore, a postulated relationship should be verified experimentally [48,49].

2. Drugs with Low Clearance and Low Protein Binding

As shown in Table 1, the different drugs which have been used to study functionalization reactions differ in their pharmacokinetic properties and correspondingly have been used for miscellaneous aims. The simplest kinetic situation is the combination of a relatively rapid distribution in body water, a low protein binding, and an almost exclusive, relatively slow elimination in the liver by metabolism independent of hepatic blood flow. These conditions lead to a so-called capacity-limited hepatic elimination and are largely fulfilled by antipyrine. The fate of this compound has been extensively investigated under a variety of circumstances [50-56]. Since antipyrine concentrations in saliva are practically identical with simultaneously determined concentrations in plasma water, sampling of saliva appears sufficient in most instances [57-59]. Aminopyrine is similar to antipyrine in many respects [48]; it has also been used to assess hepatic drug metabolism [60] in vivo, but the clearance is several times larger. Some degree of flow limitation may occur, particularly after enzyme induction [61].

3. Drugs with Low Clearance and High Protein Binding

Drugs which are tightly bound to plasma proteins may have a low hepatic clearance—less than 20% of hepatic plasma flow—because only the free or unbound fraction is available for uptake into hepatocytes. Under these circumstances, blood flow will not be rate-limiting and hepatic disposition depends mainly on plasma protein binding and on the functional capacity of the liver. For these drugs, hepatic clearance has been called "restricted" or "uptake-limited binding sensitive." Because of the prominent contribution of plasma protein binding these compounds are suitable for an assessment of hepatic drug disposition only if protein binding is studied simultaneously and if the clearance of the free drug is calculated [62,63]. In patients with liver disease, it is possible that an impairment in hepatic clearance may be counteracted by a corresponding reduction in protein binding and that the overall disposition may be normal [64,65].

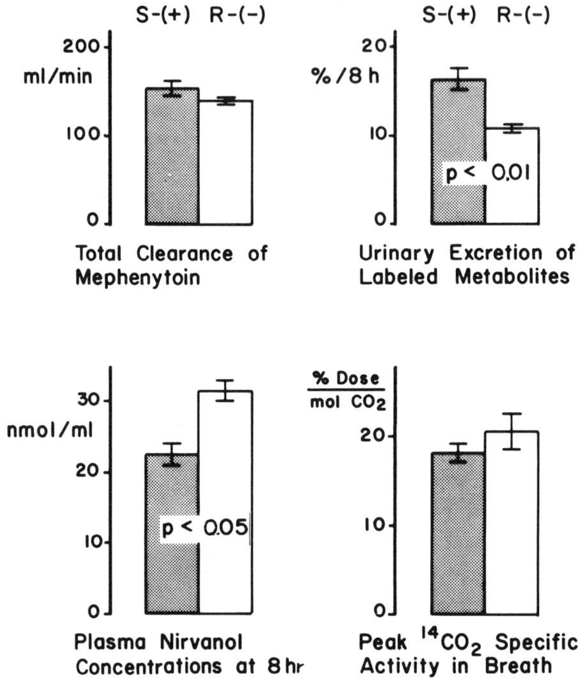

FIGURE 5 Stereoselectivity of the two metabolic pathways for mephenytoin metabolism was assessed in four dogs which had received the enantiomers intravenously according to a crossover design. The total blood clearance of the two enantiomers was practically the same. Urinary elimination of labeled metabolites, however, was highly stereoselective in favor of the (S)-(+)-enantiomer. Plasma nirvanol concentrations 8 hr after mephenytoin administration showed a stereoselectivity in favor of the (R)-(-)-enantiomer, whereas peak $^{14}CO_2$ levels in breath were not different statistically. A more complete analysis of the data has shown that the lower plasma concentrations of (S)-(+)-nirvanol resulted from a more rapid further hydroxylation of nirvanol to hydroxynirvanol, rather than from a stereoselectivity of mephenytoin demethylation. Thus mephenytoin hydroxylation—the minor metabolic pathway—seems to be stereoselective, whereas mephenytoin demethylation—the major pathway—is not. Therefore, the difference in total clearance between the two enantiomers tends to favor the more rapid hydroxylation of (S)-(+)-mephenytoin, but does not reach statistical significance. The two metabolic pathways also differ in dose dependence and in the inhibition by nirvanol, suggesting that they occur at different enzymes or enzyme sites. (From Ref. 46.)

4. Highly Extracted Drugs

If the hepatic extraction of a drug is relatively high (>0.7), hepatic clearance approaches blood or plasma flow through the liver. Hepatic elimination of such compounds has been called "flow-limited." Many of these drugs are relatively tightly bound to plasma proteins. The hepatocytes seem to be able to remove not only the free fraction, but also that portion of the drug which is protein-bound. Under these circumstances hepatic extraction has been called "nonrestrictive" [3].

In vivo methods used to study hepatic disposition of highly extracted (high-extraction) drugs present particular problems. If such compounds are administered orally, the degree of systemic availability is dependent on both intestinal and hepatic drug elimination, and these two components cannot be discriminated easily. Furthermore, in case of liver disease a fraction of the drug may bypass hepatic parenchymal cells through extra- or intrahepatic portal-hepatic venous shunts. If high-extraction drugs are administered intravenously, hepatic blood or plasma flow is likely to be the primary determinant of hepatic elimination. However, the relative contribution of hepatic blood flow and of the functional capacity of the liver for hepatic removal cannot be assessed without additional information. Either the hepatic blood flow must be measured by hepatic vein catheterization, or infusions of the drug have to be made directly into the portal vein. In either case the experiments are invasive and therefore difficult to be carried out in humans. The only noninvasive approach consists in the simultaneously combined intravenous and oral administration of the drug under study [66, 67]. Although there is hope that this experimental design may define all the pertinent physiological variables [3], this is true only if drug elimination by the gut wall can be excluded.

If the liver is abnormal, its functional capacity, its perfusion, as well as drug binding to plasma proteins may all be altered to a variable degree. It would then appear necessary to separately assess the relative contribution to hepatic clearance of each of these factors. Otherwise conclusions about the influence of disease on rate-limiting processes might be hazardous. The value of an evaluation of drug disposition which included hepatic vein catheterization and measurement of hepatic blood flow has been demonstrated by Pessayre et al. [20]. These authors compared the fate of (+)-propranolol in a group of cirrhotics and in a group of patients suffering only from liver fibrosis. Whereas the hepatic clearance averaged 18 ml/min/kg in the latter, it was 6 ml/min/kg in cirrhosis. This change was due both to a reduction in intrinsic clearance (from 72 to 12 ml/min/kg) and in hepatic blood flow (from 25 to 14 ml/min/kg) in the cirrhotic patients.

5. Nonlinear Kinetics

For many drugs linear kinetics may reasonably be assumed. There are, however, a number of reasons for nonlinearity such as saturation of first-pass elimination [68,69], of the plasma protein or tissue binding [70, 71], of hepatic elimination, and of renal tubular transport. In addition, autoinduction, accumulation of metabolites resulting in end product inhibition [46,47], enterohepatic circulation, diurnal rhythms [72], and variation in physiological functions such as hepatic blood flow in response to food [73, 74] need to be considered.

Saturation of the metabolic capacity of the liver is of practical relevance for compounds such as phenytoin [75-77], and salicylic acid [78,79]. Therapeutic plasma concentrations of these agents can be monitored and during steady-state situations V_{max} and K_m may easily be derived even as part of routine therapy by using one of the conventional linearization procedures for Michaelis-Menten kinetics [75-77]. Alternatively the plasma concentration-time curve may be followed over a sufficient range and analyzed by the integrated form of the Michaelis-Menten function [80,81].

Another example of practical consequences resulting from the study of saturation kinetics is related to biliary contrast agents. When it was recognized that short-lasting but high plasma concentrations were less useful than low concentrations for a sufficient period of time, infusion cholangiography was preferred to the previous bolus injections. Thereby the frequency of adverse effects was reduced and visualization of the biliary passages was improved [82].

Saturation kinetics have also been used to assess the maximal functional capacity of the liver: Maximal galactose elimination (Fig. 1) and maximal ethanol oxidation may be derived from simple plasma disappearance curves [1], or from more complicated kinetic calculations [83,84]. Alternatively, hepatic uptake of ICG has been assessed with a series of plasma disappearance curves after injection of varying doses of the test compound [16]. Finally, the multiple-indicator dilution technique represents a powerful albeit invasive and sophisticated method applicable to animal studies only [85,86].

In all these instances interpretation of V_{max} will be easier than that of the apparent K_m. The former represents an extrapolated maximal capacity of the liver, whereas the latter may be the consequence of several physiological and biochemical properties of the investigated subject. Among others, blood flow, transmembranous concentration gradients, protein binding, and site of sampling may be important. Interpretations of K_m values therefore require due caution.

6. Evaluation of Cytochrome P-450

Cytochrome P-450 is now known to be composed of multiple forms with differing substrate selectivities. It has been speculated that knowledge of the different forms of the system in an individual patient could be used to predict the patient's rates of metabolism of different drugs. One of the aims in the study of functionalization reactions was the development of specific tests for each form of the cytochrome P-450 system. Although this goal is as yet out of reach, the pursuit of the idea has led to some new approaches. The experimental design includes the simultaneous study of two or several chemical reactions which presumably occur at different enzyme sites, but do not differ in regard to all other variables. Only two procedures have fulfilled these criteria, namely, analysis of the stereoselectivity of chemical transformations and simultaneous determination of the formation of several metabolites from the same parent compound.

The former method has been tried with warfarin in vitro [87] and with mephenytoin in vivo [46]. Since enantiomers have similar physicochemical properties except for their steric difference, they often are handled in a similar manner by the organism except for processes which involve molecular interactions related to the chiral center (diastereoisomeric interactions). Enantiomers may have similar volumes of distribution and renal clearances with stereoselectivity being limited to enzymatic biotransformation. Thus, they may be used as molecular probes for in vivo assessment of microsomal enzymes. The validity of this approach, however, must be evaluated for each test compound (Table 3), since important exceptions have been found, such as the highly stereoselective albumin binding of oxazepam hemisuccinate [88], representing extrahepatic and nonmicrosomal stereoselectivity. Nevertheless, with the enantiomers of mephenytoin and based upon the above principles it recently has been demonstrated in vivo that stereoselectivities of two cytochrome P-450-dependent biotransformations may represent metabolism by two different enzyme sites (Figs. 4, 5) [46].

TABLE 3
Stereoselectivity of Nirvanol Disposition in the Dog
(data given as clearances in ml/min)

	(R)-(-)-nirvanol	(S)-(+)-nirvanol
Total plasma clearance	10.3	15.8
Partial clearances:		
Renal clearance	5.8	5.3
"Hepatic" clearance[a]	0.5	4.8
Unaccounted clearance[b]	4.0	5.7

[a] Calculated as ratio of the urinary output of para-hydroxynirvanol (presumably formed in the liver) to the corresponding nirvanol plasma concentration.
[b] Presumably formation of other metabolites.
Source: From Ref. 154.

If a test compound is simultaneously transformed into several primary metabolites, the ratio among the metabolites may potentially be used as an indicator for those forms of cytochrome P-450 which have carried out the reactions. Since the substrate concentration presumably is the same for the different metabolic paths, the pattern of primary metabolites may be thought to reflect the prevalence of the corresponding enzymes.

Interesting pharmacogenetic observations have already resulted from such studies [89]. In particular, hydroxylation of debrisoquine seems to be genetically determined and the reaction appears to be relevant also for the metabolism of other drugs such as guanoxan and phenacetin [90-92]. In vivo-in vitro correlations and investigation with additional compounds are needed before the potential of such investigations can be fully evaluated. Nevertheless, recent indications that the perhexiline-induced neuropathy [188] or the phenformin-induced lactic acidosis [189] may be related to the hydroxylator status point to the importance of a pharmacogenetic approach.

D. Conjugation Reactions

Functionalization and conjugation reactions have many features in common; their investigation therefore does not differ in principle but rather with respect to details. Just like the functionalization reactions of the monooxygenase system, conjugation reactions may show multiple and competing chemical pathways, localization in different organs, saturation phenomena, and the potential for toxicity [93]. Thus all the complications of in vivo investigations discussed for functionalization reactions also apply to conjugations.

It must be pointed out, however, that most conjugated metabolites are much more water-soluble than the products of functionalization reactions, and therefore may be excreted very rapidly by the kidneys. Exceptions are the acetylation and methylation reactions, the products of which have not really gained in water solubility and may accumulate in the organism due to poor renal elimination.

Conjugation reactions require endogenous compounds (e.g., amino acids, sugars, glucuronic acid) as reagents. Inasmuch as these endogenous reagents may be altered by nutritional or endocrinal factors and renal or hepatic diseases, conjugation reactions are potentially more perturbated under such conditions than functionalization reactions. Because of their more ubiquitous localization, they also may be less affected by some organ diseases than the phase I reactions. Thus, the total clearance of diazepam [5] or chlordiazepoxide [62], which are governed by functionalization reactions, are impaired in cirrhosis whereas the elimination of, e.g., oxazepam [94] which occurs by glucuronidation is not affected in such patients (Table 4). On the basis of these considerations it is difficult to understand why in vivo assessment of conjugation reactions has received less interest than investigation of biotransformation by the monooxygenase system.

When studying conjugation reactions attention should be paid to the route of administration. Since the intestinal epithelium contains other

TABLE 4
Effect of Liver Disease on Functionalization and Conjugation Reactions of Benzodiazepine Drugs ($\bar{x} \pm SD$)

	Total plasma clearance (ml/min)	
	Cirrhosis	Controls
Phase I reactions:		
Diazepam [5]	13.8 ± 2.4	26.6 ± 4.1[a]
Chlordiazepoxide [62]	7.7 ± 2.1	15.3 ± 4.4[a]
Phase II reactions:		
Oxazepam [94][b]	156 ± 32	136 ± 18
Lorazepam [187][c]	56 ± 34	64 ± 38

[a] Difference between cirrhotics and controls statistically significant $p < 0.01$.
[b] Clearance calculated after oral dose of oxazepam.
[c] Normalized for a body weight of 70 kg.

conjugation reactions may be different after oral or parenteral application. This is demonstrated for instance for isoprenaline and terbutaline which undergo O-sulfation in the gut wall. After intravenous administration this site of conjugation is bypassed [93].

Attention should also be drawn to the biliary elimination of certain conjugates. Glucuronides and glutathione conjugates of many large molecules are preferentially eliminated with the bile, whereas smaller conjugates (e.g., glycine conjugates) of the same drug may be excreted in urine. Biliary elimination may therefore lead to losses during balance calculations or may complicate drug disposition by all the vagaries of an enterohepatic circulation.

One of the most widely studied conjugation reactions is polymorphic N-acetylation. It is genetically determined and phenotyping is relatively simple. Six hours after a standard dose of sulfadimidine a blood and a urine sample are obtained and assayed before and after acid hydrolysis with the Bratton-Marshall reaction [95]. If the percentage acetylated sulfadimidine in blood and urine are then plotted against each other, a clear separation of "slow" and "rapid" acetylator phenotypes results. Interestingly, it is now well documented that all drugs which are acetylated by this polymorphic enzyme system give concordant results. Thus, the acetylator status of an individual is the same for sulfadimidine, sulfapyridine, isoniazid, procainamide, hydralazine, dapsone, and phenelzine [96,97]. For most purposes it is sufficient to phenotype an individual with one drug and to assume that the same phenotype applies to the other drugs.

E. Elimination into Bile

Although in recent years extensive work by many laboratories has been devoted to a better understanding of the biliary elimination of endogenous and exogenous compounds, much remains a mystery. Nevertheless, it is possible to outline some basic facts concerning the mechanisms of bile formation, the characterization of compounds excreted into bile, the role of different transport systems, and the ever-present problem of species differences in biliary excretion.

1. Bile Formation

Bile constitutes essentially a mixture of water, electrolytes, bile salts, phospholipids, cholesterol, and proteins. It is generally believed that the formation of bile depends upon a dual mechanism, namely, the secretion of bile acids followed by the flow of water and electrolytes along osmotic gradients ("bile acid-associated fraction" of bile) [98] and the excretion of sodium generating additional flow of water and electrolytes ("bile acid-independent fraction" of bile) [99]. After this "primary" bile is formed at the canaliculus, its quantity and content may be modified during passage through bile ductules and ducts by reabsorption of water and by net addition of a bicarbonate solution. Whereas proteins presumably enter into bile by passage between liver cells or by a transhepatocytic vesicular transport, elimination of phospholipids and cholesterol is thought to be achieved in close connection with bile acid secretion.

2. Chemical Properties and Transport Systems

In studying the biliary elimination of xenobiotics, chemists have attempted to define the chemical properties that a compound must exhibit to be excreted into bile. Thus, it was shown that not only the presence of strongly polar groups (as part of the molecule, or acquired by metabolism), but also molecular size represent important determinants for biliary excretion [100].

However, while attempting to define threshold molecular weights for biliary excretion it became clear that species differences are important barriers for reaching generalizations. Thus, in rats compounds with molecular weights below approximately 325 exhibit no appreciable biliary excretion; in guinea pigs and rabbits, on the other hand, the threshold is around 400 and 475, respectively [101].

Physiologists have been more interested in characterizing the mechanisms underlying the biliary handling of various compounds. Four separate active transport systems, three of these for organic chemicals (organic acids, bases, and neutral compounds), and one for metals, have been postulated [102]. All compounds handled in this way are characterized by a high (usually from 10:1 to 1000:1) bile/plasma concentration ratio.

Although bile acids, bilirubin, and sulfobromophthalein (BSP) have long been the prototypes used to study the transport of organic acids, it is now realized that substances of widely different chemical structures are handled by this system [103]. Since their presence as anions at the pH of plasma (or bile) is the most important prerequisite, and since many drugs fulfill this condition, it appears that this pathway represents the primary biliary transport system for xenobiotics (Table 5).

The existence of a pathway for organic bases is suggested from studies of the biliary excretion of quarternary ammonium compounds, notably procainamide ethobromide [104]. Although some drugs, such as (+)-tubocurarine, are excreted in this fashion [105], the transport system for organic bases seems to play a minor role in present-day pharmacotherapeutics.

In contrast, the pathway for neutral organic chemicals assumes importance, because it handles cardiac glycosides (ouabain, possibly digoxin and digitoxin) and steroids (corticosterone, progesterone, and testosterone) [106,107].

The fourth transport mechanism, namely, that for metals, has only recently come into focus, and presumably includes lead, copper, arsenic, and manganese [102]. Its significance for the handling of drugs is likely to be very limited.

3. Investigations of Biliary Excretion

Provided a compound is handled exclusively by the liver, its disappearance from the bloodstream may yield some—albeit limited—information concerning biliary excretion. When interpreting plasma disappearance curves, it must be kept in mind that they reflect a variety of processes. As pointed out above, these include blood flow to and uptake into the liver, intracellular binding, and "storage," where applicable, and metabolism and excretion. Nevertheless, comparison of BSP-disappearance curves with simultaneously obtained measurements of hepatic blood flow and biliary transport capacity (Tm) in humans showed that the second exponential term k_2 was closely related to the excretion of this compound in bile (Fig. 6) [17]. Since the phenomenon appears to depend upon "storage" (i.e., intracellular accumulation) and temporary saturation of biliary transport processes, this approach may be applied to other compounds handled in this fashion. Conversely, Wheeler and coworkers designed an infusion technique yielding information on the "relative storage capacity" and the biliary transport maximum of BSP [108]. This technique has subsequently also been applied to bile acids [109].

TABLE 5
Examples of Therapeutically Important Drugs Secreted into Bile

Diagnostic agents	Hormones
Sulfobromophthalein	Diethylstilbestrol
Indocyanine green	Estradiol
X-ray contrast media (iodipaide, ioglycamide, etc.)	Progesterone
	Testosterone
Diuretics	Thyroxine
Acetazolamide	Triiodothyronine
Ethacrynic acid	Hydrocortisone
Chlorothiazide	
	Antirheumatic drugs
Cardiac glycosides	Indomethacin
Lanatoside A and C	Salicylate
Ouabain	
Digitoxin	CNS drugs
Digoxin	Morphine
	Methylamphetamine
Antibiotics	Diphenylhydantoin
Tetracyclines	Glutethimide
Erythromycin	Guanethidine
Penicillin V	Imipramine
Methicillin	
Ampicillin	Miscellaneous
Nafcillin	Methotrexate
Rifomycin SV	Quarternary ammonium compounds
Oleandromycin	
Chloramphenicol	

Source: Compiled from data in Refs. 100, 102, 104.

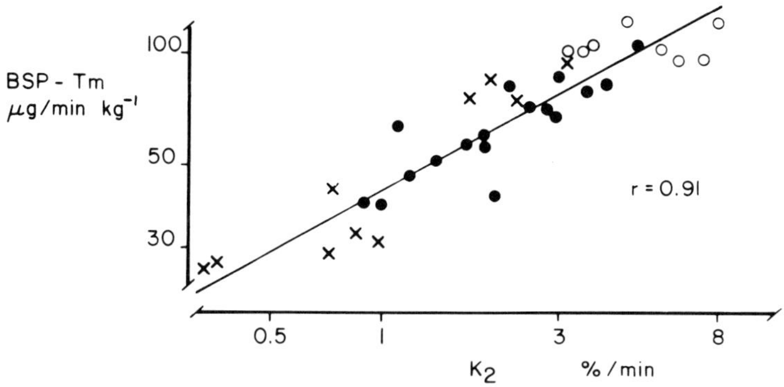

FIGURE 6 Double logarithmic correlation between BSP-Tm measured with Wheeler's multiple-infusion technique and the second exponential component (k_2) of the BSP-plasma disappearance curve. Normal control subjects are shown by open circles, patients with cirrhosis by closed circles, and a group with miscellaneous liver diseases by ×s. The regression line is described by $\log y = 0.54 \log x + 1.64$. (From Walter Häcki, Johannes Bircher, and Rudolf Preisig, A new look at the plasma disappearance of sulfobromophthalein (BSP): Correlation with the BSP transport maximum and the hepatic plasma flow in man, J. Lab. Clin. Med. 88:1019-1031, 1976.)

In this connection it is particularly noteworthy that microsomal enzyme inducers may enhance the plasma disappearance of other substances by stimulating their biliary excretion. Klaassen and Plaa demonstrated convincingly [110] that the increased plasma disappearance of BSP and of the nonmetabolized dibrominated analog DBSP following induction with phenobarbital was due to enhanced biliary excretion of these dyes. Although this particular interaction is reasonably explained by the phenobarbital-induced increment in bile salt-independent bile formation [111], other enzyme inducers may affect biliary excretion by increasing biotransformation [112] or the concentration of ligandin [113].

Due to the inaccessibility of the bile ducts, collection of bile in the intact animal or in humans is not feasible. One is forced to establish some form of biliary fistula in animals or use T-tube drainage in patients, thus interrupting the enterohepatic circulation of biliary constituents, notably bile acids. Consequently, in addition to the possible effects of surgical trauma and anesthesia, following depletion of the bile acid pool a decrease in bile flow (due to diminution of bile salt-associated fraction) is observed. Depending upon the animal species studied, bile flow may practically cease (for instance, in the dog) or continue at a reduced rate (rat, rabbit). Under these circumstances, the biliary elimination of foreign compounds is likely to be underestimated.

To overcome some of these problems, preparations with permanent biliary fistulas are in use allowing maintenance of the enterohepatic circulation during the study-free intervals (Thomas cannula) [114] or even during the investigation. Whereas the latter technique has been successfully employed for studies of bile acid metabolism in the monkey [115], considerable experience is at hand with Thomas duodenal cannulas in dogs [98,116-118]. Installation of the cannula is also feasible in pigs [119]. Since the bile duct can be catheterized under direct vision, and since compensation of the interrupted enterohepatic circulation is achieved by intravenous infusion of bile acids, studies are possible in the unanesthetized animal under near-normal physiological conditions. Between studies, the cannula is closed and the normal drainage of bile into the gut restored. This animal model can be maintained for several years. Figure 7 gives the results of investigations in the dog with Thomas cannula concerning the effect of ethacrynic acid on bile flow and erythritol clearance [120].

In humans, quantitative information concerning the biliary excretion of xenobiotics is only obtainable in patients with a T-tube. As a consequence, the results pertain exclusively to subjects who have undergone cholecystectomy and choledochotomy. The availability of balloon-equipped T-tubes permits complete collection of bile and maintenance of the enterohepatic circulation of bile acids by intraduodenal administration of (previously) collected bile [121]. Techniques have also been designed utilizing balloon-type duodenal tubes [122]. To date, however, their application has been limited to the study of biliary lipid secretion.

Once it has been established that a compound and/or its metabolites are eliminated in the bile, it is useful to consider Brauer's classification based on bile/plasma concentration ratios during excretion [123]. If a substance belongs to class A or C (ratio of 1.0 or <1.0, respectively), biliary handling is unlikely to be an important route of drug disposal for this compound. If, on the other hand, the ratio is >1.0 (usually between 10 and 1000; class B), this finding suggests active secretion of the compound into bile (Table 5); it may also indicate that the biliary route is an important determinant of drug elimination.

Regardless of classification of the compound, investigations concerning the mechanism responsible for the biliary handling of xenobiotics are of interest because they further our understanding of hepatic excretory processes. After methods became available to assess canalicular bile formation [124,125], it was shown that widely differing agents are capable of eliciting a choleresis or cholestasis by selectively stimulating (for instance theophylline, hydrocortisone) [126,127] or inhibiting (for instance estrogen, bile acids) [128,129] this mechanism. Since a similar choleresis may be observed in association with excretion of a drug in bile, the clearance technique using labeled erythritol (or mannitol) is particularly useful in characterizing the underlying events (see Figs. 8a and 8b).

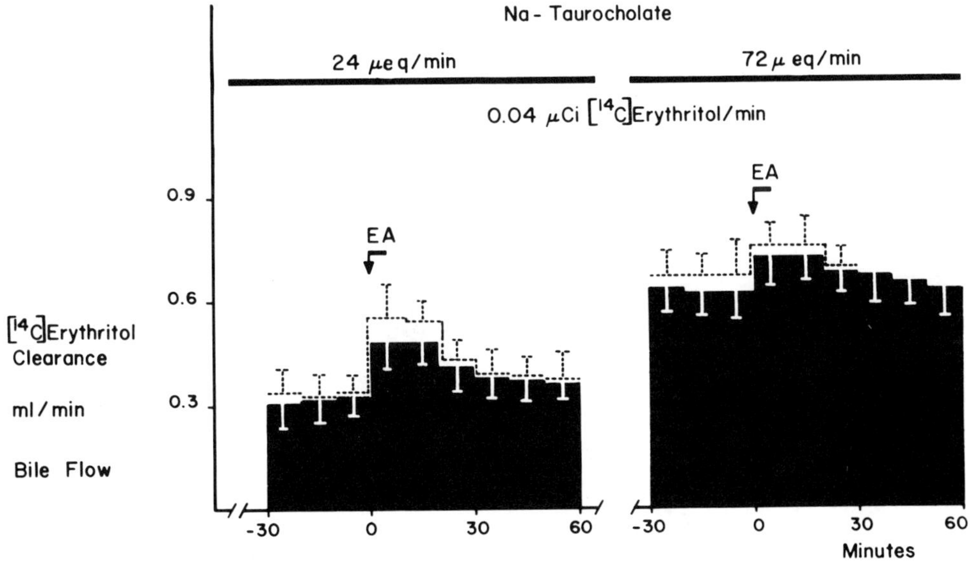

FIGURE 7 Investigations concerning the choleretic effect of ethacrynic acid (EA, 4 mg/kg body weight I.V.) in six unanesthetized dogs with Thomas duodenal cannulae. During I.V. infusion of sodium taurocholate at 24 and 72 μeq/min, respectively, ethacrynic acid injection is followed by a choleresis (bile flow indicated by black area). The choleretic response is paralleled by an increase in the biliary [^{14}C]erythritol clearance (dashed line). The vertical bars indicate standard deviations.

Pharmacotherapy often necessitates simultaneous administration of more than one drug. If two or more compounds are handled by the liver, interaction is to be expected also at the level of metabolism and/or biliary elimination. This phenomenon has been well documented for endogenous substances, where bile acids enhance the biliary excretion of bilirubin [130]. Similar effects have been established between bile acids and BSP [131]. However, little is known about interactions between exogenous compounds. Once again, our investigations of ethacrynic acid in the dog may serve as an example (Figs. 9a and 9b). When ethacrynic acid was injected during the infusion of BSP, the biliary excretion of this dye was markedly depressed. Subsequently, this phenomenon was shown to be due to an exclusive effect of the diuretic on the biliary elimination of conjugated BSP, presumably resulting from competition for the substrate glutathione (Figs. 9a and 9b).

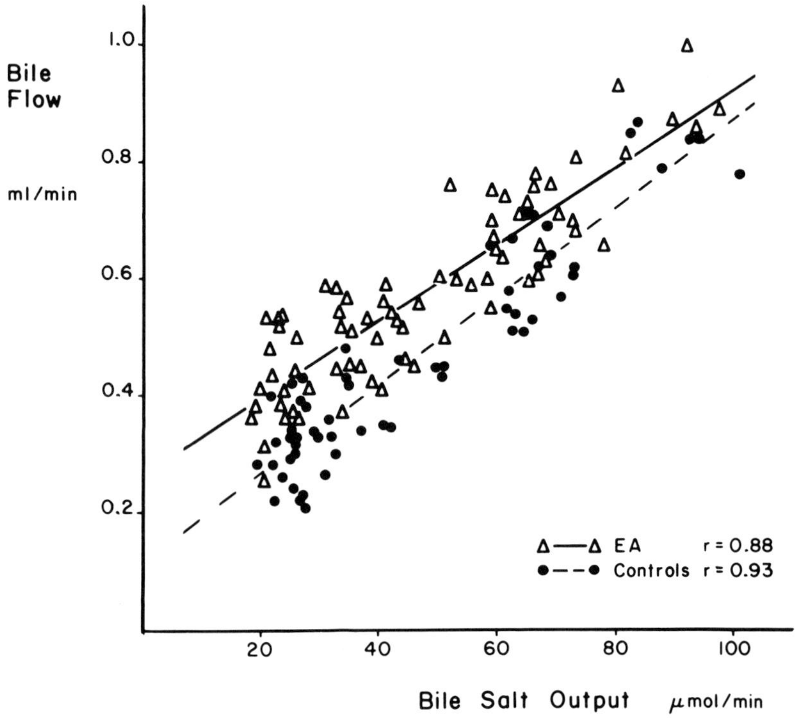

(a)

FIGURE 8 (a) All results of studies on bile formation in unanesthetized dogs with Thomas duodenal cannulae during I.V. infusion of sodium taurocholate (at 24, 45, 72, and 96 μmol/min) have been compiled. During the control period (closed circles) and following ethacrynic acid administration (open triangles), bile flow is linearly related to biliary bile salt excretion. As suggested by extrapolation of the regression lines, the ethacrynic acid-induced choleresis is bile salt-independent.

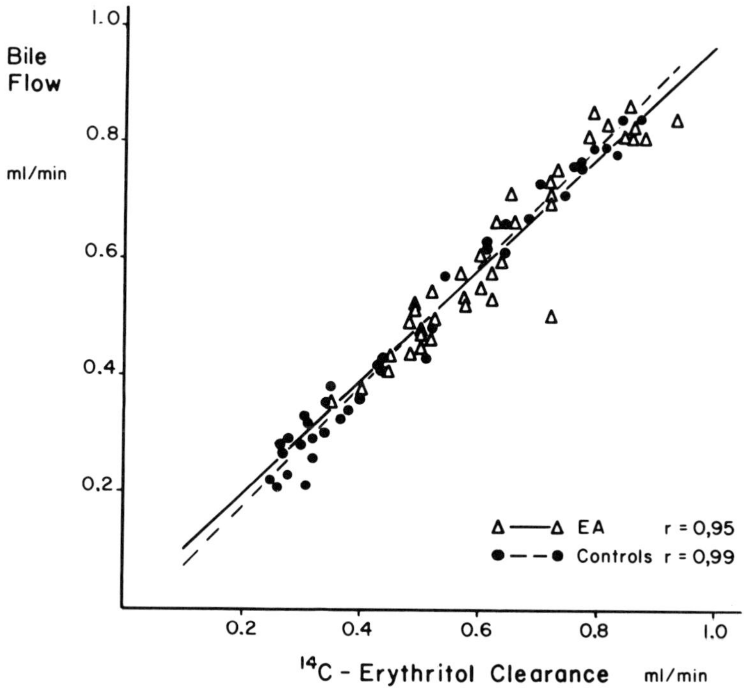

(b)

FIGURE 8 (b) Comparison of bile flow and biliary [^{14}C]erythritol clearance. Since the ethacrynic acid-induced increment in bile flow is associated with a similar increment in [^{14}C]erythritol clearance, it may be concluded that the choleresis is of canalicular origin. (Preisig et al., unpublished observations.)

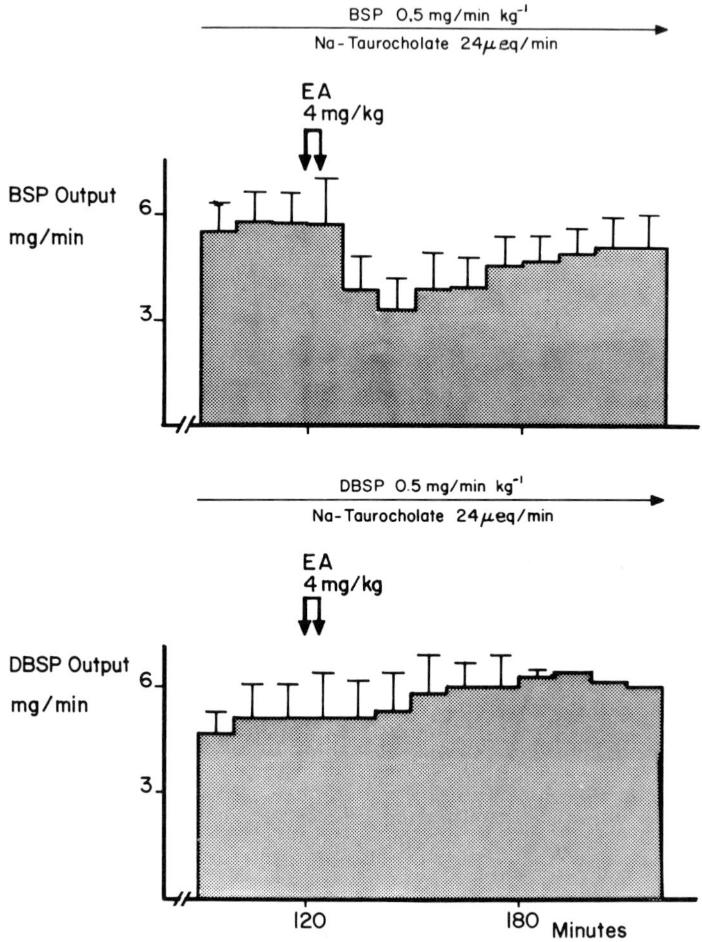

(a)

FIGURE 9 (a) In unanesthetized dogs with Thomas cannulae, sulfobromophthalein (BSP) or its dibrominated, nonmetabolized analog DBSP are administered continuously i.v. at doses sufficient to achieve biliary transport maximum. It is evident that ethacrynic acid induces a fall in biliary BSP output; the biliary elimination of DBSP, on the other hand, remains relatively unchanged.

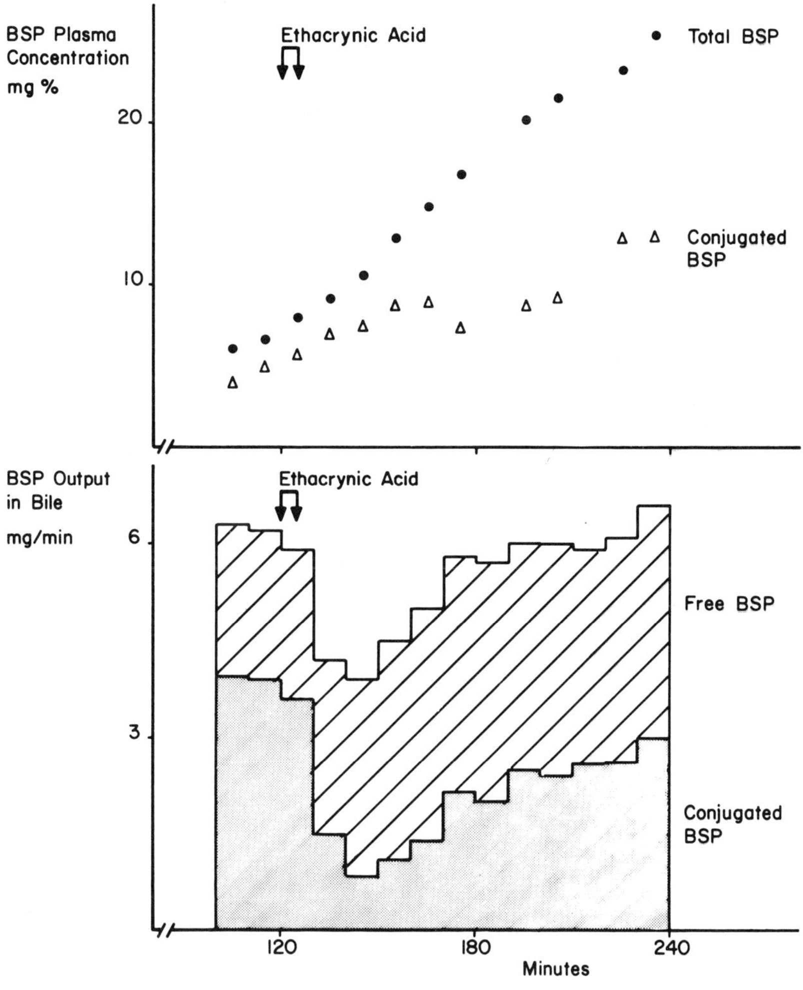

(b)

FIGURE 9 (b) Detailed analysis of the effects of ethacrynic acid on the biliary handling of BSP reveals that the decrease in biliary BSP output may be entirely accounted for by a fall in excretion of conjugated BSP. Presumably, ethacrynic acid competes for glutathione, the substrate used in conjugation for BSP and ethacrynic acid. (Preisig et al., unpublished observations.)

Recent interest concerning the formation of gallstones has focused attention on the biliary excretion of lipids. It was demonstrated that endogenous compounds such as chenodesoxycholic acid [132] and its 7β-epimer ursodesoxycholic acid [133] enhance lipid solubility in bile, thus providing a rational basis for drug therapy of cholesterol gallstones. Conversely, lipid-lowering agents of the clofibrate type have been shown to augment biliary cholesterol saturation [134], resulting in an increased incidence of gallstones following prolonged administration of these drugs [135]. In view of the importance of this finding, it appears reasonable to postulate that with compounds known to undergo hepatic handling, studies concerning the effects on biliary lipid secretion form an integral part of the preclinical and clinical investigations.

F. Elimination into Breath

Many drugs are dealkylated. The cleaved alkyl group may then be oxidized further and exhaled in part as CO_2. Consequently, the idea has been pursued to assess dealkylation reactions by labeling the alkyl groups with ^{13}C- or ^{14}C-atoms and measuring the appropriate label in the exhaled CO_2. This method has the advantage of a noninvasive sampling procedure and the disadvantage that several chemical transformations are required before the labeled ^{14}C-atom appears in breath. Precautions must therefore be taken to assure that exhalation of labeled CO_2 reflects the particular metabolic step which is to be studied, and that no other rate-limiting processes affect the results [136].

Many details of this general approach have been worked out with ([^{14}C]-dimethyl)aminopyrine as a test substance. Measuring total $^{14}CO_2$ exhalation in the rat has made it possible to study the dose-dependence of $^{14}CO_2$ output and to determine V_{max}. In several established models of altered liver function (Table 6) the changes in V_{max} corresponded to expectations [137]. Adaptation of the method for use in patients, therefore, appeared justifiable.

When performing breath tests in humans it has become customary to sample at intervals and to measure specific activity of $^{14}CO_2$ or $^{13}CO_2/^{12}CO_2$ in breath instead of total output of the label. The endogenously produced CO_2 is used as a term of reference in a similar manner to the creatinine in the urine [138,139]. It is simply assumed that CO_2 output is constant throughout the period of observation—for instance, at 9mmol/hr/kg [140, 141]. This approach circumvents potential variations in CO_2 output resulting from transient changes in alveolar ventilation which may be difficult to control. Care must be taken, however, to ensure that endogenous CO_2 production is standardized as much as possible. For this purpose the subjects should remain at rest throughout the test. Even an ordinary meal may affect CO_2 output.

TABLE 6
Experimental Evaluation of the Effects of Altered Liver Function on [^{14}C]Aminopyrine Demethylation Measured by $^{14}CO_2$ Analysis in Expired Air Using a Rat Model ($\bar{x}$ ± SEM)

			Aminopyrine demethylation	
Experimental model	n	Liver weight (g/100 g)	V_{max} (nmol/min per 100 g)	Half-saturation dose (K_m) (μmol/100 g)
Enzyme induction by phenobarbital	12	4.9 ± 0.1	745 ± 66	59 ± 9
Normal controls	16	4.0 ± 0.1	173 ± 20	26 ± 6
48-hr Bile duct ligation	12	4.3 ± 0.1	130 ± 37	36 ± 18
2/3 Hepatectomy	12	1.4 ± 0.2	80 ± 9	34 ± 7
Portacaval shunt	10	2.2 ± 0.3	45 ± 8	24 ± 6

Source: From Ref. 137.

Although the practical usefulness of the aminopyrine breath test to demonstrate abnormal liver function is now adequately demonstrated [142-145], explanation of the time course of the specific activity of $^{14}CO_2$ in breath has remained difficult. This is mainly due to the fact that aminopyrine used as test compound contains two N-methyl groups, both of which carry the label. The two demethylations probably have different kinetics [146,147] and therefore $^{14}CO_2$ exhalation representing the sum of the two reactions may not be very closely related to the disappearance of aminopyrine from the plasma [61]. The kinetics of $^{14}CO_2$ output has been investigated in more detail with [^{14}C]glycodiazine, a compound having only one [^{14}C]methyl group. In this case, the terminal disappearance of $^{14}CO_2$ from breath agreed numerically with the terminal disappearance of glycodiazine from plasma [148]. This study has demonstrated that it is possible to derive kinetic constants of an appropriately labeled test substance by analyzing the specific activity of $^{14}CO_2$ in exhaled air. The conclusions which can be drawn from a breath test, however, depend on the properties of the test compound. In the case of glycodiazine, the patient with cirrhosis had the most rapid demethylation, presumably because the effect of the disease was more marked on plasma protein binding than on the clearance of free glycodiazine. If one of the microsomal functions of the liver is to be assessed, aminopyrine is still, at the present time, the preferred test compound.

The radiation exposure due to [^{14}C] has also been evaluated with aminopyrine [149]. Balance studies have shown that about 55% of the [^{14}C]-atoms have left the organism within 48 hr. The terminal half-life was about 10 days if a pharmacological dose (9 mg/kg) and about 4 days if a tracer dose of [^{14}C]aminopyrine had been administered. Assuming an even distribution of the label throughout the organism, absorbed radiation doses of 0.6 and 1.5 mrad, respectively, could be calculated.

In considering the use of $^{14}CO_2$ breath tests as tools for in vivo assessment of a dealkylation reaction, the details of the methods should be adapted to the particular problem being investigated. For the purpose of a screening procedure it may be sufficient to take a single spot sample of $^{14}CO_2$ 2 hr after aminopyrine intake as proposed by Hepner [150] and Galizzi [145]. If more quantitative data are desired, it is preferable to establish the time course of $^{14}CO_2$ exhalation and to calculate for instance a disappearance rate constant [143]. This approach has been validated in the case of aminopyrine by a comparison of the results of breath analysis with two established quantitative tests of hepatic function [151]. For drugs which are demethylated at a slow rate (such as diazepam), it might be necessary to calculate cumulative output and to derive rate constants from there [152].

One of the potentials of the breath analysis procedures consists in the development of test compounds for specific purposes. For instance, appropriately labeled substances may be found which are demethylated by the cytochrome P-448 system, or which assess intestinal rather than hepatic drug demethylation.* Another development of CO_2 breath analysis is the use of the stable isotope ^{13}C. Although the involved methodological problems and the expense of ^{13}C-labeled test substances still limit this approach to a few laboratories, the lack of radiation and the possibility of double labeling carry a great potential [153].

G. Elimination into Blood and Urine

Following hepatic biotransformation metabolites not excreted into bile may be eliminated from the hepatocytes into the blood. Depending on their rate of urinary excretion or further metabolism, such metabolites will accumulate more or less within the organism. Consequently metabolite formation can be studied by an assessment of their plasma concentrations and/or their urinary output.

When plasma concentrations of metabolites are examined, the following aspects should be considered: Formation of a metabolite may already follow a more or less complicated time course. Its plasma concentrations will further be determined by its distribution within the organism and by its elimination, be it hepatic, renal, or both. Relatively favorable

---

*Ongoing studies in our laboratory have shown that ([^{14}C]-3 methyl) and (^{14}C]-7 methyl)caffeine may be used as indicators of the cytochrome P-448 system both in rats and in humans.

conditions exist if formation of a metabolite is much more rapid than its elimination from blood, and if its distribution within a known volume is also relatively rapid. These conditions have been reasonably well fulfilled in a study of the stereoselectivity of nirvanol formation from mephenytoin [46] (Figs. 4 and 5).

Analysis of urinary elimination of metabolites is not without risks of errors: If the unchanged drug to be tested is eliminated relatively slowly, and if its metabolite has a sufficiently high renal clearance, significant accumulation of the metabolite within the organism is unlikely. In this case the rate of urinary output of the metabolite may adequately reflect its formation in the liver. These assumptions appeared reasonable in a study of the stereoselectivity of nirvanol hydroxylation [154] (Table 3), but may not be valid for other experiments.

The above considerations are particularly pertinent, should several metabolic routes be studied simultaneously. Since different metabolites are likely to have different volumes of distribution and different renal clearances, the time course of their urinary output may be related to hepatic metabolite formation only in an indirect way. Simple calculation of ratios among different metabolites in a 12- or 24-hr urine sample may, therefore, lead to erroneous conclusions. The simultaneous administration of isotopically labeled metabolites is potentially useful to correct for variations in their distribution and renal clearance.

Another shortcoming of "metabolic ratios" in urine samples derives from the fact that each metabolic route affects the rate of disappearance of the test compound and thereby its availability for other metabolic routes. Changes in the rate of formation of a metabolite may then be secondary to changes in one of the other metabolic routes. It is not possible, therefore, to distinguish between primary and secondary changes in metabolite production, if only one of several metabolites is investigated [46].

H. Elimination into Saliva

Although salivary excretion of drugs does not represent an important mechanism for drug disposition, salivary drug concentrations were found to reflect the concentrations of the drug in blood under certain circumstances (Fig. 10). As an explanation, it is assumed that saliva formed in salivary glands equilibrates with the surrounding tissue water and that lipophilic compounds may distribute between saliva and tissue water according to prevailing physicochemical gradients. Factors which determine this distribution are the diffusion coefficient across the physiological barrier, as well as pH and protein binding on both sides of the barrier. In general, corrections for pH may be neglected with acidic drugs having a pK_a greater than 8.5 and with basic drugs having a pK_a of 5.5 or less [155]. For some drugs it has therefore been inferred that the salivary concentrations reflect concentrations of free drug in glandular tissue and correspondingly also in plasma. The number of adequately investigated compounds, however, is

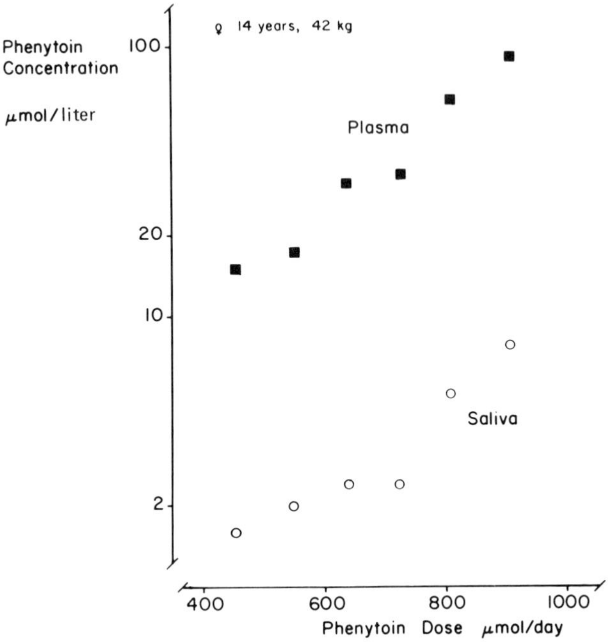

FIGURE 10 Phenytoin concentrations in saliva and in plasma plotted against the dose. The scale of the ordinate is logarithmic. The parallel changes in phenytoin concentrations in plasma and saliva imply that throughout the observed range of data their ratio has remained constant. Consequently salivary drug monitoring may be adequate in the case of phenytoin.

still relatively small and variability of the saliva to plasma concentration ratio may limit the usefulness of saliva collections. Furthermore, the more hydrophilic conjugated metabolites are unlikely to penetrate the saliva.

The optimal method of saliva collection has not as yet been defined. Although it is not difficult to sample parotid saliva with appropriate devices, it is much easier to obtain mixed saliva, by simply asking the subjects to spit into glass containers. Stimulated saliva has the advantage of a more reproducible composition than unstimulated saliva and adequate volumes may be obtained more rapidly. Care must be taken, however, that the stimulating device (paraffin, wax, parafilm, etc.) which is chewed does not adsorb the drug being studied [155].

The noninvasiveness and patient acceptance of saliva collections render this method very attractive for clinical research [48,150,156]. Consequently a large number of studies have already been carried out and further investigation of the potential of saliva as a sampling method for pharmacological research appears warranted.

IV. EVALUATION OF DRUG DISPOSITION IN LIVER DISEASES

Histologically and pathophysiologically, liver diseases are very heterogeneous and therefore difficult to classify. However, when studying drug disposition in liver patients, some simplifications seem justifiable at the present time. In particular three major types of functional abnormalities should be considered in every patient: a reduction in functioning liver cell mass, an alteration of hepatic perfusion, and/or a defect in bile formation.

The functioning mass of hepatocytes may be reduced in cirrhosis or in acute hepatitis. In these diseases it has been postulated that the remaining liver cells either function normally—"intact hepatocyte hypothesis"—or abnormally—"sick cell hypothesis" [157]. At present, there is insufficient evidence to decide between these two possibilities, and either of them may be applicable under certain circumstances.* In any case measurement of the functioning liver cell mass would be both an essential and a sufficient requirement for comparing different patients with respect to their hepatic handling of capacity-limited compounds. Thus, expression of the metabolic capacity of the liver per unit of functioning liver cell mass should normalize the findings in patients with liver disease (Fig. 11).

Several methods to assess the functioning liver cell mass have been proposed. Among them, the galactose elimination capacity is particularly interesting. If the test is performed as suggested by Tygstrup (Fig. 1) [1], results are practically independent of hepatic blood flow. The doses of galactose used for the study are well tolerated and the part of the test which involves the patient may be carried out within 45 min. Another method which has been widely used is antipyrine clearance [48,57-59]. As pointed out earlier, antipyrine may be given orally and its concentrations can be measured in saliva. The procedure therefore is noninvasive and well accepted by volunteers or patients and is also suitable for children. In view of the relatively long plasma half-life of antipyrine, particularly in liver diseases, the test lasts 1 to 2 days. The aminopyrine breath test may serve a similar purpose. It also is noninvasive and, depending on the method of analysis, it can be completed within 2 or 8 hr [142,143]. Finally the BSP-plasma disappearance curve has been empirically found to be useful for the assessment of the functioning liver cell mass [17]. Although the initial plasma disappearance of BSP is determined by both hepatic perfusion and the functioning liver cell mass, it was found to be well correlated with the galactose elimination capacity and the aminopyrine breath test. [143]. Thus, the choice among the

---

*Recently, studies were designed in our laboratory to evaluate hepatocyte function in monolayer cultures derived from rat livers after portacaval shunt. In these hepatocytes some functions were increased and other decreased, a finding incompatible with the "intact hepatocyte hypothesis" [190].

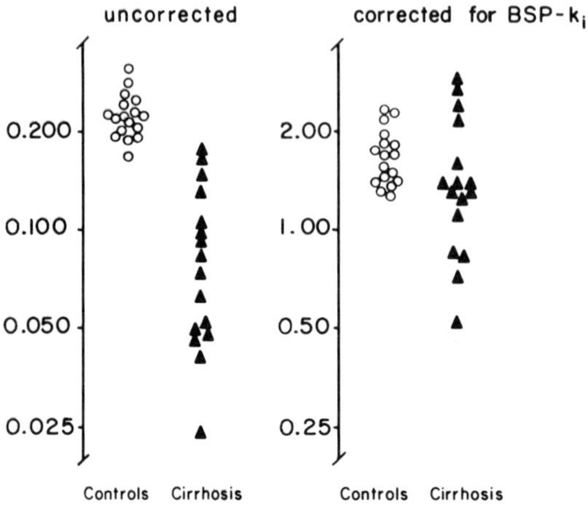

FIGURE 11 Results of the aminopyrine breath test in control subjects and in patients with cirrhosis expressed by the disappearance rate constant of $^{14}CO_2$ in breath. The data are given uncorrected (hr^{-1}) or divided by the initial plasma disappearance rate constant of BSP (BSP-k_i) determined in the same patients (hr^{-1}/min^{-1}). The figure shows that the difference between control subjects and cirrhotic patients was markedly reduced when the results of the aminopyrine breath test were corrected for the severity of the disease by another quantitative test of liver function. (Data from Ref. 143.)

The changes in hepatic perfusion occurring in liver diseases are neither stereotyped nor easy to assess [158]. Total hepatic blood flow is often decreased, but it may be normal or even increased. Various fractions of different parts of the splanchnic blood may be shunted away from the liver through hepatofugal collaterals [159]. Finally, even within the liver, blood flowing through shunts of various sizes may bypass the hepatocytes [160-163]. Perfusion of hepatic parenchyma may therefore be smaller than total hepatic blood flow.

One hypothesis to explain these observations suggests that even in cirrhosis perfusion of the functioning liver cell mass is essentially normal. This conclusion appears attractive when considering that in a group of patients with cirrhosis, severity of the impairment in hepatic handling of a capacity-limited drug (antipyrine) and of a flow-limited compound (propranolol, ICG) varied in a parallel fashion [157]. In addition, hepatocyte extraction of ICG seems to be highly correlated with the extraction of compounds being eliminated by Kupffer cells [164,165]. Therefore, an "intact functional unit" hypothesis may be postulated which implies that the "intact hepatocytes" are supplied by an "intact perfusion." Even though an "intact functional unit hypothesis" could greatly simplify the investigation of drug disposition in cirrhosis, further studies with other compounds are needed to demonstrate its applicability and its limitations. The merit of the hypothesis, however, consists of the fact that it emphasizes the importance of intrahepatic shunts: If in a cirrhotic liver the functional units are indeed intact, a reduction in hepatic extraction of drugs must be explained by portal-hepatic venous or arterial-hepatic venous shunts. The existence of such intrahepatic shunts has been demonstrated both anatomically [160] and functionally [161-163]. Unfortunately, the presently available methods to measure intrahepatic and extrahepatic shunt flow are both invasive and cumbersome. Despite their established relevance for hepatic drug disposition, their practical application has been minimal so far [166]. New and noninvasive methods are urgently needed.

For the purpose of this discussion cholestasis is defined as a reduction in hepatic excretory function which is seen in relation to the functioning liver cell mass. In cholestasis, accordingly, elimination of cholephilic compounds is reduced out of proportion to a potentially diminished liver cell mass, or it may even be completely abolished [17]. The causes for cholestasis may be mechanical obstruction of biliary passages, inflammatory changes within the portal tracts of the liver, or ill-defined processes occurring at the canalicular level. Irrespective of the cause, the consequences of cholestasis consist of a complex set of abnormalities which are as yet insufficiently understood [167-169]. The electron microscopic appearance of bile canaliculi and of the smooth endoplasmatic reticulum is changed. Bile acids accumulate in the liver and in plasma. The fate of drugs may therefore be modified by altered protein binding, abnormalities of the monooxygenase system, and an inability of the liver to eliminate cholephilic compounds in bile. Thus hepatic drug disposition in cholestasis may be normal, accelerated, or slowed [137,170,171].

Even though further studies are required to clarify how cholestasis modifies the different processes involved in hepatic drug disposition, attempts are also needed to quantitatively determine its severity. Only such an approach could render comparisons among different patients meaningful. Methods to quantitate cholestasis are scarce. Empirically, the second component of the BSP-plasma disappearance curve (k_2) was found to be promising for this purpose [17,172]. As pointed out previously, there is an excellent correlation between the excretory transport maximum for BSP (Tm) and BSP-k_2. By contrast, BSP-k_2 was independent of hepatic blood flow ($r = 0.08$, $n = 15$). The practical usefulness of BSP-k_2 for comparative purposes, however, awaits formal testing.

V. OUTLOOK

The above discussions about various aspects of in vivo assessment of hepatic drug disposition should have made it clear that investigations in healthy and diseased humans do not suffice. In order to unravel the respective role of the many mechanisms involved, these must be evaluated individually from the molecular level through the different stages of complexity—microsomal preparations, isolated cells, isolated organs, intact organism, disease models—up to the individual patient. Biochemical pharmacology, cell biology, organ physiology, and pharmacokinetics are therefore indispensible investigative tools.

Within this context, the ethical restrictions of human experimentation represent a particular problem. There appear to be two general trends to overcome these difficulties. One of them is leading to an increased use and an improvement of experimental models which allow investigation of hepatic drug disposition in the intact and nonanesthetized animal, e.g., the cholecystectomized dog with a Thomas duodenal cannula for sampling of hepatic bile, or the rabbit with permanent catheters in a peripheral artery and in the portal vein, currently under investigation in our laboratory. The other trend tries to further explore noninvasive diagnostic procedures in humans. Estimation of salivary drug concentrations, for instance, is already a commonplace. $^{14}CO_2$ breath tests hopefully can be replaced soon by $^{13}CO_2$ tests. The potential value of metabolic ratios in urine should be investigated further. Evaluation of the kinetics of a pharmacological effect may also be applied for the study of hepatic drug disposition, but with this aim it has barely been tested so far. Thus, together with the classical pharmacokinetic approach, newer techniques should make it possible to test the compatibility of hypotheses developed in animal models with the situation in humans and particularly in patients. There is good justification to believe that such a combined approach to the investigation of hepatic drug disposition may in the near future lead to concepts and procedures immediately applicable to patient care for the improvement of safety and efficacy of modern drug therapy.

REFERENCES

1. N. Tygstrup, Scand. J. Clin. Lab. Invest., Suppl. 18:118 (1966).
2. J. R. Gillette and K. S. Pang, Clin. Pharmacol. Ther. 22:623 (1977).
3. G. R. Wilkinson and D. G. Shand, Clin. Pharmacol. Ther. 18:377 (1975).
4. K. S. Pang and J. R. Gillette, Drug Metab. Dispos. 6:567 (1978).
5. U. Klotz, G. R. Avant, A. Hoyumpa, S. Schenker, and G. R. Wilkinson, J. Clin. Invest. 55:347 (1975).
6. D. J. Greenblatt, J. S. Harmatz, and R. I. Shader, Int. J. Clin. Pharmacol. 16:177 (1978).
7. H. I. Pirttiaho, E. A. Sotaniemi, J. Ahlqvist, and U. Pitkänen, Eur. J. Clin. Pharmacol. 13:61 (1978).

8. H. I. Pirttiaho, E. A. Sotaniemi, J. T. Ahokas, and U. Pitkänen, Brit. J. Clin. Pharmacol. 6:273 (1978).
9. C. G. Swift, M. Homeida, M. Halliwell, and C. J. C. Roberts, Eur. J. Clin. Pharmacol. 14:149 (1978).
10. L. Bass, S. Keiding, K. Winkler, and N. Tygstrup, J. Theor. Biol. 61:393 (1976).
11. K. S. Pang and M. Rowland, J. Pharmacokin. Biopharm. 5:625 (1977).
12. S. Keiding, S. Johansen, K. Winkler, K. Tönnesen, and N. Tygstrup, Amer. J. Physiol. 230:1302 (1976).
13. K. S. Pang and M. Rowland, J. Pharmacokin. Biopharm. 5:655 (1977).
14. K. S. Pang and M. Rowland, J. Pharmacokin. Biopharm. 5:681 (1977).
15. L. Bass, P. Robinson, and A. J. Bracken, J. Theor. Biol. 72:161 (1978).
16. G. Paumgartner, Schweiz. Med. Wschr., Suppl. 105:3 (1975).
17. W. Häcki, J. Bircher, and R. Preisig, J. Lab. Clin. Med. 88:1019 (1976).
18. G. Paumgartner, J. Reichen, and R. Preisig, Digestion 10:373 (1974).
19. G. T. Tucker, L. Wiklund, A. Berlin-Wahlen, and L. E. Mather, J. Pharmacokin. Biopharm. 5:111 (1977).
20. D. Pessayre, D. Lebrec, V. Descatoire, M. Peignoux, and J. P. Benhamou, Gastroenterology 74:566 (1978).
21. N. Tygstrup and K. Winkler, Clin. Sci. 17:1 (1958).
22. J. A. Larsen, Scand. J. Clin. Lab. Invest. 11:340 (1959).
23. R. A. Zito and P. R. Reid, N. Engl. M. Med. 298:1160 (1978).
24. S. E. Bradley, in Handbook of Physiology, Sec. 2, Circulation, Vol. 2 (W. F. Hamilton and P. Dow, Eds.). American Physiological Society, Washington, D.C., 1963, p. 1387.
25. S. E. Bradley, F. J. Ingelfinger, and G. P. Bradley, Circulation 5: 419 (1952).
26. A. H. Moreno, A. R. Burchell, L. M. Rousselot, W. F. Panke, S. F. Slafsky, and J. H. Burke, J. Clin. Invest. 46:436 (1967).
27. G. M. Fleischner and I. M. Arias, in Progress in Liver Disease, Vol. 5 (H. Popper and F. Schaffner, Eds.). Grune & Stratton, New York, 1976, p. 172.
28. D. K. F. Meijer, J. G. Weitering, and R. J. Vouk, J. Pharmacol. Exp. Ther. 198:229 (1976).
29. H. Polet, J. Pharmacol. Exp. Ther. 199:687 (1976).
30. J. G. Weitering, W. Lammers, D. K. F. Meijer, and G. J. Mulder, Naunyn-Schmiedebergs Arch. Pharmakol. Exp. Pathol. 299:277 (1977).
31. C. De Duve, V. De Barsy, B. Poole, A. Trouet, P. Tulkens, and F. Van Hoof, Biochem. Pharmacol. 23:2495 (1974).
32. R. Stegmann and M. H. Bickel, Xenobiotica 7:737 (1977).
33. J. H. Anderson, R. C. Anderson, and L. S. Iben, J. Pharmacol. Exp. Ther. 206:172 (1978).

34. M. J. Kreek, M. Oratz, and M. A. Rothschild, Gastroenterology 75: 88 (1978).
35. G. Paumgartner and J. Reichen, in The Hepatobiliary System (W. Taylor, Ed.). Plenum, New York and London, 1976, p. 287.
36. J. Reichen and G. Paumgartner, Amer. J. Physiol. 231:734 (1976).
37. D. L. Eaton and C. D. Klaassen, J. Pharmacol. Exp. Ther. 205:480 (1978).
38. K. Iwamoto, D. L. Eaton, and C. D. Klaassen, J. Pharmacol. Exp. Ther. 206:181 (1978).
39. K. Iwamoto and C. D. Klaassen, J. Pharmacol. Exp. Ther. 203:365 (1977).
40. K. Iwamoto and C. D. Klaassen, J. Pharmacol. Exp. Ther. 200:236 (1977).
41. J. G. Wagner, Eur. J. Clin. Pharmacol. 10:425 (1976).
42. M. Warner, M. V. La Marca, and A. H. Neims, Drug Metab. Dispos. 6:353 (1978).
43. W. R. Porter, R. V. Branchflower, and W. F. Trager, Biochem. Pharmacol. 26:549 (1977).
44. J. Kapitulnik, P. J. Poppers, and A. H. Conney, Clin. Pharmacol. Ther. 21:166 (1977).
45. F. Sjöqvist and C. Von Bahr, Drug Metab. Dispos. 1:469 (1973).
46. A. Küpfer and J. Bircher, J. Pharmacol. Exp. Ther. 209:190–195 (1979).
47. J. Alvin, E. Goh, and M. T. Bush, J. Pharmacol. Exp. Ther. 194: 117 (1975).
48. E. S. Vesell, G. T. Passananti, P. A. Glenwright, and B. H. Dvorchik, Clin. Pharm. Ther. 18:259 (1975).
49. B. Gradnik and L. Fleischmann, Pharm. Acta Helv. 48:181 (1973).
50. P. B. Andreasen and G. Greisen, Eur. J. Clin. Invest. 6:21 (1976).
51. D. E. Carter, R. Bressler, M. R. Hughes, M. R. Häussler, C. D. Christian, and M. W. Heine, Clin. Pharm. Ther. 18:700 (1975).
52. P. Hart, G. C. Farrell, W. G. E. Cooksley, and L. W. Powel, Brit. Med. J. 2:147 (1976).
53. M. Lichter, M. Black, and I. M. Arias, J. Pharm. Exp. Ther. 187:612 (1973).
54. P. A. Meredith, B. C. Campbell, M. R. Moore, and A. Goldberg, Eur. J. Clin. Pharmacol. 12:235 (1977).
55. E. S. Vesell, C. A. Shively, and G. T. Passananti, Clin. Pharmacol. Ther. 22:843 (1977).
56. R. E. Vestal, A. H. Norris, J. P. Tobin, B. H. Cohen, N. W. Shock, and R. Andres, Clin. Pharmacol. Ther. 18:425 (1975).
57. H. S. Fraser, J. C. Muchlow, S. Murray, and D. S. Davies, Brit. J. Clin. Pharmacol. 3:321 (1976).
58. R. L. Deangelis, M. Wingfield, and T. W. Farmer, Clin. Pharm. Ther. 18:249 (1975).

59. C. J. van Boxtel, J. T. Wilson, S. Lindgren, and F. Sjöqvist, Eur. J. Clin. Pharmacol. 9:327 (1976).
60. E. Ackermann, F. Renger, B. Dökert, and M. Walther, Z. Ges. Inn. Med. 27:849 (1972).
61. S. Scherrer, B. Haldimann, A. Küpfer, F. Reubi, and J. Bircher, Clin. Sci. Mol. Med. 54:133 (1978).
62. R. K. Roberts, G. R. Wilkinson, R. A. Branch, and S. Schenker, Gastroenterology 75:479 (1978).
63. R. L. Williams, T. F. Blaschke, P. J. Meffin, K. L. Melmon, and M. Rowland, Clin. Pharmacol. Ther. 21:301 (1977).
64. T. F. Blaschke, P. J. Meffin, K. L. Melmon, and M. Rowland, Clin. Pharmacol. Ther. 17:685 (1975).
65. R. Williams, W. L. Schary, T. F. Blaschke, P. J. Meffin, K. L. Melmon, and M. Rowland, Clin. Pharmacol. Ther. 20:90 (1976).
66. D. M. Kornhauser, A. J. J. Wood, R. E. Vestal, G. R. Wilkinson, R. A. Branch, and D. G. Shand, Clin. Pharmacol. 23:165 (1978).
67. F. Degos and J. P. Benhamou, Eur. J. Clin. Invest. 8:243 (1978).
68. G. Leopold, Arzneim.-Forsch. 27:241 (1977).
69. P. J. Murphy, R. C. Nickander, G. M. Bellamy, and W. L. Kurtz, J. Pharm. Exp. Ther. 199:415 (1976).
70. R. Gugler and J. Hartlapp, Clin. Pharmacol. Ther. 24:432 (1978).
71. M. Gibaldi and P. J. McNamara, Eur. J. Clin. Pharmacol. 13:373 (1978).
72. C. A. Shively and E. S. Vesell, Clin. Pharmacol. Ther. 18:413 (1975).
73. A. J. McLean, P. J. McNamara, P. du Souich, and M. Gibaldi, Clin. Pharmacol. Ther. 24:5 (1978).
74. A. S. Nies, D. G. Shand, and G. R. Wilkinson, Clin. Pharmacokin. 1:135 (1976).
75. A. Richens and A. Dunlop, Lancet II:247 (1975).
76. T. M. Ludden, J. P. Allen, W. A. Valutsky, A. V. Vicuna, J. M. Nappi, S. F. Hoffman, J. E. Wallace, D. Lalka, and J. L. McNay, Clin. Pharmacol. Ther. 21:287 (1977).
77. P. W. Mullen, Clin. Pharmacol. Ther. 23:228 (1978).
78. G. Levy, T. Tsuchuja, and L. P. Amsel, Clin. Pharmacol. Ther. 13:258 (1972).
79. L. K. Garretson, J. A. Procknal, and G. Levy, Clin. Pharmacol. Ther. 17:98 (1975).
80. J. G. Wagner, J. Pharmacokin. Biopharm. 1:103 (1973).
81. C. A. M. van Ginneken, J. M. van Rossum, and H. L. J. M. Fleuren, J. Pharmacokin. Biopharm. 2:395 (1974).
82. W. A. Fuchs and R. Preisig, Brit. J. Radiol. 48:539 (1975).
83. F. Lundquist and H. Walthers, Acta Pharmacol. Toxicol. 14:265 (1958).
84. P. K. Wilkinson, A. J. Sedman, E. Sakman, D. R. Kay, and J. G. Wagner, J. Pharmacokin. Biopharm. 5:207 (1977).

85. C. A. Goresky and B. E. Nadeau, J. Clin. Invest. 53:634 (1974).
86. J. Reichen and G. Paumgartner, Gastroenterology 68:132 (1975).
87. L. R. Pohl, W. R. Porter, W. F. Trager, M. J. Fasco, and J. W. Fenton, Biochem. Pharmacol. 26:109 (1977).
88. W. Müller and U. Wollert, Mol. Pharmacol. 11:52 (1975).
89. W. Kalow, D. Kadar, T. Inaba, and B. K. Tang, Clin. Pharmacol. Ther. 21:530 (1977).
90. A. Mahgoub, J. R. Idle, L. G. Dring, and R. L. Smith, Lancet II: 584 (1977).
91. T. P. Sloan, A. Mahgoub, R. Lancaster, J. R. Idle, and R. L. Smith, Brit. Med. J. 2:655 (1978).
92. J. R. Idle, A. Mahgoub, R. Lancaster, and R. L. Smith, Life Sci. 22:979 (1978).
93. J. Caldwell, in Concepts in Drug Metabolism (P. Jenner and B. Testa, Eds.). Marcel Dekker, New York, 1980, Chap. 4.
94. H. J. Shull, G. R. Wilkinson, R. Johnson, and S. Schenker, Ann. Intern. Med. 84:420 (1976).
95. D. A. Price Evans, J. Med. Genet. 6:405 (1969).
96. P. K. M. Lunde, K. Frislid, and V. Hansteen, Clin. Pharmacokin. 2:182 (1977).
97. D. E. Drayer and M. M. Reidenberg, Clin. Pharmacol. Ther. 22: 251 (1977).
98. R. Preisig, H. L. Cooper, and H. O. Wheeler, J. Clin. Invest. 41: 1152 (1962).
99. S. Erlinger, D. Dhumeaux, P. Berthelot, and M. Dumont, Amer. J. Physiol. 219:416 (1970).
100. R. L. Smith, The Excretory Function of Bile. Chapman and Hall, London, 1973.
101. P. C. Hirom, P. Millburn, R. L. Smith, and R. T. Williams, Biochem. J. 129:1071 (1972).
102. C. D. Klaassen, in Handbook of Physiology, Sec. 9, Reactions to Environmental Agents (D. H. K. Lee, Ed.). American Physiological Society, Bethesda, Md., 1977, p. 537.
103. L. S. Schanker, in Handbook of Physiology, Sec. 6, Alimentary Canal (C. F. Code, Ed.). American Physiological Society, Washington, D.C., 1968, p. 2433.
104. L. S. Schanker and H. M. Solomon, Amer. J. Physiol. 204:829 (1963).
105. D. K. F. Meijer, E. S. Bos, and K. J. van der Laan, Eur. J. Pharmacol. 11:371 (1970).
106. H. J. Kupferberg and L. S. Schanker, Amer. J. Physiol. 214:1048 (1968).
107. J. Q. Russell and C. D. Klaassen, J. Pharmacol. Exp. Ther. 186: 455 (1973).

108. H. O. Wheeler, J. I. Meltzer, and S. E. Bradley, J. Clin. Invest. 39:1131 (1960).
109. Re. Poupon, Ra. Poupon, M. Dumont, and S. Erlinger, Eur. J. Clin. Invest. 6:431 (1976).
110. C. D. Klaassen and G. L. Plaa, J. Pharmacol. Exp. Ther. 161:361 (1968).
111. P. Berthelot, S. Erlinger, D. Dhumeaux, and A. M. Preaux, Amer. J. Physiol. 219:809 (1970).
112. W. G. Levine, J. Pharmacol. Exp. Ther. 183:420 (1972).
113. H. Reyes, A. J. Levi, Z. Gatmaitan, and I. M. Arias, Proc. Nat. Acad. Sci. U.S. 64:168 (1969).
114. J. E. Thomas, Proc. Soc. Exp. Biol. 46:260 (1941).
115. R. H. Dowling, E. Mack, J. Picott, J. Berger, and D. M. Small, J. Lab. Clin. Med. 72:169 (1968).
116. R. Preisig, in Liver and Drugs (F. Orlandi and A. M. Jézéquel, Eds.). Academic, London and New York, 1972, p. 107.
117. K. Kutz, G. Paumgartner, G. Egger, and R. Preisig, Gastroenterology 67:135 (1974).
118. E. M. Grandjean, W. Zaunbauer, G. Paumgartner, and W. A. Fuchs, Schweiz. Med. Wschr. 108:1073 (1978).
119. G. Egger, K. Kutz, H. Strebel, J. Bircher, M. Weber, E. Scholl, and R. Preisig, Amer. J. Vet. Res. 35:1203 (1974).
120. G. Egger, K. Kutz, and R. Preisig, Digestion 6:273 (1972).
121. R. Preisig, H. Bucher, H. Stirnemann, and J. Tauber, Rev. Franc. Etude Clin. Biol. 14:151 (1969).
122. S. M. Grundy and A. L. Metzger, Gastroenterology 62:1200 (1972).
123. R. W. Brauer, J. Amer. Med. Ass. 169:1462 (1959).
124. E. L. Forker, J. Clin. Invest. 46:1189 (1967).
125. H. O. Wheeler, E. D. Ross, and S. E. Bradley, Amer. J. Physiol. 214:866 (1968).
126. S. Erlinger and M. Dumont, Biomedicine 19:27 (1973).
127. V. Macarol, T. Q. Morris, K. J. Baker, and S. E. Bradley, J. Clin. Invest. 49:1714 (1970).
128. J. J. Gumucio and V. D. Valdivieso, Gastroenterology 61:339 (1971).
129. R. Herz, G. Paumgartner, and R. Preisig, Scand. J. Gastroenterology 11:741 (1976).
130. C. A. Goresky, H. H. Haddad, W. S. Kluger, B. E. Nadeau, and G. G. Bach, Can. J. Physiol. Pharmacol. 52:389 (1974).
131. D. J. Ritt and B. Combes, J. Clin. Invest. 46:1108 (1967).
132. R. G. Danzinger, A. F. Hofmann, J. L. Thistle, and L. J. Schoenfield, J. Clin. Invest. 52:2809 (1973).
133. I. Makino and S. Nakawaga, J. Lipid Res. 19:723 (1978).
134. D. Pertsemlidis, D. Panveliwalla, and E. H. Ahrens, Jr., Gastroenterology 66:565 (1974).

135. M. F. Oliver, J. A. Heady, J. N. Morris, and J. Cooper, Brit. Heart J. 40:1069 (1978).
136. C. Waydhas, K. Weigl, and H. Sies, Eur. J. Biochem. 89:143 (1978).
137. B. H. Lauterburg and J. Bircher, J. Pharmacol. Exp. Ther. 196: 501 (1976).
138. A. F. Hofmann and B. H. Lauterburg, J. Lab. Clin. Med. 90:405 (1977).
139. D. A. Schoeller, J. F. Schneider, N. W. Solomos, J. B. Watkins, and P. D. Klein, J. Lab. Clin. Med. 90:412 (1977).
140. H. S. Winchell and K. Wiley, J. Nucl. Med. 12:708 (1970).
141. H. S. Winchell, H. Stahelin, and N. Kusubov, J. Nucl. Med. 12:711 (1970).
142. G. W. Hepner and E. S. Vesell, Ann. Intern. Med. 83:632 (1975).
143. J. Bircher, A. Küpfer, I. Gikalov, and R. Preisig, Clin. Pharmacol. Ther. 20:484 (1976).
144. J. Noordhoek, J. Dees, E. M. Savenij-Chapel, and J. A. P. Wilson, Eur. J. Clin. Pharmacol. 13:223 (1978).
145. J. Galizzi, R. G. Long, B. Billing, and S. Sherlock, Gut 19:40 (1978).
146. B. N. LaDu, L. Gaudette, N. Trousof, and B. B. Brodie, J. Biol. Chem. 214:741 (1955).
147. T. E. Gram, J. T. Wilson, and J. R. Fouts, J. Pharmacol. Exp. Ther. 159:172 (1968).
148. R. Platzer, R. L. Galeazzi, G. Karlaganis, and J. Bircher, Eur. J. Clin. Pharmacol. 14:293 (1978).
149. I. Gikalov and J. Bircher, Eur. J. Clin. Pharmacol. 12:229 (1977).
150. G. W. Hepner and E. S. Vesell, Clin. Pharmacol. Ther. 20:654 (1976).
151. J. Bircher, R. Platzer, I. Gikalov, A. Küpfer, and R. Preisig, in Radioaktive Isotope in Klinik und Forschung, Vol. 12 (R. Höfer, Ed.). Egermann, Vienna, 1976, p. 347.
152. G. W. Hepner, E. S. Vesell, A. Lipton, H. A. Harvey, G. R. Wilkinson, and S. Schenker, J. Lab. Clin. Med. 90:440 (1977).
153. J. F. Schneider, D. A. Schoeller, B. Nemchausky, J. L. Boyer, and P. Klein, Clin. Chim. Acta 84:153 (1978).
154. A. Küpfer, J. Bircher, and R. Preisig, J. Pharmacol. Exp. Ther. 203:493 (1977).
155. M. Danhof and D. D. Breimer, Clin. Pharmacokin. 3:39 (1978).
156. J. W. Paxton, B. Whiting, and K. W. Stephen, Brit. J. Clin. Pharmacol. 4:185 (1977).
157. R. A. Branch, D. G. Shand, Clin. Pharmacokin. 1:264 (1976).
158. J. Bircher, R. Blankart, A. Halpern, W. Häcki, J. Laissue, and R. Preisig, Eur. J. Clin. Invest. 3:72 (1973).

159. W. A. Fuchs, R. Preisig, E. Voegeli, and J. Bircher, Invest. Radiol. 7:369 (1972).
160. H. Popper and F. G. Zak, Amer. J. Med. 24:593 (1958).
161. S. Shaldon, L. Chiandussi, L. Guevara, J. Caesar, and S. Sherlock, J. Clin. Invest. 40:1346 (1961).
162. G. Gross and C. V. Perrier, N. Engl. J. Med. 293:1046 (1975).
163. G. Gross, J. F. Babel, J. Ritschard, R. Mejévand, A. Rohner, and A. Donath, in The Liver (R. Preisig, et al., Eds.). Cantor, Aulendorf, 1976, p. 159.
164. M. Horisawa, G. Goldstein, A. Waxman, and T. Reynolds, Gastroenterology 71:210 (1976).
165. P. M. Huet, D. Marlean, P. Lavoie, and A. Viallet, Gastroenterology 70:74 (1976).
166. R. Gugler, P. Lain, and D. L. Azarnoff, J. Pharmacol. Exp. Ther. 195:416 (1975).
167. V. J. Desmet, in Progress in Liver Diseases, Vol. 4 (H. Popper and F. Schaffner, Eds.). Grune and Stratton, New York and London, 1972, p. 97.
168. T. Schersten, in Progress in Liver Diseases, Vol. 4 (H. Popper and F. Schaffner, Eds.). Grune and Stratton, New York and London, 1972, p. 133.
169. F. Hutterer, H. Greim, D. Trülzsch, P. Czyan, and J. B. Schenkman, in Progress in Liver Diseases, Vol. 4 (H. Popper and F. Schaffner, Eds.). Grune and Stratton, New York and London, 1972, p. 151.
170. N. Ahmad and M. Black, J. Pharm. Exp. Ther. 203:397 (1977).
171. N. Carulli, F. Manenti, M. Ponz de Leon, A. Ferrari, G. Salvioli, and M. Gallo, Eur. J. Clin. Invest. 5:455 (1975).
172. J. Bircher and R. Preisig, Clin. Gastroenterology 7:517 (1978).
173. P. D. Thompson, K. L. Melmon, J. A. Richardson, K. Cohn, W. Steinbrunn, R. Cudihie, and M. Rowland, Ann. Intern. Med. 78:499 (1973).
174. Y. A. Weiss, M. E. Safar, J. P. Lehner, J. A. Levenson, A. Simon, and J. M. Alexandre, Brit. J. Clin. Pharmacol. 5:457 (1978).
175. A. J. Levi, S. Sherlock, and D. Walker, Lancet I:1275 (1968).
176. N. L. Benowitz and W. Meister, Clin. Pharmacokin. 3:177 (1978).
177. P. Du Souich and S. Erill, Eur. J. Clin. Pharmacol. 10:283 (1976).
178. R. Platzer, A. Küpfer, J. Bircher, and R. Preisig, Eur. J. Clin. Invest. 8:219 (1978).
179. G. A. Ellard and P. T. Gammon, Br. J. Clin. Pharmacol. 4:5 (1977).
180. K. M. Das and M. A. Eastwood, Clin. Pharmacol. Ther. 18:514 (1975).
181. L. Molin, R. Larsson, and E. Karlsson, Acta Med. Scand. 201:217 (1977).

182. I. M. Arias, L. M. Gartner, M. Cohen, J. Ben Ezzer, and A. J. Levi, Amer. J. Med. 47:395 (1969).
183. B. Combes and G. S. Stakelum, J. Clin. Invest. 40:981 (1961).
184. H. O. Wheeler, W. I. Cranston, and J. I. Meltzer, Proc. Soc. Exp. Biol. Med. 99:11 (1958).
185. V. Hoenig and R. Preisig, Biomedicine 18:12 (1973).
186. D. E. Drayer, Clin. Pharmacokin. 1:426 (1976).
187. J. W. Kraus, J. P. Marschall, R. Johnson, G. R. Wilkinson, and S. Schenker, Gastroenterology 73:1228 (1977).
188. E. Singlas, M. A. Goujet, and P. Simon, Europ. J. Clin. Pharmacol. 14:195 (1978).
189. R. R. Shah, N. S. Oates, J. R. Idle, and R. L. Smith, Lancet I:1147 (1980).
190. H. Wietholtz, S. Hottinger, and R. Preisig, World Conference on Clinical Pharmacology and Therapeutics No. 657 (1980).

Chapter 8

ALTERED DRUG DISPOSITION IN DISEASE STATES: THE FIRST PIECES OF THE JIGSAW

Peter Jenner

University Department of Neurology
Institute of Psychiatry and King's
College Hospital Medical School
London, England

Bernard Testa

School of Pharmacy
University of Lausanne
Lausanne, Switzerland

The pharmacokinetic profile of drugs can be markedly influenced by the induction of disease states. Drug-metabolizing enzyme activity as well as metabolic rates and patterns can be influenced either by diseases affecting hepatic function or by disease of nonhepatic origin which indirectly alter liver action. However, the number of disease states and substrates studied in such investigations is relatively limited; as a consequence currently available data is inadequate for the development of an overall conceptual approach. Perhaps the biggest drawback to the development of such investigations is the inadequacy of animal models with which the effect of disease on drug metabolism can be studied. It is also clear that the effect of disease states on drug metabolism is generally limited unless the disease is of sufficient severity to disrupt many endogenous enzyme systems. Indeed, it would appear that disease states may produce more pronounced effects on other pharmacokinetic parameters such as protein binding, absorption, distribution, and elimination, and that these may be of greater relevance to alterations of drug action rather than effects on drug-metabolizing enzyme activity.

I. INTRODUCTION

The development of new drugs using animal experimentation and the use of normal human volunteers ignore the abnormal pathological condition of the patients to whom such drugs are destined to be given. Disease states can alter the pharmacokinetic profiles of drugs and in some cases such alterations can be attributed to changes in drug-metabolizing activity. However, since the intensity of the desired pharmacological response or the onset of toxic side effects is often dictated by the free plasma concentration of drug, it is not usually obvious which of the many factors controlling this parameter are responsible for the change in pharmacokinetic profile. The situation is further complicated by the large individual variation in drug disposition occurring in the population and the fact that disease states seldom alter a single physiological function, thus making it extremely difficult to directly evaluate alterations in specific pharmacokinetic parameters. The present review attempts to evaluate the effects of disease states on drug disposition and in particular drug-metabolizing enzyme activity and the effect such change has on drug action in humans. We have attempted to do this in a number of ways; initially by reference to disease in humans we will examine the direct effect of hepatic disease and the indirect effect of nonhepatic disease on hepatic drug-metabolizing enzyme activity. Where possible, the extent of metabolism, the metabolic pathways, and the alteration of enzyme components will be examined. Such changes as occur will be related to the use of animal models as a means of further examining the mechanisms by which drug-metabolizing enzyme activity is altered. The discussion will then consider whether disease-mediated changes in drug-metabolizing enzyme activity are a significant factor in imposing therapy adjustments, or whether other pharmacokinetic parameters play a more important role in governing drug administration and, indeed, drug action.

It must be pointed out from the start that the major difficulty we faced in preparing this review stemmed from the large variety of disciplines and interests of the cited authors. The integration of currently available data up to a conceptual level is precluded by this assortment. We are therefore left with the hope that the critical gathering of data we have attempted will allow others to take a renewed view of this important topic and to lead us to a more conceptual approach.

II. CHANGES IN DRUG DISPOSITION RESULTING FROM DISEASE STATES

Since the ultimate level of drug achieved following administration in vivo is a result of the processes of absorption, distribution, metabolism, and excretion and since disease can affect all these processes, changes in the plasma level of drugs cannot be simply attributed to altered metabolic ability. Before discussing the effects of disease on drug-metabolizing activity it is therefore necessary to examine which physiological functions will cause alteration in the pharmacokinetic profile of a drug when modified by disease states.

Relative to disease states the most important factors to consider are changes in drug absorption, blood flow, protein binding, renal function, and hepatic activity. These have been considered in detail in a recent volume [1] and in a number of excellent reviews [2-10]. Consequently we will only briefly discuss their involvement in disease states and refer the interested reader to the original work.

A. Diseases of the Gastrointestinal Tract

Factors affecting drug absorption are numerous (see Refs. 2, 11). Relevant to the present text are the effects of food, gastrointestinal pH, gastric emptying rate, and the rate of passage of intestinal contents, which can all be altered by disease states affecting the gastrointestinal tract. Thus, impaired absorption of paracetamol occurs in patients with delayed gastric emptying and pyloric stenosis [11], and prolonged fasting in anorexia nervosa also impairs absorption of paracetamol [2]. Achlorhydria occurs in patients with pernicious anemia, gastric carcinoma, and atrophic gastritis [12] and in this disorder Aspirin was absorbed faster and salicylate levels were higher than those of control subjects [13]. Gastrointestinal motility is often abnormal in disease states and gastric stasis and pyloric stenosis impair paracetamol absorption [2,13-15]. Drug absorption may also be reduced by rapid passage of gastrointestinal contents since the absorption of nalidixic acid and ampicillin is delayed or decreased in children with acute shigella gastroenteritis [16]. Malabsorption syndromes from the gastrointestinal tract are also known, mainly affecting the absorption of nutrients, vitamins, and minerals. However, the absorption of some drugs may also be affected (cortisol, penicillin, digoxin, tetracycline) (see Ref. 2). In steathorrhea liposoluble drugs are lost in the feces [11].

Such a brief summary represents almost the sum total of our knowledge of this topic. The reasons for altered absorption are often unknown and it is obvious that much remains to be investigated in this field. Regarding other routes of drug administration even less appears known of the effects of disease states. According to Prescott [2], it is likely that the absorption of drugs administered subcutaneously or intramuscularly is accelerated in patients with peripheral vasodilation caused by fever, anemia, thyrotoxicosis, Paget's disease, hypercarbia, and hepatic disease, among others.

B. Disease States Affecting Blood Flow

Altered blood perfusion of tissues can change the absorption, distribution, and elimination of drugs and may profoundly affect the time course of these processes in humans. Alterations in the perfusion of major organs may arise because of changes in the magnitude or regional distribution of cardiac output. Using examples based on congestive heart failure and other pathological conditions compromising organ perfusion it is possible to illustrate changes occurring during disease states in humans.

Since the absorption of drug molecules from the gastrointestinal tract appears dependent on splanchnic blood flow [17-21], it is perhaps not surprising that in patients with heart failure having decreased cardiac output and consequently decreased splanchnic blood flow, decreased drug absorption occurs. Thus, impaired absorption of quinidine [22], procainamide [23,24], metolazone [25], and hydrochlorothiazide [26] occurs. The absorption of aprindine [27] and disopyramide [28] is also affected in patients with acute myocardial infarction. In contrast, the absorption of furosemide is unchanged and that of digoxin uncertain [29].

Comparison of quinidine absorption in normal subjects and in patients with congestive heart failure [22,30,31] showed peak quinidine concentrations to occur approximately 2 hr later in patients; furthermore, the estimated rate of drug absorption in this group was only one-third that in normal subjects. However, elimination rates were not different in the two groups although the volume of distribution of quinidine and its urinary excretion were reduced in patients. This later finding was interpreted as showing reduced total absorption, but has been criticized [29] since creatinine clearance had decreased by a similar amount. Indeed, Benet's work [29] contains constructive criticism of available studies on altered drug absorption in cardiac failure and outlines the pitfalls of such investigations.

Altered blood flow can affect both the magnitude and the rate at which equilibrium of distribution is achieved. Wilkinson [32] considers the distribution of lidocaine in patients with congestive heart failure to represent the classical example of this phenomenon. Thus, patients with congestive heart failure have approximately twice the plasma concentration of lidocaine compared to control subjects and this is associated with a reduction in the volume of distribution of the drug [33,34]. These changes appear due to increased cardiac output and subsequently reduced organ perfusion [35].

Similar changes in distribution have been observed for procainamide [23,24], quinidine [22], and digoxin [32].

Altered drug clearance due to decreased blood perfusion of the kidneys might also be expected. Indeed, it is clinically accepted that renal clearance of drugs is reduced when renal perfusion is impaired [32] although any body of investigative evidence for this appears lacking. Because of autoregulatory mechanisms renal blood flow and glomerular filtration are less variable than hepatic blood flow (see below) [32].

The influence of hepatic blood flow on drug clearance is now an accepted phenomenon of considerable importance [4,5,32]. It is therefore not surprising that disease states causing changes in hepatic perfusion may influence the pharmacokinetic profile of a drug without necessarily changing the activity of drug-metabolizing enzyme systems. A number of diseases alter hepatic blood flow and those investigated by drug clearance experiments are summarized in Table 1. It would be expected that drugs with high total intrinsic clearance (e.g., propranolol) would be more affected by altered liver perfusion than drugs not showing flow dependency (e.g., antipyrine). However, present evidence suggests, that in chronic liver disease at least, this expectation is not necessarily fulfilled for reasons discussed in detail by Branch and Shand [48].

C. Disease States Affecting Protein Binding

Many diseases are associated with alterations in plasma proteins that can lead to marked changes in the distribution and clearance of drugs extensively protein-bound. This topic has been the subject of a number of recent reviews [10,49,50] (see also Refs. 51-54). Three main mechanisms appear to be responsible for altered drug binding, namely, hypoalbuminemia, the competitive binding of endogenous substrates, and alteration in the size of the plasma protein pool [10,49].

TABLE 1
Diseases Affecting Hepatic Blood Flow

Disease	Drug	Change in clearance	Reference
Congestive heart failure	Lidocaine	Decreased	33,34
	N-Demethylated lidocaine	Decreased	36
	Aldosterone	Decreased	37
Shock	Indocyanine green	Decreased	38
Chronic liver disease	Lidocaine	Decreased	33,34
	Propranolol	Decreased	39
	Indocyanine green	Decreased	40-43
Acute viral hepatitis	?	Increased	44
Hypertension	?	Decreased	45
Myocardial infarction	?	Increased or decreased	46

Sources: Adapted from Refs. 32, 47, 48.

Diseases causing a decrease in plasma albumin concentration are many and the most common are summarized in Table 2. Some disease states also increase plasma albumin levels (Table 2). In either case, however, the significance of the changes in terms of pharmacokinetics is relatively poorly understood. This is illustrated by the decrease in protein binding of propranolol that occurs in parallel with the increasing severity of liver disease and the concomitant decrease in hepatic albumin synthesis [39]. The presence of abnormal concentrations of endogenous ligands in plasma may also prevent binding or cause displacement of bound drugs with or without alteration in total plasma protein concentration. For example, the reduced binding of diphenylhydantoin in patients with impaired renal function [56,57] appears to be more related to the degree of uremia than to serum albumin concentrations [57]. Changes in the size of the plasma protein pool are illustrated by the effect of ascites in chronic liver disease. Thus, the development of ascites doubles the volume of distribution of propranolol despite a similar degree of protein binding to patients without ascites [39]. Assuming the plasma and ascites contain similar protein concentrations, the increase in extravascular fluid can be estimated at 5 liters using indocyanine green. One other factor potentially able to cause altered drug binding in disease states should be noted, namely, the production of structural alterations in serum proteins (see Ref. 49). This has been documented in cystic fibrosis [58] and in rheumatoid arthritis [59]. While no alteration of pharmacokinetic profiles appears to occur as a result of these aberrations, similar effects induced by drugs are of relevance [49,60,61].

Small changes in protein binding can have a marked effect on the volume of distribution of some drugs, a phenomenon affecting acidic drugs more than basic drugs. Thus, in acute renal failure while the binding of salicylic acid, acetylsalicylic acid, phenylbutazone, diphenylhydantoin, thiopental, and sulfadiazine was found to be reduced [62], the binding of quinidine, dapsone, and desmethylimipramine was normal in uremic patients [50].

An excellent example of competition between endogenous molecules and drug molecules for binding sites arises from studies of the effect of increased levels of serum lipids as might occur in atherosclerosis and cardiovascular disease (see Ref. 63). Elevated free fatty acid concentrations are found in a number of clinical conditions including diabetes, infection, hypothyroidism, stress, and reduced calorie intake [64]. This change may be of significance in the pharmacokinetics of the hypolipidemic drug clofibrate since artificial elevation of plasma free fatty acid concentrations markedly decreased the half-life of the drug [64]. In vitro data support this displacement of clofibrate by free fatty acids [65]. Since clofibrate

TABLE 2
Disease States Altering Plasma Albumin Concentrations

Decrease	Increase
Myocardial infarction	Neuroses
Cardiac failure	Psychoses
Hepatic disease	Schizophrenia
Renal failure	Paranoia
Gastrointestinal disease	Gynecologic disorders
Neoplastic disease	Myalgia
Acute infection	Benign tumors
Chronic bronchitis	
Inflammatory disease	

Sources: Adapted from Refs. 10, 49, 55.

TABLE 3
Tissue Macromolecules Binding Drugs

Macromolecule	Example
Ligandin	Azo dyes, corticosteroids, bilirubin, bromosulfophthalein, folic acid, and carcinogens
DNA	Antineoplastic agents, antimalarials (quinacrine, chloroquine)
Melanin	Chloroquine, phenothiazines, cocaine, and ephedrine
Calcified tissues	Tetracyclines
Mucopolysaccharides	Quaternary ammonium compounds, amines
Cell fractions (microsomes, mitochondria)	Chlorpromazine, imipramine
Transcortin	Corticosteroids
Na^+/K^+ transport ATPase	Cardiac glycosides
Dihydrofolate reductase	Methotrexate

Source: Adapted from Ref. 49.

acts to reduce triglyceride synthesis continued administration should lead to an altered pharmacokinetic profile.

At this point it is also important to realize that serum albumin represents only one of a large number of serum macromolecules to which drugs may potentially bind. Of particular interest are studies indicating a role for serum lipoproteins and lipids (see Ref. 63). Excess circulating serum lipids may act as additional storage or binding sites reducing free drug concentration and drug pharmacological activity [66]. Such changes may be of particular relevance to a number of disease states.

In addition, tissue binding of drugs can occur to varying degrees to a number of tissue components (Table 3). There appears to be no reason why this type of drug binding should not also be altered during disease.

D. Disease States Affecting Renal Function

Acute or chronic renal diseases have a marked effect on the excretion of those drugs eliminated predominantly via the kidneys. As might be expected this leads in many cases to the accumulation of active compounds (parent or metabolite) and the production of toxic effects on repeated drug administration (see Refs. 2, 7, 67-69). It is therefore of importance to modify drug dosage in uremic patients and methods for this have been described [7, 70-73].

Alterations in renal function may also affect other pharmacokinetic parameters. Thus, the extent of protein binding is altered by uremia (as described above) and the activity of drug-metabolizing enzymes may also be affected (see below). In addition, the volume of distribution can be altered by accompanying edema or dehydration. Also modification of the erythrocyte concentration [7] in anemia accompanying renal insufficiency can modify the binding of drugs such as gentamycin to red blood cells [74]. Changes in function and anatomy of the gastrointestinal tract caused by uremia may affect drug absorption. For example, the serum concentration of chlorpropamide [75], deoxycycline [76], or penicillin [7] is lower in patients with renal insufficiency than in normal subjects. Finally, the reduction of renal elimination may be at least partially compensated by an increase in hepatobiliary excretion. Thus, although the proportion of digoxin or glibenclamide excreted in urine is reduced compared to control subjects, the amount detected in feces was increased with no evidence for impaired gastrointestinal absorption [7, 77].

E. Disease States Affecting Hepatic Function

Disease states of the liver are expected to alter the activity of drug-metabolizing enzyme systems and this topic forms a basis for a major portion of this chapter. It is, however, necessary to be aware of other factors altered in liver disease that might influence the pharmacokinetic profile of a drug, but without pertubating metabolic function.

The progression of liver disease is associated with abnormalities of portal blood flow as eloquently described by Branch and Shand [48]. The main consequences of the changes in vascular architecture are that only a proportion of total liver blood flow perfuses hepatic parenchymal cells [78]. In addition, increased hepatic resistance leads to the development of portal systemic vascular shunts within the liver and outside it. Such shunts can divert a significant proportion of blood flow in splanchnic and mesenteric veins from the liver [79]. Thus, in alcoholic liver disease up to 60% of mesenteric and 80% of splenic blood flow may undergo shunting [79] and up to 70% of portal blood entering liver may not perfuse the parenchyma because of intrahepatic shunts [80]. The consequences of reduced liver perfusion are the decreased clearance of drugs, particularly those with flow-limited kinetics. This effect can also be seen following the surgical introduction of portocaval anastomoses which further reduce blood flow and drug clearance [43, 81].

The reduction in hepatic blood flow would seem of particular interest when considering drugs administered orally and which undergo first-pass metabolism. Little work has been undertaken on this subject but confirmation has been obtained using a single patient receiving propranolol [82] and in the dog [83]. In addition, the increased incidence of central toxicity following administration of piridazole has been attributed to a reduction in first-pass metabolism in patients with the hepatosplenic schistozomal infection [84].

We have already discussed the effect of altered protein binding in liver disease but some points of specific relevance are to be raised here.

While a decrease in the synthesis of albumin and other serum proteins accompanies hepatic disease, this appears particularly marked only in severe liver disorders. However, while hypoalbuminemia is a major factor in decreasing protein binding of drugs, liver disorders can cause a decrease in drug binding without evidence for decreased albumin concentrations. Thus, the binding of tolbutamide and diphenylhydantoin is reduced in acute viral hepatitis despite raised plasma albumin levels [85,86]. An elevation of plasma bilirubin may partially explain this displacement but other displacing agents may also be present. In particular it should be remembered also that binding to other macromolecules may play an important role in the pharmacokinetics of some drugs (see above).

Changes in the plasma concentrations of some drugs (e.g., amobarbital, aminopyrine, phenylbutazone, and chloramphenicol) do correlate with serum albumin levels in hepatic disease [87-90]. The reason for this may not only lie in altered drug binding and distribution but in the fact that serum albumin concentrations in severe liver disease may reflect hepatic function (protein synthesis) and drug-metabolizing activity.

Liver disease may also lead to changes in body composition (including ascites) and drug binding to body tissues may consequently be altered [3]. Thus, liver disease increases the volume of distribution of lidocaine even though the extent of plasma binding of the drug is not sufficiently large to allow for such an alteration [34]. In addition the altered distribution of diazepam in cirrhotics cannot be totally explained by the observed decreases in plasma binding [91].

The consequences of a decrease in protein binding of drugs in hepatic disease are greatly dependent on the rate of drug clearance [3,6]. The changes produced can lead to erroneous conclusions concerning the effect of hepatic disease on elimination. Thus, the apparent decrease in tolbutamide half-life during acute viral hepatitis initially appears due mainly to changes in hepatic metabolism since no change in the volume of distribution occurs [47]. However, when allowance is made for the decreased plasma binding of the drug during the course of the disease no alterations in clearance are apparent. On the other hand, altered plasma binding may mask the effects of hepatic disease on drug clearance. Thus, the fall in plasma binding of amobarbital acts to offset the effect of reduced hepatic metabolizing activity such that apparently normal drug clearance is observed in chronic liver disease [89].

F. Other Factors Potentially Able to Alter Drug Disposition in Disease States

As we have seen, a single disease state may have a number of consequences of significance in determining the overall pharmacokinetic profile of a drug. In addition to this complexity it is of interest that a number of peripheral components of disease are potentially capable of altering aspects of drug absorption, drug distribution, drug binding, and blood flow in humans. Some of the more obvious parameters are summarized in Table 4. In many cases only a suspicion exists that these factors exert a significant effect but a number may place the patient in an abnormal state capable of altering the pharmacokinetic profile of drugs. Thus, it is almost certain that subjects with severe illness will undergo some stress phenomenon and from the evidence of animal experimentation alterations in drug-metabolizing activity may result. The diet of patients with severe disease states may not only differ from their normal food intake but may be restricted in one manner or another. The effects of dietary changes and deficiency on drug metabolism are numerous (see Ref. 92), and may result in significant modification of drug action. Further, disease is more likely to occur in older members of the population and as such allowance must be made for age-induced changes in pharmacokinetic parameters, particularly when using normal control subjects to detect disease-induced alterations in drug profile. For example, if the age-dependent elimination of diazepam had not been taken into account when considering the profile of this compound in liver disease a distorted picture would have emerged [91].

TABLE 4
Physiological States and Parameters which Are Modified in Diseases and Thus Potentially Able to Alter Drug Pharmacokinetic Profiles

Exercise	Body muscle mass
Posture	Fat/lean ratio
Sleep	Hemoglobinemia
Stress	Vascular permeability
Diet	Hydration state
Body size	Intestinal flora

Other, perhaps less obvious consequences of the disease state may also potentially affect the pharmacokinetic profile of drugs. For example, edema of the intestinal mucosa in patients with right-sided congestive heart failure produces malabsorption of fats [93,94]. Thus, the blood concentrations of ^{131}I-triolein were greater in normal subjects than in patients with heart failure, an effect reversed by the administration of diuretics.

G. Practical Consequences of Altered Drug Disposition

The above sections have demonstrated the complex effect of human disease on the pharmacokinetic profile of drugs. In most cases the disease does not affect a single organ nor a single factor altering drug disposition. This is not surprising since disease by definition alters the normal physiological function of the body. For example, cardiac failure produces changes in organ perfusion affecting drug absorption, distribution, and elimination. Likewise, diabetes elevates serum lipids, body metabolism is altered, altered membrane permeability occurs, and the fat/lean body ratio is changed [63]. In addition, the extent to which such changes take place depends on the severity and duration of the disease and this may fluctuate during the course of illness. Indeed, the alterations in drug pharmacokinetics measured at any one time are the sum effect of all these processes and there is probably no correlation with a single factor.

How, then, can we assess the effect of disease states on drug-metabolizing processes? The answer to this question produces arguments as complex as those determining the pharmacokinetic profile of the drug. Only a combination of approaches and data can reveal factors playing a significant role in the changes observed. In addition, a number of ethical problems affect the extent to which pharmacokinetic studies can proceed in patients with severe disease. It is not always possible to administer a preferred model drug to such subjects and indeed even if this is possible, it is seldom possible to do so without the concomitant administration of normal therapy. It can also be rightly argued that knowledge concerning the disposition of model drugs is not of relevance to a particular disease and that only drugs used to treat the disorder are of interest. Thus, investigators often find themselves undertaking studies using less than ideal conditions and resulting in the production of data requiring an almost impossible degree of interpretation. Even if these difficulties can be overcome, it is seldom possible to have determined basal levels of a parameter prior to the onset of illness. In view of the large variation in metabolizing activity that occurs in the population one can only ensure that apparently altered drug disposition in disease represents a true phenomenon by investigation of relatively large numbers of patients. This in itself can represent an almost insurmountable difficulty depending on disease severity and incidence.

Despite the vast difficulties involved our knowledge of altered drug metabolism in disease states in humans has progressed as illustrated in the following sections.

III. HEPATIC DISEASE STATES AFFECTING DRUG METABOLISM

The primary role played by the liver in the biotransformation of drugs and other xenobiotics makes alterations of its normal physiological state foremost in studies of drug metabolism in disease. But while the liver responds to insult in a limited number of ways, the intricacy of its construction and function can result in a multitude of biochemical processes being modified.

Studies of the effect of hepatic disease in humans on drug-metabolizing enzyme activity present a problem of considerable dimensions. Not only are changes in other pharmacokinetic parameters occurring (see above), but the spectrum of response to the onset of disease makes it almost impossible to obtain homogeneous patients for study. In addition, since the multiplicity of drug-metabolizing enzyme systems responsible for functionalization and conjugation pathways require different biochemical environments for activity, differential activity on different metabolic pathways is to be expected.

These difficulties are reflected in the varying effects of disease states on drug metabolism when liver disorders are considered overall (Table 5). The effects appear divided almost equally into those showing decreased drug clearance and those showing no change. It is the object of this section to look more closely at major groups of liver diseases in order to establish the direction in which change, if any, may occur and the relationship of altered activity to the abnormal physiological state of the organ.

It is clear that the classification of hepatic diseases into subclasses should alleviate some of the discrepancies that are apparent. This is seen from the elegant study of serum antipyrine half-life carried out by Branch et al. [95] (Fig. 1) which demonstrates different types of disorders to have varying effects on the clearance of this compound. The wide range of half-lives observed in all liver diseases appears due to the varied pathophysiology of the individual disorders.

Another pertinent point to be made at this time is the considerable effect of multiple-drug therapy on the change in drug clearance observed in hepatic disease. The early classical studies of Sherlock and her colleagues [88] have made it clear that the ability of some drugs to alter drug-metabolizing activity may mask the alterations occurring as a result of the progression of the disease. Thus, the half-life of phenylbutazone in patients with acute or chronic liver disease was not different from that of a control group of subjects (Table 6). However, division of both groups on the basis

TABLE 5
Examples of Drugs Whose Half-life and Clearance Are Either Altered or Not by Hepatic Disease Taken as a Whole

Decreased	
Aminopyrine	Isoniazid
Amobarbital	Lidocaine
Ampicillin	Meperidine
Antipyrine	Meprobamate
Chloramphenicol	Pentobarbital
Chlordiazepoxide	Phenobarbital
Diazepam	Phenylbutazone
Hexobarbital	
Unchanged	
Chlorpromazine	Oxazepam
Dicoumarol	Salicylic acid
Diphenylhydantoin	Tolbutamide
Lorazepam	Warfarin

Sources: Data from the work of a number of authors, but particularly Refs. 3 and 47.

TABLE 6
The Effect of Drug Pretreatment on the Half-life of Phenylbutazone in Control Subjects and in Patients with Hepatic Disease

	Half-life (hr)		
	All subjects	No pretreatment	Drug pretreatment
Control subjects (n = 55)	70.9 ± 5.0	78.1 ± 5.0	57.2 ± 8.0*
Liver disease (n = 95)	70.7 ± 6.5	100 ± 10.0	54.3 ± 5.0*

*$p < 0.05$ compared to drug-free subjects.
Source: From Ref. 88.

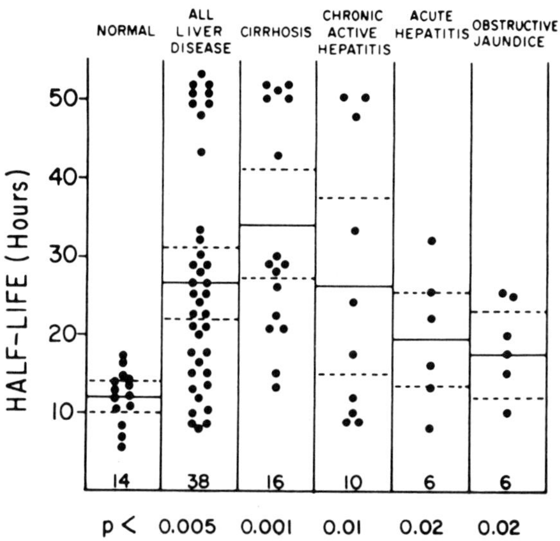

FIGURE 1 Comparison of the serum half-life (mean ± 2 SEM) of antipyrine with clinical diagnosis during hepatic disease. (From Ref. 95. Reproduced with permission of the copyright holders.)

of drug pretreatment prior to phenylbutazone administration revealed an increase in drug half-life due to hepatic disease in those subjects receiving no prior medication.

A. Acute Hepatitis

The examination of drug-metabolizing activity in acute hepatitis is almost entirely limited to the study of acute viral hepatitis. The evidence presently available would suggest the disease to cause either no change or to decrease drug clearance rates depending on the compound examined (Table 7). Since hepatic blood flow and the volume of distribution of drugs [96] are usually changed in acute viral hepatitis, changes in drug clearance can be attributed to altered metabolism by the use of compounds eliminated almost entirely by metabolism.

For example, only a small quantity of meperidine is excreted unchanged, most of the dose undergoing either demethylation to normeperidine or hydrolysis to meperidinic acid and subsequent conjugation [97]. By maintaining human urinary pH at 7.0 or greater, urinary excretion of meperidine can be minimized; under these conditions, the plasma half-life of meperidine was shown to be prolonged in patients with acute viral hepatitis compared to control subjects with no change in the volume of distribution or protein binding of the drug [97] (Table 8).

TABLE 7
Examples of the Effects of Acute Viral Hepatitis on Drug Clearance and Plasma Half-life

Decreased	
Aminopyrine	Hexobarbital
Antipyrine	Meperidine
Diazepam	Pentobarbital
Unchanged	
Diphenylhydantoin	Phenobarbital
Lidocaine	Phenylbutazone
Lorazepam	Tolbutamide
Oxazepam	

TABLE 8
Alterations of Meperidine Pharmacokinetic Parameters in Patients with Acute Viral Hepatitis

Parameter	Control subjects	Acute viral hepatitis patients
Half-life [β-phase] (hr)	3.5 ± 0.8	7.0 ± 2.7*
Plasma clearance (ml/min)	1261 ± 527	648 ± 228*
Volume of distribution (liters/kg)	5.9 ± 2.7	5.6 ± 1.8
Percentage protein binding	58.3 ± 8.7	56.0 ± 11.8

*$p < 0.05$ compared to control subjects.
Source: From Ref. 97.

Similarly, using hexobarbital, a drug completely metabolized by the human liver, the elimination half-life was increased in patients with acute viral hepatitis compared to control subjects [98] (Table 9).

Altered clearance of drugs mainly eliminated by metabolism may also be reflected in metabolite production. Thus, while the urinary excretion of unchanged hexobarbital was not different in control subjects and patients with acute viral hepatitis, the excretion of 3'-ketohexobarbital was markedly reduced in the latter group (Table 9).

TABLE 9
Alterations of Hexobarbital Disposition in Patients with Acute Viral Hepatitis

Parameter	Control subjects	Acute viral hepatitis patients
Half-life [β-phase] (hr)	4.3 ± 1.1	8.2 ± 3.1*
Plasma clearance (ml/min/kg)	3.57 ± 0.83	1.94 ± 0.85*
Volume of distribution (liters/kg)	1.10 ± 0.12	1.10 ± 0.40
Percentage 24-hr urinary excretion of hexobarbital	0.31 ± 0.13	0.33 ± 0.24
Percentage 24-hr urinary excretion of 3'-ketohexobarbital	42.3 ± 13.6	12.6 ± 6.1*

* $p < 0.05$ compared to control subjects.
Source: From Ref. 98.

Such changes can also be observed with drugs undergoing limited but significant biotransformation. Thus, the higher plasma glycoside concentrations observed in patients with acute hepatitis following β-methyldigoxin administration appear to be due to a reduced demethylation of methyldigoxin to digoxin [99]. No reduction in renal excretion of β-methyldigoxin or in protein binding was observed, but the urinary excretion of digoxin was significantly decreased. In healthy subjects approximately 25% of methyldigoxin is demethylated to digoxin after 3 days continuous administration whereas in patients with acute hepatitis only 15% is present in urine as digoxin. This apparent decrease in the metabolism of β-methyldigoxin contrasts with the situation observed following administration of digoxin itself which resulted in a more rapid clearance of plasma glycoside content in the disease state than in control subjects.

Since recovery from acute hepatitis is common, the question arises as to whether drug-metabolizing activity returns to normal as the normal physiological function of the liver is restored. The present evidence indeed suggests recovery, but requiring a longer period than normalization of liver function. Thus, the prolonged half-life of hexobarbital in acute hepatitis was lower on recovery (as judged by normal transaminase and bilirubin values) but was not normal [98] (Table 10). Similarly, the half-life of diazepam was shorter just after the return of liver function tests into the normal range than during the course of the disease but was still outside the normal range [91] (Table 10). However, the clearance of meperidine was found to be normal during recovery for acute hepatitis 1 month after normal hepatic function was restored [97]. This latter finding suggests a lag period between restoration of drug-metabolizing activity and the recovery of liver

TABLE 10
Changes in Drug Clearance upon Recovery from Acute Hepatitis

Drug	Status	Half-life [β-phase] (hr)	Plasma clearance
Hexobarbital	Normal	4.4 ± 1.2	3.57 ± 0.83 ml/min/kg
	Acute hepatitis	7.5 ± 3.0	2.04 ± 0.94 ml/min/kg
	Recovery	6.4 ± 2.1	2.32 ± 1.08 ml/min/kg
Diazepam	Normal	32.7 ± 8.9	—
	Acute hepatitis	75.7 ± 15.2	—
	Recovery	53.8 ± 6.1	—
Meperidine	Normal	3.4 ± 0.8	1261 ± 527 ml/min
	Acute hepatitis	8.2 ± 3.7	488 ± 132 ml/min
	Recovery	3.3 ± 0.8	1200 ± 555 ml/min

Sources: From Refs. 91, 97, 98.

between restoration of drug-metabolizing activity and the recovery of liver function as judged by current biochemical tests. However, as will be seen later, many of such tests do not correlate with altered drug elimination during disease states.

As already observed, acute hepatitis does not appear to alter the metabolism of many drugs. For example, no change in lorazepam clearance could be detected in patients with acute hepatitis despite the same subjects exhibiting evidence for the impaired clearance of antipyrine [100] (Table 11). However, such findings contrast with the apparent alteration of oxidative metabolism of diazepam and chlordiazepoxide in this disorder [91,101] but are consistent with the failure to find such changes with the related benzodiazepine, oxazepam [102].

The metabolism of lorazepam and oxazepam differs from that of other benzodiazepines in that it occurs almost exclusively by glucuronide formation [103,104]. It has been suggested that in contrast to oxidative pathways utilized by diazepam and chlordiazepoxide, the pathway for glucuronide formation may be resistant to the physiological lesions of hepatic disease [100]. Before such an explanation can be invoked the small decrease in protein binding of lorazepam occurring in acute hepatitis must be considered significant since this might act to mask changes in drug clearance. Such a phenomenon can be seen more clearly in cirrhotic patients where lorazepam

TABLE 11
Disposition of Lorazepam and Antipyrine in Acute Hepatitis

Drug	Status	Half-life [β-phase] (hr)	Clearance (ml/min/kg)	Volume of distribution (liters/kg)	Percentage protein binding
Lorazepam	Normal	22.1 ± 5.4	0.75 ± 0.23	19.9 ± 6.7	93.2 ± 1.9
	Acute hepatitis	25.0 ± 6.4	0.74 ± 0.34	18.1 ± 9.7	91.0 ± 1.9
Antipyrine	Normal	13.0 ± 2.1	0.50 ± 0.05	0.52 ± 0.04	—
	Acute hepatitis	29.7 ± 14.6*	0.27 ± 0.19*	0.54 ± 0.09	—

*$p < 0.05$.
Source: From Ref. 100.

protein binding is altered sufficiently to increase the volume of distribution of the drug [100]. However, this explanation cannot be the sole one since a number of drugs undergoing oxidative metabolism are also unaffected by acute hepatitis. For example, the metabolism of tolbutamide [85], diphenylhydantoin [86], warfarin [105], and phenobarbital [106] appears unchanged. It is therefore necessary to propose that the sensitivity of oxidative pathways to the acute hepatic insult differs and may be related to the heterogeneity of monooxygenase systems [11,47]. At the present time, however, little proof is available one way or the other.

Although drug-metabolizing activity may appear normal in acute hepatitis, the values provided in most studies are usually a mean for a group of patients without reference to the stage or severity of the disease. This, coupled with the individual genetic or drug-induced variations in drug-metabolizing activity, may serve to explain why the distribution of clearance values is greater in patients than in the normal population.

The study of pentobarbital hydroxylase activity in hepatic biopsy samples from patients with uncomplicated viral hepatitis has shed light on the alterations in metabolism occurring with the severity and phase of the disease [107]. No change in pentobarbital hydroxylase activity was observed in samples exhibiting localized necrosis but in specimens showing subacute autolytic necrosis (massive necrosis) a decrease in activity was observed (Fig. 2). This would suggest that altered metabolism only occurs during the more severe form of hepatitis and cannot be demonstrated in patients with only local changes. Such a situation might be explained by a relatively large reserve capacity of the liver for pentobarbital hydroxylase activity that is not compromised until massive disruption of hepatic cellular function takes place. Thus, despite fragmentation and vesiculation of endoplasmic reticulum in acute viral hepatitis the functional state of the smooth endoplasmic reticulum, as reflected by pentobarbital hydroxylase activity, is not significantly altered unless there is autolysis of hepatocytes.

In contrast to the above, a marked increase of pentobarbital hydroxylase activity was observed during the regeneration of liver parenchymal cells (as judged by Kupffer cell proliferation, hyperplasia of the smooth endoplasmic reticulum). This finding is totally unexpected since the phenomenon is unknown in vivo. Indeed, studies of pentobarbital in liver disease revealed no change in drug action or metabolism [108,109]. Further, an increase in drug-metabolizing activity is also unexpected from animal experiments where during liver regeneration decreased enzyme function is normally apparent [110,111]. Why an increase in pentobarbital hydroxylase activity occurs during cell degeneration is not clear but must be related to complex physiological and biochemical events. A decrease in bilirubin levels and transaminase was apparent during the recovery phase but these may be coincidental to the altered enzyme function. Recovery from the disease (as judged by normal histology or only focal inflammation) was accompanied by a return of enzyme activity to normal.

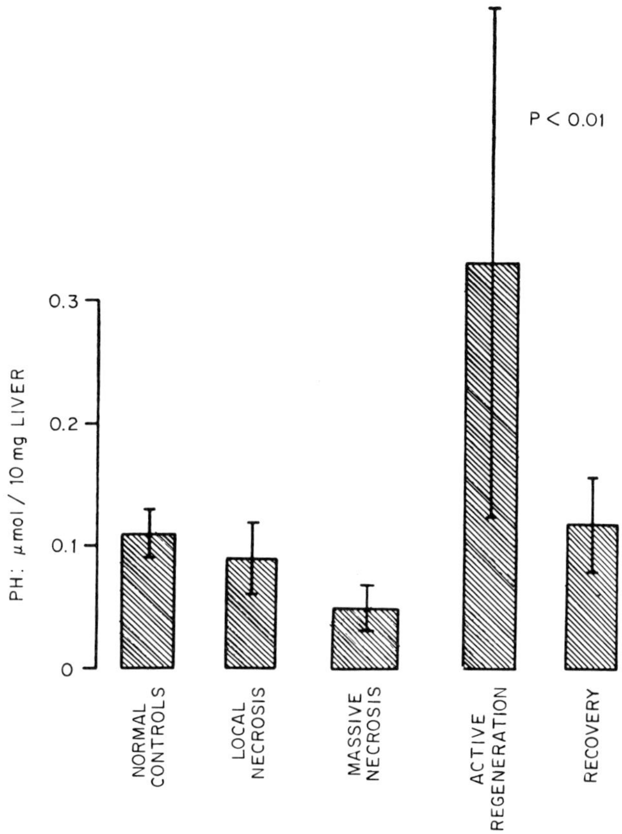

FIGURE 2 Hepatic microsomal pentobarbital hydroxylase activity in normal subjects and in patients exhibiting various stages of acute viral hepatitis. (From Ref. 107. Reproduced with permission of the copyright holders.)

To conclude this section, there is something to be gained from looking briefly at drug-induced acute hepatic necrosis. Drugs such as paracetamol or α-methyldopa induce histological changes in liver consistent with hepatitis and chronic active hepatitis. The onset of these conditions is associated with an increase in the plasma half-life of paracetamol, diphenylhydantoin, antipyrine, and barbiturates [2,112,113]. Altered drug clearance correlates well with biochemical indices of liver damage, and drug half-life in such patients provides a reliable index of the extent of liver damage. Normalization of drug clearance did accompany clinical recovery from the drug-induced injury.

B. Chronic Liver Disease

Chronic liver disease is associated with a reduction of drug-metabolizing activity (Table 12). The situation, however, is made complex by the greater likelihood of change in other pharmacokinetic parameters in such severe disease (e.g., changes in protein binding, drug distribution, hepatic perfusion, and renal clearance). In general, such factors have been considered in Sec. II but some mention will of necessity be made here.

Early studies often failed to detect changes in drug-metabolizing activity during chronic liver disease since patients were administered other drugs likely to cause enzyme induction or inhibition. Additionally, these studies failed to reveal the masking of altered metabolism resulting from other pharmacokinetic events. Thus, before such studies are used to dispute the current concept of decreased metabolism careful consideration must be given to the methodology by which they were carried out.

As a preliminary it must be stated that there are reasons to expect the metabolism of some drugs to be normal in some forms of chronic liver disease. Indeed, in contrast to the predicted loss of microsomal enzymes caused by the extensive necrosis of hepatocytes occurring with acute hepatic disease, chronic liver disease produces not only interlobular fibrosis and the accompanying disruption of hepatic architecture and blood flow, but also marked hyperplasia. This means that even if drug-metabolizing activity is reduced per tissue unit the overall capacity of the liver will be unchanged (see later). In addition, drug-metabolizing activity may actually be unaltered since the extent of change depends to a large extent on the progression of the disease (see later).

The design of drug metabolism studies in chronic liver disease must be made with greater care to ensure that sufficient parameters are measured,

TABLE 12
Drugs Whose Half-life Is Increased and Clearance Is Reduced by Chronic Liver Disease

Amobarbital [89]	Meperidine [116]
Ampicillin [114]	Paracetamol [117]
Antipyrine [95]	Phenobarbital [106]
Chloramphenicol [115]	Phenylbutazone [88]
Diazepam [91]	Procainamide [118]
Isoniazid [88]	Propranolol [39]
Lidocaine [34]	

thus unveiling changes due to reasons other than altered metabolic function. For example, the half-life of meprobamate in patients with cirrhosis or chronic hepatitis ($t_{1/2}$ = 24.3 ± 4.4 hr) is prolonged compared to control subjects (12.6 ± 2.5 hr) [119]. However, since treatment with phenobarbital did not restore the half-life toward normal values and since microsomal monooxygenase activity is normally inducible in such disease states, alterations in hepatic perfusion may be responsible for the observed change rather than altered drug-metabolizing activity. It must be noted, however, that the patients in this study were also receiving other drugs and these may have induced changes preventing an inductive effect of phenobarbital.

In other cases it is difficult to differentiate the effect of alterations in hepatic blood flow from altered drug-metabolizing activity. While a decrease in clearance and an increase in volume of distribution and plasma half-life for both lidocaine and propranolol is apparent in patients with chronic liver disease, these cannot be attributed simply to altered metabolism since the clearance of both drugs is highly dependent upon liver blood flow [34,120,121]. However, a recent comparison of the disposition of antipyrine (flow-independent) and lorcainide (flow-dependent) suggests that the elimination of drugs in cirrhotic patients is associated with relatively more impairment of enzyme activity than of hepatic blood flow [122].

Alterations in protein binding of drugs during chronic liver disease may prevent the detection of altered metabolism, it may mask the extent of the change, or it may provide an apparent change not due to altered metabolic activity. For example, examination of the plasma disappearance of chlorpromazine in patients with compensated cirrhosis compared to control subjects revealed no apparent change in the drug's pharmacokinetic profile [123] even allowing for prior drug treatment. Since chlorpromazine undergoes extensive metabolism this was interpreted as demonstrating no apparent change in drug-metabolizing activity in cirrhosis. However, a reappraisal by Wilkinson and Schenker [3] subjected individual plasma concentration time plots to pharmacokinetic analysis which demonstrated a paradoxical increase in plasma clearance and a shorter half-life in cirrhotic patients. This may be attributable to alterations of the normally extensive protein binding of chlorpromazine leading to increased drug clearance (not measured in the original study). Whether such a change occurs and whether the phenomenon compensates for a decrease in metabolic function remains unclear. It should also be noted that since the effect of chronic liver disease varies with disease state the study of chlorpromazine clearance in patients with compensated cirrhosis might not be expected to reveal a marked alteration in chlorpromazine metabolism (see later).

In alcoholic cirrhosis the plasma half-life of lorazepam was markedly increased but this was not associated with an impairment of systemic plasma clearance or urinary excretion of conjugates of lorazepam [100] (Table 13). It appears to be due entirely to a similar increase in the volume of distribution of lorazepam caused by reduction in the extent of drug plasma protein

TABLE 13
Effect of Alcoholic Cirrhosis on the Disposition of Lorazepam

Parameter	Control subjects	Patients with cirrhosis
Half-life [β-phase] (hr)	22.1 ± 5.4	31.9 ± 9.6*
Plasma clearance (ml/min/kg)	11.7 ± 4.8	10.6 ± 6.7
Volume of distribution (liters/kg)	1.28 ± 0.34	2.01 ± 0.82*
Percentage plasma protein binding	93.2 ± 1.8	88.6 ± 2.5*
Urinary recovery (% of administered dose)	52.4 ± 14.1	53.3 ± 15.8

*$p < 0.05$
Source: From Ref. 100.

binding. Again why the metabolism of lorazepam (and indeed oxazepam [102]) should not be affected by hepatic disease (acute or chronic) is by no means clear.

Investigation of diazepam disposition in chronic liver disease contains several aspects worthy of discussion. Thus, in patients with alcoholic cirrhosis, chronic active hepatitis, or liver fibrosis, the half-life and clearance of the drug was prolonged compared to normal healthy individuals [91, 124,125] (Table 14). This change can largely be attributed to altered hepatic metabolism since virtually no diazepam is excreted unchanged in urine and the clearance of diazepam is not dependent on hepatic perfusion. Altered clearance was accompanied by an increase in the volume of distribution due predominantly to decreased plasma protein binding. This led to a marked increased fraction of unbound drug in plasma which consequently implies that the degree of hepatic impairment measured by total clearance of drug underestimates the decrease in drug-metabolizing activity [3,8].

The impairment of hepatic metabolism of diazepam in chronic liver disease is substantiated by the delayed appearance and achievement of peak levels of desmethyldiazepam following diazepam administration. Since the peak plasma levels of metabolite achieved are similar to those in normal subjects, it appeared likely that the further metabolism of desmethyldiazepam by hydroxylation to oxazepam is also impaired. This was confirmed following administration of desmethyldiazepam to patients with hepatic disease and to healthy volunteers where the half-life of the compound was prolonged and the total plasma clearance reduced [124].

A further difference between normal subjects and patients with chronic liver disease is apparent on repeated diazepam administration. Thus, the elimination half-life of diazepam is prolonged in normal subjects receiving repeated diazepam administration for 7 days [126] whereas in patients with chronic liver disease no significant increase is apparent and other pharmacokinetic parameters remain unchanged [124].

In normal subjects the prolongation has been attributed to feedback inhibition of diazepam metabolism by desmethyldiazepam. Two explanations have been put forward to explain the lack of change in the disease state. It may be that the generally lower levels of desmethyldiazepam reached in liver patients are not sufficient to cause feedback inhibition. Alternatively, and perhaps a more attractive hypothesis, is the possibility that the already extensively impaired metabolism of diazepam cannot be inhibited further.

The investigation of drugs cleared mainly by metabolism appears particularly useful in investigating altered drug-metabolizing activity in chronic liver disease particularly if such compounds are not extensively protein bound or affected by changes in hepatic blood flow and if changes in levels of metabolites can also be demonstrated. Obviously, such a statement is idealistic, but a number of drugs go some way toward meeting these criteria.

For example, meperidine elimination (under conditions of controlled urinary pH) occurs predominantly by hepatic metabolism. In cirrhotic patients the half-life of elimination is increased and total plasma meperidine clearance reduced [116] (Table 15). Although the drug is bound to plasma proteins to a marked degree no alteration in binding due to the disease state was apparent and the volume of distribution was unchanged. This would

TABLE 14
Effect of Alcoholic Cirrhosis on the Disposition of Diazepam

Parameter	Control subjects	Patients with cirrhosis
Half-life [β-phase] (hr)	46.6 ± 14.2	105.6 ± 15.2*
Volume of distribution (liters/kg)	1.13 ± 0.28	1.74 ± 0.21*
Elimination rate constant ($k_{1,3}$; hr^{-1})	0.08 ± 0.04	0.03 ± 0.01*
Plasma clearance (ml/min)	26.6 ± 4.1	13.8 ± 2.4*
Percentage protein binding	97.8 ± 1.0	95.3 ± 1.8*
Percentage free drug	2.2 ± 1.0	4.7 ± 1.8*

*$p < 0.05$.
Source: From Ref. 91.

TABLE 15
Effect of Cirrhosis on the Disposition of Meperidine

Parameter	Normal subjects	Cirrhotic patients
Half-life [β-phase] (hr)	3.2 ± 0.8	7.0 ± 0.9*
Elimination rate constant ($k_{1,3}$; hr^{-1})	0.67 ± 0.24	0.24 ± 0.06*
Plasma clearance (ml/min)	1316 ± 383	664 ± 293*
Volume of distribution (liters/kg)	4.17 ± 1.33	5.76 ± 2.55
Percentage plasma protein binding	64.3 ± 13.5	64.9 ± 5.8

*$p < 0.05$.
Source: From Ref. 116.

suggest the occurrence of impairment of meperidine metabolism (normally by demethylation or hydrolysis). No metabolite levels were reported.

Amobarbital is also cleared predominantly by hepatic metabolism [127], a major urinary metabolite in humans being the 3'-hydroxy derivative [128]. In cirrhotic patients the elimination of this drug was found to be reduced in those subjects with hypoalbuminemia but unchanged in patients with normal serum albumin concentrations [89]. Since a decrease in hepatic protein synthesis, particularly albumin, occurs as the disease progresses these data suggest that the metabolism of amobarbital is only affected when the synthesis of microsomal monooxygenases is impaired in the more severe forms of chronic liver disease. Thus, during the early compensated stages of the disease such effects may be of little significance. However, as the disease progresses ascites, hypoalbuminemia, portocaval shunting, and the accumulation of endogenous materials occur, all complicating normal drug profiles. The decrease in plasma albumin caused a consequential decrease in amobarbital binding. By basing drug clearance on the free serum drug concentration, a twofold reduction in plasma clearance was estimated. That this reflects decreased metabolism of amobarbital was confirmed by a decrease in urinary excretion of 3'-hydroxyamobarbital.

The disposition of the related barbiturate hexobarbital is also impaired in cirrhotic disorders [129] as shown by the increased half-life and decreased clearance compared to healthy volunteers in both compensated and decompensated cirrhosis (Table 16). These changes were, however, more marked in the more severe stages of the disease. In addition, while the volume of distribution was unchanged in compensated cirrhosis a marked increase was apparent in patients with decompensated cirrhosis. Unlike amobarbital no change in plasma protein binding was apparent. Again the decreased half-life

TABLE 16
Effect of Compensated and Decompensated Cirrhosis on Hexobarbital Disposition

Parameter	Control subject	Patients with compensated cirrhosis	Patients with decompensated cirrhosis
Half-life [β-phase] (hr)	5.7 ± 1.8	8.5 ± 2.9*	17.0 ± 7.5*
Plasma clearance (ml/min/kg)	3.32 ± 0.99	1.88 ± 0.70*	1.26 ± 0.49*
Volume of distribution (liters/kg)	1.25 ± 0.24	1.14 ± 0.26	1.57 ± 0.64
24-hr excretion of hexobarbital (% dose)	0.30 ± 0.14	0.33 ± 0.19	
24-hr excretion of 3'-ketohexobarbital (% dose)	39 ± 18	5.2 ± 5.3*	

*$p < 0.05$.
Source: From Ref. 129.

of hexobarbital may be attributed to a decrease in hepatic metabolism, a finding corroborated by the decreased 24-hr urinary excretion of 3'-keto-hexobarbital.

Finally, mention must be made of the use of antipyrine since this compound possesses almost all the properties required to allow examination of altered drug-metabolizing activity in chronic liver disease. Thus, antipyrine is readily absorbed, almost entirely metabolized by the liver, virtually unbound to plasma proteins, and is only distributed in body water. In addition and perhaps more important is the fact that this drug is virtually nontoxic. In chronic liver disease antipyrine elimination half-life is prolonged and this effect is even more pronounced in cirrhotic patients with hypoalbuminemia [95]. No correlation was apparent with the estimated volume of distribution or with the presence of portosystemic anastomosis or encephalopathy confirming the lack of dependence of metabolism on hepatic perfusion.

C. Alterations in Components of the Drug-metabolizing Enzyme System during Acute and Chronic Liver Disease

Although we have now seen that the metabolism of at least some drugs can be reduced in liver disease, little evidence has been presented to show whether such changes are due to a reduction in size of the functional liver mass or to a reduction in the level of activity of drug-metabolizing enzymes themselves. This relatively short section will look at the evidence currently available to decide between those alternatives.

The few studies devoted to this topic have fortunately reached convergent conclusions (Table 17). Thus, it is clear that only in severe hepatitis or severe cirrhosis is the level of cytochrome P-450 reduced [130-133].

TABLE 17
Effect of Hepatic Disease on Cytochrome P-450 Concentrations

Histological definition of disease	Cytochrome P-450 (nmol/g) Ref. 130	Ref. 131	Ref. 132	Ref. 133
Normal	11.1 ± 2.6	10.6 ± 1.6	11.4 ± 1.7	11.1 ± 2.1
Slight	—	6.9 ± 3.3*	8.6 ± 3.6*	7.3 ± 2.7*
Severe	7.0 ± 1.9*	5.1 ± 2.4*	5.8 ± 1.7*	5.1 ± 1.9*

*$p < 0.05$.

TABLE 18
Relationship between Altered Hepatic Histology, Cytochrome P-450 Levels, and Antipyrine Half-life

Hepatic histology	Cytochrome P-450 (nmol/g)	Antipyrine half-life [β-phase] (hr)
Normal parenchyma	11.1 ± 2.1	7.7 ± 1.5
Slight changes	7.3 ± 2.7*	10.3 ± 2.4*
Severe changes	5.1 ± 1.9*	24.6 ± 10.1*

*$p < 0.05$ compared to subjects with normal parenchyma.
Source: From Ref. 133.

This correlates with a reduction in functional enzyme activity as shown by a decrease in aminopyrine and para-nitroanisole demethylation [130]. In mild forms of parenchymal liver disease, less marked alteration in cytochrome P-450 levels or enzyme activity can be observed. However, even severe liver disease did not alter the level of NADPH-cytochrome c reductase [130]. The question immediately arises as to whether such changes mirror alterations in in vivo drug-metabolizing activity. A comparison of cytochrome P-450 levels in biopsy specimens with antipyrine half-life has shown that in general alterations in liver histology are related to altered drug metabolism (Table 18). Thus, patients with severe disease had a prolonged half-life and low cytochrome P-450 levels whereas the changes in those with slight parenchymal alterations were less pronounced [131]. Such an approach, however, ignores the fact that hepatic size may change during the disease, and allowance for this must be made relative to the unit drug-metabolizing activity of biopsy specimen. In patients with alcoholic hepatitis or cirrhosis the cytochrome P-450 content of tissue is low and correlates with increased antipyrine half-life, while in cirrhotic subjects the increase in hepatic size is largely compensatory, causing an almost normal total cytochrome P-450 content [132]. Similarly, while the cytochrome P-450 content and antipyrine clearance were decreased in patients with parenchymal alterations observed at biopsy, the alteration in liver size restored total cytochrome P-450 levels to or above normal [133] (Fig. 3). These data would indicate that the apparent in vivo change in drug-metabolizing activity observed are not reflected in its total cytochrome P-450 content. This might indicate that factors other than cytochrome P-450 control the level at which activity takes place. It should be especially remembered that the values obtained from a single biopsy sample may not reflect the overall activity of the organ particularly since large areas of histological change may be present. Alternatively it may indicate that it is not a

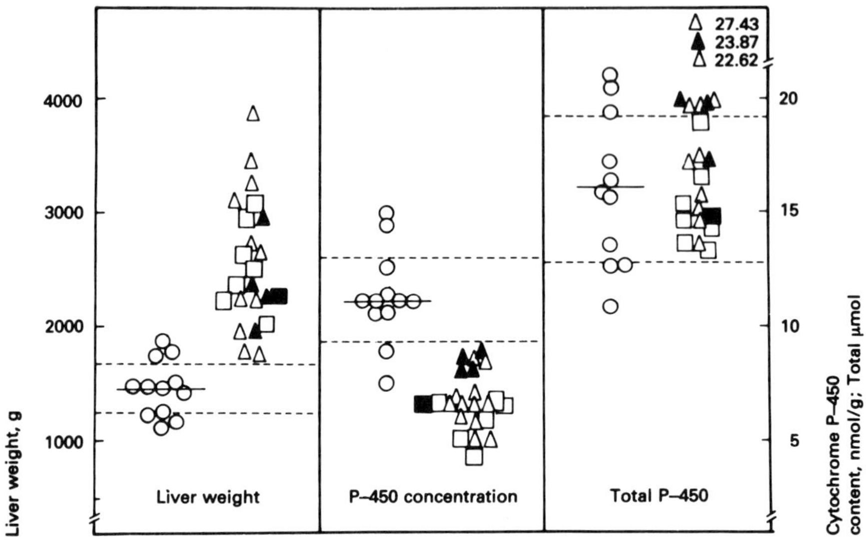

FIGURE 3 Compensatory effect of liver enlargement on the total amount of cytochrome P-450 in subjects with parenchymal alterations and decreased cytochrome P-450 concentration due to liver disease. ○ = normal parenchyma; △ = slight changes; □ = severe changes. Closed symbols indicate a history of inducing drugs. The solid and dotted horizontal lines represent the mean and standard deviation respectively for subjects with normal parenchyma. (From Ref. 133. Reproduced with permission of the copyright holders.)

deficiency in drug-metabolizing enzyme function that is responsible for the altered in vivo clearance of drugs. Changes in hepatic architecture and hepatic perfusion may therefore be the limiting factors governing the overall disposition of the drug.

Why the level of cytochrome P-450 is low is not known. Presumably such a change will reflect a deficiency of protein synthesis. However, a functional deficit is not evident since the administration of enzyme inducers to patients with severe hepatic dysfunction can increase cytochrome P-450 levels and decrease drug half-life [95,109,131,133] (Table 19). Perhaps the deficit is due to a disruption of the normal biochemical function of hepatocytes during the course of the disease, an effect which can be overcome by stimulation of intact protein synthesis. However, since in general protein synthesis is deficient in liver disease, this might seem unlikely. Alternatively perhaps the disruption of blood flow may deprive the system of endogenous factors (e.g., hormones) required to keep the drug-metabolizing system operant at the normal level.

TABLE 19
Effect of Enzyme Induction on Cytochrome P-450 Levels and Antipyrine Half-life in Hepatic Disease

	Cytochrome P-450 (nmol/g)		Antipyrine half-life [β-phase] (hr)	
Hepatic histology	Before	After	Before	After
Normal parenchyma	10.6 ± 1.6	18.2 ± 4.1*	7.9 ± 2.1	4.1 ± 1.9*
Slight changes	6.9 ± 3.3	15.9 ± 7.2*	10.8 ± 3.1	7.4 ± 3.1*
Severe changes	5.1 ± 2.4	10.0 ± 4.2*	21.3 ± 10.1	11.6 ± 5.1*

*$p < 0.05$ compared to drug-free controls.
Source: From Ref. 131.

Obviously little is known of the effect of disease on monooxygenases, while even less appears known of other hepatic microsomal enzyme systems. Thus, while cirrhosis appeared to decrease N,N-dimethylaniline N-oxidase (but interestingly not aminopyrine N-demethylase activity) in biopsy samples, other hepatic disease (alcoholic liver disease, viral hepatitis, etc.) did not affect either parameter [132]. Similarly, patients with hepatitis or cirrhosis exhibited normal bilirubin uridine diphosphate (UDP)-glucuronyltransferase activity although a marked fall was apparent in patients with Gilbert's syndrome [135]. This is somewhat difficult to explain in view of the apparent decrease in in vivo glucuronide formation of chloramphenicol and N-acetyl-para-aminophenol occurring in chronic hepatitis and cirrhosis [90,136]. This may, however, reflect the heterogeneity of the group of glucuronyltransferase enzymes in hepatic tissue. Whether other conjugation pathways are affected remains unknown. Despite some evidence for a decrease in drug acetylation in vivo [88,118], no in vitro corroboration of this change is apparent.

Animal models of hepatic parenchymal disease have not been widely employed perhaps because of the difficulties of reproducing the human diseases, in particular the time course of chronic disorders. The effect of murine hepatitis virus was to initially increase in vitro hexobarbital and strychnine metabolism up to 24 hr but to subsequently decrease activity [137]. This early study, unfortunately, only continued for some 8 days and did not measure components of the drug-metabolizing enzyme system. Further attempts to mimic hepatitis do not seem to have been forthcoming. Perhaps these would be of little use since, as already pointed out, the enhanced pentobarbital hydroxylase activity apparent in humans during liver regeneration after hepatitis would not be observed in animals where such a condition is accompanied by decreased drug-metabolizing activity. Little appears to have been done to model cirrhosis. This is somewhat puzzling since many of the changes observed can be seen following induction of carbon tetrachloride hepatotoxicity in animals [138]. Indeed, induction of CCl_4-induced liver disease caused a prolongation of desmethyldiazepam half-life [91].

D. Hepatic Tumors

Despite the prevalence of malignant tumors in the human population surprisingly little information is available on the effect of hepatic tumors on drug-metabolizing activity. Currently available data is from basically one group and concerns only the metabolism of aminopyrine. The answer obtained, however, appears quite clear. Thus, in patients with hepatic malignancy, aminopyrine demethylation, as judged by $^{14}CO_2$ production from ([^{14}C]methyl)-aminopyrine, is reduced compared to control subjects (Fig. 4) [87,139]. This is reflected also in altered aminopyrine clearance rates (32.4 ml/min in hepatic malignancy; 103.4 ± 18.8 ml/min in patients without; $p < 0.05$ [140]. The use of [^{14}C]aminopyrine provides a sensitive index of hepatic malignancy. A comparison of patients with malignant disease having and not having diagnosed hepatic neoplasm showed the excretion of $^{14}CO_2$ to correctly identify hepatic involvement in up to 90% of patients even if abnormal serum biochemistry was not present [140]. No decreases in $^{14}CO_2$ values were seen in patients without hepatic involvement. Although perhaps a sensitive test of hepatic malignancy, this technique tells us little of the changes that may occur in drug-metabolizing activity during the progress of the disease. Indeed, it may not even reflect a general decrease in demethylation if a greater reserve enzymatic capacity exists for substrates other than aminopyrine.

There is a small amount of other evidence to support a decrease in drug-metabolizing activity in hepatic carcinoma. Thus, the relative importance of competitive metabolic pathways in the metabolism of methaqualone (hydroxylation and N-oxidation) appeared reduced in two patients with secondary hepatomas as judged by urinary metabolite excretion [141]. Obviously the study lacks a sufficient number of patients and was inadequately controlled with regard to normal subjects and competing drug therapy. However, if such a change in pathway importance occurs, it may have considerable consequence to drug therapy.

At the enzymatic level, also, little appears to be known. A reduction in the in vitro reductive cleavage of potentially cytotoxic azo compounds has been reported in biopsy specimens of hepatocellular carcinoma (normal liver 61.2 ± 17.4 nmol dye reduced/100 mg protein/min; hepatocellular carcinoma 15.4 ± 7.5 nmol dye reduced/100 mg protein/min; $p < 0.05$) [142]. In addition, biopsy specimens from a small number of patients with other various forms of carcinoma showed a decrease in components of the

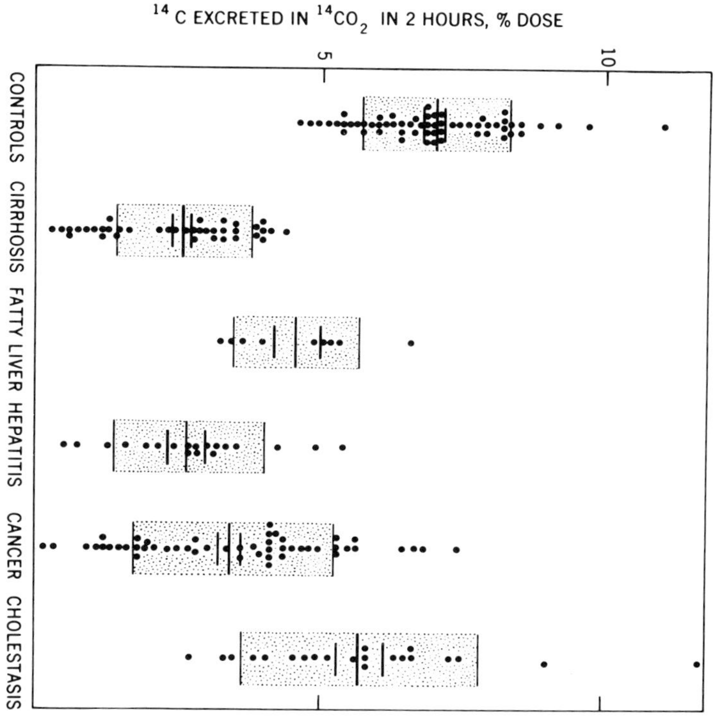

FIGURE 4 Percentage of orally administered [^{14}C]aminopyrine excreted as $^{14}CO_2$ in breath 2 hr after drug administration. Transverse lines represent the mean ± 1 SE and the hatched areas represent the standard deviation. (From Ref. 87. Reproduced with permission of the copyright holders.)

microsomal drug-metabolizing system as the histological evidence of hepatic malignancy clarified (Table 20) [143]. Thus, although some evidence exists to suggest decreased hepatic drug-metabolizing activity in hepatic malignancy, there is no evidence as to why such a change occurs. It is clear from malignancy of other organs that some endogenous factor can cause a decrease in hepatic metabolism (see later) and it is perhaps probable that a similar explanation applies to hepatic neoplasms. It must also be considered, however, that the extent of formation of tumor tissue may play a role since drug-metabolizing activity in the tumor itself is lower than in the immediate neighboring areas and in normal tissue [144,145]. This is accompanied by a lower cytochrome P-450 and NADPH-cytochrome P-450 reductase activity than in normal liver [146]. Although the components of the hepatoma drug-metabolizing enzyme systems appear comparable

TABLE 20
Alteration in Components of the Drug-metabolizing Enzyme Systems in Malignant Disease

Disease classified by hepatic histology	Cytochrome P-450 (nmol/mg protein)	Cytochrome b_5 (nmol/mg protein)	NADPH-cytochrome c reductase (nmol/mg/min)	Benzpyrene hydroxylase (pmol/g liver/min)	Aminopyrine demethylase (nmol/g liver/min)	Aniline hydroxylase (nmol/g liver/min)
All patients	0.43 ± 0.21	0.19 ± 0.07	67 ± 15	104 ± 43	30.9 ± 19.4	72 ± 3.5
Normal histology	0.60 ± 0.29	0.26 ± 0.04	71 ± 19	173 ± 102	46.2 ± 31.1	9.2
Inflammatory and degenerative changes	0.43 ± 0.13	0.18 ± 0.04	70 ± 14	63 ± 24	26.8 ± 14.8	9.0 ± 2.9
Clearly malignant picture	0.27 ± 0.10	0.17; 0.22	61 ± 13	73 ± 37	23.7 ± 6.7	5.3 ± 0.6
Normal values (patients with cholecystolithiasis)	0.53 ± 0.33	0.22 ± 0.08	78 ± 21	141 ± 65	48.2 ± 34.4	8.7 ± 6.8

Source: From Ref. 143.

to those of normal liver, the hepatoma reductase requires an order of magnitude more NADPH to support reduction than does liver reductase [146]. It is suggested that the binding site for NADPH may be altered in such a way as to reduce the affinity of the hepatoma reductase for the electron donor and this may represent a major reason for the lowered level of activity of the tumor drug-metabolizing system.

The effect of malignancy on drug-metabolizing enzyme activity will be considered further in Sec. IV.F.

E. Correlation of Altered Drug Metabolism with Liver Function Tests

If alterations in drug-metabolizing enzyme activity and function occur during hepatic disease other biochemical indices of hepatic function might also be expected to be impaired. This, however, presumes similar functional capacity and susceptibility to the alteration occurring during the progression of the disease state. Indeed, the evidence presently available generally suggests little correlation between alteration in drug metabolism and altered liver function tests (serum albumin, prothrombin time, SGOT, serum bilirubin, and alkaline phosphatase). None of these function tests is thus a successful index of the progress of the disease or the degree of impairment. It is also clear that none of the commonly used liver function tests provides a readily interpretable index of hepatic capacity (see Refs. 3, 6).

While the above statement is correct within its limits, it by no means corresponds to the entire picture. Thus, while no relationship exists between liver function tests and altered diazepam, meperidine, lidocaine, and tolbutamide metabolism [34,91,97,147] other strong correlations exist. For example, the prolongation of antipyrine half-life in patients with liver disease was most marked in those with hypoalbuminemia and hypoprothrombinemia [95]. Similarly, antipyrine clearance was found to be significantly correlated with galactose elimination capacity, serum albumin, and prothrombin values [148] (Table 21). Galactose elimination has been suggested from this and other studies (see Ref. 149) as a useful index of drug-metabolizing capacity. However, although a similar correlation of galactose elimination with phenylbutazone clearance has been demonstrated [150] further intensive investigation is required to evaluate the predictive value of this index, especially since it utilizes an invasive technique.

Even those correlations established between drug clearance and liver function suffer from serious shortcomings. In general, there is no continuity of effect, meaning that while the greatest alterations in clearance are associated with the greatest changes in liver function tests other subjects having normal function tests still show altered drug clearance (see Refs. 89, 95). Further, the lag in recovery of normal values between liver function tests and drug clearance described in hepatitis [91,98] again suggests the poor relationship between these parameters. The attempts to establish

TABLE 21
Relationship between Alterations in Liver Function Tests and Pharmacokinetic Parameters of Antipyrine in Hepatic Disease

Parameter	Control subjects	Patients with liver disease
Antipyrine plasma clearance (ml/min)	58.6 ± 16.6	18.5 ± 11.8*
Antipyrine half-life [β-phase] (hr)	31.8 ± 19.5	7.9 ± 1.7*
Antipyrine volume of distribution (liters)	36.9 ± 9.3	38.5 ± 7.3
Galactose elimination (mg/min)	406 ± 91	232 ± 60
Serum albumin (μmol/liter)	560 ± 111	363 ± 98*
Percentage prothrombin	93 ± 17	61 ± 23

*$p < 0.05$.
Source: From Ref. 148.

such correlations appear ambitious since they are usually based only on plasma drug clearance and do not in general take into account other alterations in pharmacokinetic parameters which may act to distort the time relationship. Where a correlation is established between drug clearance and liver function tests it should at present be considered as being only of relevance to that particular drug.

A recent approach utilizing measurement of serum zinc levels may provide a more realistic means of measuring altered drug metabolism in hepatic disease [151]. Indeed, it is known that a deficiency of trace elements such as zinc and copper produces profound alterations in drug-metabolizing capacity in animals [152-154]. In humans altered serum levels of these elements are found in cirrhosis, malignant states, and thyrotoxicosis and this may be of relevance to the altered metabolism of drugs occurring in such syndromes (see Ref. 151). Measurement of serum zinc levels in alcoholics with normal, mild, or severe liver histology showed a significant correlation between hepatic cytochrome P-450 levels and antipyrine half-life (Table 22). No such correlation existed for serum copper levels. Obviously, the application of this examination to other hepatic (and perhaps nonhepatic) disease states requires rigorous investigation utilizing alterations in the clearance of a number of drugs.

TABLE 22
Alterations in Serum Zinc and Copper Levels and Indices of Drug Metabolism in Alcoholics with Various Histological Lesions of the Liver

Disease state judged by liver histology	Serum zinc (μg/100 ml)	Serum copper (μg/100 ml)	Antipyrine half-life [β-phase] (hr)	Cytochrome P-450 levels (nmol/g)
Normal	161 ± 39	237 ± 33	6.5 ± 1.9	14.4 ± 6.6
Fatty liver	141 ± 31	168 ± 43	9.5 ± 1.9	8.2 ± 4.0*
Alcoholic hepatitis	105 ± 18*	206 ± 33	24.6 ± 15.6*	5.5 ± 2.6*
Cirrhosis	84 ± 13*	215 ± 54	24.1 ± 9.6*	6.2 ± 1.4*

*$p < 0.05$ compared to alcoholics with normal hepatic histology.
Source: From Ref. 151.

Perhaps the use of a model drug such as antipyrine provides as good an index of liver function as is currently available (although this of course would not be predictive of altered metabolism for all drugs) and may in fact provide a useful diagnostic aid to the detection of hepatic disorders. We have already seen the predictive value of measurement of $^{14}CO_2$ excretion following administration of [^{14}C]aminopyrine in hepatic carcinoma; this technique has found further application in the detection of other hepatic disorders.

The idea of utilizing measurement of expired $^{14}CO_2$ following administration of [^{14}C]aminopyrine as an in vivo index of monooxygenase activity arose from studies of Lauterberg and Bircher [155] in rats. Adaptation of the technique to humans demonstrated that the rate of clearance of aminopyrine correlated with $^{14}CO_2$ output and that since the drug is eliminated almost entirely by metabolism such parameters can be utilized as an index of metabolic function [156]. This was further demonstrated by the ability of the monooxygenase system inducer phenobarbital and the enzyme inhibitor disulfiram to produce increases and decreases, respectively, in aminopyrine clearance and $^{14}CO_2$ output.

Subsequent comparison of $^{14}CO_2$ output in normal subjects and in patients with various forms of hepatic disorders demonstrated first the impairment of aminopyrine metabolism of such disorders and secondly the use of measuring $^{14}CO_2$ output as a relatively sensitive and accurate technique for diagnosis. Thus, following oral administration of labeled aminopyrine the drug clearance and $^{14}CO_2$ output are reduced in hepatitis, cirrhosis, fatty liver, schistozomal infection, and hepatic malignancy [87,139, 140,156-158] (Fig. 4). The decrease in $^{14}CO_2$ output does not, however, provide an overall picture of change in drug-metabolizing activity since no significant correlation with altered antipyrine clearance was observed.

It would seem nevertheless that alteration in $^{14}CO_2$ output may be a fairly selective tool in the diagnosis of hepatocellular disease. Thus, while radioactivity excretion falls in liver disease with cellular disruption, no change is observed in patients exhibiting cholestasis. Indeed, the use of aminopyrine clearly distinguished between patients with hyperbilirubinemia due to hepatocellular disease and those with cholestasis [139].

The advantages of the aminopyrine breath test from both a drug metabolism and clinical diagnostic viewpoint are readily apparent. It is noninvasive, quick, easy, and sensitive. It provides by means of metabolite formation a simple measure of drug clearance, which in this case reflects predominantly alterations in liver drug-metabolizing activity, that may be of use in defining parenchymal liver disorders (see also Ref. 159). There is, however, evidence to suggest that the absorption of the labeled drug may be impaired in some cirrhotic patients and that this may provide an additional factor decreasing $^{14}CO_2$ output. Also, it would appear that the formation of $^{14}CO_2$ may not only reflect demethylation of aminopyrine but also the subsequent metabolism of primary metabolites. Thus, Noordhoek et al. [158] demonstrated that $^{14}CO_2$ levels declined 1.8 times more slowly than aminopyrine plasma levels and that $^{14}CO_2$ production continued after the disappearance of aminopyrine from plasma at a time when marked amounts of monomethylaminoantipyrine were present. This, taken with the lack of correlation of aminopyrine demethylation with antipyrine clearance would suggest that although useful the aminopyrine breath test can perhaps not be regarded as a pure index of altered metabolic function.

F. Biliary Obstruction and Cholestasis

The effect of biliary obstruction and cholestasis on drug metabolism in humans is at present unclear. One major reason for this is the variable degree of stasis involved, the extent of liver cell injury, and the small number of substrates examined. While Branch et al. [95] found a modest increase in antipyrine half-life in biliary obstruction in six patients, no marked alteration in antipyrine half-life could be detected in cholestasis [160]. Additionally, no alteration in antipyrine half-life resulted from the occurrence of gallstones or cholecystectomy [87]. The slight effect of cholestasis on antipyrine clearance was confirmed by measurement of $^{14}CO_2$ following administration of [^{14}C]aminopyrine [139]. Thus, aminopyrine metabolism was normal in 70% of patients with cholestasis-associated hyperbilirubinemia and only grossly abnormal in 1 of 40 subjects. This contrasted with the severely abnormal values obtained in 70% of patients with hyperbilirubinemia due to hepatocellular disease. In those cholestatic patients undergoing surgery for extrahepatic biliary obstruction a normalization of $^{14}CO_2$ values was observed, indicating that some initial impairment of aminopyrine metabolism does indeed occur [87].

Using meprobamate, pentobarbital, or tolbutamide as test substrates some evidence to confirm a decrease in drug clearance during cholestasis has been obtained [161]. We shall for our purpose ignore the data generated for tolbutamide since the complications caused by its displacement from plasma binding sites by bile salts only further confuse the issue. Division of patients into clinically and histologically distinct categories of cholestasis revealed different effects on drug clearance and in vitro metabolism (Table 23). Thus, in recurrent cholestasis the half-life of meprobamate and pentobarbital was unchanged and this correlated with the normal liver structure observed on histological examination. However, in patients with cholestatic hepatitis showing inflammation and necrosis of liver lobules the half-life of these drugs was significantly increased. Extrabiliary obstruction in contrast produced a differential effect only prolonging pentobarbital half-life and was accompanied by less pronounced liver cell involvement. This in vivo prolongation was associated with reduced in vitro metabolism of pentobarbital and correlated with the 40% decrease in hexobarbital metabolism found in biopsy specimens from patients with acute or chronic cholecystitis and obstructive jaundice [162].

TABLE 23
Changes in Drug Clearance and In Vitro Metabolism During Cholestasis

Diagnosis	Half-life [β-phase] (hr)		In vitro pentobarbital metabolism (nmol metabolite found/g liver/min)
	Meprobamate	Pentobarbital	
Control subjects	7.4 ± 0.6	25.4 ± 1.1	0.57
Intrahepatic recurrent cholestasis	7.2 ± 1.6	25.6 ± 3.2	—
Cholestatic hepatitis	13.8 ± 7.0*	39.7 ± 6.5*	—
Extrabiliary obstruction	8.4 ± 3.2	31.2 ± 2.5*	0.26*

*$p < 0.05$.
Source: From Ref. 161.

It would therefore appear that cholestasis can indeed produce some alterations of the drug-metabolizing enzyme system. These changes appear to depend very much on the substrate examined and the extent to which hepatic anatomy is affected. Supportive evidence is found in the human metabolism of diazepam and antipyrine which is not altered by the different categories of cholestasis outlined above (see Ref. 139). It is perhaps surprising that substrates requiring mainly biliary mechanisms for elimination do not appear to have been studied. It is also somewhat puzzling that the changes observed are relatively small since deoxycholic acid and other bile acids have a marked effect on in vitro drug metabolism in lower species.

Thus, two decades ago McLuen and Fouts [163] demonstrated that ligation of the bile duct of rabbits caused a depression of drug-metabolizing activity in vitro that paralleled the severity of hepatic damage (Table 24). This study led to the suggestion that bile acids may be responsible for the observed depression since it was reduced by perfusion of jaundiced livers with KCl while the addition of deoxycholic acid to preparations of normal liver inhibited drug metabolism. At this time the depression was attributed to a solubilization action of the bile acids.

Subsequent investigation in the rat, however, revealed that while in vitro aminopyrine (a type I substrate) metabolism was markedly decreased 4 days following bile duct ligation, aniline (a type II substrate) hydroxylase activity, cytochrome P-450 levels, and NADPH-cytochrome P-450 reductase were only slightly reduced [164]. The inhibition of aminopyrine

TABLE 24
Effect of Bile Duct Ligation in Rabbits on In Vitro Drug Metabolism

	Amount metabolized (μmol/g)		
Substrate	Normal liver[a]	Mild damage[b]	Severe damage[c]
Chlorpromazine	3.1 ± 0.4	1.7 ± 0.6	0.6 ± 0.4
Hexobarbital	2.8 ± 0.8	1.4 ± 0.4	0.3 ± 0.3
(-)-Amphetamine	2.6 ± 0.5	0.5 ± 0.5	0.07 ± 0.12
Codeine	2.0 ± 0.8	0.3 ± 0.2	0.3 ± 0.2
Acetanilide	1.4 ± 0.6	0.4 ± 0.2	0.3 ± 0.2
Aminopyrine	0.8 ± 0.3	0.09 ± 0.08	0.04 ± 0.02

[a] Histological assessment.
[b] Assessed 4 days after ligation.
[c] Assessed 15 days after ligation.

metabolism in the presence of adequate cytochrome P-450 concentrations appeared due to the inhibition of the binding of the type I substrate to the terminal oxidase, which in turn leads to a reduction in the rate of cytochrome P-450 reduction. Presumably this represents an action of bile acids since treatment of control tissue with taurochenodeoxycholate produced a selective impairment of type I binding.

This latter conclusion was substantiated by the fact that conjugated and free dihydroxy acids such as taurochenodeoxycholic acid interact with drug-metabolizing enzyme in three progressive stages [165]:

Stage 1. Taurochenodeoxycholic acid produces a type I binding spectrum with cytochrome P-450 and competitively inhibits the metabolism of other type I substrates. Type II substrates and the concentration of cytochrome P-450 are unaffected.

Stage 2. Both the binding and metabolism of type I substrates are noncompetitively inhibited. Type II substrates and the concentration of cytochrome P-450 remain unaffected (as seen 4 days after bile duct ligation).

Stage 3. Noncompetitive inhibition of the binding and metabolism of type I and II substrates accompanied by significant loss of cytochrome P-450 (as seen 15 days after bile duct ligation).

The prolonged ligation of the bile duct in rats is associated with hepatic enlargement, bile duct proliferation, and hyperplasia of the smooth endoplasmic reticulum [166]. This fact, taken together with evidence for decreased microsomal enzyme activity, would indicate a hypoactivity of the smooth endoplasmic reticulum (see Ref. 167). The effect is, however, reversible since enzyme-inducing agents restore the biochemical values to normal [166,168]. It is necessary to point out that the evidence for hyperplasia of the smooth endoplasmic reticulum is equivocal, since 48 hr following total biliary obstruction no proliferation but in fact a decrease in smooth endoplasmic reticulum has been observed [169]. Hyper- and hypoplasia may represent extremes of a spectrum of little-known changes which require further investigation. No reason can be put forward why the same arguments should not be applied also to humans.

As we have already seen, there is little evidence for the selective impairment of metabolism of type I substrates during cholestasis in humans. In addition, liver biopsy samples from patients with cholestasis showed no marked alteration in microsomal protein, NADPH-cytochrome c reductase, cytochrome P-450 or cytochrome b_5 [170]. This was reflected in unchanged ethylmorphine N-demethylase activity. Further, prolonged cholestasis in humans produces little evidence for altered synthetic function of hepatic cells and no gross changes in drug metabolism. It would therefore seem that the animal models do not truly reflect the human condition, a situation at least partially due to the differences in microsomal bile salt metabolism that exist in different species.

IV. DISEASES OF NONHEPATIC ORGANS AFFECTING HEPATIC DRUG METABOLISM

Most human diseases do not affect, at least directly, the normal functioning of the liver. Nevertheless, the diseases of major organs other than the liver, perturbations of the endocrine system, and nonhepatic tumors can bring about detectable changes in hepatic drug-metabolizing activity. These effects will now be examined together with our present knowledge of the manner in which infectious disease states can affect drug disposition in humans.

A. Cardiac Disease

Determination of changes in drug-metabolizing activity in patients suffering from cardiac disease are difficult to assess since the disease state affects other pharmacokinetic parameters altering the level of drug and/or metabolites in plasma or urine (see Sec. II). Most of the drugs so far studied have been compounds active directly on the heart, such as procainamide, quinidine, or lidocaine, or compounds such as diuretics frequently administered to cardiac patients. Many changes in drug clearance have been reported but these have been interpreted in a number of ways. Thus, decreased clearance has been attributed to an altered volume of distribution [33,34], decreased renal function [36], or decreased hepatic metabolism secondary to reduced hepatic perfusion [33].

There is, however, some evidence that at least part of the changes observed may be due to actual alterations in drug-metabolizing activity. The reduced plasma clearance of lidocaine observed in patients with acute myocardial infarction occurs without the presence of cardiac failure or hypotension and therefore is not attributable to a decreased hepatic of renal perfusion (see Ref. 2). Further, in patients with heart failure where the excretion of procainamide and its metabolites is decreased compared to normal subjects, presumably due to reduced drug absorption, a number of changes occurred which may indicate altered metabolic function [171]. Thus, there was a relative increase in the proportion of the dose undergoing urinary excretion as N-acetylprocainamide and N-acetyl-para-aminobenzoic acid compared to normal subjects. Altered renal function or hepatic perfusion would produce the opposite effect and therefore cannot explain this change. It might appear that altered acetylation of drugs occurs in cardiac disease. There was, however, also an apparent decrease in procainamide hydrolysis but this was only marked in patients having biventricular heart failure involving hepatic dysfunction.

Obviously such studies are totally unsatisfactory for determining whether altered metabolism does actually occur. No correlation is found in the measurement of cytochrome P-450 concentration in biopsy specimens from patients with congestive heart failure [172]. Thus, although decreased benzo[a]pyrene hydroxylase activity and cytochrome P-450 levels were observed, the patients' average age was much greater than that of the control group and no allowance was made for this discrepancy.

In a similar manner the animal studies carried out so far utilizing the genetically bred cardiomyopathic hamster [173,174] have done nothing to solve this problem. Despite decreased levels of cytochrome P-450, aminopyrine N-demethylase activity, and aniline hydroxylase activity in all stages of the disease (Table 25), such experiments can only be controlled by comparison to a normal strain of hamster. It is therefore impossible to determine whether the alterations in drug-metabolizing parameters occur as a consequence of the disease state or whether they occur because of common genetic traits predisposing to heart failure.

B. Pulmonary Disease

In view of the incidence of pulmonary disease in the population and the drug exposure of pulmonary patients it is more than surprising that the effect of such disease states on drug-metabolizing activity has barely been investigated. This is perhaps even less understandable if one takes into account the interest that has centered on the lung as an organ potentially important in extrahepatic metabolism.

Only one recent study is available to illustrate the potential changes [171]. The hydrolysis of procainamide and procaine were found to be reduced in patients with chronic respiratory insufficiency; a similar situation occurs in cardiac insufficiency. Division of patients into those showing chronic obstructive pulmonary disease and those with a diagnosis of cor pulmonale revealed, however, that these changes were only of relevance in those patients exhibiting more severe cardiac and hepatic involvement.

Changes in drug metabolism would be expected following chronic respiratory failure due to the decrease in arterial partial oxygen tension. Thus, the metabolism of zoxazolamine and hexobarbital is decreased in the rat when arterial partial oxygen tension falls below 45 mm Hg [175-177]. This is perhaps unexpected since drug metabolism by microsomal monooxygenases is not affected until very low oxygen tension is reached which under normal circumstances is incompatible with life in the intact animal. However, the use of isolated perfused liver preparations has shown the whole organ to be more sensitive than subcellular preparations to altered oxygen tension. Similarly, decreased metabolic activity in rats breathing oxygen-poor atmospheres causes a marked fall in hexobarbital clearance [176].

A similar situation would appear to exist in humans. In patients with various pulmonary disorders and having arterial partial oxygen tension values of 55 torr or below, the half-life of antipyrine is markedly increased (18.4 ± 3.5 hr in patients; 8.4 ± 1.0 hr in control subjects; $p < 0.005$) [178]. This suggests that altered dosage schedules might be advisable under such conditions, but further studies would obviously be an enormous advantage.

TABLE 25

Alterations in Drug-metabolizing Parameters in the Cardiomyopathic Hamster

Disease state and animal age (days)	Normal or diseased	Cytochrome P-450 (nmol/mg protein)	Aminopyrine N-demethylation (nmol/mg protein/min)
30 days: prenecrotic stage	Normal	0.86 ± 0.05	418 ± 28
	Diseased	0.64 ± 0.05*	344 ± 15*
60 days: moderate to severe myocardial degeneration	Normal	1.03 ± 0.04	585 ± 51
	Diseased	0.72 ± 0.04*	408 ± 31*
120 days: cardiac enlargement, mild to moderate liver congestion	Normal	1.14 ± 0.04	477 ± 30
	Diseased	0.80 ± 0.04*	340 ± 27*
>180 days: advanced signs of heart failure, liver degeneration	Normal	1.12 ± 0.06	440 ± 40
	Diseased	1.08 ± 0.11	396 ± 38

*$p < 0.05$.

<u>Source</u>: From Ref. 174.

C. Vascular and Blood Disorders

Alterations in blood flow due to changes in arterial pressure influence a number of physiological parameters pertaining to drug disposition. Of particular interest are changes in plasma volume, vascular permeability, renal vascular resistance, and renal plasma flow, all of which may exert a rate-limiting impairment on drug elimination. For example, in severe arterial hypertension the serum clearance of furosemide is reduced compared to normal subjects (1.83 ml/min/kg in patients compared to 2.96 ml/min/kg in control subjects; $p < 0.05$) with no change in drug-protein binding [179]. In general, however, no change in drug metabolism is apparent except in changes due to alterations in hepatic perfusion. Thus, although in severe arterial hypertension there is a significant negative correlation between furosemide serum clearance and the amount of its glucuronide conjugate excreted in urine, this is likely to be due to either competition during renal excretion or more probably to the retention of the parent molecule allowing more extensive conjugation. Other examples to illustrate the effect of vascular disease in humans appear lacking.

Although altered drug metabolism is not apparent in humans during vascular disease, there is some evidence from animal experiments to suggest changes in cytochrome P-450 levels. Thus, in a strain of spontaneously hypertensive rats the levels of cytochrome P-450 and adrenal ferredoxin were 35% lower in the adrenals of hypertensive animals than in normotensive controls [180]. This difference is due to a decreased concentration of these proteins in mitochondria, the observation being consistent with the suggestion of an altered pattern of steroidogenesis in the adrenals of spontaneously hypertensive rats. This study, however, suffers from the same deficit as studies of cardiomyopathic hamsters in that it assumes that the normotensive control rats are adequate to allow comparison of adrenal protein content and that the genetic trait causing hypertension is not simply coincidental with other genetic factors resulting in lowered cytochrome P-450 and ferredoxin levels.

Blood disorders in man have a more profound effect on drug-metabolizing activity than the vascular diseases discussed above. To illustrate the influence we shall look mainly at the effects of sickle cell anemia (and hereditary hemolytic anemia) and hepatic porphyria. In each case loss of red blood cells is encountered which might be thought to decrease arterial oxygen tension. More important appears the fact that sickle cell anemia leads to an increase in hepatic heme levels, while hepatic porphyria is associated with a reduction.

In subjects suffering from sickle cell anemia the plasma excess of heme is degraded by uptake into hepatic parenchymal cells. This is of importance to drug metabolism since heme serves as the prosthetic group for cytochrome P-450. The pathway for heme biosynthesis is controlled by the rate-limiting enzyme γ-aminolevulinic acid synthetase which is sensitive to inhibition by product heme. Indeed, the hepatic cytochrome P-450 content can be reduced by administration of small amounts of heme to phenobarbital-treated rats [181]. There is therefore some reason to expect a decrease in drug metabolism in patients with hemolytic disease. In patients with sickle cell anemia, however, no significant alteration was found in antipyrine half-life compared to normal subjects although the half-life of phenylbutazone was shortened (Table 26) [182]. These data suggest that there is at least no apparent deficit in heme biosynthetic pathways, a conclusion confirmed by the ability of phenobarbital pretreatment to increase the metabolism of both antipyrine and phenylbutazone in this group of patients (Table 26). Why a difference is apparent between antipyrine and phenylbutazone is not clear. It must, however, be pointed out that both the volume of distribution and metabolic clearance rate for phenylbutazone were increased, suggesting enhanced extravascular distribution as well as more rapid hepatic metabolism. Indeed, phenylbutazone is extensively protein-bound and it may be displacement of drug by endogenous factors that leads to more rapid clearance.

It would appear that there is no impairment of the monooxygenase system in such hemolytic disorders, as confirmed by the finding of unaltered or shortened antipyrine serum half-life in patients with β-thalassemia major [183]. In addition, phenobarbital treatment of patients with hemolytic disorders leads to a fall in serum bilirubin concentrations presumably indicating UDP-glucuronyltransferase to remain inducible [182,184].

Patients with sickle cell anemia exhibit decreased plasma hemopexin concentrations (plasma heme binding protein) suggesting increased heme uptake into the hepatocytes, which would from animal experiments be expected to lead to repression of cytochrome P-450 synthesis and a subsequent decrease in drug metabolism. However, it should be remembered that the disease state in man is relatively long-term compared to the acute administration of heme to rodents that causes synthesis repression. This might suggest the existence of compensatory mechanism preventing the repression of heme synthesis. It is conceivable that compensation could occur due to an increase in the level of hepatocellular heme oxygenase which is an inducible enzyme [185,186]. Indeed, mice with hereditary hemolytic anemia [187] exhibit a continuous excess production of heme and bilirubin, but possess normal levels of microsomal cytochrome P-450 and show no impairment of ethylmorphine N-demethylase or benzo[a]pyrene hydroxylase activity in liver compared to control animals. This is reflected by normal hepatic levels of γ-aminolevulinic acid synthetase but is accompanied by increased specific activity of heme oxygenase.

This lack of effect on drug-metabolizing activity contrasts with the inhibition of increased synthesis of γ-aminolevulinic acid synthetase and cytochrome P-450 in response to phenobarbital caused by a single injection of hemin [181,188]. Thus, it appears that an adaptive response can indeed develop during chronic hemolysis which prevents excess free heme from

TABLE 26
Altered Drug Clearance in Sickle Cell Anemia

Drug	Parameter	Before phenobarbital		After phenobarbital	
		Sickle cell anemia	Controls	Sickle cell anemia	Controls
Antipyrine	Half-life [β-phase] (hr)	10.0 ± 1.2	11.6 ± 2.4	5.5 ± 0.9*	7.5 ± 1.4*
	Volume of distribution (liters/kg)	0.66 ± 0.03	0.61 ± 0.03	0.70 ± 0.03	0.67 ± 0.03
	Metabolic clearance rate (ml/min/kg)	0.87 ± 0.20	0.77 ± 0.14	1.64 ± 0.24*	1.19 ± 0.23*
Phenylbutazone	Half-life [β-phase] (hr)	2.2 ± 0.2**	3.2 ± 0.4	1.7 ± 0.2*	2.0 ± 0.1*
	Volume of distribution (liters/kg)	0.20 ± 0.01**	0.13 ± 0.01	0.20 ± 0.01	0.14 ± 0.01
	Metabolic clearance rate (ml/min/kg)	0.049 ± 0.005**	0.021 ± 0.002	0.060 ± 0.011	0.034 ± 0.002*

*$p < 0.05$ compared to no phenobarbital treatment.
**$p < 0.05$ compared to control subjects.
Source: From Ref. 182.

repressing heme biosynthesis and formation of microsomal cytochrome P-450.

Sassa et al. [187] have proposed a scheme which may explain the difference between the acute and chronic effects of heme (Fig. 5). Thus, in the acute situation the excess heme represses drug-mediated induction of

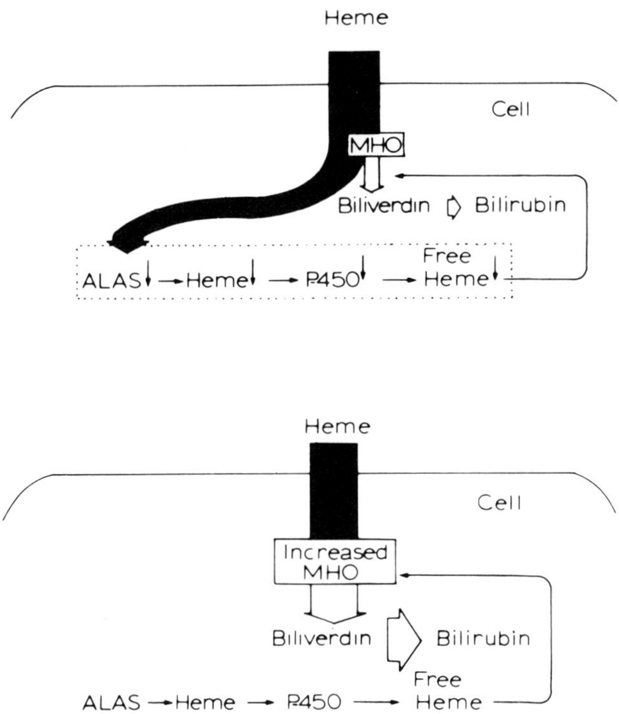

FIGURE 5 Hypothesis to explain the acute and chronic effects of heme on the heme biosynthetic pathway: (a) An acute injection of heme results in repression of the formation of γ-aminolevulinic acid synthetase, heme, and cytochrome P-450 since the capacity of acutely induced microsomal heme oxygenase is insufficient to metabolize excess heme. (b) In contrast, excess heme produced chronically by hemolysis leads to sustained induction of heme oxygenase activity which can metabolize excess heme and thereby prevents heme from acting on the formation of γ-aminolevulinic acid synthetase, heme, and cytochrome P-450. MHO = microsomal heme oxygenase; ALAS = γ-aminolevulinic acid synthetase. (From Ref. 187. Reproduced by permission of the copyright holders.)

γ-aminolevulinic acid synthetase and microsomal cytochrome P-450 since the capacity of acutely induced heme oxygenase is insufficient to metabolize excess heme. In contrast, chronic production of excess heme induces heme oxygenase to a level which can metabolize excess substrate and therefore can prevent the changes seen in the short term. It is thus evident that the markedly increased level of heme oxygenase is critical.

In contrast to hemolytic disease acute intermittent porphyria is characterized by a genetically determined reduction in uroporphyrinogen I synthetase and an increase in γ-aminolevulinic acid synthetase [189]. It has been hypothesized that the decrease in the activity of uroporphyrinogen I synthetase results in a decrease in hepatic heme synthesis (although this has never been measured) and this in turn may result in a reduction in cytochrome P-450 levels. Indeed, reduced metabolism of antipyrine and salicylamide (but not phenylbutazone) has been reported in patients with porphyria [190,191]. This is understandable if cytochrome P-450 levels are reduced but there is as yet no supportive evidence. Indeed, since γ-aminolevulinic acid synthetase levels are increased (presumably due to derepression by the low heme levels), then the heme concentration must have fallen sufficiently for the step no longer to be rate-limiting. However, other reasons for the change in drug-metabolizing activity must also be considered since the plasma antipyrine half-life is not altered in patients who are completely latent carriers of this disease even though they exhibit a deficit of uroporphyrinogen I synthetase (and no apparent alteration in γ-aminolevulinic acid synthetase). Whatever the nature of the biochemical disturbance it is also reflected in a defect of hepatic steroid Δ^4-5α-reductase activity [192].

D. Renal Disease

As might be expected, renal disease results in a considerable impairment of the elimination of water-soluble drugs and/or their metabolites. The reduction in glomerular filtration rate observed may parallel the increase in plasma drug levels or drug half-life under such conditions. For example, the acetylated metabolite of procainamide accumulates in renal failure [193, 194]. Also, the renal clearance of the glucuronide conjugate of oxazepam was correlated to creatinine clearance [195] and accordingly the plasma concentration of conjugates were related to the severity of the uremic condition. The accumulation of drugs and pharmacologically active metabolites might lead to enhanced pharmacological action and indeed patients with renal dysfunction often react abnormally or unpredictably to a number of drugs (see Ref. 7). This is particularly true for drugs having urinary excretion as a major elimination pathway (Table 27).

Most drugs, however, are not excreted unchanged and to a greater or lesser extent undergo metabolism to more water-soluble products. The possibility exists that the accumulation of potentially toxic body waste matter might be expected to inhibit hepatic function. It is of interest, therefore,

TABLE 27
Drugs Having Urinary Excretion as a Major Elimination Pathway

Anticholinergics (quaternary ammonium)	Methotrexate
Barbital	Methyldopa
Carboxicillin	Neomycin
Chlorpropamide	Phenformin
Colistin	Phenobarbital
Cycloserine	Procainamide
Digoxin	Streptomycin
Ethambutol	Sulfinpyrazone
5-Fluorocytosine	Tetracycline
Gentamycin	Tobramycin
Kanamycin	Vancomycin

Source: From Ref. 196.

that in many cases of drugs undergoing oxidation no alterations in drug metabolism are observed in renal disease (Table 28). Perhaps this is to be expected since overall the function of the liver would not seem to be grossly impaired by renal failure. For example, timolol is 80% metabolized by hydrolytic cleavage and subsequent oxidation and no apparent impairment of timolol elimination is observed in patients with chronic renal insufficiency [197] (Table 29).

The situation surely cannot be as simple as suggested by the above examples. Indeed, most drugs are not exclusively metabolized but are also eliminated via renal excretion. For example, 40% of a dose of pindolol is normally excreted unchanged in urine yet the plasma half-life of this drug is not affected by renal disease [198]. It may therefore be that compensatory mechanisms exist to control the potential accumulation of drug in renal failure, and some evidence exists to support this hypothesis.

Thus, the plasma half-life of antipyrine is normal or shortened in patients with chronic renal failure [199,200]. This difference is not due to a change in the volume of drug distribution or in the limited protein binding of antipyrine since no change in half-life is apparent in patients with hypoalbuminemia secondary to nephrotic syndrome but with relatively normal renal function. It therefore appears that the change is due to altered drug metabolism.

TABLE 28
Effect of Renal Failure on the Apparent Elimination Rate of Drugs

Route of metabolism	Drug	Activity
Oxidation	Antipyrine	Normal or rapid
	Diphenylhydantoin	Rapid
	Lidocaine	Normal
	Meperidine	Normal
	Pentobarbital	Normal
	Phenacetin	Normal
	Phenobarbital	Normal
	Propranolol	Normal or slowed
	Quinidine	Normal
	Tolbutamide	Normal
Reduction	Cortisol	Slowed
Glucuronide conjugation	Chloramphenicol	Normal
	Lorazepam	Normal
	Paracetamol	Normal
Sulfate conjugation	Paracetamol	Normal
Acetylation	p-Aminosalicylate	Slowed
	Isoniazid	Normal or slowed
	Sulfasoxazole	Slowed
Glycine conjugation	Salicylate	Normal
Hydrolysis	Cephalothin	Slowed
	Insulin	Slowed
	Procaine	Slowed

Source: From Ref. 196.

TABLE 29
Effect of Chronic Renal Insufficiency on Timolol Elimination

	Control subjects	Chronic renal insufficiency
Peak concentration (ng/ml)	84.3 ± 33.8	87.1 ± 22.8
Time to peak (hr)	0.83 ± 0.37	1.67 ± 1.15
Area under curve 0-24 (hr·ng/ml)	432 ± 249	493 ± 229
Half-life [β-phase] (hr)	5.2 ± 2.6	4.0 ± 1.2
Elimination rate constant	0.172 ± 0.094	0.189 ± 0.059

Source: From Ref. 197.

Similar changes are also observed with drugs having more complex pharmacokinetic profiles than antipyrine. For example, patients with impaired renal function exhibit lower serum levels of digoxin and a shorter drug half-life coupled with an increase in cardioactive metabolites [201]. This occurs despite less renal excretion of digitoxin and its cardioactive metabolites in uremic patients than in control subjects. The altered metabolism of digitoxin appears due to the production of more hydroxylated and hydrolyzed metabolites while sulfate and glucuronide conjugation is unchanged. For details of the complex changes occurring the reader is referred to Storstein's original paper [201].

Such changes may also occur with the diuretic furosemide in functionally anephric patients [202]. Furosemide differs from our other examples in that it is normally 90% excreted unchanged by renal mechanisms. Thus, in functionally anephric patients drug half-life is increased (29.5 min in control subjects compared to 80.7 min in anephric patients) and drug clearance is reduced (162 ml/min in control subjects compared to 105 ml/min in anephric patients). This might at first be thought to be due purely to decreased renal elimination. However, if this were so, the elimination rate constant should have decreased to 10% of normal values (that is, from 0.024 min^{-1} to 0.0024 min^{-1}) but instead it averaged 0.00926 min^{-1}. This would suggest that non-renal elimination mechanisms are clearing the drug 4 times as fast as normal and that this probably represents hepatic metabolism [202].

If the changes we have described are indeed due to increased metabolism, the question then arises as to the causative mechanism. Reidenberg [196] suggests that some factor inducing hepatic monooxygenases may be leached out of dialysis equipment, but this appears unlikely since such changes are apparent or indeed may be more pronounced [199] in nondialyzed patients. This latter finding might suggest the presence of an endogenous circulating factor causing induction. Certainly dialysis restores a normal digitoxin metabolite pattern suggesting prevention of altered metabolism [201]. However, the effect on antipyrine clearance was variable showing no overall effect (Table 30) [199]. Thus, the mechanism concerned remains unknown and no direct measurements of hepatic drug-metabolizing components have been made. It is clear, however, that the drug-metabolizing enzyme system is responsive to inducing agents since glutethimide induces antipyrine metabolism in renal patients [199]. Perhaps the metabolic alterations in renal disease are only apparent and principally due to alterations of other pharmacokinetic parameters. In particular alterations in the volume of drug distribution may play an important role in determining drug disposition in renal disease [Balant, personal communication].

The human data on drug metabolism in renal failure is somewhat surprising since experimental animal models of renal failure point to exactly the opposite conclusion. Thus, in rats with renal failure induced by ligation of the ureters (2 days) or intravenous injection of the nephrotoxic agent uranyl nitrate (5 days), although the concentration of cytochrome P-450 and aniline hydroxylase activity were not significantly reduced, aminopyrine N-demethylase activity was decreased (Table 31) [203]. Other techniques give slightly different answers: some authors found that subtotal nephrectomy decreased cytochrome P-450 as well as both aminopyrine N-demethylase

TABLE 30
Effect of Hemodialysis on Antipyrine Metabolism

	Plasma half-life [β-phase] (hr)	
Patient	Before dialysis	After dialysis
1	11.3	12.5
2	7.6	13.2
3	9.0	6.6
4	6.1	7.5
5	15.3	4.8
Mean ± SD	9.9 ± 3.2	8.9 ± 3.3
	$p > 0.10$	

Source: From Ref. 199.

TABLE 31
Effect of Experimental Renal Failure on the In Vitro Drug-metabolizing Activity in the Rat

	Ligation of ureters		Uranyl nitrate	
	Sham	Uremic	Sham	Uremic
Serum urea (mg %)	32.0 ± 6.0	482.0 ± 19.0*	51.0 ± 8.0	222.0 ± 7.0*
Cytochrome P-450 (nmol/g liver)	19.3 ± 0.7	14.2 ± 2.8	27.3 ± 1.6	22.2 ± 1.4
Aminopyrine N-demethylase (nmol/g liver/min)	34.8 ± 2.6	25.4 ± 2.9*	45.1 ± 2.3	34.0 ± 1.8*
Aniline hydroxylase (nmol/g liver/min)	12.2 ± 0.9	11.1 ± 1.9	15.4 ± 1.4	12.4 ± 1.4

*$p < 0.05$.
Source: From Ref. 203.

and acetanilide hydroxylase activity [204,205], while other authors [206] reported a decrease in cytochrome P-450 but no change in aminopyrine N-demethylase or aniline hydroxylase activity (in addition see also Refs. 207-209).

We have until now made only passing reference to routes of drug metabolism other than oxidation. In general, such pathways appear to be either normally active or slowed (Table 28). Thus, while glucuronide formation and glycine and sulfate conjugation appear normal, some acetylation reactions are slowed while hydrolysis appears consistently slowed.

The amount of work designed to establish why this should be so is surprisingly little. It is, however, clear that the deficit in hydrolysis, at least, is due to a low level of enzyme rather than competitive inhibition since serum dialysis does not restore enzyme activity. Also, in vivo studies which demonstrate decreased activity are somewhat puzzling since the higher drug levels present due to renal impairment would presumably result in enhanced formation of conjugated or hydrolyzed metabolites, unless saturation occurs.

Obviously, it is necessary to unravel these changes and at present the lack of good animal models prevents a basic investigation. Perhaps part of the answer lies in the acute nature of the animal experimentation compared to the relatively long period over which renal disease develops in humans.

E. Diseases Affecting Endocrine Function

The prime controlling influence of endocrine organs on normal body function makes them primary candidates for disordered activity causing changes in the drug-metabolizing capacity of the organisms. While this is certainly true in animals (see later) it has yet to be clearly established whether or not altered endocrine function has an active function in controlling drug-metabolizing activity in humans.

Thyroid disease has been most intensively investigated but even here the effect on drug metabolism is not clearcut (Table 32). While the half-life of drugs such as antipyrine and methimazole is altered by thyroid dysfunction, the clearance of other drugs is unaffected. It is, however, clear that those changes which do occur appear to be in the same direction, dependent on the level of thyroid function.

For example, the half-life of antipyrine is increased in hypothyroidism and decreased in hyperthyroidism (Table 33) [211-216]. This change is accompanied by corresponding changes in drug clearance but not in the volume of distribution or plasma protein binding. The disposition of antipyrine also was normalized on return of thyroid function to control values. Considering the close correlation that exists between the change in circulating thyroid hormone levels and altered antipyrine half-life it appears likely that such changes in thyroid function exert a controlling function on the drug-metabolizing activity for antipyrine.

TABLE 32
Effect of Thyroid Disease on Drug Half-life

Substrate	Hypothyroidism	Hyperthyroidism
Aminopyrine	Unchanged?	Unchanged?
Antipyrine	Increased	Decreased
Dicoumarol	Unchanged	Unchanged
Digoxin	Increased	Decreased
Diphenylhydantoin	Unchanged	Unchanged
Methimazole	Increased	Decreased
Practolol	Increased	Decreased
Propranolol	Unchanged	Unchanged
Propylthiouracil	Unchanged or increased	Unchanged or decreased
Tolbutamide	—	Decreased

Sources: From the work of several authors, in particular Ref. 210.

However, it remains a subject for conjecture why the metabolism of antipyrine (which undergoes N-demethylation and hydroxylation) should be clearly altered while changes in the metabolism of dipyrone (an aminopyrine derivative) are more obscure [217] and no changes in the disposition of diphenylhydantoin are apparent [218]. It could be argued that the actual routes of metabolism of these compounds differ or that each is reliant on a different monooxygenase system. However, the reasons probably relate to different hormonal sensitivity of the individual components of the drug-metabolizing system.

Not all changes in drug disposition in thyroid disease, however, can be attributed to altered drug-metabolizing activity. Thus, it is clear that the plasma levels of cardiac glycosides achieved following administration of digoxin are higher in hypothyroidism and lower in hyperthyroidism than that observed in control subjects [219-221]. The close correlation observed between creatinine clearance, serum digoxin, concentration and half-life suggests that the changes are due to the altered renal function known to occur in thyroid disorders. This is confirmed by the higher cumulative 24-hr urinary excretion of digoxin in hyperthyroid patients than occurs on normalization of thyroid function and the parallel changes observed in renal digoxin clearance [221] (Table 34).

TABLE 33
Effect of Thyroid Dysfunction on the Disposition of Antipyrine

Parameter	Normal subjects	Hypothyroid patients	Hyperthyroid patients	Normalized patients
Half-life [β-phase] (hr)	10.8 ± 0.4	16.2 ± 2.3*	7.9 ± 0.6*	11.2 ± 1.2
Volume of distribution (liters)	33.1 ± 0.8	36.5 ± 2.1	28.2 ± 0.8*	—
Clearance (liters/kg)	2.2 ± 0.1	2.0 ± 0.2	2.6 ± 0.2*	—

*$p < 0.05$.
Source: From Ref. 212.

TABLE 34
Disposition of Digoxin in Patients with Hyperthyroidism and on Normalization of Thyroid Function

Parameter	Hyperthyroid patients	Normalized patients
Half-life [β-phase] (hr)	24 ± 6	39 ± 15*
Elimination rate constant (hr^{-1})	0.0305 ± 0.0085	0.0200 ± 0.0066*
Volume of distribution (liters)	849 ± 240	586 ± 136*
Renal clearance (ml/min)	120 ± 38	70 ± 43*

*$p < 0.05$.
Source: From Ref. 221.

Changes in drug-metabolizing activity occurring in thyroid dysfunction are of particular importance if they influence the disposition of those drugs used to treat the disease. This certainly appears to be the case for methimazole (half-life: normal subjects 9.3 ± 1.4 hr; hyperthyroid patients 6.9 ± 0.6 hr; $p < 0.05$; hypothyroid patients 13.6 ± 4.8 hr, $p < 0.05$) [216]. Administration of the antithyroid drug carbimazole to hyperthyroid patients restores methimazole half-life to normal (7.9 ± 0.4 hr vs. 11.2 ± 1.2 hr) [212]. In the case of propylthiouracil, however, the situation is not clear; two groups have reported the half-life and clearance of this compound to be unchanged in hyperthyroid states [222-224] while Vesell and colleagues [216] have demonstrated a decrease in half-life of propylthiouracil in hyperthyroidism and an increase in hypothyroid states. Obviously this is an important problem which requires resolving.

Thyroid dysfunction also appears to interfere with the metabolism of a number of endogenous substrates. While hyperthyroid states result in increased cortisol production, the plasma half-life of cortisol is decreased with increased urinary excretion of 11-keto metabolites present in urine [225,226]. Hypothyroidism produces the opposite effects. Furthermore, hyperthyroidism produces a decrease in testosterone clearance and conversion of testosterone to androstenedione [227], resulting in increased plasma levels of testosterone in both sexes. Again the exact opposite is observed in hypothyroidism.

There is virtually no direct evidence available to suggest the type of change occurring in components of the drug-metabolizing enzyme system in patients with thyroid disorders. It would appear that the increase in the metabolism of some compounds occurring in hyperthyroidism is accompanied by a hypertrophy of the hepatic smooth endoplasmic reticulum, as observed at biopsy [228]. This dearth of information differs radically from the situation in animal experimentation where the effect of altered thyroid function on components of the drug-metabolizing enzyme has been examined in detail.

The situation in animals is, however, complex and will only be surveyed where relevant to the human disorders (for a review see Ref. 9 and references contained therein). In the rat administration of thyroxine to male animals leads to a decrease in in vitro hexobarbital and aminopyrine metabolism but an increase in aniline oxidation accompanied by increased NADPH-cytochrome c reductase activity and decreased cytochrome P-450 levels [229,230]. In female rats, however, thyroxine increased hexobarbital and aminopyrine as well as aniline metabolism, but this also was accompanied by decreased NADPH-cytochrome c reductase activity while cytochrome P-450 levels were unaltered. Since castration of male animals and the subsequent administration of thyroxine did not result in a further decrease of hexobarbital or aminopyrine metabolism (an effect reversed by administration of methyltestosterone) an androgen-dependent system appears involved.

These data suggest that the variable effects of thyroxine are due to the overall effects of altered electron-transport chain components, altered amounts of terminal oxidase, and the involvement of androgen-dependent monooxygenase enzymes altering cytochrome P-450 substrate binding capacity [231,232].

In hypothyroidism produced by thyroidectomy in rats the situation is less complex. Animals of both sexes exhibit a decrease in the in vitro metabolism of hexobarbital, aminopyrine, and aniline with a decrease in NADPH-cytochrome c reductase activity but no marked change in cytochrome P-450 levels or NADPH-cytochrome P-450 reductase or spectral binding [230,231,233]. These changes can be reversed by pretreatment with triiodothyronine.

Whether such data can be applied to the human thyroid disorders is unknown. Although there is some evidence for humans possessing drug-metabolizing enzyme systems which are under sex hormone control, their involvement in thyroid malfunction has not been investigated. It is, however, clear that the effects of manipulating thyroid function on drug-metabolizing enzyme systems are species-dependent, the rat, mouse, and rabbit showing differing responses [234,235] (Fig. 6). As a result it is premature to extrapolate such data to humans. In addition, although altered biochemical parameters are reported from animal studies, the actual mechanisms involved still await assessment.

Despite the relatively common occurrence of diabetes in the population, little appears known of the effects of insulin deficiency on drug-metabolizing activity in humans although diabetes alters hepatic function and structure [236,237]. The plasma half-life of antipyrine is not different

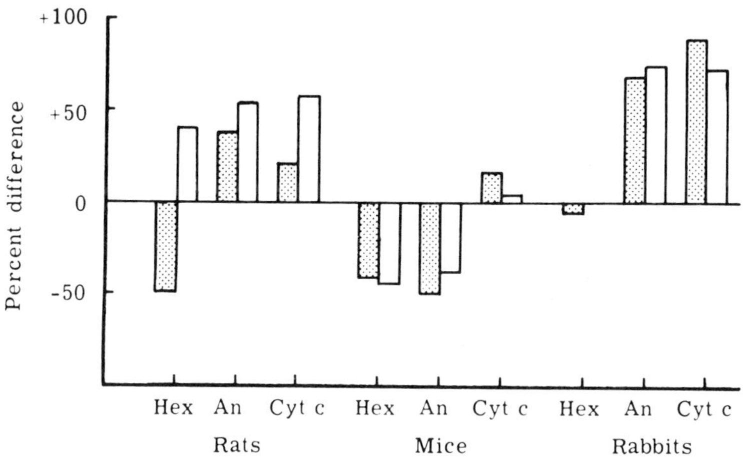

FIGURE 6 The effect of thyroxine on hexobarbital hydroxylase (Hex), aniline hydroxylase (An), and NADPH-cytochrome c reductase activity (Cyt c) by liver microsomes from rats, mice, and rabbits. Rats, mice, and rabbits were treated intraperitoneally with thyroxine (1.0, 1.6, and 0.2 mg/kg, respectively) for 10 days. Dotted columns represent male animals and open columns female animals. (From Ref. 9. Reproduced with permission of the copyright holders.)

from control values in diabetic patients (diet maintained) and in those receiving tolbutamide, but insulin and chlorpropamide administration increases drug clearance [238] (Table 35). Similarly, the half-lives of tolbutamide and phenylbutazone are unaltered in diabetes [239,240] although the metabolism of phenacetin appears diminished [241]. Studies of conjugation reactions in diabetic patients have focused on acetylation reactions but increases, decreases, and lack of change have all been reported [9], suggesting the need for more careful study.

As with thyroid disorders more appears known from animal models of diabetes than from the patient population, but the situation appears equally complex. The induction of diabetes by various means (alloxan, streptozotocin, and 6-aminonicotinamide) has been shown in male rats to produce a decrease in aminopyrine N-demethylase, hexobarbital biotransformation, and aryl hydrocarbon hydroxylase activity, but an increase in aniline hydroxylase activity and no change or an increase in cytochrome P-450 content [229,242-248]. Such changes not only occur in vitro but can also be demonstrated in isolated perfused liver preparations [249]. In female rats, on the other hand, the chemical induction of diabetes results in an increase in aminopyrine, hexobarbital, aniline, aryl hydrocarbon, and biphenyl metabolism and an increase in cytochrome P-450 levels. Once

TABLE 35
Effect of Diabetes in Humans and Its Therapy on Antipyrine Disposition

Parameter	Control subjects	Diet-maintained diabetics	Insulin-treated diabetics	Chlorpropamide-treated diabetics	Tolbutamide-treated diabetics
Plasma antipyrine half-life [β-phase] (hr)	12.6 ± 0.7	11.9 ± 2.2	7.7 ± 0.8*	8.6 ± 1.2*	11.3 ± 0.6
Volume of distribution (liters)	42.7 ± 1.5	50.2 ± 6.4	43.8 ± 2.9	36.2 ± 3.1	32.4 ± 5.1*
Clearance (liters/kg)	2.5 ± 0.1	3.3 ± 0.6	4.5 ± 0.8*	3.4 ± 0.6*	2.0 ± 0.3

*$p < 0.05$.
Source: From Ref. 238.

again these differences are interpreted as being due to interference with androgen-dependent monooxygenase pathways.

The changes induced by the induction of a diabetic state are all reversed by the administration of insulin in either male or female rats [242, 243, 247]. However, the administration of insulin alone has little or no effect on drug metabolism in normal animals [243, 247], suggesting that its major action is to correct the insulin deficient state of diabetic animals.

It would appear, therefore, that the diabetic state in animals has marked effects on drug metabolism although this has yet to be observed in humans. It is clear, however, that the administration of insulin can potentially reverse such changes as do occur. The question then arises as to whether a deficiency of insulin directly affects monooxygenase systems to cause its effects or whether the changes produced are due to the elevation of blood glucose. Since N-methylacetamide, which causes an insulin-resistant state (and thus no decrease in blood glucose) but no insulin deficiency, does not affect the in vitro metabolism of hexobarbital or aniline this would appear unlikely [246]. In addition, the lack of effect on in vitro drug metabolism of hyperglycemia induced by glucose infusion would support this conclusion. It must presently be assumed, therefore, that insulin has a direct effect on drug-metabolizing enzyme systems, the mechanism of which is at present unknown. Two thoughts should, however, be borne in mind. First, the diabetic state is accompanied by hyperglucagonemia and an increased blood glucagon/insulin ratio which may be of significance since glucagon also induces alteration in drug-metabolizing activity [250]. In addition both insulin deficiency and administration of glucagon cause an increase in hepatic cyclic AMP levels [251, 252]. Since this nucleotide has been demonstrated to indirectly cause both an inhibition of drug-metabolizing activity [253] and to be involved in enzyme induction phenomena (see Ref. 254 and references contained therein) such changes may be of primary importance in determining the effect of the disease state on monooxygenase activity. It must be remembered, however, that molecules such as glucagon affect many systems including pituitary and thyroid function which might equally alter hepatic function.

As far as other endocrine disturbances are concerned we can find virtually no reports of investigations of such states on drug metabolism in humans despite evidence from animal experimentation to indicate potential alterations in drug clearance.

Thus, in general, adrenalectomy of male rats reduces the in vitro metabolism of hexobarbital, aminopyrine, and ethylmorphine, but not that of aniline or zoxazolamine, and decreases cytochrome P-450, NADPH-cytochrome c reductase, and NADPH-cytochrome P-450 reductase and the magnitude of the spectral change induced with cytochrome P-450 [229, 255-258] (Table 36). No such changes, however, appear to occur in female rats. The administration of cortisone or prednisolone to adrenalectomized male rats has been found to reverse the decrease in drug-metabolizing activity

TABLE 36
Effect of Adrenalectomy in Male Rats on Components of the Drug-metabolizing Enzyme System[a]

Parameter	Sham-operated	Adrenalectomized	Adrenalectomized and cortisone
Ethylmorphine N-demethylation (nmol HCHO formed/mg protein/10 min)	45 ± 1	24 ± 3*	53 ± 4
Cytochrome P-450 (nmol/mg protein)	1.27 ± 0.04	1.03 ± 0.06*	0.96 ± 0.05*
NADPH-cytochrome c reductase (nmol/mg protein/min)	113 ± 5	78 ± 3*	127 ± 9
NADPH-cytochrome P-450 reductase (nmol/mg protein/min)	7.36 ± 0.40	4.97 ± 0.34*	10.30 ± 0.08*
Ethylmorphine maximum spectral change (Δ O.D./mg $\times 10^3$)	9.0 ± 0.6	6.6 ± 0.3*	6.8 ± 0.7*

* $p < 0.05$ compared to sham-operated animals.
[a] NADPH-cytochrome c reductase and NADPH-cytochrome P-450 reductase may be the same enzyme but differ in the former being measured following the addition of cytochrome c whereas the latter measures the rate of reduction of endogenous cytochrome P-450.
Source: From Ref. 255.

[255, 259] although the decrease in cytochrome P-450 levels appears to be unaffected [255, 260]. This latter fact has been interpreted as demonstrating that the decrease in drug-metabolizing activity in adrenalectomized male rats is not due to a decrease in cytochrome P-450 levels or to the extent of drug binding to cytochrome P-450, but to alterations in reductase components of the electron-transport chain [255].

The potential effect of adrenal cortical hormones on drug metabolism in humans comes from a single study carried out some 20 years ago. Thus, the in vivo acetylation of para-aminobenzoic acid was found to be increased in patients with hyperadrenocorticoidism and in patients treated with cortisone but decreased in patients with Addison's disease [261].

Hypophysectomy of rats also reduces drug-metabolizing activity [262, 263]. This is perhaps not unexpected because of the controlling influence of the pituitary on other endocrine systems (thyroid, adrenals, gonads). In particular the pituitary appears to play an important role in the control of sexually differentiated hepatic monooxygenases [263-265]. Obviously disturbance of pituitary function leads to a change in circulating levels of a number of hormonal substances (TSH, ACTH, LH, FSH, GH, PL, MSH, oxytocin, and vasopressin). The effects of most of these hormones on drug-metabolizing activity appears unknown but may be of considerable direct or indirect significance. For example, it would seem logical to expect TSH to exert actions on the thyroid which would in turn lead to alteration in hepatic drug metabolism. Further, ACTH might well be expected to cause effects on drug metabolism via the adrenals and in this case some evidence exists to support this hypothesis. Thus, the administration of ACTH to male rats caused a decrease in the in vitro metabolism of hexobarbital and aminopyrine but not aniline and zoxazolamine [229]. In contrast, only aminopyrine metabolism was altered in female rats but this was increased. These effects, however, are somewhat difficult to reconcile with the ability of ACTH to elevate ethylmorphine N-demethylase activity in hypophysectomized male rats [263], but perhaps indicate that in the normal animal ACTH effects are dependent on the presence of other pituitary factors.

In contrast to the effects of most pituitary hormones, the actions of growth hormone on drug-metabolizing activity have been extensively investigated. Thus, growth hormone decreases drug metabolism in male rats, an effect not inhibited by adrenalectomy, castration, or induction of diabetes [266-268]. The decrease in drug metabolism is accompanied by a reduction of cytochrome P-450 levels and a decrease in NADPH-cytochrome c reductase and NADPH-cytochrome P-450 reductase activity [269] (Table 37). In female rats growth hormone appears to exert no action of drug-metabolizing parameters [267] and there appears to be some relationship between gonadal hormones and the effect of growth hormone on drug metabolism in the rat [264].

Whether or not growth hormone exerts similar actions in hypophysectomized animals remains open to question. While it has been reported that

TABLE 37
Effects of Growth Hormone Administration to Male Rats on Hepatic Drug Metabolism Parameters[a]

Parameter	Control animals	Growth hormone
Hexobarbital metabolism (nmol/mg protein/min)	11.2 ± 0.3	8.4 ± 0.4*
Aniline metabolism (nmol/mg protein/min)	1.5 ± 0.05	1.2 ± 0.04*
Cytochrome P-450 (nmol/mg protein)	0.56 ± 0.01	0.49 ± 0.01*
NADPH-cytochrome c reductase (nmol/mg protein/min)	91 ± 6	69 ± 5*
NADPH-cytochrome P-450 reductase (nmol/mg protein/min)	7.88 ± 0.24	6.58 ± 0.30*

*$p < 0.05$.
[a] NADPH-cytochrome c reductase and NADPH-cytochrome P-450 reductase may be the same enzyme but differ in the former being measured following the addition of cytochrome c whereas the latter measures the rate of reduction of endogenous cytochrome P-450.
Source: From Ref. 269.

the inhibition of drug metabolism by growth hormone occurs even after hypophysectomy [266] other studies have refuted this. Thus, in hypophysectomized rats of either sex, growth hormone increases ethylmorphine demethylation [264] but not aminopyrine metabolism [268] and may or may not increase aniline metabolism [264,268]. There is, therefore, some evidence to suggest that the effects of growth hormone in the intact animal are also dependent on other pituitary-induced phenomena and it is probable that the effect of such hormones is dependent on a net balance between pituitary factors.

Although there is presently little or no evidence to demonstrate altered drug metabolism in humans due to pituitary malfunction, the potential for such changes is apparent. Whether or not this extends to gonadal hormones is unknown for it is not clear whether such sex-dependent enzyme systems occur in humans. That evidence presently available to indicate such systems comes mainly for altered metabolism during pregnancy and in women utilizing oral contraceptives (although it should be remembered that such compounds are irreversible inhibitors of cytochrome P-450 in that such compounds are irreversible inhibitors of cytochrome P-450 in their own right). Whether this can be extrapolated to disease states associated with altered levels of androgens and estrogens remains to be determined.

F. Nonhepatic Tumors

Present evidence is insufficient to allow a decision as to whether nonhepatic tumors can affect hepatic drug metabolism activity in humans. Thus, using the elimination of $^{14}CO_2$ following oral administration of labeled aminopyrine as an index of drug-metabolizing activity in subjects with a variety of malignant disorders, a decrease in drug clearance was only apparent in those with hepatic involvement [140]. In contrast, the elimination half-life of aminopyrine was found to be reduced in patients with lung cancer compared to normal volunteers [270] particularly when the involvement of hepatic metastases could be demonstrated. This latter study appears inadequately controlled and in turn contrasts with a more recent definitive study which has carefully examined the disposition of antipyrine in lung cancer patients [271]. No significant difference could be observed in the plasma clearance or half-life of antipyrine or in 48-hr urinary excretion of its two major metabolites (Table 38). However, the trend was for a decrease in drug clearance, a finding corroborating many animal studies.

Dependent on the tumor line employed, the implantation of tumors into animals in general causes a depression of hepatic drug-metabolizing activity. Thus, in male or female rats there is a decrease in aminopyrine N-demethylase, aniline hydroxylase, benzo[a]pyrene hydroxylase, and ring

TABLE 38
Effect of Lung Cancer on the Disposition of Antipyrine in Humans

Parameter	Patients with lung cancer	Matched control subjects
Half-life [β-phase] (hr)	9.5 ± 1.3	7.7 ± 1.3
Volume of distribution (liters/kg)	0.56 ± 0.02	0.57 ± 0.02
Plasma clearance (liters/hr/kg)	0.048 ± 0.009	0.056 ± 0.007
48-hr urinary excretion of 4-hydroxyantipyrine (% dose)	19.6 ± 2.1	16.4 ± 2.0
48-hr urinary excretion of N-demethylantipyrine (% dose)	17.2 ± 1.8	18.2 ± 2.1

Source: From Ref. 271

and N-hydroxylation of 2-acetylaminofluorene [272-275]. This decrease is accompanied by alteration in microsomal electron-transport chain components. For example, there is a decrease in NADPH-cytochrome c reductase activity and in the levels of cytochrome P-450 or cytochrome b_5 with an accompanying decrease in magnitude of hexobarbital- or aniline-induced spectral change [276,277]. The changes in components of the drug-metabolizing system are accompanied by morphological changes in the hepatocytes including disruption and degranulation of the rough endoplasmic reticulum and hypertrophy of smooth endoplasmic reticulum [278,279]. That such changes are of functional significance is indicated by the decrease in the in vivo metabolism of amphetamine and pentobarbital [280,281].

It is apparent from such animal studies that tumor size is an important factor governing the depression of drug-metabolizing activity. It requires a tumor of approximately 2% body weight to produce a significant depression of activity and approximately 10% of body weight to induce a maximal suppression [272,274]. Since tumors of this size are seldom found in humans this may explain the only slight decrease in metabolism observed in patients with malignant disease.

The mechanism by which nonhepatic tumors can alter hepatic drug metabolism is not understood. However, this mechanism clearly involves the secretion of an inhibitory factor into the circulation which can influence drug-metabolizing activity. Thus, surgical removal of the tumor reverses the observed inhibition [282,283]. In addition, the implantation of a tumor into one of a pair of parabiotic rats induces a decrease in drug-metabolizing activity in both animals [284]. This is substantiated by the finding that perfusion of normal liver with blood from a tumor-bearing animal caused a decrease in pentobarbital metabolism [285].

Two mechanisms for the suppression of drug-metabolizing activity according to tumor type have been proposed. Thus implanted tumors may exert their action by the secretion of toxohormones [286] which on injection into animals decrease the activity of drug-metabolizing enzymes and reduce the level of components of the microsomal enzyme system [9,287]. However, the components of the substance remain unknown although it is reported to occur in urine from patients with malignant disease but not in control subjects [288]. Since the effects of tumors on drug metabolism are not apparent when grown as free ascites cells in the peritoneal cavity compared to solid implantation sites, it has been proposed that toxohormones are only produced during necrosis of malignant cells, a phenomenon occurring less commonly in the free ascites form [289].

The exception to the above hypothesis of tumor effect concerns animals bearing pituitary mammotropic tumors. The presence of such tumors is associated with elevated blood levels of prolactin, ACTH, and growth hormone which are also found in the tumor brei [290]. Injection of tumor brei or growth hormone or implantation of such tumors causes a decrease in drug-metabolizing activity [291-297]. Since implanted tumors affect drug metabolism at a size below that at which other tumors are active [283] it is conceivable that their secretion of pituitary hormones may be responsible for their adverse effect on drug-metabolizing activity.

Although the studies carried out in animals do not closely parallel the picture of malignant disease in humans, they serve to indicate the potential activity of tumors in producing substances that inhibit drug-metabolizing enzyme systems. That a decrease in drug metabolism may occur in malignant disease should therefore be given further consideration.

G. Fever, Infection, and Bacterial Extracts

We have so far examined dysfunction of major organ components responsible for the maintenance of normal body homeostasis. However, there is some evidence to suggest that a variety of other disorders found in humans, or components of such disorders, can lead to an alteration in hepatic drug-metabolizing activity.

For example, alterations in body temperature can occur as short-term or prolonged components of numerous disease states. In humans fever induced by the administration of etiocholanolone or other pyrogens is generally associated with a decrease in drug-metabolizing activity. Thus, plasma antipyrine half-life was increased and drug clearance decreased in subjects developing fever after administration of etiocholanolone [298] (Table 39). However, the effect observed may to a large extent depend on the substrate and route of metabolism. For example, the proportion of salicylamide metabolized by the predominant pathway to the glucuronide conjugate is reduced during pyrogen-induced fever as opposed to an increased urinary

TABLE 39
Effect of Etiocholanolone-induced Fever on Antipyrine Clearance in Humans

Parameter	Basal levels in subjects prior to fever	Levels in subjects during fever
Half-life [β-phase] (hr)	9.2 ± 0.8	11.7 ± 1.1*
Plasma clearance rate (ml/min)	51.6 ± 5.0	43.3 ± 5.5*
Volume of distribution (liters)	38.0 ± 3.0	39.9 ± 3.9

*$p < 0.05$.
Source: From Ref. 298.

excretion of other metabolites, namely the sulfate conjugate and gentisamide glucuronide [299]. Also, while altered disposition of sulfobromophthalein occurs in pyrogen-induced fever no change is observed in indocyanine green clearance [300]. The latter compound indeed reflects a lack of change in hepatic perfusion while the alteration in bromosulfophthalein kinetics appears due to modified metabolism since both compounds have high intrinsic hepatic clearance.

In general, the changes in drug clearance during artificially induced fever are small and reasons other than altered metabolism due to the febrile state must also be considered. For example, the agents administered to induce fever, particularly steroids, may exert direct actions on hepatic drug-metabolizing enzymes. In addition, changes in drug distribution are also apparent during fever in humans [300,301], which may be of significance in altered drug disposition. Thus, in fever induced in rats by the intracerebroventricular administration of prostaglandin E_1 the half-life of antipyrine and the volume of drug distribution were increased but overall did not result in any significant change in drug clearance [302]. Interestingly, the in vitro metabolism of antipyrine in suspensions of isolated rat hepatocytes was unaltered by temperature changes between 29 and 39°C confirming the overall in vivo finding. However, conjugation of paracetamol in this system was decreased.

The common occurrence of febrile states warrants the further investigation of changes occurring in drug metabolism in a number of disease states, using other substrates before it can be clearly established that the variations already observed are indicative of a common situation. In particular, it would be of considerable interest to determine whether altered metabolism occurs as a result of the fever frequently accompanying the common cold or influenza.

If increased body temperature decreases drug-metabolizing activity it is also to be expected that hypothermia altering homeostasis may exert an adverse effect. Indeed, studies of in vitro drug metabolism have demonstrated a decrease in the metabolism of drugs including propranolol and procaine [303,304]. This is reflected by the altered disposition of propranolol in patients undergoing hypothermic cardiopulmonary bypass or in dogs subjected to systemic cooling to 26°C by immersion in water [305] (Table 40). The increase in plasma propranolol levels and decreased half-life observed may, however, also be attributed to the decreased volume of drug distribution or alternatively to altered hepatic perfusion which may alter the high intrinsic hepatic clearance of this drug.

Febrile states often accompany infectious disorders and may be responsible for alterations in drug-metabolizing activity. In experimentally induced malaria, the plasma levels of quinine and the ratio of quinine to total drug (parent drug and metabolites) were found to be increased compared to values obtained in the same subjects prior to infection [306]. Since no change in urinary excretion of quinine was apparent the effects

TABLE 40
Effect of Hypothermia on the Disposition of Propranolol in Dogs

Parameter	Normothermia (37°C)	Hypothermia (26°C)
Half-life [β-phase] (min)	73.6 ± 15.2	45.0 ± 10.2*
Plasma clearance (liters/min/kg)	0.0644 ± 0.01110	0.0323 ± 0.0072*
Elimination rate constant (min^{-1})	0.0098 ± 0.0020	0.0161 ± 0.0040*
Volume of distribution (liters/kg)	6.78 ± 1.65	2.08 ± 0.58*

*$p < 0.05$.
Source: From Ref. 305.

appear to be due to changes in quinine oxidation to 2-hydroxyquinine and a 6-hydroxyquinuclidine derivative. This effect is, however, maximal during the acute stages of malaria when fever and other disease manifestations are most intense. Indeed, a survey of quinine therapy in chloroquine-resistant malaria showed the highest plasma levels of drug to occur in those patients exhibiting fever during therapy [307]. This would perhaps suggest the febrile state to be responsible for the observed changes in metabolism. However, experimentally induced etiocholanolone fever generally produces a smaller change in quinine levels than observed during malaria [306]. In addition, malaria is associated with altered liver function as judged by liver biopsy studies and by increased serum transaminase levels [308,309]. Measurement of in vitro components of the hepatic drug-metabolizing enzyme system may throw more light on this problem.

Other infections have also been reported to decrease drug-metabolizing activity (e.g., hepatitis virus, schistozomal infections; see Sec. III) but only where involvement of hepatic function is observed. Nothing appears known of the ability of the many other infectious disorders afflicting humans and associated with febrile states to cause altered drug disposition.

It would also appear that vaccination against infection utilizing live or killed preparations may exert actions on drug-metabolizing enzyme systems. Thus, treatment of mice with whooping cough vaccine (killed Bordettela pertussis cells) decreases aminopyrine and ethylmorphine N-demethylase activity, aniline hydroxylase activity, NADPH-cytochrome c reductase levels, and cytochrome P-450 and b_5 concentrations [310] (Table 41). This effect of vaccines is seemingly not due to general hepatotoxicity since other liver functions are unimpaired (see Ref. 310). Apart from illustrating that even bacterial extracts may be able to cause altered drug metabolism it is of considerable interest that pertussis vaccination of infants is associated with histamine sensitivity and other effects reminiscent of the changes observed in vaccinated mice [311]. Confirmation of altered metabolism has yet to be obtained.

The ability of mycobacterial extracts to decrease drug-metabolizing activity is observed in adjuvant-induced arthritis in rodents [312-315] (Table 42). Such changes appear not to be due to the induction of the arthritic state but to a direct action of the adjuvant on hepatic function (see Ref. 313 for discussion). In particular, mycobacterial extracts having no arthritis-inducing activity still cause profound decrease in drug-metabolizing activity. Also, while administration of phenobarbital can reverse the effects of adjuvant administration on drug metabolism, this does not prevent the onset of the arthritic condition. Human data would also suggest no alteration in drug metabolism in arthritic conditions [316,317].

TABLE 41
Effect of Pertussis Vaccination on In Vitro Drug-metabolizing Activity in Mice

Parameter	Control animals	Vaccinated animals
Aminopyrine N-demethylase (μmol HCHO/mg protein/hr)	0.668 ± 0.045	0.432 ± 0.049*
Ethylmorphine N-demethylase (μmol HCHO/mg protein/hr)	0.714 ± 0.006	0.418 ± 0.043*
Aniline hydroxylase (nmol p-aminophenol/mg protein/hr)	47.5 ± 0.72	29.2 ± 0.74*
Cytochrome P-450 (nmol/mg protein)	1.03 ± 0.04	0.55 ± 0.06*
Cytochrome b_5 (nmol/mg protein)	0.41 ± 0.02	0.29 ± 0.03*
NADPH-cytochrome c reductase (nmol reduced/mg protein/min)	182 ± 5	141 ± 8*

*$p < 0.05$.
Source: From Ref. 310.

TABLE 42
Effect of Adjuvant (Killed Mycobacterium butyrium Suspension in Light Mineral Oil) Administered 15 Days Previously on Hepatic In Vitro Drug-metabolizing Parameters in Rats

Parameter	Control animals	Adjuvant-treated animals
Aniline hydroxylase (nmol para-aminophenol formed/mg protein/15 min)	7.88 ± 0.36	2.44 ± 0.36*
Aminopyrine N-demethylase (nmol 4-aminoantipyrine/mg protein/30 min)	7.56 ± 0.37	1.71 ± 0.04*
para-nitroanisole O-demethylase (nmol product/mg protein/min)	10.8 ± 0.7	7.7 ± 1.1*
Cytochrome P-450 (nmol/mg protein)	0.73 ± 0.01	0.16 ± 0.01*
Cytochrome P-420 (nmol/mg protein)	0	0.04 ± 0.01*

*$p < 0.05$.
Source: From Ref. 313.

V. DISCUSSION

It is clear from the currently available literature that the study of altered drug disposition in disease states is still in its infancy. Although much recent interest has centered on this topic, it is as yet impossible to reach any gross generalizations concerning the effect of disease on drug disposition and, in particular, drug metabolism. We have therefore adopted a factual approach to this topic in order to bring to the fore the most prominent features of the investigations so far undertaken. Our choice of such a factual topic in a volume devoted to the development of a more conceptual approach to drug disposition was intentional. Realizing the potential importance of altered drug disposition during the course of disease states it seemed to us that this was a topic of direct relevance to those investigating the development of novel drugs or trying to improve the therapeutic use of existing drugs. We have therefore tried, primarily from a drug metabolism viewpoint, to evaluate the currently available data on the effect of disease on drug disposition. This approach has emphasized the areas of current interest but has also revealed the sources of weakness which prevent us from being able with any degree of conviction to predict the direction or intensity of change in drug disposition that may occur during the course of the disease or on recovery from disease.

Investigations of the effects of disease on drug disposition have naturally centered on diseases of the liver. Since this organ represents the major component of the body's drug-metabolizing capacity, its dysfunction would be expected to lead to changes in drug disposition. In addition, it is clear from the studies which we have discussed that other organs can indirectly affect the capacity of the liver to metabolize drugs. What is perhaps worrying, however, is the fact that the number of disease states so far studied is relatively small and the number of patients studied in many of such diseases is also less than one would ideally envisage. In particular, little has been done to assess the impact of acute disease requiring rapid treatment where a knowledge of alteration of drug disposition would be an advantage in designing therapy. In this context acute illnesses which regularly affect large numbers of the population (colds, influenza, migraine, bronchitic disorders), and where a number of common drugs are taken with alarming regularity without medical supervision, have received little or no attention. For the interested investigator it would appear a more feasible proposition to investigate altered drug disposition in such relatively normal members of the population rather than to study much rarer diseases in small numbers of patients under clinical conditions. But perhaps the reason for this lack of interest in such common ailments is apparent from the data presently at hand, considering that the effects of disease on drug disposition are minimal except where the disease condition is particularly advanced and severe. Therefore in less severe disease states from which rapid recovery can be expected, increases in drug half-life as a result of a decreased drug metabolism seldom exceed more than 20-30% whereas in chronic disease, particularly irreversible disorders, a two- to threefold increase in drug half-life can occur. It is therefore probable that in the more acute illnesses which affect the general population minimal alterations in drug metabolism would be expected. However, it is still necessary to undertake studies to prove this point since the number of humans involved in some diseases of epidemic proportions is sufficient to justify the investigative effort. When assessing the effect of disease on drug disposition it must also be remembered that patients do not lead normal lives. Rather they spend much of their time prostrate, with little exercise, their food intake is low and their diet often abnormal, and in the more severe diseases there may be a significant decrease in body fat depots, all such factors providing sufficient physiological abnormality as to potentially alter drug disposition. One is therefore left to wonder whether such parameters may be of equal or perhaps even greater importance than the progress of the disease state itself.

From the viewpoint of drug metabolism it is clear that the number of substrates examined in disease states is as yet insufficient to allow construction of general rules explaining the quantitative and qualitative changes that occur. For obvious reasons there are advantages in using model drugs such as antipyrine to investigate alterations in drug metabolism, keeping in mind that the number of such compounds available and the number of routes of metabolism undergone are limited. In addition it could be argued that since such drugs are not used to treat the particular disease state under investigation, alterations in their metabolism are not of relevance to that disorder and therefore studies should be confined to those drugs therapeutically used to treat the disease. This is a difficult problem which might benefit from a more rigorous examination of a number of drug substrates using in vitro investigation of liver samples taken at biopsy. However, in many cases such tissue is not available and it is arguable whether the information gained would be sufficient to justify the use of this invasive procedure.

While information is available on alterations in functionalization reactions during disease, the current data on conjugation mechanisms is limited and as yet no clear picture can be assembled of whether these routes are similarly affected. But even when a change can be demonstrated in the extent of a given functionalization reaction the causative mechanisms generally remain poorly understood. The use of hepatic biopsy samples can often show that a decrease in metabolism correlates with decreased amounts either of electron-transport chain components or of the terminal oxidase. However, the underlying cause of these deficits, be it disruption of hepatic architecture, alterations in subcellular components, or deficits in protein synthesis, has yet to be conclusively identified. In particular, a number of examples have arisen where substrates undergoing apparently identical routes of metabolism are differentially affected by the disease state. In in vivo studies this may be attributed to differences in other pharmacokinetic parameters such as hepatic perfusion, but where reflected in in vitro studies can only at the present time be attributed to the multiplicity of monooxygenases known to exist. However, the evidence that this is actually the reason for the differential effect on different substrates is as yet open to considerable doubt. The question then arises as to the selectivity of various disease states in altering components of the monooxygenase system such as to cause rather discrete changes in drug-metabolizing activity that might be reflected in altered metabolism undergone by certain substrates.

One of the major reasons that our present knowledge of the effect of disease states on the components of the drug-metabolizing enzyme system is relatively poor is the fact that the animal models of such diseases are in general inadequate. While it is often difficult using animals to mimic the disease states occurring in humans, other causes of the discrepancies we have discussed are more apparent. It would appear to us that one of the major reasons for the poor correlation observed lies in the fact that the animal models try to acutely mimic disease states whose onset in humans occurs over protracted periods. The animal models, therefore, do not allow for adaptive changes that may occur in humans as the disease slowly progresses. Development of more representative animal models of human disease would be a trememdous asset in understanding alterations occurring during the disease state, particularly at the subcellular level.

Although the liver represents the major site of drug metabolism the growing awareness of the importance of extrahepatic metabolism should not be forgotten. Thus, while we have some knowledge of the effect of disease on hepatic drug-metabolizing activity we appear to know little or nothing about the effects of disease on extrahepatic drug metabolism. The information currently available is based to a large extent on alterations in plasma enzymes (esterases, amidases) but since the latter are reliant on the liver for protein synthesis this is hardly a true indication of extrahepatic metabolism. The only direct evidence of an alteration in extrahepatic drug-metabolizing activity caused by local disease of that tissue comes from the studies of monooxygenase activity in skin preparations from subjects with psoriasis [318]. It is somewhat surprising that studies of altered metabolism in lung tissue have not been carried out since its structure and function can be dramatically altered by a number of respiratory and other disease states and since tissue from some such disorders may be readily available after routine surgery. It would seem, therefore, that there is a place for some basic investigations of changes in extrahepatic metabolism using, of necessity, in vitro techniques.

Finally, the question must be asked as to whether the studies so far carried out have yielded information of use in modifying drug therapy in disease states. The answer to this is probably no, since drug therapy is still largely carried out on a cause-and-effect basis. Therefore, even though the half-life of a drug may have been greatly increased by the evolution of a disease state, continuous drug administration can be adjusted to produce the desired effect based on initial response or previous experience. Even if the effect of disease on drug disposition and its pharmacological activity is known, it may not be of any therapeutic consequence. Indeed, the latter will depend largely on the therapeutic index of the drug and the safety margin subsequently involved. Thus, doubling of antipyrine half-life is unlikely to be of any significance whereas, of course, a similar increase in digoxin half-life may have more severe consequences. One is led to wonder, therefore, whether changes in pharmacokinetic parameters other than biotransformation itself may be of greater significance in governing the therapeutic use of drugs in disease. For example, it would seem that alterations in organ perfusion may be of greater consequence since this may affect not only the extent of the metabolism of substrates showing high intrinsic clearance, but it can also affect the rate of drug absorption, the extent of distribution, and to some extent the renal clearance of drugs. Similarly, it is clear that small changes in the plasma protein binding of highly bound drugs may result in a greater rise in free plasma levels of drug than would be observed following severe impairment of hepatic drug-metabolizing activity. In addition it must not be forgotten that for a given drug the alterations in the pharmacokinetic profile occurring during disease may be accompanied by profound changes in the sensitivity of the receptors responsible for the drug's pharmacological actions. This is particularly apparent in renal disease where a number of commonly used drugs have a much more marked clinical effect than is observed in normal subjects. When assessing the influence of disease on drug disposition it is therefore clear that alterations in drug metabolism must be considered alongside a number of other factors and that changes in metabolism may be less important than other pharmacokinetic or pharmacodynamic alterations.

In conclusion, disease states can, indeed, alter the ability of the liver to metabolize drugs. The extent of this alteration varies with the severity of the disease, and to a large extent may represent the reserve capacity of the liver for carrying out this function. But a great deal of further investigation is obviously required before fundamental principles governing the effect of disease on drug metabolism and drug disposition can be satisfactorily established. Nevertheless, with the utilization of a unified approach involving both clinical investigation and animal experimentation our knowledge of this subject will be enhanced to a point where further reviews of the subject will result in the formulation of guiding principles both for the clinician and for those involved in the development of novel drug molecules.

REFERENCES

1. L. Z. Benet (Ed.), The Effect of Disease States on Drug Pharmacokinetics. American Pharmaceutical Association and Academy of Pharmaceutical Sciences, Washington, D.C., 1976.

2. L. F. Prescott, in Handbook of Experimental Pharmacology, Vol. 28 (J. R. Gillette and J. R. Mitchell, Eds.). Springer-Verlag, Berlin, 1975, p. 234.
3. G. R. Wilkinson and S. Schenker, Drug Metab. Rev. 4:139 (1975).
4. G. R. Wilkinson, Ann. Rev. Pharmacol. 15:11 (1975).
5. G. R. Wilkinson and D. G. Shand, Clin. Pharmacol. Ther. 18:377 (1975).
6. G. R. Wilkinson and S. Schenker, Biochem. Pharmacol. 25:2675 (1976).
7. J. Fabre and L. Balant, Clin. Pharmacokin. 1:99 (1976).
8. U. Klotz, Eur. J. Drug Metab. Pharmacokin. 3:129 (1976).
9. R. Kato, Xenobiotica 7:25 (1977).
10. J. P. Tillement, F. Lhoste, and J. F. Giudicelli, Clin. Pharmacokin. 3:144 (1978).
11. E. S. Vesell, in Microsomes and Drug Oxidations (V. Ullrich, I. Roots, A. Hildebrandt, R. W. Estabrook, and A. H. Conney, Eds.). Pergamon Press, Oxford, 1977, p. 628.
12. S. Andersson, Acta Pharmacol., Suppl. 3, 29:103 (1971).
13. L. F. Prescott, Med. Clin. N. Amer. 58:907 (1974).
14. R. C. Heading, J. Nimmo, L. F. Prescott, and P. Tothill, Brit. J. Pharmacol. 47:415 (1973).
15. J. Nimmo, R. C. Heading, P. Tothill, and L. F. Prescott, Brit. Med. J. 1:587 (1973).
16. J. D. Nelson, S. Shelton, H. T. Kusmiesz, and K. C. Haltalin, Clin. Pharmacol. Ther. 13:879 (1972).
17. L. Ther and D. Winne, Ann. Rev. Pharmacol. 11:57 (1971).
18. D. Winne, J. Theor. Biol. 53:145 (1975).
19. D. Winne and J. Remischovsky, J. Pharm. Pharmacol. 22:640 (1970).
20. W. G. Crouthamel, L. Diamond, L. W. Dittert, and J. T. Doluisio, J. Pharm. Sci. 64:661 (1975).
21. A. Haass, H. Lüllmann, and T. Peters, Eur. J. Pharmacol. 19:366 (1972).
22. W. G. Crouthamel, Amer. Heart J. 90:335 (1975).
23. J. Koch-Weser and J. W. Klein, J. Amer. Med. Ass. 215:1454 (1971).
24. J. Koch-Weser, Ann. N.Y. Acad. Sci. 179:370 (1971).
25. W. J. Tilstone, H. Dargie, E. N. Dargie, H. G. Morgan, and A. C. Kennedy, Clin. Pharmacol. Ther. 16:322 (1974).
26. K. V. Anderson, H. R. Brettell, and J. K. Aikawa, Arch. Intern. Med. 107:168 (1961).
27. F. Hagemeijer, Eur. J. Clin. Pharmacol. 9:21 (1975).

28. J. W. Ward and G. R. Kinghorn, J. Int. Med. Res., Suppl. 1, 4:49 (1976).
29. L. Z. Benet, A. Greither, and W. Meister, in The Effect of Disease States on Drug Pharmacokinetics (L. Z. Benet, Ed.). American Pharmaceutical Association and Academy of Pharmaceutical Sciences, Washington, D.C., 1976, p. 33.
30. S. Bellet, L. R. Romand, and A. Boza, Amer. J. Cardiol. 27:368 (1971).
31. W. G. Crouthamel, N. Engl. J. Med. 290:1379 (1974).
32. G. R. Wilkinson, in The Effect of Disease States on Drug Pharmacokinetics (L. Z. Benet, Ed.). American Pharmaceutical Association and Academy of Pharmaceutical Sciences, Washington, D.C., 1976, p. 13.
33. P. D. Thomson, M. Rowland, and K. Melmon, Amer. Heart J. 82:417 (1971).
34. P. D. Thomson, K. L. Melmon, J. A. Richardson, K. Cohn, W. Steinbrunn, R. Cudihee, and M. Rowland, Ann. Intern. Med. 78:499 (1973).
35. N. Benowitz, R. P. Forsyth, K. L. Melmon, and M. Rowland, Clin. Pharmacol. Ther. 16:99 (1974).
36. H. Halkin, P. Meffin, K. Melmon, and M. Rowland, Clin. Pharmacol. Ther. 17:669 (1975).
37. C. A. Camargo, A. J. Dowdy, E. W. Hancock, and J. A. Luetscher, J. Clin. Invest. 44:356 (1965).
38. R. Ritz, J. Cavanilles, S. Michaels, H. Shubin, and M. H. Weil, Surg. Gynecol. Obstet. 136:57 (1973).
39. R. A. Branch, J. James, and A. E. Read, Brit. J. Clin. Pharmacol. 3:243 (1976).
40. J. Caesar, S. Shaldon, L. Chiandussi, L. Guevera, and S. Sherlock, Clin. Sci. 21:43 (1961).
41. C. M. Leevy, C. L. Mendenhall, W. Leska, and M. M. Howard, J. Clin. Invest. 41:1169 (1962).
42. J. N. Cohn, I. M. Khatri, R. J. Groszmann, and B. Kotelanski, Amer. J. Med. 53:704 (1972).
43. R. A. Branch, J. James, and A. E. Read, Clin. Pharmacol. Ther. 20:81 (1976).
44. P. Lundberg, Scand. J. Infect. Dis. 6:297 (1974).
45. F. H. Messerli, J. Genest, W. Nowaczynski, O. Kuchel, M. Honda, Y. Latour, and G. Dumont, Circulation 51:1114 (1975).
46. O. L. Wade, J. M. Bishop, and K. W. Donald, Cardiac Output and Regional Blood Flow. Blackwell, Oxford, 1962.

47. M. Rowland, T. F. Blaschke, P. J. Meffin, and R. L. Williams, in The Effect of Disease States on Drug Pharmacokinetics (L. Z. Benet, Ed.). American Pharmaceutical Association and Academy of Pharmaceutical Sciences, Washington, D.C., 1976, p. 53.
48. R. A. Branch and D. G. Shand, in The Effect of Disease States on Drug Pharmacokinetics (L. Z. Benet, Ed.). American Pharmaceutical Association and Academy of Pharmaceutical Sciences, Washington, D.C., 1976, p. 77.
49. W. J. Jusko, in The Effect of Disease States on Drug Pharmacokinetics (L. Z. Benet, Ed.). American Pharmaceutical Association and Academy of Pharmaceutical Sciences, Washington, D.C., 1976, p. 99.
50. M. M. Reidenberg and M. Affrime, Ann. N.Y. Acad. Sci. 226:115 (1973).
51. L. Dettli, Clin. Pharmacokin. 1:126 (1976).
52. M. M. Reidenberg, Clin. Pharmacokin. 1:121 (1976).
53. T. F. Blaschke, Clin. Pharmacokin. 2:32 (1977).
54. R. Gugler and D. L. Azarnoff, Clin. Pharmacokin. 1:25 (1976).
55. E. A. Casey, F. E. Gilbert, J. F. Graulce, and E. L. Downey, Alabama J. Med. Sci. 8:168 (1971).
56. A. H. Anton and W. T. Corey, Acta Pharmacol. Toxicol., Suppl. 3, 29: 134 (1971).
57. M. M. Reidenberg, I. Odar-Cederlof, C. von Bahr, O. Borga, and F. Sjöqvist, N. Engl. J. Med. 285:264 (1971).
58. G. B. Wilson, T. L. Jahn, and J. R. Fonseca, Clin. Chim. Acta 49: 79 (1973).
59. R. T. Reid and R. S. Farr, Arthritis Rheum. 7:747 (1964).
60. D. Hawkins, R. N. Pinckard, and R. S. Farr, Science 160:780 (1968).
61. R. S. Farr, R. T. Reid, and P. Minden, J. Clin. Invest. 45:1006 (1966).
62. F. Andreasen, Acta Pharmacol. Toxicol. 32:417 (1973).
63. W. G. Crouthamel, in The Effect of Disease States on Drug Pharmacokinetics (L. Z. Benet, Ed.). American Pharmaceutical Association and Academy of Pharmaceutical Sciences, Washington, D.C., 1976, p. 1.
64. W. G. Crouthamel and R. J. Cenedella, Pharmacology 13:465 (1975).
65. A. A. Spector, E. C. Santos, J. D. Ashbrook, and J. E. Fletcher, Ann. N.Y. Acad. Sci. 226:247 (1973).
66. R. J. Cenedella, W. G. Crouthamel, G. C. Bierkamper, and D. P. Westfall, Arch. Int. Pharmacodyn. Ther. 218:229 (1975).

67. P. G. Welling and W. A. Craig, in The Effect of Disease States on Drug Pharmacokinetics (L. Z. Benet, Ed.). American Pharmaceutical Association and Academy of Pharmaceutical Sciences, Washington, D.C., 1976, p. 155.
68. T. P. Gibson, E. Matusik, and W. A. Briggs, in The Effect of Disease States on Drug Pharmacokinetics (L. Z. Benet, Ed.). American Pharmaceutical Association and Academy of Pharmaceutical Sciences, Washington, D.C., 1976, p. 189.
69. P. A. Michelson, W. A. Miller, J. F. Warner, L. A. Ayers, and H. G. Boxenbaum, in The Effect of Disease States on Drug Pharmacokinetics (L. Z. Benet, Ed.). American Pharmaceutical Association and Academy of Pharmaceutical Sciences, Washington, D.C., 1976, p. 207.
70. L. Dettli, Med. Clin. N. Amer. 58:977 (1974).
71. L. C. Dettli, Clin. Pharmacol. Ther. 16:274 (1974).
72. W. M. Bennett, I. Singer, and C. H. Coggin, J. Amer. Med. Ass. 223:991 (1973).
73. M. M. Reidenberg, Renal Function and Drug Action. Saunders, Philadelphia, 1971.
74. L. J. Riff and G. G. Jackson, J. Infect. Dis., Suppl. 124:98 (1971).
75. B. Pititpierre and J. Fabre, Schweiz. Med. Wschr. 102:590 (1972).
76. J. Fabre, J. S. Pitton, C. Virieux, F. L. Laurencet, J. P. Bernhardt, and J. C. Godel, Med. Wschr. 97:915 (1967).
77. P. M. Bloom and W. P. Nelp, J. Med. Sci. 251:133 (1966).
78. H. Popper, H. Elias, and D. E. Petty, Amer. J. Clin. Path. 22:717 (1954).
79. R. Groszman, B. Kotelanski, J. N. Cohn, and I. M. Khatri, Amer. J. Med. 53:715 (1972).
80. G. Gross and C. V. Perrier, N. Engl. J. Med. 293:1046 (1975).
81. A. G. Redeker, H. M. Geller, and T. B. Reynolds, J. Clin. Invest. 37:606 (1958).
82. D. G. Shand and R. E. Rangno, Pharmacology 7:159 (1972).
83. R. Gugler, P. Lain, and D. L. Azarnoff, J. Pharmacol. Exp. Ther. 195:416 (1975).
84. R. W. Faigle, Acta Pharmacol. Toxicol., Suppl., 29:233 (1971).
85. R. L. Williams, T. F. Blaschke, P. J. Meffin, K. L. Melman, and M. Rowland, Clin. Pharmacol. Ther. 21:301 (1977).
86. T. F. Blaschke, P. J. Meffin, K. L. Melmon, and M. Rowland, Clin. Pharmacol. Ther. 17:685 (1975).
87. G. W. Hepner and E. S. Vesell, Ann. Int. Med. 83:632 (1975).
88. A. J. Levi, S. Sherlock, and D. Walker, Lancet i:1275 (1968).
89. G. E. Mawer, N. E. Miller, and L. A. Turnberg, Brit. J. Pharmacol. 44:549 (1972).

90. F. Azzollini, A. Gazzaniga, E. Lodola, and R. Natangelo, Int. J. Clin. Pharmacol. Ther. Toxicol. 6:130 (1972).
91. U. Klotz, G. R. Avant, A. Hoyumpa, S. Schenker, and G. R. Wilkinson, J. Clin. Invest. 55:347 (1975).
92. T. K. Basu and J. W. T. Dickerson, Chem. Biol.-Interact. 8:193 (1974).
93. D. Berkowitz, M. N. Croll, and W. Likoff, Amer. J. Cardiol. 11:43 (1963).
94. J. Hakkila, T. E. Makela, and P. I. Halonen, Amer. J. Cardiol. 5: 295 (1960).
95. R. A. Branch, C. M. Herbert, and A. E. Read, Gut 14:569 (1973).
96. R. Preisig, J. G. Rankin, J. Sweeting, and S. E. Bradley, Circulation 34:188 (1966).
97. T. S. McHorse, G. R. Wilkinson, R. F. Johnson, and S. Schenker, Gastroenterology 68:775 (1975).
98. D. D. Breimer, W. Zilly, and E. Richter, Pharmacol. Ther. 18:433 (1975).
99. W. Zilly, E. Richter, and N. Rietbrock, Clin. Pharmacol. Ther. 17: 302 (1975).
100. J. W. Kraus, P. V. Desmond, J. P. Marshall, R. F. Johnson, S. Schenker, and G. R. Wilkinson, Clin. Pharmacol. Ther. 24:411 (1978).
101. R. K. Roberts, G. R. Wilkinson, R. A. Branch, and S. Schenker, Gastroenterology 75:479 (1978).
102. H. J. Shull, G. R. Wilkinson, R. Johnson, and S. Schenker, Ann. Int. Med. 84:420 (1976).
103. S. F. Sisenwine, C. O. Tio, S. R. Schrader, and H. W. Ruelius, Arzneim.-Forsch. 22:632 (1972).
104. J. A. Knowles, W. H. Comer, and H. W. Ruelius, Arzneim.-Forsch. 21:1055 (1971).
105. R. L. Williams, W. L. Schary, T. F. Blaschke, P. J. Meffin, K. L. Melmon, and M. Rowland, Clin. Pharmacol. Ther. 20:90 (1976).
106. J. Alvin, T. McHorse, A. Hoyuma, M. T. Bush, and S. Schenker, J. Pharmacol. Exp. Ther. 192:224 (1975).
107. J. Doshi, A. Luisada-Opper, and C. M. Leevy, Proc. Soc. Exp. Biol. Med. 140:492 (1972).
108. J. T. Sessions, H. P. Minkel, J. C. Bullard, and F. J. Ingelfinger, J. Clin. Invest. 33:1116 (1954).
109. D. Singh, R. Vijayvargiya, and A. L. Kakrani, Indian J. Med. Res. 66:832 (1977).
110. T. E. Gram, A. M. Guarino, F. E. Greene, P. L. Gigon, and J. R. Gillette, Biochem. Pharmacol. 17:1769 (1968).

111. P. Th. Henderson and K. J. Kersten, Biochem. Pharmacol. 19:2343 (1970).
112. L. F. Prescott, N. Wright, P. Roscoe, and S. S. Brown, Lancet i: 519 (1971).
113. E. A. Sotaniemi, O. T. Hokkanen, J. T. Ahokas, R. O. Pelkonen, and J. Alqvist, Eur. J. Clin. Pharmacol. 12:429 (1977).
114. G. P. Lewis and W. J. Jusko, Clin. Pharmacol. Ther. 18:475 (1975).
115. C. M. Kunin, A. J. Glazko, and M. Finland, J. Clin. Invest. 38: 1498 (1959).
116. U. Klotz, T. S. McHorse, G. R. Wilkinson, and S. Schenker, Clin. Pharmacol. Ther. 16:667 (1974).
117. M. Shamszad, H. Solomon, S. Mobarhan, and F. L. Iber, Gastroenterology 69:865 (1975).
118. P. du Souich and S. Erill, Clin. Pharmacol. Ther. 22:588 (1977).
119. H. Held and H. F. von Oldershausen, Klin. Wschr. 48:565 (1970).
120. R. E. Stenson, R. T. Constantino, and D. C. Harrison, Circulation 43:205 (1971).
121. R. A. Branch, J. James, and A. E. Read, Gut 15:837 (1974).
122. U. Klotz, C. Fischer, P. Müller-Seydlitz, J. Schulz, and W. A. Müller, Clin. Pharmacol. Ther. 26:221 (1979).
123. J. D. Maxwell, M. Carrella, J. D. Parkes, R. Williams, G. P. Mould, and S. H. Curry, Clin. Sci. 43:143 (1972).
124. U. Klotz, K. H. Antonin, H. Brügel, and P. R. Bieck, Clin. Pharmacol. Ther. 21:430 (1977).
125. P. B. Andreasen, J. Hendel, G. Greisen, and E. F. Hvidberg, Eur. J. Clin. Pharmacol. 10:115 (1976).
126. U. Klotz, K. H. Antonin, and P. R. Bieck, Eur. J. Clin. Pharmacol. 10:121 (1976).
127. J. J. Kamm and E. J. van Loon, Clin. Chem. 12:789 (1966).
128. E. W. Maynert, J. Pharmacol. Exp. Ther. 150:118 (1965).
129. W. Zilly, D. D. Breimer, and E. Richter, Clin. Pharmacol. Ther. 23:525 (1978).
130. B. Schoene, R. A. Fleischmann, H. Remmer, and H. Oldershausen, Eur. J. Clin. Pharmacol. 4:65 (1972).
131. E. A. Sotaniemi, R. O. Pelkonen, J. Ahokas, J. Ahlqvist, and O. T. Hokkanen, Arch. Toxicol., Suppl. 1:339 (1978).
132. H. I. Pirttiaho, E. A. Sotaniemi, J. Ahlqvist, U. Pitkanen, and R. O. Pelkonen, Eur. J. Clin. Pharmacol. 13:61 (1978).
133. H. Pirttiaho, Int. J. Clin. Pharmacol. Biopharm. 17:271 (1979).

134. M. S. Gold and D. M. Ziegler, Xenobiotica 3:179 (1973).
135. M. Black and B. H. Billing, N. Engl. J. Med. 280:1266 (1969).
136. C. H. Hammer and W. Prellwitz, Klin. Wschr. 44:1010 (1966).
137. R. Kato, Y. Nakamura, and E. Chiesara, Biochem. Pharmacol. 12: 365 (1963).
138. N. Heni and H. Remmer, Arch. Toxicol. 28:1 (1971).
139. G. W. Hepner and E. S. Vesell, Clin. Pharmacol. Ther. 21:620 (1977).
140. G. W. Hepner, S. R. Uhlin, A. Lipton, H. A. Harvey, and G. V. Rohrer, J. Amer. Med. Ass. 236:1587 (1976).
141. D. Burnett, C. N. Reynolds, and K. Wilson, Eur. J. Clin. Pharmacol. 15:57 (1979).
142. H. Autrup, B. J. Thurlow, and G. P. Warwick, Biochem. Pharmacol. 23:2341 (1974).
143. O. Pelkonen, N. T. Kärki, and T. K. I. Larmi, Chirurgia Gastroenterolica 7:436 (1973).
144. A. H. Conney and J. J. Burns, Advan. Enzyme Regul. 1:189 (1963).
145. L. A. Rogers, H. P. Morris, and J. R. Fouts, J. Pharmacol. Exp. Ther. 157:227 (1963).
146. Ṡ. E. Saine and H. W. Strobel, Mol. Pharmacol. 12:649 (1976).
147. H. Ueda, T. Sakurai, M. Ota, A. Nakajima, K. Kamii, and H. Maezawa, Diabetes 12:414 (1963).
148. P. B. Andreasen, L. Ranek, B. E. Statland, and N. Tygstrup, Eur. J. Clin. Invest. 4:129 (1974).
149. P. B. Andreasen, Arch. Toxicol., Suppl. 1:131 (1978).
150. E. F. Hvidberg, P. B. Andreasen, and L. Ranek, Clin. Pharmacol. Ther. 15:171 (1974).
151. T. R. Hartoma, E. A. Sotaniemi, O. Pelkonen, and J. Ahlqvist, Eur. J. Clin. Pharmacol. 12:147 (1977).
152. G. C. Becking, Med. Clin. N. Amer. 60:813 (1976).
153. A. E. Moffitt, Jr., and S. D. Murphy, Biochem. Pharmacol. 22:1463 (1973).
154. M. A. Peters and J. R. Fouts, Biochem. Pharmacol. 19:533 (1970).
155. B. Lauterberg and J. Bircher, Gastroenterology 65:556 (1973).
156. G. W. Hepner and E. S. Vesell, N. Engl. J. Med. 291:1384 (1974).
157. J. Bircher, A. Küpfer, I. Gikalov, and R. Preisig, Clin. Pharmacol. Ther. 20:484 (1976).
158. J. Noordhoek, J. Dees, E. M. Savenije-Chapel, and J. H. P. Wilson, Eur. J. Clin. Pharmacol. 13:223 (1978).
159. J. Bircher and R. Preisig, in Concepts in Drug Metabolism, Part B (P. Jenner and B. Testa, Eds.). Marcel Dekker, New York, 1981, pp. 406-408.

160. J. Elfstrom and S. Lindgren, Eur. J. Clin. Pharmacol. 7:467 (1974).
161. N. Carulli, F. Manenti, M. Porz de Leon, A. Ferrari, G. Salvioli, and M. Gallo, Eur. J. Clin. Invest. 5:455 (1975).
162. A. Auranen, Acta Chir. Scand., Suppl. 424:1 (1972).
163. E. F. McLuen and J. R. Fouts, J. Pharmacol. Exp. Ther. 131:7 (1961).
164. F. Hutterer, P. G. Bacchin, I. H. Raisfeld, J. B. Schenkman, F. Schaffner, and H. Popper, Proc. Soc. Exp. Biol. Med. 133:702 (1970).
165. F. Hutterer, H. Denk, P. G. Bacchin, J. B. Schenkman, F. Schaffner, and H. Popper, Life Sci. 9(2):877 (1970).
166. B. Solymoss and G. Zsigmond, Proc. Soc. Exp. Biol. Med. 147:430 (1974).
167. F. Schaffner and H. Popper, Lancet ii:355 (1969).
168. M. Mackinnon and F. Simon, Biochem. Pharmacol. 24:748 (1975).
169. A. L. Jones, D. L. Schmucker, J. S. Mooney, R. D. Adler, and R. K. Ockner, Gastroenterology 71:1050 (1976).
170. N. Ahmad and M. Black, J. Pharmacol. Exp. Ther. 203:397 (1977).
171. P. du Souich and S. Erill, Eur. J. Clin. Pharmacol. 14:21 (1978).
172. O. Tokola, O. Pelkonen, N. T. Kärki, and P. Luoma, Brit. J. Clin. Pharmacol. 2:429 (1975).
173. M. Beaudoin-Jacob and C. Marchand, Eur. J. Drug Metab. Pharmacokin. 2:3 (1977).
174. K. W. Renton, J. C. Baker, and L. E. Bailey, Can. J. Physiol. Pharmacol. 57:302 (1979).
175. M. R. Montgomery and R. J. Rubin, J. Appl. Physiol. 35:505 (1973).
176. J. F. Cumming and G. J. Mannering, Biochem. Pharmacol. 19:973 (1970).
177. R. A. Roth, Jr., and R. J. Rubin, Drug Metab. Dispos. 4:460 (1976).
178. J. F. Cumming, Clin. Pharmacol. Ther. 19:468 (1976).
179. F. Andreasen, O. Lederballe Pedersen, and E. Mikkelsen, Eur. J. Clin. Pharmacol. 14:237 (1978).
180. D. K. Hartle, G. F. Kapke, and J. Baron, Biochem. Biophys. Res. Commun. 77:953 (1977).
181. H. S. Marver, in Microsomes and Drug Oxidations (J. R. Gillette, A. H. Conney, G. J. Cosmides, R. W. Estabrook, J. R. Fouts, and G. J. Mannering, Eds.). Academic, New York, 1969, p. 495.
182. K. E. Anderson, C. M. Peterson, A. P. Alvares, and A. Kappas, Clin. Pharmacol. Ther. 22:580 (1977).
183. A. B. Rifkind, V. Canale, and M. I. New, Clin. Pharmacol. Ther. 20:476 (1976).
184. G. Perona, R. Corrocher, M. Frezza, G. C. Falezza, R. Cellerino, C. Tiribelli, A. Fusaro, and G. De Sandre, Brit. J. Haematol. 25:723 (1973).

185. M. D. Maines and A. Kappas, Proc. Nat. Acad. Sci. U.S. 71:4293 (1974).
186. R. Tenhunen, H. S. Marver, and R. Schmid, J. Lab. Clin. Med. 75: 410 (1970).
187. S. Sassa, A. Kappas, S. E. Bernstein, and A. P. Alvares, J. Biol. Chem. 254:729 (1979).
188. B. A. Schacter, E. B. Nelson, H. S. Marver, and B. S. S. Masters, J. Biol. Chem. 247:3601 (1972).
189. S. Sassa, S. Granick, D. R. Bickers, H. L. Bradlow, and A. Kappas, Proc. Nat. Acad. Sci. U.S. 71:732 (1974).
190. K. E. Anderson, A. P. Alvares, S. Sassa, and A. Kappas, Clin. Pharmacol. Ther. 19:47 (1976).
191. C. S. Song, H. L. Bonkowsky, and D. P. Tschudy, Clin. Pharmacol. Ther. 15:431 (1974).
192. A. Kappas, H. L. Bradlow, P. N. Gillette, and T. F. Gallagher, J. Exp. Med. 136:1043 (1972).
193. E. Karlsson, L. Molin, B. Norlander, and F. Sjöqvist, Brit. J. Clin. Pharmacol. 1:467 (1974).
194. M. M. Reidenberg, Clin. Nephrol. 4:83 (1975).
195. I. Odar-Cederlof, J. Vessman, G. Alvan, and F. Sjöqvist, Acta Pharmacol. Toxicol., 1, 40:52 (1977).
196. M. M. Reidenberg, Amer. J. Med. 62:482 (1977).
197. D. T. Lowenthal, J. M. Pitone, M. B. Affrime, J. Shirk, P. Busby, K. E. Kim, J. Nancarrow, C. D. Swartz, and G. Onesti, Clin. Pharmacol. Ther. 23:606 (1978).
198. E. E. Ohnhaus, Brit. J. Pharmacol. 47:620 (1973).
199. M. Lichter, M. Black, and I. M. Arias, J. Pharmacol. Exp. Ther. 187:612 (1973).
200. J. L. Maddocks, C. J. Wake, and M. J. Harber, Brit. J. Clin. Pharmacol. 2:339 (1975).
201. L. Storstein, Clin. Pharmacol. Ther. 21:536 (1977).
202. R. E. Cutler, A. W. Forrey, T. G. Christopher, and B. M. Kimpell, Clin. Pharmacol. Ther. 15:588 (1974).
203. A. P. van Peer and F. M. Belpaire, Arch. Int. Pharmacodyn. Ther. 228:180 (1977).
204. H. W. Leber, P. Streitzig, M. Kayser, and G. Schutterle, Klin. Wschr. 49:944 (1971).
205. H. W. Leber and G. Schutterle, Kidney Int. 2:152 (1972).
206. E. Mezey, R. E. Vestal, J. J. Potter, and J. W. Rowe, J. Lab. Clin. Med. 86:931 (1975).
207. A. P. van Peer, F. M. Belpaire, and M. G. Bogaert, Arch. Int. Pharmacodyn. Ther. 234:346 (1978).
208. A. van Peer, F. Belpaire, and M. Bogaert, Pharmacology 17:307 (1978).
209. Y. Ishizuka and T. Ariyoshi, Yakugaku Zasshi 96:1049 (1976).

210. M. Eichelbaum, Clin. Pharmacokin. 1:339 (1976).
211. C. MacNee, A. J. Headley, D. G. Adamson, and J. Crooks, Israel J. Med. Sci. 8:42 (1972).
212. J. Crooks, A. J. Headley, C. MacNee, and I. H. Stevenson, Brit. J. Pharmacol. 49:156P (1973).
213. M. Eichelbaum, G. Bodem, and Ch. Schneider-Deters, Naunyn-Schmiedebergs Arch. Pharmakol. Exp. Pathol., Suppl. 277:R14 (1973).
214. M. Eichelbaum, G. Bodem, Ch. Schneider-Deters, and H. J. Dengler, N. Engl. J. Med. 290:1040 (1974).
215. R. Gugler, M. Eichelbaum, Ch. Schneider-Deters, G. Bodem, and H. J. Dengler, Verhandl. Deutsch. Gesellsch. Inn. Med. 79:1230 (1973).
216. E. S. Vesell, J. R. Shapiro, G. T. Passananti, H. Jorgensen, and C. A. Shively, Clin. Pharmacol. Ther. 17:48 (1975).
217. S. F. Brunk, S. P. Combs, J. D. Miller, M. Delle, and W. R. Wilson, J. Clin. Pharmacol. 14:271 (1974).
218. J. M. Hansen, L. Skovsted, J. P. Kampmann, B. I. Lumholtz, and K. Siersbaek-Nielsen, Acta Pharmacol. Toxicol. 42:343 (1978).
219. W. Eickenbusch, Hg. Lahrtz, U. Seppelt, and P. A. van Zwieten, Klin. Wschr. 48:270 (1969).
220. M. S. Croxson and H. K. Ibbertson, Brit. Med. J. 3:566 (1975).
221. J. Bonelli, H. Haydl, K. Hruby, and G. Kaik, Int. J. Clin. Pharmacol. Biopharm. 16:302 (1978).
222. D. Schuppan, S. Riegelman, B. von Lehmann, A. Pilbrandt, and C. Becker, J. Pharmacokin. Biopharm. 1:307 (1973).
223. J. Kampmann and L. Skovsted, Acta Pharmacol. Toxicol. 35:361 (1974).
224. J. Kampmann and L. Skovsted, Acta Pharmacol. Toxicol. 37:201 (1975).
225. R. E. Peterson, J. Clin. Invest. 37:736 (1958).
226. T. F. Gallagher, L. Hellman, J. Finkelstein, K. Yoshida, E. D. Weitzman, H. D. Roffwarg, and D. K. Fukushima, J. Clin. Endocrinol. Metab. 34:919 (1972).
227. G. G. Gordon, A. L. Sonthern, S. Tochimoto, J. J. Rand, and J. Olivo, J. Clin. Endocrinol. Metab. 29:164 (1969).
228. F. M. Klion, R. Segal, and F. Schaffner, Amer. J. Med. 50:317 (1971).
229. R. Kato and J. R. Gillette, J. Pharmacol. Exp. Ther. 150:285 (1965).
230. R. Kato and A. Takahashi, Mol. Pharmacol. 4:109 (1968).
231. R. Kato, A. Takanaka, and A. Takahashi, J. Biochem. (Tokyo) 66:613 (1970).
232. R. Kato and K. Onoda, Biochem. Pharmacol. 19:1649 (1970).

233. J. V. Aranda, K. W. Renton, G. Kunous, G. Boyd, and E. Colle, Pediat. Res. 7:317 (1973).
234. R. Kato, A. Takanaka, A. Takahashi, and K. Onoda, Jap. J. Pharmacol. 19:5 (1969).
235. C. S. Catz, M. R. Juchau, and S. J. Yaffe, J. Pharmacol. Exp. Ther. 174:197 (1970).
236. V. M. Pain, J. Lanoix, J. J. M. Bergeron, and J. C. Michael, Biochem. Biophys. Acta 353:487 (1974).
237. D. L. Topping and M. E. Targ, Horm. Res. 6:129 (1975).
238. H. Daintith, I. H. Stevenson, and K. O'Malley, Int. J. Clin. Pharmacol. 13:55 (1976).
239. H. Ueda, T. Sakurai, M. Ota, A. Nakajima, K. Kamii, and H. Maezawa, Diabetes 12:414 (1963).
240. K. Yamashita, Acta Hepat. Jap. 8:119 (1967).
241. R. M. Dajani, S. Kayyali, S. E. Saheb, and B. Birbari, Comp. Gen. Pharmacol. 5:1 (1974).
242. R. L. Dixon, L. G. Hart, L. A. Rogers, and J. R. Fouts, J. Pharmacol. Exp. Ther. 142:312 (1963).
243. R. L. Dixon, L. G. Hart, and J. R. Fouts, J. Pharmacol. Exp. Ther. 133:7 (1961).
244. R. Kato, A. Takanaka, and K. Onoda, Jap. J. Pharmacol. 18:516 (1968).
245. R. Kato, K. Onoda, and A. Takanaka, Jap. J. Pharmacol. 20:546 (1970).
246. M. D. Ackerman and K. C. Leibman, Drug Metab. Dispos. 5:405 (1977).
247. L. A. Reinke, S. J. Stohs, and H. Rosenberg, Xenobiotica 8:611 (1978).
248. L. A. Reinke, S. J. Stohs, and H. Rosenberg, Xenobiotica 8:769 (1979).
249. D. E. Cook and M. R. Past, Res. Commun. Chem. Path. Pharmacol. 24:389 (1979).
250. J. V. Aranda and K. W. Renton, Can. J. Physiol. Pharmacol. 53:873 (1975).
251. C. R. Clark, S. B. Lewis, and J. H. Exton, Diabetes 21:439 (1972).
252. E. W. Sutherland, G. A. Robinson, and R. Butcher, Circulation 37:279 (1968).
253. M. Weiner, G. G. Buterbaugh, and D. A. Blake, Res. Commun. Chem. Path. Pharmacol. 6:551 (1973).
254. M. Costa, E. R. Costa, C.-A. Manen, I. G. Sipes, and D. H. Russell, Mol. Pharmacol. 12:871 (1976).
255. J. A. Castro, F. E. Greene, P. Gigon, H. Sasame, and J. R. Gillette, Biochem. Pharmacol. 19:2461 (1970).
256. R. Kato, A. Takanaka, and K. Onoda, J. Biochem. (Tokyo) 66:739 (1969).

257. R. Kato, A. Takanaka, and K. Onoda, Biochem. Pharmacol. 20:447 (1971).
258. W. J. Marshall, Biochem. Pharmacol. 20:1723 (1971).
259. H. Remmer, Naunyn-Schmied. Arch. Exp. Path. Pharmakol. 236:7 (1959).
260. S. Orrenius, Y. Gnosspelius, M. L. Das, and L. Ernster, in Structure and Function of the Endoplasmic Reticulum in Animal Cells (P. N. Campbell, Ed.). Universitetsborlaget, Oslo, 1968, p. 81.
261. E. A. Nikkila, Ann. Med. Intern. Fenn. 49:269 (1960).
262. V. Nair and D. Bau, Proc. Soc. Exp. Biol. Med. 126:853 (1967).
263. R. E. Kramer, J. W. Greiner, W. J. Canady, and H. D. Colby, Biochem. Pharmacol. 24:2097 (1975).
264. R. E. Kramer, J. W. Greiner, R. C. Rumbaugh, T. O. Sweeney, and H. D. Colby, J. Pharmacol. Exp. Ther. 204:247 (1978).
265. J. A. Gustafsson and A. Stenberg, Proc. Nat. Acad. Sci. U.S. 73:1462 (1976).
266. E. Wei and J. T. Wilson, J. Pharmacol. Exp. Ther. 177:227 (1971).
267. J. T. Wilson, Fed. Proc. 30:281 (1971).
268. D. E. Cook and C. K. Phares, Experientia 33:1110 (1977).
269. J. T. Wilson, Biochem. Pharmacol. 22:1717 (1973).
270. J. Ambre, F. Butes, D. Haupt, D. Graeff, and K. Deason, Clin. Res. 22:598A (1974).
271. C. Tschanz, C. E. Hignite, D. H. Huffman, and D. L. Azarnoff, Cancer Res. 37:3881 (1977).
272. R. Kato, A. Takanaka, A. Takahashi, and K. Onoda, Jap. J. Pharmacol. 18:224 (1968).
273. R. Kato, A. Takanaka, and T. Oshima, Jap. J. Pharmacol. 18:245 (1968).
274. M. Watanabe, V. R. Potter, and H. P. Morris, Cancer Res. 30:263 (1970).
275. P. D. Lotlikar, Biochem. J. 118:513 (1970).
276. R. Kato, A. Takanaka, and A. Takahashi, Gann 59:83 (1968).
277. R. Kato, A. Takanaka, and A. Takahashi, Gann 61:359 (1970).
278. J. D. Khandekar, D. Dardachiti, B. D. Garg, B. Tuchweber, and K. Kovacs, Cancer 29:738 (1972).
279. K. Kovacs, J. D. Khandekar, D. Dardachiti, B. D. Garg, and B. Tuchweber, Experientia 27:1068 (1971).
280. R. Rosso, L. Dolfini, and G. Franchi, Biochim. Pharmacol. 17:633 (1968).
281. R. Rosso, E. Dolfini, and M. G. Donelli, Eur. J. Cancer 4:133 (1968).
282. B. M. Boulos and C. Sirtori, Clin. Toxicol. 4:361 (1971).
283. J. T. Wilson, Endocrinology 88:185 (1971).
284. B. M. Boulos, M. MacDougall, D. W. Shoeman, and D. L. Azarnoff, Proc. Soc. Exp. Biol. Med. 139:1353 (1972).

285. I. Bartosek, A. Guaitani, and M. G. Donelli, Biochem. Pharmacol. 21:2359 (1972).
286. W. Nakahara and H. Fukuoka, Jap. J. Med. 1:271 (1948).
287. A. Takahashi and R. Kato, J. Biochem. (Tokyo) 65:325 (1969).
288. W. Nakahara, in Methods in Cancer Research, Vol. 2 (H. Busch, Ed.). Academic, New York, 1967, p. 203.
289. N. E. Sladek, B. E. Domeyer, R. L. Merriman, and G. T. Brophy, Drug Metab. Dispos. 6:412 (1978).
290. R. W. Bates, S. Milkovic, and M. M. Garrison, Endocrinology 71: 943 (1962).
291. J. T. Wilson, J. Pharmacol. Exp. Ther. 160:179 (1968).
292. J. T. Wilson, Biochem. Pharmacol. 17:1449 (1968).
293. J. T. Wilson, Biochem. Biophys. Res. Comm. 32:903 (1968).
294. J. T. Wilson, Proc. Soc. Exp. Biol. Med. 128:445 (1968).
295. J. T. Wilson, J. Natl. Cancer Inst. 43:1067 (1969).
296. J. T. Wilson, Life Sci. 8:1095 (1969).
297. J. T. Wilson, Biochem. Pharmacol. 18:2029 (1969).
298. R. J. Elin, E. S. Vesell, and S. M. Wolff, Clin. Pharmacol. Ther. 17:447 (1975).
299. C. S. Song, N. A. Gelb, and S. M. Wolff, J. Clin. Invest. 51:2959 (1972).
300. T. F. Blaschke, R. J. Elin, P. D. Berk, C. S. Song, and S. M. Wolff, Ann. Intern. Med. 78:221 (1973).
301. J. R. Pennington, D. C. Dale, H. Y. Reynolds, and J. D. MacLowry, J. Infect. Dis. 132:270 (1975).
302. J. Aarbakke, G. Gadeholt, and H. Olsen, Eur. J. Pharmacol. 49:31 (1978).
303. S. C. Kalser, E. J. Kelvington, R. Kunig, and M. M. Randolph, J. Pharmacol. Exp. Ther. 164:396 (1968).
304. R. G. McAllister, Jr., T. G. Tan, and E. P. Todd, Clin. Pharmacol. Ther. 23:121 (1978).
305. R. G. McAllister, Jr., D. W. Bourne, T. G. Tan, J. L. Erickson, C. C. Wachtel, and E. P. Todd, Clin. Pharmacol. Ther. 25:1 (1979).
306. G. M. Trenholme, R. L. Williams, K. H. Rieckmann, H. Frischer, and P. E. Carson, Clin. Pharmacol. Ther. 19:459 (1976).
307. R. D. Powell and J. V. McNamara, Proc. Helminth. Soc. Wash. 39: 331 (1972).
308. J. J. Deller, P. S. Cifarelli, and S. Berque, Milit. Med. 132:614 (1967).
309. L. G. White and A. Doermer, J. Amer. Med. Ass. 155:637 (1954).
310. J. F. Williams and A. Szentivanyi, Eur. J. Pharmacol. 43:281 (1977).
311. D. K. Sen, S. Arora, S. Gupta, and R. K. Sanyal, J. Allergy Clin. Immunol. 54:25 (1974).
312. D. M. Morton and D. H. Chatfield, Biochem. Pharmacol. 19:473 (1970).

313. P. P. Mathur, R. D. Smyth, C. M. Witmer, G. S. Carr, and N. H. Reavey-Cantwell, J. Pharmacol. Exp. Ther. 203:169 (1977).
314. P. P. Mathur, R. D. Smyth, C. Witmer, G. W. Nuss, and G. Carr, Fed. Proc. 35:537 (1976).
315. P. P. Mathur, G. S. Carr, and R. D. Smyth, Biochem. Pharmacol. 27:1379 (1978).
316. M. L. Selley, J. Glass, E. J. Triggs, and J. Thomas, Clin. Pharmacol. Ther. 17:599 (1975).
317. D. E. Furst and H. E. Paulus, Clin. Pharmacol. Ther. 17:622 (1975).
318. P. H. Chapman, M. D. Rawlins, and S. Shuster, Brit. J. Clin. Pharmacol. 7:499 (1979).

Chapter 9

XENOBIOTIC METABOLISM: NECESSITY, CHANCE, MISHAP, OR NONE OF THE ABOVE?

Bernard Testa

School of Pharmacy
University of Lausanne
Lausanne, Switzerland

Frederick J. Di Carlo

Environmental Protection Agency
Washington, D.C.

Peter Jenner

University Department of Neurology,
Institute of Psychiatry and King's College
Hospital Medical School
London, England

"There is no permanence to scientific concepts because they are only our interpretations of natural phenomena."

—Jacob Bronowski, 1967*

---

*In The Origins of Knowledge and Imagination, Yale University Press, New Haven, 1978, p. 96.

I. INTRODUCTION

Science is imprinted and dominated by the Aristotelian logic of the excluded middle, or the "black-white" dichotomy. Consider in biology the division between living and nonliving matter, and in drug metabolism consider such discriminations as endogenous versus exogenous substrates, functionalization (phase I) versus conjugation (phase II) pathways, enzymatic versus chemical processes. Such logic is certainly very useful, and also mind-pleasing. However, by ignoring intermediate cases, it is a mental trap (e.g., Ref. 1). Black and white are just extreme cases in the very rich scale of (grey) colors.

In drug metabolism, the discrimination just mentioned are of high convenience and universal use. Here again, the trap is well hidden—and wide open. Consider the division of pathways into phase I and phase II; in some cases, the division varies with the criteria applied and is somewhat arbitrary. Thus, methylation reactions have properties of both functionalization and conjugation reactions [2]. Similarly when distinguishing between endogenous and exogenous substrates, strong mental reservations must be made because their definitions intertwine and forbid sharp discrimination. For example, histamine is certainly an endogenous substrate, while the fate of endogenous and exogenous histamine in rodents is not identical. Thus endogenous histamine is metabolized by both diamine oxidase and histamine N-methyltransferase whereas exogenous histamine is almost exclusively metabolized by the transferase [3]. Comparably, isotopomers of neurotransmitters, e.g., (2R)- and (2S)-^{3}H-dopamine, are undoubtedly exogenous compounds, yet they so much resemble an endogenous substrate that they can be used to gain information on the metabolism of the latter [4].

Much of what follows will make use of the discrimination between exogenous and endogenous substrates, but the shortcomings and dangers of such a simplifying classification must be constantly remembered. This is especially significant in view of the provocative ideas and concepts presented hereafter. Indeed, we aim in this concluding chapter at critically reconsidering some of the classical beliefs and opinions implicit in many texts. That such ideas may later be proven correct or wrong by future advances is irrelevant to our goal. We cannot and will not offer definitive answers to the problems raised, and restrict ourselves to the hope of generating some intellectual stimulation.

II. XENOBIOTIC METABOLISM: A NECESSITY?

From a thermodynamic point of view, living entities are open systems, exchanging both energy and matter with their environment. This exchange of matter cannot be stopped without precipitating death, but in itself it presents a permanent threat to life should the homeostatic equilibrium of the living entity be disrupted. This applies particularly to chemical compounds which enter the organism and do not serve as nutrients or other essential factors. Such xenobiotics cannot be allowed to concentrate beyond limits in a living system, but must be eliminated by excretion.

Xenobiotic metabolism appears as a logical evolutionary acquisition in this context since it generates metabolites which as a rule are more easily excreted than the parent compound. Almost all conjugates are more hydrosoluble than their parent compound, and so are most metabolites generated by functionalization reactions. Products of carbon oxidation are classical examples of metabolites with enhanced hydrosolubility and more rapid urinary excretion, and for several years products of nitrogen oxidation have been recognized in the same role [5].

Xenobiotic metabolism occurs with minimal energy expenditure, and this again can be considered as a logical result of natural selection. Minimum use of energy is apparent from the fact that easily excreted (highly water-soluble) compounds undergo little or no metabolism; such xenobiotics include saccharin, guanazole, and cromolyn sodium [6]. Furthermore, a limited number of metabolic steps usually precede excretion, as opposed to the extensive exothermic degradation (yielding mainly CO_2 and urea) of nutrients.

Increased excretability alone does not appear sufficient to consider xenobiotic metabolism as an evolutionary necessity. Additional drive could be provided by another benefit, namely, decreased toxicity. For many decades, biotransformation had been considered as synonymous with detoxication, and examples abound where this is true. A representative case is that of As(III), an ubiquitous and natural "contaminant" of the environment, which in mammals is oxidized to As(V) and then methylated, each of these steps representing a genuine detoxifying process [7-9].

These arguments each afford fractional evidence to consider xenobiotic metabolism as a necessity in terms of evolutionary gain. In this evolutionary perspective, let us consider the monooxygenases, which are recognized as the most important xenobiotic-metabolizing enzyme systems, and more specifically cytochrome P-450. An enlightening paper by Wickramasinghe and Villee [10] presents good evidence that "a form of cytochrome P-450 has been present in life forms for billions of years, and probably before the advent of free oxygen and the development of other respiratory hemoproteins." Its low redox potential could have allowed cytochrome P-450 to function enzymatically in a reducing atmosphere. Upon the progressive appearance of molecular oxygen, cytochrome P-450 provided an early line of defense. And when its protective value in detoxifying oxygen was superseded by the development of aerobic organisms, its other activities retained their usefulness in the degradation of various molecules [10]. Today, cytochrome P-450s are known to exist in microorganisms, plants, and animals. Quite impressive are the similarities in the metabolism of drugs, mutagens, and other xenobiotics carried out by cytochrome

P-450s from microorganisms and mammals (see Ref. 11 and references therein).

While several lower organisms possess soluble forms of cytochrome P-450 which can be purified without loss of activity, mammalian tissues yield cytochrome P-450s which are closely associated with membranes [12]. Indeed, mammalian monooxygenases are highly organized multienzymatic systems [13-17], consisting of two electron-transport chains and the terminal oxidase. The deep significance of this organizational complexity is far from being understood, but may be related to the functional involvement of monooxygenase constituents in other activities. Thus, NADPH-cytochrome P-450 reductase also reduces cytochrome c [18]. Similarly, cytochrome b_5, the biological significance of which is being actively investigated after many years of neglect, is involved in fatty acid desaturation and likely also in other synthetic processes besides its role as donor of the second electron to cytochrome P-450 [19,20].

The highly organized state of mammalian monooxygenases is certainly consistent with an evolutionary pressure for efficient xenobiotic-metabolizing activity. Several advantages are apparent for such systems, including increased efficiency of electron transport, as well as multiplied possibilities of control, feedback, and functional links with other biological processes. These advantages should be of particular significance for a system designed to handle compounds whose concentrations vary widely over a given period of time. Indeed, as opposed to endogenous substrates and nutrients whose concentrations vary over relatively narrow ranges, some xenobiotics may invade the organism in great amounts at a given time, and become negligible later. Such variations imply a considerable adaptability of monooxygenases as regards their level of activity, and functional links can allow electrons to be diverted to other systems in the absence of exogenous substrates. The marked influence of nutritional factors on the regulation of human drug metabolism [21,22] may be explainable in part as a result of these functional links. However, the in vivo assessment of functional interrelationships between lipid-carbohydrate metabolism and drug metabolism comes up against methodological difficulties, and currently available data are disappointing (e.g., Ref. 23).

Enzymes metabolizing endogenous compounds are usually known for their very high substrate and product selectivity. An aptly illustrative example is afforded by the chick vitamin D endocrine system, which is unable to 1α-hydroxylate the synthetic compound 24-nor-25-hydroxyvitamin D_3 [24]. In contrast, the endogenous substrate 25-hydroxyvitamin D_3 is readily hydroxylated to its active metabolite 1α,25-dihydroxyvitamin D_3. It thus appears that shortening the side chain of the natural substrate by a single methylene group dramatically reduces enzyme affinity. Such a high substrate selectivity implies strict spatial relationships between the various binding groups within the enzymatic active site, resulting in a highly selective recognition of the substrate (binding selectivity). The other aspect of enzyme selectivity is recognition of the transition state by catalysis (catalytic, or kinetic, selectivity) [25,26] resulting in product selectivity [27,28]. The product selectivity of endobiotic-metabolizing enzymes is generally observed to be high, or even as complete as the methods of examination can reveal [29].

Another characteristic of endobiotic-metabolizing enzymes is to be found in their rates of reaction. Often, these have been found to correspond to the rates of diffusion-controlled reactions, meaning that every collision between enzyme and substrate is an effective one [30].

The conjunction of high selectivity and fast reaction rates generally characterizing endobiotic-metabolizing enzymes is not observed with xenobiotic-metabolizing enzymes. In particular, substrate selectivity is usually quite low. Indeed, what would be the protective utility of an enzyme able to metabolize a given xenobiotic but completely inactive toward its homologs? If this were the case, the number of enzymes required for an efficient protection would be immense. It is therefore easily understandable that natural selection should favor enzymes active toward large varieties of substrates.

Low substrate selectivity means the ability to bind and metabolize sustrate varying not only in size and shape, but also in the nature of functional groups. While size and shape variations can be accommodated to a certain extent by increased conformational adaptability of the enzyme, the variety in functional groups (i.e., potential haptophores) would call for impossibly versatile binding sites. Rather, one would expect the driving force binding xenobiotics to their metabolizing enzymes to be provided mainly by hydrophobicity. Such an interacting force is relatively nonspecific in structural terms, as opposed to the accurate fit typically displayed by endobiotic-enzyme complexes. Indeed, monooxygenases are consistently found to behave as a lipophilic phase extracting the substrates from the aqueous environment. This partition model demonstrates hydrophobic interactions to be the greatest single factor in the binding of substrates to cytochrome P-450 [31], as assessed by the consistent role played by the partition coefficient in structure-metabolism relationship studies [32]. In this context, it is important to discriminate the hydrophobicity-driven substrate binding to cytochrome P-450 from the metabolically inactive ligand binding of type II and modified type II compounds where electronic factors, namely, the availability of an electron lone pair, influence the interaction with the ferric ion [33]. Ligand binding results in inhibition of substrate metabolism, and its physiological significance remains unassessed.

The above discussion convincingly suggests a low substrate selectivity to be a prerequisite for versatile xenobiotic-metabolizing enzymes. But the gain in versatility has to be compensated somehow, and may well have been obtained at the cost of a dramatic decrease in reaction rates as compared to the anabolism and catabolism of endogenous compounds. Ferreira [30] reports that the rate constants of many bimolecular enzymatic reactions lie in the range of 10^7 to 10^9 M^{-1} sec^{-1}. On the other hand, bimolecular rate constants for cytochrome P-450-catalyzed oxidation of xenobiotics can be approximated from many in vitro data to lie close to 10^0 to 10^3 M^{-1} sec^{-1}. Such a difference raises numerous questions as to its origin. One explanation could be that hydrophobicity-driven binding precludes substrate activation by the enzyme. The latter process indeed requires a close fit between the activating groups(s) of the active site and the activated moiety or moieties in the substrate molecule. An interesting model has been proposed to explain the extremely high activity of endobiotic-metabolizing enzymes, namely, that the latter act as orbital symmetry adapters [30].

As far as we are aware, direct substrate activation by monooxygenases has never been detected, while overwhelming evidence indicates these enzymes to activate oxygen [34] and transfer it to the bound and "passive" substrate. Alternatively, one of the forms of the activated oxygen may in turn activate the substrate, e.g., by hydrogen abstraction. These points have been discussed in detail by Trager in Part A of this work [35]. Briefly, the main mechanism of action of cytochrome P-450 involves reduction and cleavage of molecular oxygen resulting in the formation of an oxenoid species, followed by transfer of the latter electrophilic species to the substrate. Such a transfer is certainly not expected to occur at random, i.e., to be equally distributed to all possible accepting moieties in the substrate. Rather, selective oxene transfer is expected to occur to moieties more receptive than others.

Quantum calculations can be useful at this stage to help clarify these mechanistic aspects. If the hypothesis of oxene transfer to an unactivated substrate is correct, then those moieties calculated to be electron-rich should indeed be found to be selective sites of oxene attack. We have shown in Part A [32] that this is indeed the case for regioselective carbon hydroxylation. These results provide additional evidence for the great substrate versatility of monooxygenases.

The product selectivity resulting from regio- and stereoselective oxene transfer although high is far from complete. Interestingly, the overall product selectivity for the metabolism of a given substrate is often decreased after enzyme induction. This fact provided one of the earliest indications that the product selectivity of monooxygenase-mediated reactions is higher than experimentally detected due to enzyme multiplicity.

Recently, impressive evidence has accumulated proving the simultaneous presence of several individual forms of cytochrome P-450 in the endoplasmic reticulum, each displaying its own product selectivity (e.g., Ref. 36) as well as substrate selectivity [37]. For example, liver microsomes from phenobarbital-treated mice have yielded four distinct cytochrome P-450 fractions (A_1, A_2, C_1, and C_2) [38]. In rat liver microsomes, four antigenically different forms of cytochrome P-450 have been demonstrated in the PB-P450 preparation, and two different forms in the MC-P448 preparation [39]. More recently, preliminary evidence has been obtained for the presence of more than eight forms of cytochrome P-450 in liver microsomes from untreated rats [40]. Rabbit liver microsomal fractions yield the following forms of cytochrome P-450: LM_2 and LM_x (PB-treated animals), LM_{4a} and LM_{4b} (β-naphthoflavone-treated animals), and LM_1 and LM_7 (untreated animals) [41].

The recent discovery that liver nuclear membranes contain cytochrome P-450s opens fascinating avenues of research, particularly as to the biological significance of such enzymes in nuclei. The question arises whether novel forms of cytochrome P-450s, distinct from the microsomal ones, will be found in nuclei. Spectrally, hepatic nuclear cytochrome P-450 from uninduced, phenobarbital-induced, and 3-methylcholanthrene-induced rats differ from the corresponding microsomal species [42]. In contrast, hepatic nuclear cytochrome P-448 was found to be immunochemically identical with microsomal cytochrome P-448 [42a].

Enzyme multiplicity is not restricted to monooxygenases. For example, two forms of catechol-O-methyltransferase can be isolated from rat liver displaying different meta/para methylation ratios [43,44]. Similarly, glutathione S-transferases exist in human liver as multiple enzymatic species with somewhat distinct substrate selectivities [45].

Low substrate selectivity is incompatible with high enzyme affinity, the latter resulting in relatively low rates of biotransformation. Low substrate selectivity can thus be considered both favorable and unfavorable to the efficiency of lipophilic xenobiotic elimination in vivo. In this context, enzyme multiplicity is a clear and considerable evolutionary advantage since it allows for markedly increased enzyme affinity without loss of substrate versatility. This is achieved by a set of distinct yet overlapping substrate selectivities each characterizing a given form of the enzyme. Each of these forms, because of its own not too broad substrate selectivity, may thus display an affinity high enough to metabolize xenobiotics present in low concentrations, as for environmental contaminants. Ullrich and Kremers have commented along these lines [37].

Such effects are magnified when metabolites of the same class are generated by unrelated enzyme systems. An even greater number of substrates can then be metabolized without a decrease in enzyme affinity. The classical example is provided by the N-oxidation of amines. Nonbasic amines are N-oxidized by cytochrome P-450 systems, while basic amines are not, probably due in part to strong ligand binding. In contrast, basic amines are N-oxidized by a flavoprotein-dependent mixed-function amine oxidase, while weak bases such as aromatic amines are substrates for both systems [46,47].

As in the case of enzyme multiplicity, the functional multiplicity of monooxygenases has been unraveled by recent discoveries and is still much of a terra incognita, in particular regarding its overall in vivo biological significance. Monooxygenases function as oxene transferases in the context of oxygen rather than substrate activation discussed earlier [34,35,48]. The chemical products resulting from oxene transfer are many indeed, depending on the functional moiety or moieties of the substrate. Furthermore, the chemical or biochemical reactivity of several of these primary products results in a variety of secondary metabolites. In this context, consider the products resulting from oxene transfer to carbon atoms (various stable or unstable epoxides, stable or unstable C-hydroxylated metabolites, some of the latter generating N-, O-, or S-dealkylated products, or products of deamination), to nitrogen atoms (N-oxides, hydroxylamines, nitroso derivatives), to sulfur atoms (sulfoxides, sulfones, sulfines, sulfenes, oxathiiranes, oxathiaphosphiranes, etc.), as well as to other heteroatoms (silanols, phosphine oxides, arsenoxides, etc.) [49,49a]. Multiplicity of oxidative routes for a single substrate is partly due to enzyme multiplicity, but is not a priori related to any beneficial effect to the organism since the probability of generating toxic products is increased. This point will be developed in Sec. IV

Besides their main—and considered physiological—role as oxene transferases, cytochrome P-450s also act as NADPH oxidases. In the latter reaction, NADPH is oxidized to $NADP^+$ in the presence of O_2 and upon release of hydrogen peroxide [50,50a]. Such a reaction is the product of uncoupling, that is, it occurs due to a lack of transfer of oxene to the (pseudo)substrate caused by chemical or steric hindrance, or occurs in the absence of exogenous substrates. The mechanism of H_2O_2 production appears related to the known release of superoxide anion [50b], and would then involve dismutation of the latter [51]; however, oxene transfer to a molecule of water is a possible yet neglected mechanistic candidate.

The physiological significance of this oxidase activity is far from being established, but should be linked to a discharge of activated oxygen. However, the extreme complexity of oxygen chemistry and the high reactivity of several activated and reduced oxygen derivatives make oxidase activity potentially harmful. The metabolism of 9,10-dimethyl-1,2-benzanthracene to its transannular 9,10-peroxide [52] is a very rare example of a reaction which may be related to the oxidase activity, and whose beneficial or detrimental effects have yet to be assessed. In contrast, lipid peroxidation is clearly related to superoxide and/or hydrogen peroxide generation. Its consequences are detrimental to the organism resulting in a loss of functional membrane integrity and monooxygenase activity [53].

Two additional activities of cytochrome P-450 demonstrate its versatility and multiplicity of function, namely, peroxidase and reductase activity. Organic peroxides are decomposed by the cytochrome P-450 system, and the peroxide anion binding to the iron atom is cleaved to hydroxylate a substrate. The peroxidase activity thus represents a shunt of the normal O_2 binding and two-electron reduction preceding oxene transfer [54,55]. Also intriguing is the reductase activity of cytochrome P-450, which reduces such substrates as arene oxides, amine oxides, and nitro derivatives [56-58].

A remarkable and much studied property of monooxygenase is their inducibility, a property shared with such enzymes as uridine diphosphate

(UDP)-glucuronyltransferase and glutathione S-transferases. The pharmmacological and more specifically in our context the toxicological consequences of enzyme induction [59] clearly suggest the phenomenon to represent a considerable evolutionary gain. This is emphasized by the link between enzyme multiplicity and inducibility. Schematically, the two main groups of inducers (lipophilic drugs such as phenobarbital, and the polycyclic hydrocarbons) each induce the class of cytochrome P-450s for which they are main substrates, cytochrome P-450 and P-448, respectively [60]. In this context, a highly interesting finding is the increase of in vitro benzo[a]-pyrene monooxygenase activity when UDP-glucuronic acid is present, an effect further enhanced by the addition of UDP-N-acetylglucosamine, an allosteric activator of UDP-glucuronyltransferase [61]. This would suggest a physiological coupling between the two enzyme systems which may assist xenobiotic elimination [61].

The mechanisms of monooxygenase induction are presently undergoing exhaustive investigations but have already allowed fascinating insights. Thus, the induction of the cytochrome P-448-linked aryl hydrocarbon hydroxylase is genetically controlled [62], and the chain of reactions is initiated by the interaction of the inducer with a cytosolic receptor; the inducer-receptor complex, translocated into the nucleus, becomes the effector [63]. As regards phenobarbital and analogous compounds, a relationship has been demonstrated between their inducing ability and their affinity for the type I binding site of cytochrome P-450 [64]; these drugs have no affinity for the cytosolic receptor of polycyclic hydrocarbons [63]. Paine [65] has put forward the far-reaching hypothesis that inducers act by uncoupling electron flow from substrate oxidation permitting a leak of activated oxygen (see earlier). The common endogenous inducer would be the superoxide anion or another form of activated oxygen. Highly seductive in this theory is its presentation of induction as a protective mechanism compensating for the detrimental effects of superoxide leakage discussed earlier. The fact that lipid peroxides also act as inducers led Paine to believe that the cytochrome P-450 system evolved to protect organisms from the toxic effects of these as well as other naturally occurring dietary anutrients [65]. In view of the discussion above, such a mechanism does not appear as directly acceptable for the inducers of the polycyclic hydrocarbon type. In contrast, there is good evidence to support such a mechanism for induction elicited by phenobarbital and analogs.

The functional aspects of monooxygenases which have been considered in the present section are increased excretion and decreased toxicity of products as compared to substrates, an evolutionary perspective of cytochrome P-450, functional links between monooxygenases and general metabolism, slow reaction rates, relatively low substrate selectivity, activation of oxygen rather than substrate, enzyme multiplicity, functional multiplicity, and inducibility. All these aspects would indicate that monooxygenases, as the principal xenobiotic-metabolizing enzymes, are highly complex and efficient systems. Because of their clear evolutionary advantages, xenobiotic-metabolizing enzymes may be viewed as an evolutionary necessity. But are there truly xenobiotic-metabolizing enzymes per se, or is the biotransformation of xenobiotics a series of chance reactions carried by endobiotic-metabolizing enzymes? And are not the global consequences of xenobiotic metabolism in reality more detrimental than beneficial to the organism due to the generation of numerous reactive and toxic metabolites? Evidence sustaining these controversial views constitutes the matter of the next sections.

III. XENOBIOTIC METABOLISM: A CHANCE PHENOMENON?

Microsomes prepared from endoplasmic reticulum form the classical xenobiotic-metabolizing systems used for in vitro studies. However, a huge amount of information has now accumulated demonstrating the biotransformation of endogenous compounds by microsomes of liver and other organs, as aptly reviewed by Brenner [66]. Such in vitro data provide evidence for the central role of the endoplasmic reticulum in the anabolism and catabolism of many physiological constituents..

In this context, a daring and thus stimulating question is the following: Are the enzyme systems mediating this endobiotic metabolism distinct from xenobiotic-metabolizing enzymes? And is a yes or no answer inadequate, by what criteria and how much are they distinct? The following discussion of the enzymes encountered in xenobiotic transformation should demonstrate the difficulty of obtaining clear answers, not to mention definitive ones. Such enzymes are conveniently classified as endobiotic-metabolizing ones (fortuitously acting also on xenobiotics), and the properly xenobiotic-metabolizing ones (also transforming physiological compounds). We attempt to judge by what criteria these systems differ, and whether the differentiation is realistic or not.

Steroidogenic tissues contain mitochondrial cytochrome P-450 systems which display properties quite distinct from systems present in the liver endoplasmic reticulum. Thus, adrenocortical cytochrome P-450 is coupled to adrenodoxin which functions as an electron-transferring enzyme; although this system is responsible for the hydroxylation of several steroids, it also binds xenobiotics [67, 68]. Testis mitochondrial and human placenta microsomal and mitochondrial cytochrome P-450s also appear as highly substrate- and product-selective, yet the latter possess a marked ability to bind xenobiotics [69-71]. The significance of the placenta as a xenobiotic-metabolizing organ is well recognized [72], and it is of considerable interest to determine whether the cytochrome P-450s involved in steroidogenesis in this organ are identical with the xenobiotic-metabolizing systems. Should this be so, then xenobiotic-metabolizing activity could indeed be regarded as being due to chance factors.

The steroidogenic cytochrome P-450s have certainly not evolved as a protection against exogenous anutrients. The same can reasonably be postulated for liver nuclear cytochrome P-450. This enzyme is inducible like its microsomal analogs and activates aromatic hydrocarbons to metabolites binding to DNA, but is spectrally distinct from microsomal cytochrome P-450s [42]. Again this could appear as a monooxygenase which metabolizes xenobiotics by chance.

Cytochrome P-450s in the hepatic endoplasmic reticulum (commonly referred to as liver microsomal cytochrome P-450s are involved in the metabolism of several groups of endogenous compounds. For example, they are the main enzymes responsible for the biosynthesis and metabolism of bile acids [73]. They also hydroxylate steroid hormones such as testosterone [74, 75] and prostaglandins [76]. Whether these microsomal monooxygenases are distinct from those enzymes metabolizing xenobiotics remains to be answered. Using such criteria as inducibility, circadian rhythm, and sex differences, it has been shown that among rat liver microsomal monooxygenases cholesterol-7A-hydroxylase behaves differently from drug-metabolizing enzymes, while progesterone-16α-hydroxylase behaves comparably [77]. Utilizing linoleic acid hydroperoxide, Mannering and collaborators [78] have demonstrated that this compound has a distinct destructive effect on cytochrome P-450s. The labile form [designated cytochrome $P\text{-}450_{(1l)}$] is phenobarbital-induced and is associated with almost all drug-metabolizing activities; in contrast, the stable form [cytochrome $P\text{-}450_{(1s)}$] is induced by 3-methylcholanthrene and functions in the metabolism of endogenous substrates. The two forms were thus found to be essentially independent of each other. However, the metabolism of polycyclic aromatic hydrocarbons was not taken into account in this study, but since aryl hydrocarbon hydroxylase (cytochrome P-448) is 3-methylcholanthrene-inducible, it should belong to the $P\text{-}450_{(1s)}$ group.

As mentioned earlier, the early phases in the time course of induction of cytochrome P-450s and P-448s appear different [63, 65], perhaps indicating a further dissimilarity between the two groups of enzymes. In the light of the available evidence, the following schematic view can reasonably be postulated: two groups of cytochrome P-450s exist in liver microsomes, namely, the phenobarbital-inducible $P\text{-}450_{(1l)}$ forms which metabolize drugs and the 3-methylcholanthrene-inducible $P\text{-}450_{(1s)}$ forms which metabolize endogenous substrates. In addition, the $P\text{-}450_{(1s)}$ forms, or at least the subgroup containing cytochrome P-448, also metabolize aryl hydrocarbons and other xenobiotics, while the $P\text{-}450_{(1l)}$ forms are perhaps involved in some endobiotic metabolism. If this is correct, then the metabolism of xenobiotics and endobiotics by the cytochrome $P\text{-}450_{(1l)}$ and $P\text{-}450_{(1s)}$ groups, respectively, represent their true physiological activity imposed by evolution, while the metabolism of polycyclic hydrocarbons and other xenobiotics by the $P\text{-}450_{(1s)}$ forms is merely fortuitous (a chance phenomenon). The same would apply to endobiotic metabolism by $P\text{-}450_{(1l)}$ forms, if this occurs. Such rationalizations, however, although stimulating, fall into the trap of Aristotelian logic and as such are suspicious oversimplifications.

If two functionally distinct groups of cytochrome P-450s do exist, it is of interest to determine whether these arise by convergent or divergent evolution. The answer to such a question may well help to unify our views on the biological significance of monooxygenases.

Having considered cytochrome P-450s at length, let us briefly turn our attention toward other xenobiotic-metabolizing enzymes. These are classified in Table 1 according to the endogenous or exogenous nature of their major substrates. This classification is based on currently available evidence and may change in further investigations. Table 1 nevertheless serves our purpose by showing how frequently xenobiotics undergo chance metabolism simply because structural similarities with the endogenous substrate(s) render them recognizable by class A enzymes.

The major xenobiotic-metabolizing enzymes, however, are to be found in class B, which encompasses in particular most conjugating enzymes. For example, glucuronyltransferases act on a variety of endogenous substrates, e.g., steroids [96] and bilirubin. For glucuronidation of xenobiotics to be a fortuitous pathway, the same enzymes should be operative toward both endogenous and exogenous substrates. This does not appear to be the case despite incomplete evidence. Thus, based on various responses, it has been concluded that the form of UDP-glucuronyltransferase conjugating bilirubin differs from that responsible for the glucuronidation of para-nitrophenol, ortho-aminophenol, and ortho-aminobenzoate [97]. Furthermore, the glucuronidation of tertiary amines, a pathway found almost exclusively in humans [98], has no apparent endogenous counterpart, a specialized form of the enzyme being involved.

Based on the evidence for cytochrome P-450s and UDP-glucuronyltransferases the conclusion must be that drug metabolism by class B enzymes is not fortuitous, but rather is attributable to genuine xenobiotic-metabolizing forms of the enzymes. Such a conclusion, however, is at best tentative. Our understanding of drug metabolism is clearly too fragmentary to decide whether drug-metabolizing enzyme systems have arisen out of necessity or by chance.

IV. XENOBIOTIC METABOLISM: A MISHAP?

Xenobiotic metabolism has numerous physiological implications to the cell [99], in particular to hepatocytes. The idea most frequently referred to in this chapter is that of a protective mechanism against toxic effects on cellular function; such an effect can result from genuine chemical detoxication and/or by the facilitated elimination of toxic material.

TABLE 1
Conjectural Classification of Representative Enzymes Acting on Xenobiotics

Enzymes	Examples of exogenous substrates
Class A: Endobiotic-metabolizing enzymes "fortuitously" acting on a limited number of xenobiotics	
Catalase	Methanol [79]
Dopamine-β-hydroxylase	Phenylethylamines [80]
Aldehyde oxidase	Aromatic N-heterocycles [81,82,82a]
Xanthine oxidase	Nitrofuran derivatives (reduction) [82a,83]
Aldo sugar reductase	Daunorubicin [84]
Dihydropyrimidinases	Hydantoins, succinimides, cyclic imides [85]
Phenylethanolamine N-methyltransferases	Phenylethanolamine derivatives [80] and nonaromatic analogs [86]
Catechol-O-methyltransferases	Catechol derivatives [87]
NADases	Nicotine [88]
Class B: Enzymes existing in multiple forms, or families of distinct enzymes, a part of which may be predominantly xenobiotic metabolizers, while others may be essentially endobiotic metabolizers	
Cytochrome P-450s	Drugs, hydrocarbons, insecticides (see text)
Flavoprotein monooxygenases	Basic amines [88a]
Dehydrogenases	Alcohols, aldehydes, ketones [89]
Epoxide hydrases	Oxiranes [89a]
Esterases	Esters [90]
Acylases	Primary amines, aromatic acids [91]
Sulfotransferases	Phenols, alcohols, hydroxylamines [92]
UDP-glucuronyltransferases	Alcohols, phenols, hydroxylamines, carboxylic acids, amines, amides [93]
Glutathione transferases	Alkyl sulfates, organic nitrates, epoxides, α,β-unsaturated carbonyls [94,95]

For many decades, drug metabolism was identified with detoxication [100], until other implications to the cell became apparent. Competition with endogenous substrates for enzymes, cofactors, and oxygen is known to occur but the physiological significance of such metabolic interactions is poorly understood. In contrast, the formation of reactive and toxic metabolites has recently become a major object of interest and concern (e.g., Ref. 49a). Some mechanisms of toxicity that occur following metabolic activation are outlined below.

Not infrequently, drugs are activated to toxic metabolites acting in a more or less unique and often unpredictable manner. For example, a major metabolite of thalidomide accounting for most or all teratological activity has been found to be a phthalimide derivative containing a glutamyl moiety [101,102]. Similarly, 4-hydroxyglutethimide is more active than the parent compound in inducing ataxia, particularly at high doses, when conjugation pathways appear saturated and the metabolite accumulates in plasma [103].

Of more concern are those classes of xenobiotics which after biotransformation undergo covalent binding and incorporation into endogenous molecules, thereby initiating the cytotoxic effects of mutagenicity and carcinogenicity. Relevant xenobiotics include in particular polycyclic aromatic hydrocarbons and other epoxide-generating structures, aromatic amines and amides [49a], nitrosamines [49a,104], hydrazines and hydrazides [49a] and thiocarbonyl derivatives [49a]. So much has been written on the many aspects of covalent binding and carcinogenicity that lengthy discussions would be superfluous; the reader is referred to two authoritative works [105,106].

Epoxide-forming xenobiotics are of particular interest due to the intermingling and complexity of activating and detoxifying pathways. A major factor in determining the relative and sequential significance of these routes is certainly the chemical structure of the substrates. For example, vinyl chloride after activation by epoxidation is mainly inactivated by glutathione conjugation [107], while some aflatoxin epoxides are so reactive that little protection seems to exist against their covalent binding [108].

The generation of toxic and reactive metabolites is a clear failure from the point of view of metabolism-assisted elimination of xenobiotics—hence, the title of this section. Some protection, however, exists resulting in the subsequent detoxication of potentially harmful intermediates, as is the case for the glutathione trapping of epoxides. Such reactions of deactivation can in tactical terms be viewed as a "second line of defense," should the first protection, namely, the functionalization reaction, yield aberrant results.

Adding much weight to a dark image of xenobiotic metabolism is the fact that the "second line of defense" may also act to transform a potenially harmful metabolite to an ultimate toxic derivative. For example, glucuronyl- and sulfotransferases by conjugation of dihydrodiols may reduce the formation of dihydrodiol-epoxides. In contrast, sulfates and glucuronides of some aromatic hydroxylamines are markedly more reactive than the parent compounds. This dual role of glucuronyl- and sulfotransferases in converting metabolites to either reactive or biologically inactive compounds has been emphasized by Bock [109].

A similar dual role is seen for epoxide hydrase. While hydration of benzo[a]pyrene 4,5-epoxide is a true detoxication, the hydration of the 7,8-epoxide is a step toward the ultimate carcinogen, benzo[a]pyrene 7,8-dihydrodiol-9,10-epoxide [110].

A series of metabolic steps leading to the production of toxic metabolites is an obvious drawback to the idea of the protective role of xenobiotic-metabolizing enzymes. Perhaps such examples should be viewed as exceptions to the rule, as so many mishaps. Alternately, if xenobiotic metabolism is accepted as a chance phenomenon, activation or inactivation would have been equally likely prior to an evolution-driven restraint of harmful pathways.

The characterization of pathways of toxification is rather recent, implying that much remains to be uncovered. The activation of xenobiotics to "free" radicals in particular appears worthy of further investigations [111]. "Free" radicals are involved in polycyclic hydrocarbons metabolism and carcinogenesis [106], as well as for example in the activation of catechols to covalent binding species [112]. This entire field is connected to the biology of oxygen radical, another domain of considerable toxicological significance [113].

V. XENOBIOTIC METABOLISM: NONE OF THE ABOVE?

The preceding sections illustrate the failure of Aristotelian logic, at least as applied by us, to resolve an apparently simple question about the basic nature of xenobiotic metabolism. The reason for the failure may be that cells do not observe such logic. Many facets of xenobiotic metabolism do indeed suggest that the cell cannot always discriminate between black and white in terms of deploying mechanisms which favor survival rather than death. So let us finally consider the view that the cell does not discriminate at all, but simply reacts. Whether or not the cellular capabilities transcend discrimination is a philosophical question, which fortunately lies beyond the scope of this chapter.

The cellular capabilities under considerations here involve interactions between small and large molecules. The large molecules specifically mentioned so far have been proteins with enzymatic activity. Not mentioned specifically were the macromolecules which serve as receptors for the subsequent expression of pharmacological activity. Also covered by implication were the DNA macromolecules which are alkylated by reactive metabolites with resultant mutagenesis, teratogenesis, or carcinogenesis. It is now appropriate to cite reactions with other macromolecules so as to consider a broader question.

It is well known that metabolites of xenobiotics alkylate proteins as well as nucleic acids, and that they are also capable of acylation, arylation, and arylamidation. Of these reactions, the highest level of current interest is focused upon the alkylation of hemoglobin [114-117]. The reasons are that hemoglobin is so plentiful in higher species and that it acts as a nucleophilic trap. This combination qualifies hemoglobin as a major detoxifier of epoxide intermediates.

The broader question is whether the scientist might not be well advised to postpone discrimination and to consider that the cell does not discriminate at all. Differently worded, this view states that alkylated and acylated macromolecules are simply metabolites of xenobiotics. Whether a given alkylated DNA can or cannot be detoxified (by excision repair, for example) is a separate and specific question which may be expected to yield opposite answers in different situations. The view goes further and states that cellular activity subsequent to the formation of alkylated and acylated macromolecules should also be regarded as xenobiotic metabolism. The situation differs from those considered in the preceding sections only by virtue of the macromolecular nature of the substrate. Macromolecular substrates of course are commonplace and are attacked readily. Excision repair mechanisms are also enzymatic activities which appear to proceed with vigorous kinetics. Are these reactions not components of xenobiotic metabolism? Deletion and replacement of amino acids occur in proteins of humans and other species. Is it not possible that these "natural" modifications are due to xenobiotics which intercalate between the bases in DNA strands to cause nucleotide deletion?

Xenobiotics impact macromolecules with resultant changes to either or both, and this seems to be the essence of xenobiotic metabolism. Therefore, this chapter generates two equally acceptable answers to the question posed in its title. These answers are: none of the above and all of the above. It might not be stretching too far to conclude that the organism never responds by discriminating black from white, but always selects an intermediate point according to circumstances. This viewpoint has at least the merit of being consistent with the rich spectrum of activities associated with xenobiotic metabolism which were so aptly described by the other authors of Part A and Part B of this work.

REFERENCES

1. C. Ponnamperuma, Chemistry 51(9):6 (1978).
2. B. Testa and P. Jenner, Drug Metabolism: Chemical and Biochemical Aspects. Marcel Dekker, New York, 1976, p. 173.
3. R. W. Schayer and M. A. Reilly, J. Pharmacol. Exp. Ther. 184:33 (1973).

4. A. R. Battersby, P. W. Sheldrake, J. Staunton, and D. C. Williams, J. Chem. Soc. P.T.I., 1056 (1976).
5. P. Jenner, Xenobiotica 1:399 (1971).
6. B. Testa and P. Jenner, Drug Metabolism: Chemical and Biochemical Aspects. Marcel Dekker, New York, 1976, pp. 267-269.
7. V. Bencko, B. Benes, and M. Cikrt, Arch. Toxicol. 36:159 (1976).
8. S. A. Peoples and J. U. Lakso, Proc. West. Pharmacol. Soc. 16:244 (1973).
9. J. U. Lakso and S. A. Peoples, Agr. Food Chem. 23:674 (1975).
10. R. H. Wickramasinghe and C. A. Villee, Nature 256:509 (1975).
11. D. F. Callen and R. M. Philpot, Mutat. Res. 45:309 (1977).
12. B. W. Griffin, J. A. Peterson, J. Werringloer, and R. W. Estabrook, Ann. N.Y. Acad. Sci. 244:107 (1975).
13. J. W. DePierre and G. Dallner, Biochim. Biophys. Acta 415:411 (1975).
14. C. S. Yang, Life Sci. 21:1047 (1977).
15. K. Ruckpaul, Pharmazie 33:310 (1978).
16. J. A. Peterson, R. E. Ebel, D. H. O'Keeffe, T. Matsubara, and R. W. Estabrook, J. Biol. Chem. 251:4010 (1976).
17. V. Ullrich, I. Roots, A. Hildebrandt, R. W. Estabrook, and A. H. Conney (Eds.), Microsomes and Drug Oxidations. Pergamon, Oxford, 1977.
18. J. L. Vermilion and M. J. Coon, J. Biol. Chem. 253:2694 (1978).
19. J. B. Schenkman, I. Jansson, and K. M. Robie-Suh, Life Sci. 19:611 (1976).
20. N. Oshino, Pharmacol. Ther., Ser. A 2:477 (1978).
21. A. P. Alvares, K. E. Anderson, A. H. Conney, and A. Kappas, Proc. Nat. Acad. Sci. U.S. 73:2401 (1976).
22. A. Kappas, A. P. Alvares, K. E. Anderson, W. A. Garland, E. J. Pantuck, and A. H. Conney, in Microsomes and Drug Oxidations (V. Ullrich, I. Roots, A. Hildebrandt, R. W. Estabrook, and A. H. Conney, Eds.). Pergamon, Oxford, 1977, pp. 703-708.
23. E. Fellenius, K. O. Borg, B. Eklund, K. J. Hoffmann, B. M. Magnusson, I. Skånberg, M. Wallborg, and B. Wallin, in Microsomes and Drug Oxidations (V. Ullrich, I. Roots, A. Hildebrandt, R. W. Estabrook, and A. H. Conney, Eds.). Pergamon, Oxford, 1977, pp. 610-614.
24. A. Mouriño, P. Blair, W. Wecksler, R. L. Johnson, A. W. Norman, and W. H. Okamura, J. Med. Chem. 21:1025 (1978).
25. K. Dalziel, Phil. Trans. Roy. Soc., Ser. B 272:109 (1975).
26. H. R. Bosshard, Experientia 32:949 (1976).
27. P. Jenner and B. Testa, Drug Metab. Rev. 2:117 (1973).
28. B. Testa and P. Jenner, J. Pharm. Pharmacol. 28:731 (1976).
29. K. R. Hanson and I. A. Rose, Acc. Chem. Res. 8:1 (1975).

30. R. Ferreira, J. Theor. Biol. 39:665 (1973).
31. W. J. Canady, D. A. Robinson, and H. D. Colby, Biochem. Pharmacol. 23:3075 (1974).
32. B. Testa and P. Jenner, in Concepts in Drug Metabolism, Part A (P. Jenner and B. Testa, Eds.). Marcel Dekker, New York, 1980. pp. 53-176
33. B. Testa, Chem.-Biol. Interact. 34:287 (1981).
34. R. W. Estabrook and J. Werringloer, in Mic somes and Drug Oxidations (V. Ullrich, I. Roots, A. Hildebrandt, R. W. Estabrook, and A. H. Conney, Eds.). Pergamon, Oxford, 1977, pp. 748-757.
35. W. F. Trager, in Concepts in Drug Metabolism, Part A (P. Jenner and B. Testa, Eds.). Marcel Dekker, New York, 1980, pp. 177-209.
36. F. J. Wiebel, J. K. Selkirk, H. V. Gelboin, D. A. Haugen, T. A. van der Hoeven, and M. J. Coon, Proc. Nat. Acad. Sci. U.S. 72:3917 (1975).
37. V. Ullrich and P. Kremers, Arch. Toxicol. 39:41 (1977).
38. M. T. Huang, S. B. West, and A. Y. H. Lu, J. Biol. Chem. 251:4659 (1976).
39. P. E. Thomas, A. Y. H. Lu, D. Ryan, S. B. West, J. Kawalek, and W. Levin, Mol. Pharmacol. 12:746 (1976).
40. M. Warner, M. Vella LaMarca, and A. H. Neims, Drug Metab. Dispos. 6:353 (1978).
41. F. P. Guengerich, Biochem. Biophys. Res. Commun. 82:820 (1978).
42. E. Rogan and E. Cavalieri, Mol. Pharmacol. 14:215 (1978).
42a. P. E. Thomas, D. Korzeniowski, E. Bresnick, W. A. Bornstein, C. B. Kasper, W. E. Fahl, C. R. Jefcoate, and W. Levin, Arch. Biochem. Biophys. 192:22 (1979).
43. G. Marzullo and A. J. Friedhoff, Life Sci. 17:933 (1975).
44. M. M. O. Huh and A. J. Friedhoff, J. Biol. Chem. 254:299 (1979).
45. W. H. Habig, K. Kamisaka, J. N. Ketley, M. J. Pabst, I. M. Arias, and W. B. Jacoby, in Glutathione: Metabolism and Function (I. M. Arias and W. B. Jacoby, Eds.). Raven, New York, 1976, pp. 225-232.
46. J. W. Gorrod, Chem.-Biol. Interact. 7:289 (1973).
47. P. Hlavica and M. Kehl, Biochem. J. 164:487 (1977).
48. F. Lichtenberger, W. Nastainczyk, and V. Ullrich, Biochem. Biophys. Res. Commun. 70:939 (1976).
49. B. Testa and P. Jenner, Drug Metabolism: Chemical and Biochemical Aspects. Marcel Dekker, New York, 1976, Sec. 1.1.1.
49a. B. Testa and P. Jenner, Drug Metab. Rev. 7:325 (1978).
50. A. G. Hildebrandt, M. Tjoe, and I. Roots, Biochem. Soc. Trans. 3:807 (1975).
50a. G. D. Nordblom and M. J. Coon, Arch. Biochem. Biophys. 180:343 (1977).
50b. C. Auclair, D. de Prost, and J. Hakim, Biochem. Pharmacol. 27:355 (1978).

51. J. Werringloer, in Microsomes and Drug Oxidations (V. Ullrich, I. Roots, A. Hildebrandt, R. W. Estabrook, and A. H. Conney, Eds.). Pergamon, Oxford, 1977, pp. 261-268.
52. C. Chen and M. H. Tu, Biochem. J. 160:805 (1976).
53. G. L. Plaa and H. Witschi, Ann. Rev. Pharmacol. 16:125 (1976).
54. R. W. Estabrook, J. Werringloer, E. G. Hrycay, P. J. O'Brien, A. D. Rahimtula, and J. A. Peterson, Soc. Trans. 3:811 (1975).
55. G. D. Nordblom, R. E. White, and M. J. Coon, Arch. Biochem. Biophys. 175:524 (1976).
56. P. Jenner and B. Testa, Xenobiotica 8:1 (1978).
57. M. Sugiura, K. Iwasaki, and R. Kato, Mol. Pharmacol. 12:322 (1976).
58. B. Testa and P. Jenner, Drug Metabolism: Chemical and Biochemical Aspects. Marcel Dekker, New York, 1976, pp. 304-307.
59. A. H. Conney, Pharmacol. Rev. 19:317 (1967).
60. B. Testa and P. Jenner, Drug Metabolism: Chemical and Biochemical Aspects. Marcel Dekker, New York, 1976, Sec. 2.2.1.
61. K. W. Bock, N. S. Arch. Pharmacol. 304:77 (1978).
62. A. Jori, in Concepts in Drug Metabolism, Part B (P. Jenner and B. Testa, Eds.). Marcel Dekker, New York, 1981, pp. 265-305.
63. T. M. Guenthner and D. W. Nebert, J. Biol. Chem. 252:8981 (1977).
64. A. N. Latham and G. D. Sweeney, Can. J. Physiol. Pharmacol. 54:844 (1976).
65. A. J. Paine, Biochem. Pharmacol. 27:1805 (1978).
66. R. R. Brenner, Drug Metab. Rev. 6:155 (1977).
67. H. Honeck, Pharmazie 33:317 (1978).
68. I. C. Gunsalus, T. C. Pederson, and S. G. Sligar, Ann. Rev. Biochem. 44:377 (1975).
69. J. I. Mason and G. S. Boyd, Biochem. Soc. Trans. 3:832 (1975).
70. J. A. Canick and K. J. Ryan, Mol. Cell. Endocrinol. 6:105 (1976).
71. E. Hodgson and M. R. Juchau, J. Steroid Biochem. 8:669 (1977).
72. B. Testa and P. Jenner, Drug Metabolism: Chemical and Biochemical Aspects. Marcel Dekker, New York, 1976, Sec. 2.4.
73. I. Björkhem, H. Danielsson, and K. Wikvall, Biochem. Soc. Trans. 3:825 (1975).
74. A. Y. H. Lu, W. Levin, S. West, M. Jacobson, D. Ryan, R. Kuntzman, and A. H. Conney, Ann. N.Y. Acad. Sci. 212:156 (1973).
75. A. Y. H. Lu and S. B. West, Pharmacol. Ther., Ser. A 2:337 (1978).
76. D. Kupfer and J. Navarro, in Microsomes and Drug Oxidations (V. Ullrich, I. Roots, A. Hildebrandt, R. W. Estabrook, and A. H. Conney, Eds.). Pergamon, Oxford, 1977, pp. 370-376.
77. J. E. Gielen, J. Van Cantfort, and P. Kremers, Arch. Toxicol. 36:255 (1976).
78. E. Jeffery, A. Kotape, R. el Azhary, and G. J. Mannering, Mol. Pharmacol. 13:415 (1977).

79. B. Testa and P. Jenner, Drug Metabolism: Chemical and Biochemical Aspects. Marcel Dekker, New York, 1976, Sec. 1.1.1.1.
80. T. Fujita and T. Ban, J. Med. Chem. 14:148 (1971).
81. C. Stubley, L. Subryan, J. G. P. Stell, R. H. Perrett, P. B. H. Ingle, and D. W. Mathieson, J. Pharm. Pharmacol., Suppl. 29:77P (1977).
82. J. J. McCormack, B. A. Allen, and C. N. Hodnett, J. Heterocycl. Chem. 15:1249 (1978).
82a. T. A. Krenitsky, Biochem. Pharmacol. 27:2763 (1978).
83. K. Tatsumi, S. Kitamura, and H. Yoshimura, Arch. Biochem. Biophys. 175:131 (1976).
84. R. L. Felsted, M. Gee, and N. R. Bachur, J. Biol. Chem. 249:3672 (1974).
85. J. H. Maguire and K. H. Dudley, Drug Metab. Dispos. 6:140, 601 (1978).
86. G. L. Grunewald, J. M. Grindel, W. C. Vincek, and R. T. Borchardt, Mol. Pharmacol. 11:694 (1975).
87. B. Testa and P. Jenner, Drug Metabolism: Chemical and Biochemical Aspects. Marcel Dekker, New York, 1976, Sec. 1.2.1.
88. W. C. Shen and H. Van Vunakis, Res. Commun. Chem. Pathol. Pharmacol. 9:405 (1974).
88a. T. P. Singer (Ed.), Flavins and Flavoproteins. Elsevier, Amsterdam, 1976.
89. B. Testa and P. Jenner, Drug Metabolism: Chemical and Biochemical Aspects. Marcel Dekker, New York, 1976, Secs. 1.1.1.1, 1.4.2.3, and 1.4.3.2
89a. G. T. Brooks, Gen. Pharmacol., Ser. A 8:221 (1977).
90. B. Testa and P. Jenner, Drug Metabolism: Chemical and Biochemical Aspects. Marcel Dekker, New York, 1976, Sec. 1.1.3.1.
91. B. Testa and P. Jenner, Drug Metabolism: Chemical and Biochemical Aspects. Marcel Dekker, New York, 1976, Secs. 1.2.2 and 1.2.5.
92. K. S. Dodgson, in Drug Metabolism: From Microbe to Man (D. V. Parke and R. L. Smith, Eds.). Taylor and Francis, London, 1977, pp. 91-104.
93. G. J. Dutton, G. J. Wishart, J. E. A. Leakey, and M. A. Goheer, in Drug Metabolism: From Microbe to Man (D. V. Parke and R. L. Smith, Eds.). Taylor and Francis, London, 1977, pp. 71-90.
94. P. L. Grover, in Drug Metabolism: From Microbe to Man (D. V. Parke and R. L. Smith, Eds.). Taylor and Francis, London, 1977, pp. 105-122.
95. I. M. Arias and W. B. Jacoby (Eds.), Glutathione: Metabolism and Function. Raven, New York, 1976.
96. T. Gessner, Biochem. Soc. Trans. 4:532 (1976).
97. D. A. Vessey, J. Goldenberg, and D. Zakim, Biochim. Biophys. Acta 309:75 (1973).

98. H. B. Hucker, S. C. Stauffer, A. J. Balletto, S. D. White, A. G. Zacchei, and B. H. Arison, Drug Metab. Dispos. 6:659 (1978).
99. S. Orrenius, P. Moldéus, H. Thor, and J. Högberg, in Microsomes and Drug Oxidations (V. Ullrich, I. Roots, A. Hildebrandt, R. W. Estabrook, and A. H. Conney, Eds.). Pergamon, Oxford, 1977, pp. 292-306.
100. R. T. Williams, Detoxication Mechanisms. Chapman and Hall, London, 1st ed., 1947; 2nd ed., 1959.
101. W. Meise, H. Ockenfels, and F. Köhler, Experientia 29:423 (1973).
102. H. Koch and F. Köhler, Arch. Toxicol. 35:63 (1976).
103. J. J. Ambre and L. J. Fischer, Drug Metab. Dispos. 2:151 (1974).
104. P. N. Magee, J. Toxicol. Environ. Health 2:883 (1977).
105. J. R. Gillette and L. R. Pohl, J. Toxicol. Environ. Health 2:849 (1977).
106. P. O. P. Ts'o, J. Toxicol. Environ. Health 2:1305 (1977).
107. T. Green and D. E. Hathway, Chem.-Biol. Interact. 11:545 (1975).
108. T. C. Campbell and J. R. Hayes, Toxicol. Appl. Pharmacol. 35:199 (1976).
109. K. W. Bock, Arch. Toxicol. 39:77 (1977).
110. P. Bentley, F. Oesch, and H. Glatt, Arch. Toxicol. 39:65 (1977).
111. R. L. Willson, Chem. Ind. (London) 183 (1977).
112. E. Dybing, S. D. Nelson, J. R. Mitchell, H. A. Sasame, and J. R. Gillette, Mol. Pharmacol. 12:911 (1976).
113. I. Fridovich, Science 201:875 (1978).
114. S. Osterman-Golkar, L. Ehrenberg, D. Segerbäck, and I. Hällström, Mutation Res. 34:1 (1976).
115. S. Osterman-Golkar, D. Hultmark, D. Segerbäck, C. J. Callerman, R. Göthe, L. Ehrenberg, and C. A. Wachtmeister, Biochem. Biophys. Res. Commun. 7:259 (1977).
116. D. Segerbäck, C. J. Calleman, L. Ehrenberg, G. Löfroth, and S. Osterman-Golkar, Mutation Res. 49:71 (1978).
117. L. Truong, J. B. Ward, Jr., and M. S. Legator, Mutation Res. 54:271 (1978).

AUTHOR INDEX

Numbers in brackets are reference numbers and indicate that an author's work is referred to although his name is not cited in the text. Underlined numbers give the page on which the complete reference is listed.

SUBJECT INDEX